Audiology: Clinical Aspects of Hearing

Audiology: Clinical Aspects of Hearing

Edited by Hannah Cummins

hayle
medical

New York

Hayle Medical,
750 Third Avenue, 9th Floor,
New York, NY 10017, USA

Visit us on the World Wide Web at:
www.haylemedical.com

ISBN: 978-1-63241-726-8

The publisher's policy is to use permanent paper from mills that operate a sustainable forestry policy. Furthermore, the publisher ensures that the text paper and cover boards used have met acceptable environmental accreditation standards.

Printed in China.

Cataloging-in-Publication Data

Audiology : clinical aspects of hearing / edited by Hannah Cummins.
p. cm.
Includes bibliographical references and index.
ISBN 978-1-63241-726-8
1. Audiology. 2. Hearing disorders--Treatment. 3. Deafness--Prevention. I. Cummins, Hannah.
RF290 .A83 2019
617.8--dc23

Table of Contents

Preface

The main aim of this book is to educate learners and enhance their research focus by presenting diverse topics covering this vast field. This is an advanced book which compiles significant studies by distinguished experts in the area of analysis. This book addresses successive solutions to the challenges arising in the area of application, along with it; the book provides scope for future developments.

The branch of science which is concerned with the study of hearing and related disorders is called audiology. The doctors who specialize in treating those with hearing loss and other hearing ailments are known as audiologists. Hearing tests, like Weber test and Rinne test, otoacoustic emission measurements, and electrophysiologic tests are commonly used to assess a person's hearing abilities. Hearing aid and cochlear implant are two of the most common devices that assist in hearing disorders. Hearing aid is a device which improves a person's hearing by making sound audible to the indivisual. A surgically implanted neuroprosthetic device which provides a sense of sound to a person having severe hearing loss is known as a cochlear implant. This book elucidates the concepts and innovative models around prospective developments with respect to audiology. It studies, analyses and upholds the pillars of audiology and its utmost significance in modern times. This book includes contributions of experts and doctors which will provide innovative insights into this field.

It was a great honour to edit this book, though there were challenges, as it involved a lot of communication and networking between me and the editorial team. However, the end result was this all-inclusive book covering diverse themes in the field.

Finally, it is important to acknowledge the efforts of the contributors for their excellent chapters, through which a wide variety of issues have been addressed. I would also like to thank my colleagues for their valuable feedback during the making of this book.

Editor

1

Noise-Induced Hearing Loss in Korean Workers: Co-Exposure to Organic Solvents and Heavy Metals in Nationwide Industries

Yoon-Hyeong Choi[1], **KyooSang Kim**[2*¤]

1 Department of Preventive Medicine, Gachon University Graduate School of Medicine, Incheon, Korea, 2 Occupational Safety and Health Research Institute, Korea Occupational Safety and Health Agency, Incheon, Korea

Abstract

Background: Noise exposure is a well-known contributor to work-related hearing loss. Recent biological evidence suggests that exposure to ototoxic chemicals such as organic solvents and heavy metals may be additional contributors to hearing loss. However, in industrial settings, it is difficult to determine the risks of hearing loss due to these chemicals in workplaces accompanied by excessive noise exposure. A few studies suggest that the effect of noise may be enhanced by ototoxic chemicals. Therefore, this study investigated whether co-exposure to organic solvents and/or heavy metals in the workplace modifies the risk of noise exposure on hearing loss in a background of excessive noise.

Methods: We examined 30,072 workers nationwide in a wide range of industries from the Korea National Occupational Health Surveillance 2009. Data on industry-based exposure (e.g., occupational noise, heavy metals, and organic solvents) and subject-specific health outcomes (e.g., audiometric examination) were collected. Noise was measured as the daily 8-h time-weighted average level. Air conduction hearing thresholds were measured from 0.5 to 6 kHz, and pure-tone averages (PTA) (i.e., means of 2, 3, and 4 kHz) were computed.

Results: In the multivariate linear model, PTA increment with occupational noise were 1.64-fold and 2.15-fold higher in individuals exposed to heavy metals and organic solvents than in unexposed individuals, respectively.

Conclusion: This study provides nationwide evidence that co-exposure to heavy metals and/or organic solvents may exacerbate the effect of noise exposure on hearing loss in workplaces. These findings suggest that workers in industries dealing with heavy metals or organic solvents are susceptible to such risks.

Editor: Jonathan I. Matsui, Harvard University, United States of America

Funding: These authors have no support or funding to report.

Competing Interests: The authors have declared that no competing interests exist.

* E-mail: kyoosang@daum.net

¤ Current address: Department of Occupational Environmental Medicine, Seoul Medical Center, Seoul, Korea

Introduction

Work-related hearing loss is a critical issue in workplace safety and health. The U.S. National Institute for Occupational Safety and Health (NIOSH) and the occupational safety and health community designated hearing loss as one of the 21 priority research areas in the 21st century [1]. Loud noise is a major risk factor for work-related hearing loss, and audiologists are well aware of the need for monitoring and protecting against noise in the workplace [2–4]. In fact, many countries have conducted surveillance and/or compensation programs to monitor workplace noise and identify occupational noise-induced hearing loss [5–8].

Evidence accumulated over recent decades suggests that exposure to neurotoxic chemicals is an additional contributor to occupational hearing loss. Some organic solvents, heavy metals, asphyxiants, and pesticides fall within this category and are widely used in many industries and occupations [9–11]. Organic solvents such as toluene (C_7H_8), styrene (C_8H_8), xylene (C_8H_{10}), isopropyl alcohol (C_3H_8O), and ethyl benzene (C_8H_{10}) have been widely studied for their ototoxicity. Indeed, animal experiments demonstrate sensorineural hearing loss with cochlear damage as a result of exposure to these chemicals [12–16]. Furthermore, several workplace studies suggest that such solvents are associated with an increased risk of hearing loss [17–22]. Heavy metals such as cadmium, lead, mercury, and manganese are reported to impair inner ear cells, leading to auditory function disorders in animal studies [23–27]. There is further evidence for their ototoxicity in human studies as well [28–30].

However, the effects of organic solvents and/or heavy metals on hearing loss in industrial settings are difficult to distinguish from the effect of noise [31]. In fact, many studies in workplaces involving exposure to both solvents and noise commonly assume noise to be the sole contributor to hearing loss; but, they could not observe the effects of solvents despite scientific plausibility that both noise and solvents have biological effects. A possible reason for the null findings of the ototoxic effects of solvents include diluted observation due to the dominant effect of noise; this is because workplaces using these chemicals are likely to be accompanied by excessive noise as well [32,33]. A few recent studies suggest that the effect of noise can be enhanced by ototoxic chemical exposure [34–38].

The Korea National Occupational Health Surveillance (KNOHS), also known as Korean Occupational Medical Examination Program [39], is a nationwide annual surveillance program designed to monitor problematic industries and their workers, including work-related hearing loss. The program includes audiometric testing, industrial-based noise measurement, and assessment of exposure to ototoxic chemicals (e.g., organic solvents and heavy metals).

Thus, the present study estimated the national burdens of occupational noise exposure on work-related hearing loss using nationwide data from various industries from the KNOHS 2009 and evaluated the hypothesis that co-exposure to heavy metals and/or organic solvents in the workplace modifies the risk of occupational noise exposure on hearing loss in a background of excessive noise.

Methods

Study population

The final study sample consisted of 30,072 employees aged 18 to 77 years registered in 1,935 industries from the KNOHS 2009; this program was established by the Ministry of Labor of Korea as part of a government program aimed at preventing and compensating for work-related hearing loss.

Data on industry-based exposure and subject-specific health outcomes were collected. The Occupational Safety and Health Research Institute (OSHRI) of the Korea Occupational Safety and Health Agency (KOSHA) compiled a list of all available industries registered with the Korea Ministry of Labor and administered the industries particularly in which the noise exposure level was ≥80 decibels of ambient noise (dBA). These industries were assigned to the KNOHS, which assessed noise exposure levels. All employees who have worked in these industries underwent audiometric examinations and interviews to obtain demographic and physical information. The initial sample included 300,741 participants for primary audiometric examination at limited frequencies (necessarily including 1 kHz) from the KNOHS 2009. From the initial sample, all employees who worked in the industries where the noise level was ≥85 dBA underwent an advanced audiometric examination at various frequencies.

For the present study, we selected participants who had measures in all available frequencies (i.e., 0.5, 1, 2, 3, 4, and 6 kHz); therefore, 64,974 subjects were eligible for inclusion in data analyses. We further excluded participants with missing information for covariate variables ($n = 33,782$), and additional participants were excluded for non-Korean ($n = 1,120$) (see Figure S1). The final analysis included 30,072 participants in the analysis.

Ethics Statement

The KNOHS is a national dataset collected by the OSHRI that followed the Korean Occupational Safety and Health (OSH) Act [8]. The study protocol was approved by the Occupational Safety and Health Research Institute institutional review board, and written informed consent was provided by study participants.

Occupational Noise Measures

For each industry, occupational noise exposure assessment was conducted at various onsite spots (1 to 2,109 spots depending on each industry's scale). Exposure was measured as a daily eight-hour time-weighted average (8HR TWA) using a sound level meter (SLM) and was based upon 5 dB exchange rate for calculating noise dose as a function of exposure time and level [40]. The mean noise value from these spot measurements for each industry was computed. All individuals who have worked in the industries with 8HR TWA ≥85 dBA (i.e., noisy industries) were selected to participate in an advanced audiometric examination component.

Hearing Threshold Examination

An advanced audiometric examination was conducted at various frequencies in a silent room by health technicians trained by a KOSHA-certified audiologist. For standardized measurements, audiometric components, including an audiometer and headphones, and measurement environment followed the guidelines of the Korean Audiometric Quality Control Program [41]. Pure tone air conduction hearing thresholds were obtained for both ears at each frequency over intensity range of −10 to 120 dB and computed as a pure-tone average (PTA) of 2, 3, and 4 kHz following the definition of standard threshold shift of the Occupational Safety and Health Administration. Hearing loss was defined as PTA >25 dB in one or both ears. The details of audiometric examination have been described elsewhere [42]. Hearing thresholds at1 kHz were obtained only in a primary audiometric examination from an initial sampling stage and were not attained in advanced examination in a silent room by trained technicians.

Ototoxic Chemical Exposures

Non-noise source exposures to organic chemicals and heavy metals were classified based on industries-database compiled by the OSHRI. The OSHRI administered a list of problematic industries exposed to occupational agents (i.e., organic chemicals and heavy metals) among all available industries registered with the Korea Ministry of Labor, similar to a list of problematic noisy industries. Each industry was classed as exposure or not to organic solvents and heavy metals, respectively. Organic solvent exposure was considered for toluene, isopropyl alcohol, and/or xylene (a mixture and individual elements); heavy metal exposure was considered for lead, cadmium, mercury, chrome, and/or manganese (a mixture). Exposure to a mixture was defined as exposure to one or more of the individual elements.

We modeled organic solvent exposure or heavy metal exposure as an exposure to a mixture, because workplaces are not solely exposed to any individual chemical but commonly exposed to a mixture. Instead, sensitivity analyses were examined in all individual organic solvents including toluene, isopropyl alcohol, and xylene. No data regarding individual types of heavy metals were available. Further details are available elsewhere (see File S1).

Demographic and Potential Risk Variables

Data on demographic and potential risk variables were obtained through physical examinations and extensive interviews. Body mass index (BMI) was computed as weight in kilograms/height in meters squared. Hypertension was classified based on either systolic blood pressure ≥140 mmHg or diastolic blood pressure ≥ 90 mm Hg at the time of the examination.

Statistical Analysis

All regression analyses began with univariate analyses to identify outliers and influential points. The statistically significant level was set as P values less than 0.05. Linear regression was fit for the association of hearing thresholds in PTA and individual frequencies with occupational noise measures. To identify the influence of potential confounders, we developed a sequence of models — initially crude model; adjusted for age, age-squared, and sex; and further adjusted for BMI and hypertension. We also fit multivariate-adjusted linear regressions in subgroups stratified by age, sex, BMI, and hypertension as well as occupational exposures to organic solvents and heavy metals, in order to evaluate whether these factors modify the association of PTA with occupational noise exposure. Logistic regression was used to estimate odds ratio (ORs) for the hearing loss. All statistical analyses were performed using SAS (version 9.1) and R (2.13.1).

Results

The KNOHS estimated that 64,974 Korean workers in 7,394 industries were exposed to a daily occupational noise ≥80 dB and that 77% of them had hearing loss (PTA > 25 dB in one or both ears) in 2009 (see Figure S1). Table 1 shows the characteristics of the 30,072 study participants, eligible for the analyses. Their mean ± standard deviation (SD) age was 44.4±9.3 years. Because hearing ability is strongly correlated with age, we computed age-adjusted means for hearing thresholds and other continuous variables. The age-adjusted mean PTA was 28.1±14.7 decibels hearing level (dBHL). The age-adjusted mean of occupational noise exposure was high at 88.6±5.3 dBA, which is unsurprising considering that participants were originally collected from the industries with problematic noise levels. Table 2 shows the occupational noise exposure levels by subject characteristics. Occupational noise exposure was higher for women, older workers, those more exposed to organic chemicals, those less exposed to heavy metals, and those with hypertension and a BMI <25 kg/m^2 (Table 2).

Table 3 presents the associations between occupational noise exposure and hearing thresholds on PTAs and at each frequency in covariate-adjusted models. In the crude model, occupational noise was significantly associated with elevated hearing thresholds at all frequencies and PTAs (Model A). After adjusting for age and sex, although the associations were attenuated over all frequencies and PTAs, their significance remained, except at 0.5 kHz (Model B). After further adjustment for BMI and hypertension, similar associations between occupational noise and increased hearing thresholds were observed (Model C). In the multivariate-adjusted Model C, the average increase in hearing thresholds in PTAs was 2.35 dBHL (95% confidence interval [CI], 2.05–2.64 dBHL) for an interquartile range (IQR) increase in occupational noise exposure. Further adjustment for occupational exposure to organic solvents and heavy metals did not alter the results (Model D). In all models, the largest rate increase in hearing thresholds with occupational noise exposure was observed at 3 kHz.

Table 4 shows the multivariate-adjusted associations of PTAs with occupational noise exposure in groups stratified according to participant status listed in Table 1. There was a significant increase in the associations of PTAs with occupational noise exposure with increasing age ($p_{interaction}$ = 0.004) and a marginally stronger association in women than in men ($p_{interaction}$ = 0.055).

We also evaluated whether the association between occupational noise exposure and hearing outcome is modified by co-exposure to ototoxic chemicals. Table 5 shows the multivariate-adjusted associations of PTA with occupational noise levels in groups stratified according to occupational organic solvent or heavy metal exposure. The PTA increment with the IQR increase in occupational noise was significantly higher in subjects exposed to organic solvents (versus non-exposed subjects, 4.43 dBHL [CI, 3.43–5.42] vs. 2.06 dBHL [CI, 1.75–2.37]) as well as in subjects exposed to heavy metals (vs. non-exposed subjects, 3.25 dBHL [CI, 2.58–3.92] vs. 1.98 dBHL [CI, 1.65–2.31]). When individual frequencies were examined, similar higher increments were observed in the organic solvent-exposed group at 3, 4, and 6 kHz as well as in the heavy metal-exposed group at 2 and 3 kHz compared to the respective non-exposed reference groups (see Table S1).

Logistic regression models revealed significantly greater odds of hearing loss with occupational noise levels in groups exposed to heavy metals and organic solvents than in the respective non-exposure reference groups (Table S2).

Table 1. General characteristics of study participants (N = 30,072[a]).

Characteristic	Mean[b] ± SD
Occupational noise[c]	88.6±5.3
Age *(y)*	44.4±9.3
BMI *(kg/m^2)*	23.6±3.0
Sex [male; *n (%)*]	27,857 (92.6)
Hypertension [*n (%)*]	4,873 (16.2)
Hearing Thresholds *(dBHL)*	
PTA at 2, 3, 4 Khz[d]	28.1±14.7
0.5 kHz	15.6±11.1
1 kHz[e]	15.8±12.2
2 kHz	18.8±14.3
3 kHz	28.4±17.4
4 kHz	37.3±18.3
6 kHz	41.6±20.3
Hearing Loss[f] *(PTA>25dBHL, %)*	20461, 68%

[a]Participants (N = 33,072) are the individuals having all interest variables in this study: advanced audiometric measurements, age, occupational noise, sex, BMI, and hypertension.
[b]Age-adjusted means were presented.
[c]Occupational noise (a daily 8-hour time weighted average level in each industry).
[d]PTA (pure tone average) of standard threshold at 2, 3, 4 kHz frequencies.
[e]Hearing thresholds at 1 kHz were obtained from primary audiometric tests.
[f]Hearing Loss (PTA at 2, 3, 4 KHz frequencies > 25 dBHL).
SD, standard deviation.

Discussion

The present study of a nationwide working population demonstrates association of occupational noise exposure with poorer hearing outcomes, and that individuals working in industries that particularly involve exposure to organic solvents and/or heavy metals are susceptible to an increased risk of hearing loss due to occupational noise, suggesting noise–organic solvent interaction and noise–heavy metal interaction.

Work-related hearing loss is one of the most common occupational hazards [1]. Noise is a well-known contributing factor. Thus, many researchers suggest the need to control noise exposure in order to reduce the burden of work-related hearing loss. Although many countries have implemented national programs to monitor and control noise levels in various industries, it is difficult to reduce noise exposure in many industries. Therefore, identifying susceptibility-related factors in conjunction

Table 2. Means and 95% confidence intervals of occupational noise exposure by participants characteristics.

Characteristic	No.	Occupational noise (dBA), mean (95% C.I.)	*p-value*[a]
Age *(year)*			<0.001
10–29	2356	85.8 (85.6–86.0)	
30–39	6995	87.9 (87.8–88.1)	
40–49	10062	89.2 (89.1–89.3)	
≥50	10659	90.7 (90.6–90.8)	
Sex			<0.001
Male	27857	89.0 (89.0–89.1)	
Female	2215	90.8 (90.5–91.0)	
Body mass index *(kg/m²)*			<0.001
<25	20991	89.3 (89.3–89.4)	
≥25	9081	88.7 (88.6–88.8)	
Hypertension			<0.001
No	25199	89.1 (89.0–89.1)	
Yes	4873	89.6 (89.5–89.8)	
Occupational exposure to heavy metals			<0.001
Non exposure	27382	89.4 (89.4–89.5)	
Exposure	2690	86.1 (85.9–86.3)	
Occupational exposure to organic solvents			<0.001
Non exposure	22164	89.0 (88.9–89.0)	
Exposure	7908	89.7 (89.6–89.8)	

CI, confidence interval
[a]*t*-test for binominal groups and *trend-P* for ordinal categorical groups were used.

with the avoidance of noise (the major risk factor) is important for effectively preventing occupational noise-induced hearing loss.

Despite biological evidence of the ototoxicity of industrial chemicals, previous studies in occupational settings assume noise to be the sole contributor to hearing loss and observed little effects of ototoxic chemicals. The dominant effect of loud noise in workplaces may explain why such previous studies did not find effects of ototoxic chemicals. Interestingly, 2 recent studies in a general population [43,44] report adverse effects of lead and cadmium exposure on hearing outcomes not in the group exposed to higher noise levels, but only in those exposed to lower or mid-noise levels; these findings support the notion that the observed risk due to heavy metals may be diluted by the greater risk due to noise. In fact, consistent with previous studies, the present sensitivity analysis stratified according to noise levels revealed that organic solvent exposure adversely affected hearing thresholds in a group exposed to mid-noise levels but found no effect of organic solvent exposure in a group exposed to more noise (Table S3). This suggests that noise exposure is basically the greatest contributing factor to hearing loss while ototoxic chemicals may have additive effects in low-noise environments (that is, when there remains room for additional damage) and should be approached as a modifiable factor in workplaces involving regular high noise levels.

The current study provides evidence of effect modification by the exposure to heavy metals and organic solvents. Individuals exposed to heavy metals and organic solvents had a higher risk of hearing loss in relation to noise than unexposed individuals. The effect sizes of PTA increment with occupational noise were 1.64-fold and 2.15-fold higher in individuals exposed to heavy metals and organic solvents than in unexposed individuals, respectively (3.25 vs. 1.98 dBHL and 4.43 vs. 2.06 dBHL, respectively; see Table 5). Such effect modifications were roughly comparable to estimated effect modification by sex (1.36-fold higher in women [3.19 dBHL] than in men [2.23 dBHL]) and age over 20 years (1.36-fold higher in subjects aged ≥50 years [2.79 dBHL] than in subjects in their 30s [2.05 dBHL]; see Table 4).

Few studies have evaluated the effect modification (i.e., interaction) by organic solvents or heavy metals on the risk of occupational noise towards hearing outcomes. Several small-scale workplace studies compared noise-only exposure cases and noise- and solvent-exposure cases with a control group (i.e., non-exposure). One such study examining 1,117 employees in the yacht, shipping, paint and lacquer, plastics, and footwear industries found an increased risk of hearing loss by co-exposure to solvents; the odds ratios (ORs) of hearing loss were 3.8 and 6.7–21.5 in the cases of noise only, and noise and solvents (i.e., mixtures, styrene, *n*-hexane plus toluene, or styrene plus toluene) compared to a control group, respectively [36]. Another study analyzing the responses of 701 dockyard workers to a questionnaire on exposure revealed that the OR of hearing loss increased approximately 3-fold in the group exposed to only noise but almost 5-fold in the group exposed to both noise and solvent [35]. Although these studies do not provide evidence of multiplicative interaction by solvents on the risk of noise towards hearing loss, they are broadly compatible with the present findings. A previous study of case-control design supported a potential interaction between noise and toluene; the risk of hearing loss was 11 times greater for noise- and toluene-exposure group compared with unexposed group. The estimated effects were larger than the sums of the individual effects [noise-only (4 times) and solvent-only (5 times)] [45]. To our knowledge, this is the first epidemiologic study

Table 3. Effect estimates (95% CI) of hearing thresholds (dBHL) with IQR increment in occupational noise exposure (dBA).

Frequency	Model A[a]		Model B[b]		Model C[c]		Model D[d]	
	Per noise IQR[e]		Per noise IQR[e]		Per noise IQR[e]		Per noise IQR[e]	
	Estimate	(95% CI)	Estimate	(95% CI)	Estimate	(95% CI)	Estimate	(95% CI)
PTA[f]	6.06	(5.73, 6.39)*	2.33	(2.03, 2.62)*	2.35	(2.05, 2.64)*	2.24	(1.94, 2.54)*
0.5 kHz	0.54	(0.32, 0.76)*	−0.10	(−0.33, 0.12)	−0.12	(−0.35, 0.11)	−0.14	(−0.37, 0.09)
1 kHz	1.97	(1.73, 2.22)*	0.62	(0.37, 0.87)*	0.64	(0.39, 0.89)*	0.64	(0.39, 0.89)*
2 kHz	4.22	(3.92, 4.52)*	1.72	(1.43, 2.01)*	1.71	(1.43, 2.00)*	1.65	(1.36, 1.95)*
3 kHz	7.21	(6.82, 7.59)*	2.97	(2.63, 3.32)*	3.01	(2.66, 3.36)*	2.88	(2.52, 3.23)*
4 kHz	6.75	(6.34, 7.16)*	2.29	(1.93, 2.65)*	2.32	(1.96, 2.69)*	2.19	(1.82, 2.56)*
6 kHz	6.90	(6.45, 7.34)*	2.67	(2.26, 3.07)*	2.70	(2.29, 3.11)*	2.54	(2.13, 2.95)*

CI, confidence interval.
[a]Model A was a crude model.
[b]Model B was adjusted for age, age^2, sex.
[c]Model C: Model B + further adjusted for BMI, hypertension.
[d]Model D: Model C + further adjusted for occupational exposures to organic solvents and heavy metals.
[e]Hearing Thresholds (dBHL) change per interquartile range (IQR) of occupational noise, 94.26 dBA - 84.74 dBA: 9.52 dBA.
[f]PTA (pure tone average at 2, 3, 4 kHz).
*$p<0.05$.

Table 4. Multivariate-adjusted effect estimates (95% CI) of hearing thresholds (dBHL) with IQR increment in occupational noise exposure (dBA), stratified according to participant status.

		Per noise IQR[a]	*p*-value for
Stratification variable	**No.**	**Estimate (95% CI)**	**interaction**
Overall	30072	2.35 (2.05, 2.64)*	
Age *(year)*			*0.004*
≤29	2356	0.93 (0.17, 1.68)*	
30–39	6995	2.05 (1.51, 2.58)*	
40–49	10062	2.10 (1.58, 2.62)*	
≥50	10659	2.79 (2.23, 3.35)*	
Sex			*0.055*
Male	27857	2.23 (1.92, 2.54)*	
Female	2215	3.19 (2.28, 4.09)*	
BMI *(kg/m)*			*0.573*
<25	20991	2.35 (1.99, 2.70)*	
≥25	9081	2.31 (1.78, 2.84)*	
Hypertension			*0.375*
No	25199	2.26 (1.93, 2.58)*	
Yes	4873	2.61 (1.91, 3.31)*	

Models were adjusted for age, age^2, sex, BMI, and hypertension, defined in Model C, Table 3.
CI, confidence interval.
[a]PTA (dBHL) change per interquartile range (IQR) of occupational noise, 94.26 dBA - 84.74 dBA: 9.52 dBA.
**p*<0.05.*

to evaluate effect modifications by heavy metals on the association between noise and hearing outcomes in the workplace, although there is existing evidence for a main effect of heavy metals on hearing outcomes [4,28,46]. Nevertheless, the precise mechanisms underlying the observed effect modifications by heavy metals and organic solvents remain unclear. Previous animal experiments show that solvents such as toluene, styrene, xylene, isopropyl alcohol, and ethyl benzene damage the cochlea (predominantly the supporting and outer hair cells) and provoke irreversible sensorineural hearing loss [12–16]. Furthermore, heavy metals such as cadmium, lead, mercury, and manganese induce the impairment (i.e., apoptosis and/or degeneration) of inner ear receptor cells, leading to auditory neuronal function disorders [23–27]. These findings provide a possible explanation that heavy metals and/or organic solvents condition the cochlea for damage triggered by oxidative stress produced by noise exposure. In addition, heavy metals and organic solvents are associated with the regulation of intracellular calcium homeostasis [47,48], and thus, they may play an additional role in auditory hair cell death.

In the present study, the associations between occupational noise and poorer hearing outcomes were stronger, particularly at middle-to-high frequencies. In addition, effect modifications by heavy metals and organic solvents on the associations between noise and hearing outcomes were strong at middle-to-high

Table 5. Multivariate-adjusted effect estimates (95% CI) of hearing thresholds (dBHL) with IQR increment in occupational noise exposure (dBA), stratified according to occupational exposure to ototoxic chemicals.

Stratification variable		**Per noise IQR[a]**	***p-value* for interaction**
	No.	**Estimate (95% CI)**	
Overall	30072	2.35 (2.05, 2.64)*	
Heavy metals			*<.001*
Non exposure	22164	1.98 (1.65, 2.31)*	
Exposure	7908	3.25 (2.58, 3.92)*	
Organic solvents			*<.001*
Non exposure	27382	2.06 (1.75, 2.37)*	
Exposure	2690	4.43 (3.43, 5.42)*	

Models were adjusted for age, age^2, sex, BMI, and hypertension, defined in Model C, Table 3.
CI, confidence interval.
[a]PTA (dBHL) change per interquartile range (IQR) of occupational noise, 94.26 dBA - 84.74 dBA: 9.52 dBA.
**p*<0.05.*

frequencies. These frequencies are known to be sensitive to noise [49,50]; therefore, the present observations suggests that heavy metals and organic solvents act as effect modifiers regulating "noise"-induced hearing loss.

This study investigated the effect caused by mixtures of organic solvent(s) or heavy metal(s) on the association between noise and hearing. Indeed, models including an individual organic solvent (e.g., toluene, isopropyl alcohol, and xylene) confirmed similar effect modifications to findings from models including a mixture of organic solvents (data not shown). However, there are no data for different types of heavy metals. Occupational environments do not expose workers solely to any given chemical; instead, workers are commonly exposed to a mixture of chemicals. Furthermore, molecular mechanisms involved in toxicity due to individual solvents (also, metals) are similar. Therefore, this study did not consider individual effects separately.

This study used a hearing outcome with a PTAs of 2, 3, and 4 kHz on a "standard threshold shift" as defined by the Occupational Safety and Health Administration rather than the most commonly used method of PTA definition at speech frequencies (i.e., 0.5, 1, 2, and 4 kHz) as defined by the World Health Organization (WHO). This is because hearing data at 1 kHz were collected only through a primary audiometric test and subsequently without an advanced examination by trained technicians in a silent room. Instead, sensitivity analyses were examined at all individual frequencies including 0.5 and 1 kHz.

The main strength of this study is its large sample population, which included over 30,000 available subjects in industries with problematic noise selected from an initial sample drawn from all industries registered with the Korean Department of Labor. In addition, the present data support the on-site measurement of noise exposure in all industries. Therefore, the present results extend the partial observations of previous epidemiological studies on work-related hearing loss, which are limited to certain occupations and particularly by the difficulty in assessing exposure, to a nationwide scale including a wide range of occupations/industries. In turn, this enabled us to observe co-exposure to noise and ototoxic chemicals in the workplace.

This study has several limitations that should be considered. First, occupational organic solvent and heavy metal exposure are classed as exposure or not, but no data regarding instrumental measured levels were available; thus, the present study may not account for variability in exposure levels of organic solvents and heavy metals. Moreover, noise and other ototoxic exposure were assigned only at the industrial level; exposure variation among different jobs/tasks within the same industry was not accounted for. Second, the present data do not provide information on various potential confounding factors such as smoking or exposure to non-occupational noise (e.g., residential and recreational). Therefore, the true associations of occupational noise and other ototoxic factors with hearing thresholds may be weaker than those reported in the present study. Third, it can be argued that the present findings regarding the effect modification by ototoxic chemicals on the association between noise and hearing loss are due to the correlation between ototoxic chemical exposure and high-level noise. However, the present results demonstrate the risk of hearing loss due to noise is higher in individuals exposed to heavy metals (see Table 5) even if they are exposed to less noise (see Table 2). Finally, although a nationwide representative sample of noise-exposed workers in Korea increased power to our findings, the observed effect modification may not apply to the general population. Because the present data were collected only from industries that have considerable noise levels, and therefore a majority of subjects may have work-related hearing loss and were male, our observations could be different from general populations exposed to low-level noise and who reflect half male and half female. We suggest more research is needed to confirm our evidence using a large sample of general adults.

The present study based on the Korea National Occupational Health Surveillance program estimates that more than 7,000 Korean industries involve occupational daily exposure to levels exceeding 85 dB. These industries include over 60,000 workers, 77% of whom have hearing loss attributable to their work. Indeed, it is difficult to control noise levels for all potentially problematic industries in a country. In addition, noise exposure is common in certain industries and occupations. Therefore, with the need for cost-effective control of noise, the present study provides data for establishing criteria for priority industries to implement monitoring and reduce occupational noise and chemicals to effectively lessen the national burden of work-related hearing loss.

Conclusion

In conclusion, the present study supports the hypothesis that co-exposure to organic solvents and heavy metals may increase the risk of hearing loss due to noise exposure. The present findings suggest that the risk of noise-induced hearing loss may vary by industry. Furthermore, employees in industries dealing with heavy metals and/or organic solvents are susceptible to such risks, and these industries should prioritize noise and chemicals reduction to prevent work-related hearing loss.

Supporting Information

Figure S1 Study participants profile.

Table S1 Multivariate-adjusted effect estimates (95% CI) of hearing thresholds (dBHL) at individual frequencies with IQR increment in occupational noise exposure (dBA), stratified according to occupational exposure to ototoxic chemicals.

Table S2 Multivariate-adjusted ORs (95% CIs) of hearing loss[a] with IQR increment in occupational noise exposure (dBA), stratified according to occupational exposure to ototoxic chemicals.

Table S3 Multivariate-adjusted effect estimates (95% CIs) of hearing thresholds (dBHL) attributable to occupational exposure to ototoxic chemicals, stratified according to noise exposure levels (dBA).

File S1 Methods: Ototoxic Chemical Exposures, References.

Author Contributions

Conceived and designed the experiments: YC KK. Performed the experiments: YC. Analyzed the data: YC. Contributed reagents/materials/analysis tools: YC KK. Wrote the paper: YC.

References

1. CDC (2001) Work Related Hearing Loss. Atlanta, GA: Centers for Disease Control and Prevention.
2. Palmer KT, Griffin MJ, Syddall HE, Davis A, Pannett B, et al. (2002) Occupational exposure to noise and the attributable burden of hearing difficulties in Great Britain. Occupational and Environmental Medicine 59: 634–639.
3. Stanbury M, Rafferty AP, Rosenman K (2008) Prevalence of Hearing Loss and Work-Related Noise-Induced Hearing Loss in Michigan. Journal of Occupational and Environmental Medicine 50: 72–79.
4. Choi Y-H, Hu H, Tak S, Mukherjee B, Park SK (2012) Occupational Noise Exposure Assessment using O*NET and Its Application to a Study of Hearing Loss in the US General Population. Occupational and Environmental Medicine 69: 176–183.
5. CDC (2013) Occupational Hearing Loss Surveillance. Atlanta, GA: Centers for Disease Control and Prevention.
6. Meyer JD, Chen Y, McDonald JC, Cherry NM (2002) Surveillance for work-related hearing loss in the UK: OSSA and OPRA 1997-2000. Occup Med 52: 75–79.
7. Wu TN, Liou SH, Shen CY, Hsu CC, Chao SL, et al. (1998) Surveillance of noise-induced hearing loss in Taiwan, ROC: a report of the PRESS-NHL results. Prev Med 27: 65–69.
8. OSHRI (2010) Research on Occupational Exposures-Related Disease (I): the Korea National Occupational Health Surveillance 2009 on occupational audiological disorders. Incheon, Republich of Korea: The Occupational Safety and Health Research Institute, The Korea Occupational Safety and Health Agency.
9. Wallhagen MI, Strawbridge WJ, Cohen RD, Kaplan GA (1997) An increasing prevalence of hearing impairment and associated risk factors over three decades of the Alameda County Study. Am J Public Health 87: 440–442.
10. Fuente A, McPherson B (2006) Organic solvents and hearing loss: The challenge for audiology. International Journal of Audiology 45: 367–381.
11. Morata TC (2003) Chemical Exposure as a Risk Factor for Hearing Loss. Journal of Occupational and Environmental Medicine 45: 676–682.
12. Śliwinska-Kowalska M, Prasher D, Rodrigues C, Zamysłowska-Szmytke E, Campo P, et al. (2007) Ototoxicity of Organic Solvents - From Scientific Evidence to Health Policy. International Journal of Occupational Medicine and Environmental Health 20: 215–222.
13. Crofton K, Lassiter T, Rebert C (1994) Solvent-induced ototoxicity in rats: An atypical selective mid-frequency hearing deficit Hearing Research 80: 25–30.
14. Campo P, Lataye R, Loquet G, Bonnet P (2001) Styrene-induced hearing loss: a membrane insult. Hearing Research 154: 170–180.
15. Spandow O, Anniko M, Moller AR (1988) The round window as access route for agents injurious to the inner ear. American Journal of Otolaryngology 9: 327–335.
16. Cappaert NLM, Klis SFL, Muijser H, Kulig BM, Smoorenburg GF (2001) Simultaneous exposure to ethyl benzene and noise: synergistic effects on outer hair cells. Hearing Research 162: 67–79.
17. Sliwinska-Kowalska M, Zamyslowska-Szmytke E, Szymczak W, Kotylo P, Fiszer M, et al. (2001) Hearing loss among workers exposed to moderate concentrations of solvents. Scand J Work Environ Health 27: 335–342.
18. Sliwinska-Kowalska M, Zamyslowska-Szmytke E, Szymczak W, Kotylo P, Fiszer M, et al. (2003) Ototoxic Effects of Occupational Exposure to Styrene and Co-Exposure to Styrene and Noise. Journal of Occupational and Environmental Medicine 45: 15–24.
19. Abbate C, Giorgianni C, Munaò F, Brecciaroli R (1993) Neurotoxicity induced by exposure to toluene. International Archives of Occupational and Environmental Health 64: 389–392.
20. Varney NR, Kubu CS, Morrow LA (1998) Dichotic Listening Performances of Patients with Chronic Exposure to Organic Solvents. The Clinical Neuropsychologist 12: 107–112.
21. Morata TC, Fiorini AC, Fischer FM, Colacioppo S, Wallingford KM, et al. (1997) Toluene-induced hearing loss among rotogravure printing workers. Scandinavian Journal of Work, Environment and Health 23: 289–298.
22. Fuente A, Slade MD, Taylor T, Morata TC, Keith RW, et al. (2009) Peripheral and central auditory dysfunction induced by occupational exposure to organic solvents. J Occup Environ Med 51: 1202–1211.
23. Yamamura K, Terayama K, Yamamoto N, Kohyama A, Kishi R (1989) Effects of acute lead acetate exposure on adult guinea pigs: Electrophysiological study of the inner ear. Fundamental and Applied Toxicology 13: 509–515.
24. Lasky RE, Maier MM, Snodgrass EB, Hecox KE, Laughlin NK (1995) The effects of lead on otoacoustic emissions and auditory evoked potentials in monkeys. Neurotoxicology and Teratology 17: 633–644.
25. Jones LG, Prins J, Park S, Walton JP, Luebke AE, et al. (2008) Lead exposure during development results in increased neurofilament phosphorylation, neuritic beading, and temporal processing deficits within the murine auditory brainstem. The Journal of Comparative Neurology 506: 1003–1017.
26. Kim S-J, Jeong H-J, Myung N-Y, Kim M-C, Lee J-H, et al. (2008) The Protective Mechanism of Antioxidants in Cadmium-Induced Ototoxicity *in Vitro* and *in Vivo*. Environ Health Perspect 116: 854–862.
27. Ozcaglar H, Agirdir B, Dinc O, Turhan M, Kilinçarslan S, et al. (2001) Effects of cadmium on the hearing system. Acta Otolaryngol 121: 393–397.
28. Chuang H-Y, Kuo C-H, Chiu Y-W, Ho C-K, Chen C-J, et al. (2007) A case-control study on the relationship of hearing function and blood concentrations of lead, manganese, arsenic, and selenium. Science of The Total Environment 387: 79–85.
29. Choi YH, Hu H, Mukherjee B, Miller J, Park SK (2012) Environmental cadmium and lead exposures and hearing loss in u.s. Adults: the national health and nutrition examination survey, 1999 to 2004. Environ Health Perspect 120: 1544–1550.
30. Shargorodsky J, Curhan SG, Henderson E, Eavey R, Curhan GC (2011) Heavy metals exposure and hearing loss in US adolescents. Arch Otolaryngol Head Neck Surg 137: 1183–1189.
31. Sliwinska-Kowalska M (2008) Organic solvent exposure and hearing loss. Occupational and Environmental Medicine 65: 222–223.
32. Jacobsen P, Hein HO, Suadicani P, Parving A, Gyntelberg F (1993) Mixed solvent exposure and hearing impairment: an epidemiological study of 3284 men. The Copenhagen male study. Occup Med 43: 180–184.
33. Sass-Kortsak AM, Corey PN, Robertson JM (1995) An investigation of the association between exposure to styrene and hearing loss. Annals of Epidemiology 5: 15–24.
34. Vyskocil A, Truchon G, Leroux T, Lemay F, Gendron M, et al. (2011) A weight of evidence approach for the assessment of the ototoxic potential of industrial chemicals. Toxicology and Industrial Health 28:796–819.
35. Sliwinska-Kowalska M, Zamyslowska-Szmytke E, Szymczak W, Kotylo P, Fiszer M, et al. (2004) Effects of Coexposure to Noise and Mixture of Organic Solvents on Hearing in Dockyard Workers. Journal of Occupational and Environmental Medicine 46: 30–38.
36. Sliwinska-Kowalska M, Zamyslowska-Szmytke E, Szymczak W, Kotylo P, Fiszer M, et al. (2005) Exacerbation of noise-induced hearing loss by co-exposure to workplace chemicals. Environmental Toxicology and Pharmacology 19: 547–553.
37. Johnson A-C, Morata TC (2010) 142. Occupational exposure to chemicals and hearing impairment. The Nordic Expert Group for Criteria Documentation of Health Risks from Chemicals. Nordic Expert Group. Arbete och Hälsa; 44(4): 177 pp.
38. EU-OSHA (2009) Combined exposure to noise and ototoxic substances. Luxembourg: European Agency for Safety and Health at Work
39. Park J, Kim Y, Kim KS (1999) Remodeling of the occupational medical examination program in South Korea. Int Arch Occup Environ Health 72: 411–417.
40. OSHRI (2009) Occupational Health Surveillance Standard Methods: Noise. Incheon, Republic of Korea: The Occupational Safety and Health Research Institute, The Korea Occupational Safety and Health Agency.
41. Kim K-S (2007) Development of Korean Audiometric Quality Control Program for the Special Health Examination. Audiology 3: 9–16.
42. OSHRI (2009) Standard Methods for Manual Pure Tone Threshold Audiometry. Incheon, Republich of Korea: The Occupational Safety and Health Research Institute, The Korea Occupational Safety and Health Agency.
43. Park SK, Elmarsafawy S, Mukherjee B, Spiro Iii A, Vokonas PS, et al. (2010) Cumulative lead exposure and age-related hearing loss: The VA Normative Aging Study. Hearing Research 269: 48–55.
44. Choi Y-H, Hu H, Mukherjee B, Miller J, Park SK (2012) Environmental Cadmium and Lead Exposures and Hearing Loss in US Adults: the National Health and Nutrition Examination Survey, 1999 to 2004. Environ Health Perspectives Under review.
45. Morata TC, Dunn DE, Kretschmer LW, Lemasters GK, Keith RW (1993) Effects of occupational exposure to organic solvents and noise on hearing. Scand J Work Environ Health 19: 245–254.
46. Discalzi G, Fabbro D, Meliga F, Mocellini A, Capellaro F (1993) Effects of occupational exposure to mercury and lead on brainstem auditory evoked potentials. International Journal of Psychophysiology 14: 21–25.
47. Maguin K, Campo P, Parietti-Winkler C (2009) Toluene can perturb the neuronal voltage-dependent Ca2+ channels involved in the middle-ear reflex. Toxicol Sci 107: 473–481.
48. Sabolić I (2006) Common Mechanisms in Nephropathy Induced by Toxic Metals. Nephron Physiology 104: 107–114.
49. Rabinowitz PM, Galusha D, Slade MD, Dixon-Ernst C, Sircar KD, et al. (2006) Audiogram Notches in Noise-Exposed Workers. Ear and Hearing 27: 742–750.
50. Beckett WS (2003) Noise Induced Hearing Loss-Evidence Based Statement. Journal of Occupational and Environmental Medicine 45: 1029.

2

Age-Related Hearing Loss in Rhesus Monkeys is Correlated with Cochlear Histopathologies

James R. Engle[1,3], Steve Tinling[2], Gregg H. Recanzone[3,4]*

1 Evelyn F. McKnight Brain Institute and ARL Division of Neural Systems, Memory and Aging, University of Arizona, Tucson, Arizona, United States of America, **2** Department of Otolaryngology, University of California Davis, Davis, California, United States of America, **3** Center for Neuroscience, University of California Davis, Davis, California, United States of America, **4** Department of Neurobiology, Physiology and Behavior, University of California Davis, Davis, California, United States of America

Abstract

Audiometric hearing deficits are a common symptom of age-related hearing loss (ARHL), as are specific histopathological changes in the cochlea; however, very little data have been collected in non-human primates. To examine this relationship further, we collected auditory brainstem responses (ABRs) from rhesus monkeys spanning in age from 10 to 35 years old, and examined four different morphological features of their cochleae. We found significant correlations between ABR thresholds and the loss of outer hair cells and spiral ganglion cells, but not with the loss of inner hair cells or a reduced thickness of the stria vascularis. The strongest correlation with ABR thresholds was the number of different pathologies present. These findings show that while aged rhesus monkeys experience audiometric hearing deficits similar to that seen in humans, they are not correlated with a single peripheral deficit, but instead with a number of different underlying cochlear histopathologies, indicating that similar histopathologies may exist in geriatric humans as well.

Editor: Joel Snyder, UNLV, United States of America

Funding: Funded by National Institute on Aging (NIA) R21AG024372, R01AG034137 (GHR), and National Institute on Deafness and Other Communication Disorders (NIDCD) T32DC008072 (JRE) and R01DC008649 (ST). The funders had no role in study design, data collection and analysis, decision to publish, or preparation of the manuscript.

Competing Interests: The authors have declared that no competing interests exist.

* E-mail: ghrecanzone@ucdavis.edu

Introduction

Age-related hearing loss (ARHL), or presbycusis, is a complex auditory disorder that impairs spectral, temporal and spatial auditory perceptions in the aged. One of the more common deficits is a shift in the audiometric thresholds, which is most likely to be manifested peripherally due to pathological changes in the cochlea. It has been hypothesized that different patterns of ARHL emerge in the human as the result of distinct cochlear pathologies [1–4], although this dataset is necessarily limited. Subsequent studies in humans have indicated that while there are examples where a single cochlear pathology can account for changes in audiometric thresholds, there are approximately 25% of cases that result from mixed cochlear pathologies [4], and in most cases there are complex interactions between different elements of the cochlea (e.g. see [5]). This is similar to studies in rodents, where either single or multiple pathologies can exist depending on the strain (reviewed by [6]).

How these rodent models can relate to human ARHL remains unclear, and how to relate the results from the different species relies heavily on the questions being addressed and the strain of animals being used. One advantage of broadening the animal models to non-human primates is that the ascending auditory nervous system, particularly the cerebral cortex, is more similar between humans and monkeys compared to humans and rodents, allowing for a better understanding of the cortical contributions to central processing deficits [7,8]. Accumulating evidence from behavioral and electrophysiological studies suggests that rhesus monkeys also experience ARHL [9–13]. Bennett et al. [9] reported age-related changes in both their middle-aged and old groups of monkeys that were primarily due to high-frequency hearing loss. The auditory brainstem response has been used to assess auditory thresholds to clicks [10] and high frequency tones [11,14] in macaque monkeys. In their most recent study, Fowler et al., [11] found that high-frequency hearing loss increases with age, and that hearing impairments at mid frequencies increased after 21 years of age. These combined results strongly suggest that rhesus monkeys experience at least one form of ARHL. To our knowledge, there has been only one publication on the age-related histopathological changes in the cochlea of the rhesus monkey, and the results from that study were inconclusive. Hawkins et al. [15] showed a progressive loss of hair cells that extended from both the lower base and upper apex with increasing age. They also reported a decrease of spiral ganglion cells that appeared to be primarily restricted to the base of the cochlea, but this pattern was not quantified.

Recently, we have found age-related broadening of spatial tuning curves and impaired gap processing in auditory cortex in two aged rhesus monkeys [12,13]. This suggests that the age-related histopathological changes in the cochlea of the rhesus monkey may be more extensive that what was previously reported by Hawkins et al [15]. To test this hypothesis and to gain a better understanding of the potential origin of acoustic processing deficits, we directly related auditory brainstem response (ABR) thresholds to clicks and pure tones to the histopathological changes in the cochlea in order to investigate how aging influences audiometric changes in rhesus monkeys. We found that normal aging is strongly associated with decreasing ABR sensitivity and extensive changes across multiple cochlear histopathologies in rhesus monkeys.

Materials and Methods

Ethics Statement

All experimental procedures conformed to the National Institutes of Health guidelines for animal use, and were approved by the UC Davis Institutional Animal Care and Use Committee (Protocol number 15783).

Animals

We used a combination of gross electrophysiological techniques (auditory brainstem response; ABR) and light microscopy to probe the peripheral auditory system for age-related changes in cochlear function and histopathology in 9 rhesus monkeys (*Macaca mulatta*). The age of the monkeys ranged from 10–35 years old. The 10 and 15 year old monkeys were male, while the remaining monkeys were female. These animals were sampled at random from a larger study that is examining the incidence and degree of hearing loss [16]. Six of the nine monkeys were housed at the California Regional Primate Research Center at the University of California of Davis, and were euthanized for unrelated medical reasons. The other three had participated in unrelated experiments and their cochleae were harvested upon completion of a terminal study. All animals were maintained on *ad libitum* food and free access to water. The inclusion criteria were: 1) No known history of receiving ototoxic drugs; 2) No known history of loud noise exposure or traumatic injury to the ear; 3) Auditory brainstem response recorded within 6 months of euthanasia; and 4) Otoscopic examination found no outer ear occlusions or signs of otitis media.

Auditory Brainstem Response Procedure and Analysis

Each animal was anesthetized with ketamine (10 mg/kg, IM) and medetomidine (0.3 ml/10 kg, IM) and placed in the prone position with their head slightly elevated. The animal's ear canals were then inspected and cleaned of debris if necessary and to determine the condition of the tympanic membrane. Neither large debris nor otitis media was detected in any of the animals tested. Each animal was given additional injections of ketamine to maintain chemical restraint throughout the procedure, which ranged from 1–3 hours. Following sedation, the skin was wiped clean with alcohol wipes and 0.22 gauge skin electrodes were placed subcutaneously behind each ear, on the forehead, and on the back of the neck [10,11,17,18]. Electrode impedance was checked after placement into the skin, and was below 1 k ohm for all recordings. ABR recordings were obtained by using an Intelligent Hearing System (Smart EP Win USB, Version 3.97) controlled by a laptop computer. Evoked responses were amplified at 100 K times, and our physiological filters were set to pass at 100–1500 Hz. Soft insert earphones were placed in both the left and right ear and connected to a pair of etymotic ER3A transducers for delivery of low frequency stimuli, and then to high-frequency transducers for the 12 and 16 kHz frequency stimuli. The audible range of the rhesus monkeys extends from 26 Hz –42 kHz [12,19]. We obtained ABRs to clicks and tone bursts (10 msec duration; 2 msec rise/fall trapezoidal envelope) at frequencies of 0.5 kHz, 1 kHz, 2 kHz, 4 kHz, 8 kHz, 12 kHz and 16 kHz. All stimuli were presented binaurally at a rate of 50 stim/sec. ABR waveforms were averaged over a minimum of 1000 repetitions. Clicks and tone bursts were presented at 80 dB pSPL (peak sound pressure level) and decreased in 10 dB pSPL increments until the ABR response was no longer visually identifiable, and then increased by 5 dB pSPL to obtain an estimated hearing threshold. All recordings were obtained in a quiet electrically shielded room or in a double-walled sound booth, and stored for offline analysis. ABR threshold, peak, and latency measurements of waves II and IV were manually scored by two independent raters who were blind to the identity and age of the monkeys. There was greater than 95% agreement between the two raters.

Histological Processing

Each animal was anesthetized with ketamine (30 mg/kg, IM), and euthanized with a lethal dose of sodium pentobarbital (60 mg/kg, IV). Each animal was then transcardially perfused with saline followed by two fixatives. The first fixative contained a mixture of 4% paraformaldehyde in 0.1 M phosphate buffer (PB; pH 7.4) or 4% paraformaldehyde and 0.5% glutaraldehyde in 0.1 M PB (pH 7.4), and the second fixative contained a mixture of 4% paraformaldehyde and 10% sucrose. The brain was removed from the cranial vault, and then the temporal bone was chipped free. The middle ear was then exposed to puncture the round and oval windows. Each specimen was then submerged in 2% paraformaldehyde and 2% glutaraldehyde in 0.1 M PB and stored in a refrigerator at 4°C. Each cochlea was gently infused through the oval window with 1% osmium tetroxide for 2–4 minutes to reveal the location of the Organ of Corti and to facilitate precise trimming of the remaining temporal bone until only a thin layer of bone remained [20,21]. Each cochlea was then decalcified in 0.35% EDTA and microwave accelerated [22]. This procedure took 4–8 weeks to reach an acceptable level of decalcification. Following decalcification and additional trimming, one cochlea was randomly selected from each monkey and prepared for whole mount examination, while the opposing cochlea was dehydrated through an ascending series of acetone and then embedded in epon-araldite. Following polymerization, each cochlea was mounted onto a plastic stub and cut in the mid-modiolar plane in 400 µm blocks with a 75 µm thick diamond blade on a radial arm bone saw. Mid-modiolar sections were then cut semi-thinly at 1 µm. Four mid-modiolar sections were collected every 10 µm over 40 µm, mounted on 1×3 glass slides, stained for toluidine blue and basic fuscin for bright field microscopy, cover slipped, and then examined on a Nikon D8000 microscope which was equipped with an MD3-plot x/y stage encoding system (Accustage Inc., Shoreview, MN) and moticam camera which was attached to the computer.

Data Analysis

We characterized each audiogram based upon the pattern of the ABR threshold shift as a function of age. This was accomplished by calculating the difference between each monkey and the youngest monkey. We then calculated a seven frequency pure tone average (PTA) and a pure tone average loss (PTAL) as a function of age to quantify age-related changes in the ABR threshold functions, and to classify the type of spectral impairment. Next, we used conservative cutoff values that have been assigned to humans [23] to define mild (>30 dB) or moderate to severe (>55 dB) spectral impairments across the low (0.5 kHz), mid (1–8 kHz), and high (12–16 kHz) frequency ranges. Standard light microscopy techniques were used in conjunction with unbiased stereological counting procedures and computerized planimetry to quantify the histopathological changes in each cochlea. We randomly sampled each cochlea due to slight deviations in the angle and position of the mid-modiolar blocks. This strategy, however, hindered our ability to consistently measure the upper apical turn (A3) on every cochlea. We therefore only analyzed the lower and upper turns of the base (B1 and B2), middle (M1 and M2) and the apex (A1 and A2). We measured the density of spiral ganglion cells (SGCs), counted inner (IHC) and outer hair cells (OHCs), and measured the thickness of the stria vascularis (SV). The packing density of SGCs was calculated in each section by randomly overlaying a grid with points that were spaced at 75 µm. A 75 µm unbiased counting frame [24] was then used at every point within the boundary of Rosenthal's canal throughout the entire modiolus. This strategy allowed us to randomly sample approximately 90–100% of Rosenthal's canal. Spiral ganglion cells were counted if the nucleolus was present and the nucleus was within and not touching the rejection region of the counting frame. Packing density was expressed as the number of cells per point. IHC and OHC counts were performed on complete or partial hair cell profiles, which included either the cell body or stereocilia. The thickness of the stria vascularis was averaged over 10 orthogonal measurements across the entire extent of the stria vascularis at each level of the cochlea. All values were normalized to the data collected from the youngest monkey to reveal age-related changes in cochlear pathologies. Lastly for each monkey, we quantified the number of pathological features (i.e., density of SGC, IHCs, OHCs, and SV thickness) that were significantly different from the youngest monkey (t-test, $p<0.05$). This additional assessment accounted for individual variation across animals.

Statistical analyses were performed on the original ABR and the age-normalized data with SPSS, version 19 (Chicago, IL). We used Pearson product moment correlations to examine the relationships between age, ABR thresholds at each stimulus, ABR threshold loss, classified type of spectral impairment, PTA, the density of SGCs, IHC and OHCs counts, and the thickness of the SV. We used stepwise multiple regression analysis to separate the contribution of the cochlear histopathologies on the original and age-normalized ABR, PTA, and classified type of spectral impairment. Explanatory variables were entered in a hierarchical and stepwise manner when appropriate. We used a criterion of $p<0.05$ to enter and a $p>0.10$ to remove predictors from the model. We also used t-tests when necessary. Statistically significant relationships and differences were considered significant at $p<0.05$.

Results

Age-related Increases in ABR Thresholds Reveal Multiple Spectral Impairments in Monkeys

We recorded auditory brainstem responses (ABR) to clicks (Figure 1A) and tones in nine rhesus monkeys aged 10 years and 3 months to 35 years and 3 months. Rhesus monkeys age at approximately three times that of humans, so these animals were roughly equivalent to 30 and 105 human years of age. ABR threshold was defined as the lowest stimulus intensity at each specified stimulus to generate an observable wave II and/or IV in the ABR waveform (see Table S1). We found that the ABR thresholds to clicks and pure tones increased with age (see Table 1). Next, we plotted ABR thresholds as a function of the clicks and pure tone frequencies to determine the pattern of loss across the frequencies tested (Figure 1B). Our initial impression of these data was the appearance of increasing thresholds across frequencies, which is a pattern of loss that has been associated with age-related hearing loss in humans and in different strains of rodents [4,25]. Next, we created ABR hearing loss functions by subtracting the evoked ABR thresholds of the youngest monkey from every other evoked ABR threshold in our study as a function of the stimulus type (Figure 1C). This procedure revealed age-related hearing loss across the frequencies tested, but not as a simple shift of the same audiometric profile across frequencies. What is clear from this analysis is that the higher frequencies were affected to a greater degree compared to lower frequencies, and these deficits also increased with age. Furthermore, we classified the type of spectral impairment as mild if any ABR threshold shift was greater than 30 dB (light gray region of Figure 1C), or moderate-to-severe if the ABR threshold shift was greater than 55 dB (dark gray region of Figure 1C). For example, the 15 year old monkey was classified as having mild high-frequency hearing loss, whereas the 35 year old monkey was classified as the only monkey that had threshold increases that extended from moderate-to-severe for mid and high frequency tones to mild hearing loss for low frequency tones. We found that the remaining monkeys had mild hearing loss for most low and mid-frequency tones, and most had moderate-to-severe hearing loss for the high-frequency tones.

One caveat with the above analysis is that it is relatively qualitative. We therefore quantified the type of spectral impairment by calculating the pure tone average (PTA) across the seven tested frequencies and the pure tone average loss (PTAL) on the age-normalized threshold values, and then examined PTAL as function of age (Figure 1D) compared to the qualitative classified type of hearing loss. We found that PTAL was strongly correlated with age ($r = 0.88$, $p<0.01$). These combined qualitative and quantitative results strongly suggest that rhesus monkeys experience a pattern of hearing loss that progresses across the audiometric range and increases in severity with age, similar to what is seen in humans.

Qualitative Observations of the Primate Cochlea

Figure 2 illustrates an extracted cochlea from the temporal bone of a rhesus monkey before whole mount dissection (Figure 2A, 2B) and mid-modiolar sectioning (Figure 2C). We gently infused each cochlea with osmium to reveal the location of the Organ of Corti. Whole mount preparations of the opposing cochlea revealed putative myelinated spiral ganglion cell axons that traverse the osseous spiral lamina from the base to apex (Figure S1). This pattern was observed from the base to apex in all nine cochlea specimens. This result suggests that this methodology does not reveal a significant thinning of axons that traverse the osseous spiral lamina, which has been found to be a characteristic of neuritic presbycusis [26]. Additionally, prolonged noise-exposure in monkeys has been shown to result in a frequency specific loss of spiral ganglion cell axons that extends through the osseous spiral lamina [27]. We did not expect to see such degeneration in our sample since one of our inclusion criteria, along with no known administration of ototoxic drugs, was that there was not a significant noise exposure event noted in their medical records. This result suggests that any of the observed pathologies in the cochlea can be attributed to aging and not to significant noise-induced trauma at a single frequency band.

Our initial impression of the mid-modiolar semi-thin sections was that many of the selected features within our analysis deteriorated with age in one or more animals, for example in the Organ of Corti (Fig. 2D) and the stria vascularis (Fig. 2E). One potential caveat with semi-thin sections, however, is that cross sections often appear fractured [28], which may potentially bias hair cell counts. This was accounted for by counting complete or partial hair cells, which included either hair cells or stereocilia (see methods).

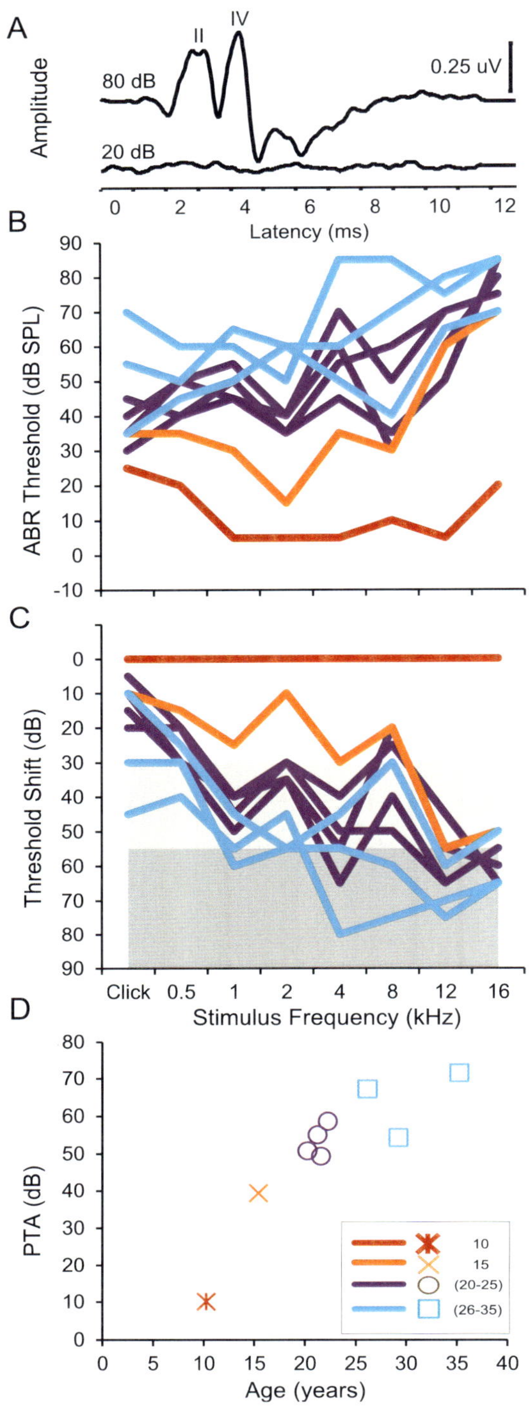

Figure 1. Auditory brainstem response (ABR) measurements of age-related hearing loss. Panel A shows two representative ABR waveforms from the youngest monkey. Waves II and IV are marked. The top trace shows the response to click stimuli presented at 80 dB SPL, which was well above threshold, and the bottom trace shows the response in the same monkey to a 20 dB SPL click stimulus. No obvious response was noted at this stimulus intensity. Panels B-D show the data from each monkey organized by symbols and colorized to represent different age-groups. ABR thresholds (B) and age-related shift in threshold (C) as a function of stimulus and age of the monkey. The seven frequency pure tone average loss (PTAL; Panel D) increases as a function of age, $r = 0.88$, $p < 0.01$.

Age-related Decrease of Inner Hair Cells does not Correlate with Changes in ABR Threshold

In five out of nine cochleae, we found IHC profiles (Figure 2D) in 95–100% of the sections examined. In the remaining four cochleae, we found reductions of IHCs up to approximately 50% in some of the sections examined. In the next level of the analysis, we analyzed IHCs at different levels of the cochlea to determine if the IHCs deteriorate with age in a selective manner in a particular region of the cochlea, which may ultimately influence the PTA. Figure 3 shows the relationship between the age-normalized counts of IHCs in the lower base, upper base and lower apex as a function of age (left panels) and PTA (right panels; see Table S2 for values for the youngest animal). We found that the number of IHCs in the lower base decreases with age ($r = -0.73$, $p < 0.05$). The reduction was fairly small with an average IHC reduction of about 12.5% across the sample. We found that the correlations between age and the number of IHCs in the lower base ($r = -0.66$, $p = 0.054$) and the upper apex ($r = -0.60$, $p = 0.08$) did not meet our criterion for significance. The reductions of IHCs in the lower base and upper apex were also small with an average loss of 9.4% and 6.25%, respectively. Next, we examined the relationship between IHC counts and PTA to determine if the above age-related decreases in counts influenced the degree of spectral deficit. We found that the IHC counts were unrelated with PTA at all levels of the cochlea (lowest $r = -0.56$, $p > 0.05$). This result suggests that the observed age-related loss of IHCs had, if any, only a negligible effect on the identified audiometric impairments. The contribution of IHCs loss on frequency-specific deficits will be reconsidered in a section below.

Age-related Decrease of Outer Hair Cells is Associated with Changes in ABR Threshold

We performed OHC counts to determine the relationship between OHC counts, age and PTA. In six out of nine cochleae, we found complete or partial OHC profiles in 94–100% of the sections examined. In the three remaining cochleae, we found approximate reductions of 45%, 21% and 40% of OHCs in the oldest, second oldest and third oldest monkeys, respectively. We then examined each level of the cochlea independently to determine if the loss of OHCs with age was selective to a particular region of the cochlea. Figure 4 shows the relationship between the age-normalized OHC counts with age (left column) and PTA (right column). Interestingly, the only significant correlation we found between OHC counts and age was in the upper apex, where OHC counts were significantly decreased with age ($r = -0.80$, $p < 0.05$). The effect was moderately small with an average OHC reduction of about 16.7% across the sample. In the upper base there was a non-significant trend for OHC counts to decrease with age ($r = -0.65$, $p = 0.06$). The effect was also small with an average OHC reduction in the upper base of about 10.5% over the sample. Even though we did not find a significant correlation in the lower base, it is noteworthy to mention that the average OHC reduced by approximately 25% across the sample. Next, we examined the relationship between OHC counts and PTA to determine if the above age-related decrease in OHCs in the upper apex influenced the degree of the hearing deficit. Again, we found that decreasing OHC counts in the upper apex was correlated with increasing PTA ($r = -0.70$, $p < 0.05$). This result suggests that the observed age-related decrease of OHCs is likely to contribute to the identified frequency-specific audiometric impairments in monkeys.

Table 1. Correlation matrix between age and ABR thresholds to clicks and tones.

	Age	Click	0.5 kHz	1 kHz	2 kHz	4 kHz	8 kHz	12 kHz	16 kHz
Age	1.00								
Click	0.79*	1.00							
0.5 kHz	0.89**	0.76*	1.00						
1 kHz	0.84**	0.71*	0.91**	1.00					
2 kHz	0.87**	0.57	0.79*	0.90**	1.00				
4 kHz	0.84**	0.75*	0.90**	0.91**	0.75*	1.00			
8 kHz	0.83**	0.96**	0.82**	0.85**	0.70*	0.84**	1.00		
12 kHz	0.74**	0.67*	0.8	0.93**	0.78*	0.87**	0.80*	1.00	
16 kHz	0.69*	0.59	0.86**	0.89**	0.71*	0.83**	0.67*	0.89**	1.00

Note: ** = p<.01, * = p<.05.

Age-related and Threshold Related Decreases of Spiral Ganglion Cells

The third cochlear morphological feature that we investigated was the packing density of the spiral ganglion cells (SGCs). Figure 5 shows several examples of the observed packing density of SGCs in the lower base and the modiolus of the 10, 21.5 and 35 year old monkeys. The packing density of the SGCs in Rosenthal's canal appeared to be full in both the lower base and in the modiolus of the 10 year old monkey. However, the packing density was much lower in the base in both the 21.5 and the 35 year old monkey. Quantification of this age-related effect is shown in Figure 6, which along with Figure 5 shows that the packing density clearly

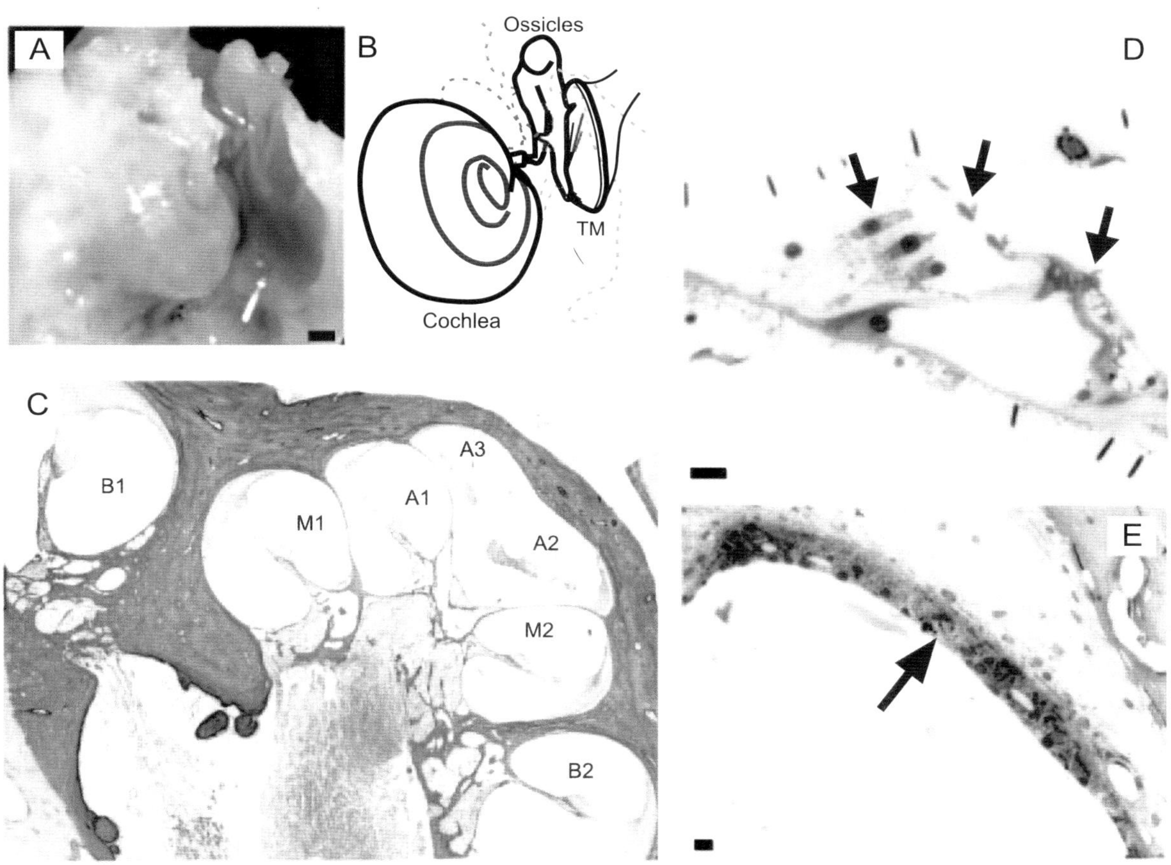

Figure 2. Histology of the rhesus monkey cochlea. This specimen came from the 15 year old monkey. Whole mount (A), illustration (B) and semi-thin mid-modiolar section (C) of the rhesus monkey cochlea. Semi-thin section revealing inner and outer hair cells are shown in D. Arrows indicate stereocilia or soma of inner and outer hair cells. Semi-thin section revealing the stria vascularis are shown in E. Different levels of the base (B1,2), middle (M1,2) and apical (A1,2,3) turns are indicated in panel C. TM = tympanic membrane. Scale bar 1 mm (A), 10 μm (D,E).

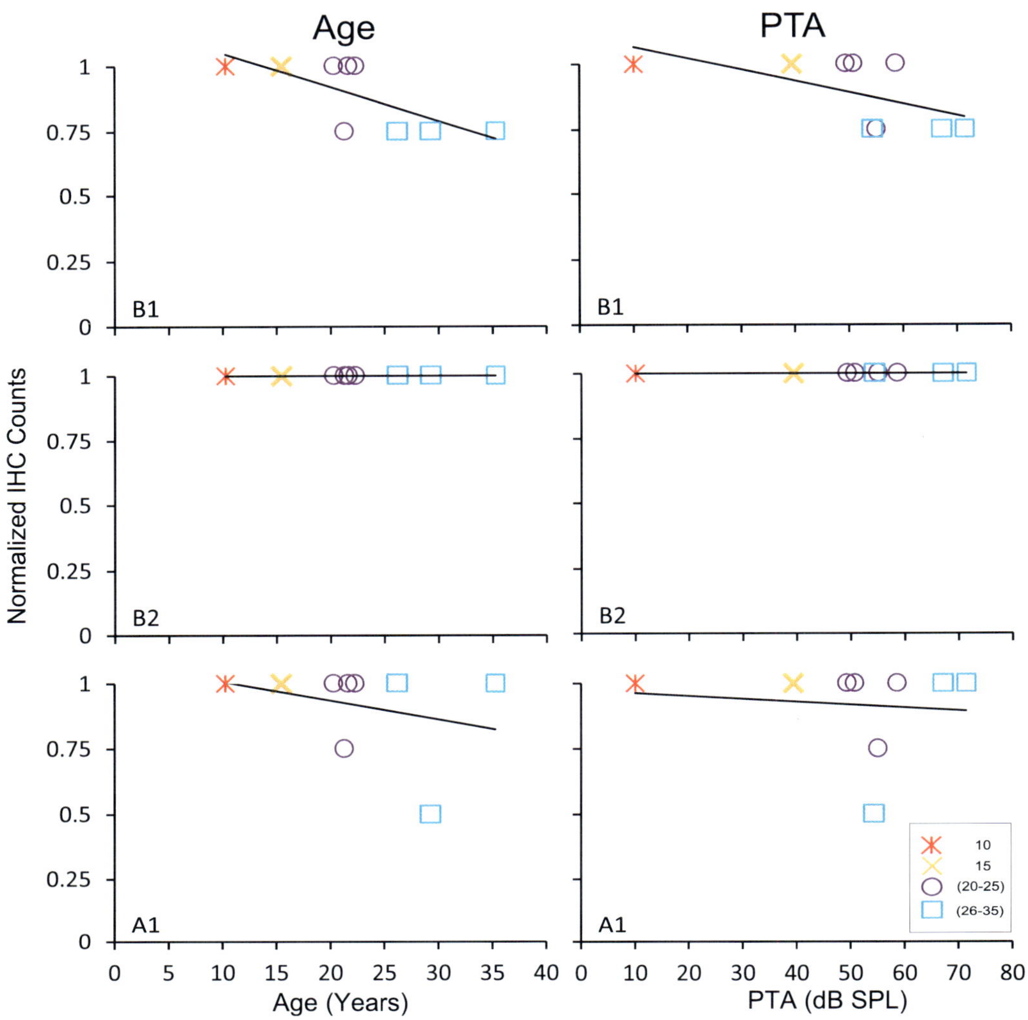

Figure 3. Effect of age and PTA on inner hair cells. Age-normalized inner hair cell counts as a function of age (left) and PTA (right) in the lower base (top), upper base (middle), and lower apex (bottom). A few monkeys had decreased inner hair cells in the lower base and apex, but all were normal in the upper base.

decreases with age. In the lower base we found that the density of SGCs significantly decreases with age ($r = -0.76$, $p < 0.05$), where the packing density was reduced on average by approximately 61%. The packing density of SGCs in the upper base ($r = -0.65$, $p = 0.058$) showed a non-significant trend in the same direction as the lower base, with reductions of 32% on average. In the modiolus ($r = -0.48$, $p > 0.05$), the correlation was not significant although the average reduction in SGC density was 40%. These results suggest that a major age-related effect on the packing density of SGCs is the disproportionate rate of loss of SGCs across the cochlea.

The previous analysis revealed that the packing density of SGCs in the lower base was associated with age, but not in the other regions of the cochlea. It is possible that the packing density of SGCs in the upper base and modiolus are more indicative of changes in threshold across the frequencies tested. Figure 6 shows the relationship between the PTA and age normalized counts of SGCs in the lower base, upper base and modiolus. This analysis showed that that the packing density of SGCs in the lower ($r = -0.78$, $p < 0.05$) and upper ($r = -0.073$, $p < 0.05$) base decreases with increasing PTA. This suggests that decreases in the packing density of the SGCs in the lower and upper base, but not at higher levels of the modiolus, are likely to contribute to the identified spectral impairments.

We also investigated whether the age-related decrease in the packing density of SGCs degenerated in parallel with the degeneration of the IHCs and OHCs. Figure 7 shows the relationship between the age-normalized inner and outer hair counts as a function of the age-normalized packing density of the SGCs. The solid diagonal line represents the unity line. A value of 0 indicates the equal loss of either hair cells or SGCs, respectively. Values greater than 1 indicate more cells for that animal compared to the youngest animal, which was usually in the form of either a higher packing density of SGCs or a fourth row of OHCs. Points that land on the unity line indicate that both hair cells and SGCs degenerated at the same rate. Points that fall above the unity line indicate that hair cells degenerated at a slower rate than SGCs and those that fall below indicate the reverse. The majority of points fall above the unity line for both IHCs and OHCs. This indicates that SGCs degenerate at a faster rate than their associated IHCs and OHCs.

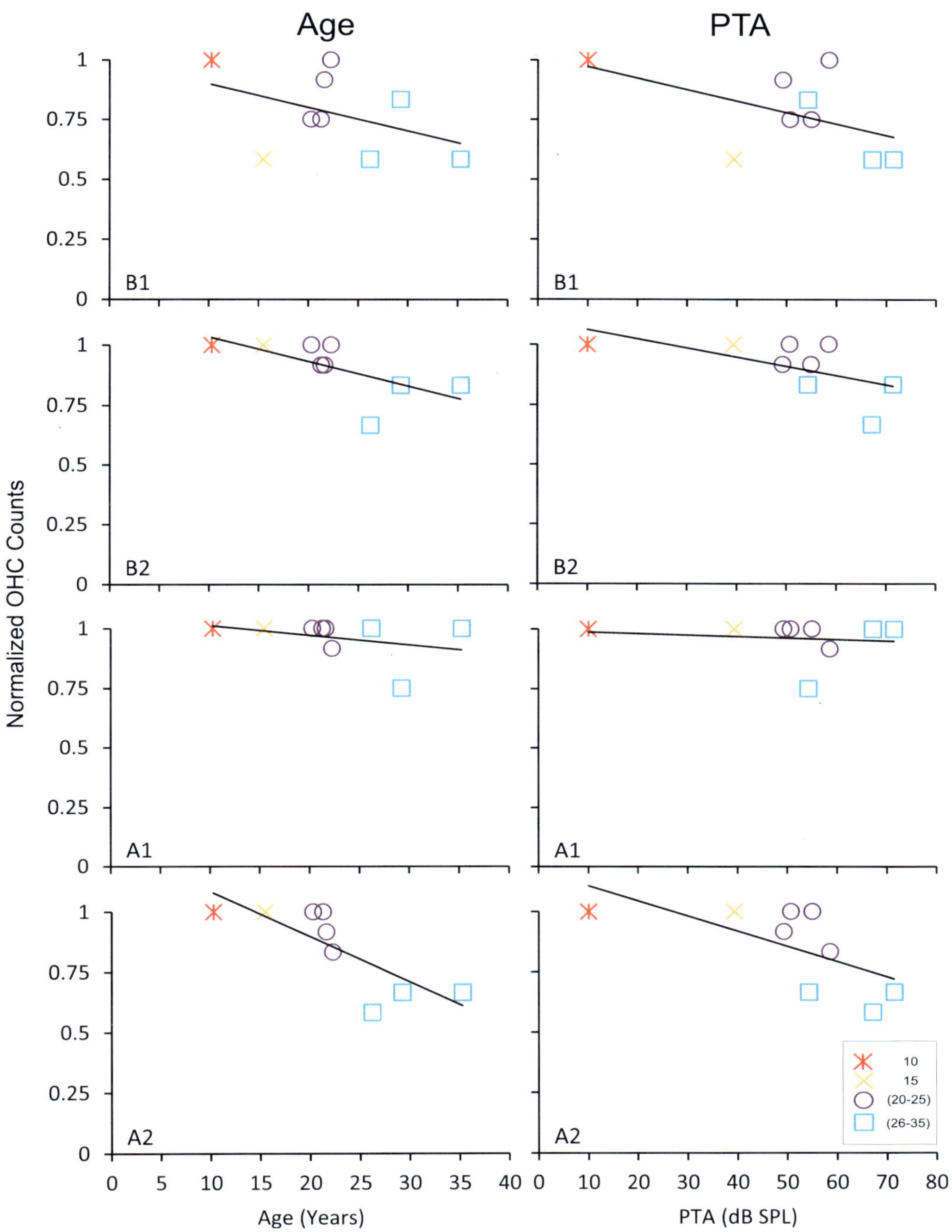

Figure 4. Effects of age and PTA on outer hair cells. Age-normalized outer hair cell counts as a function of age (left) and PTA (right) in the lower base (B1), upper base (B2), lower apex (A1) and upper apex (A2). Many monkeys had decreased outer hair cells, particularly at the lower base and upper apex.

The Thickness of the Stria Vascularis does not Decrease with Age or Spectral Impairment

Finally, we measured the thickness of the SV to determine if a pathological change in the SV is associated with age and PTA. The endocochlear potential has been shown to be inversely associated with the thickness of the SV in the lower base and lower apex [29]. Figure 8 shows the relationship between the thickness of the SV with age and PTA in the lower base, upper base and lower apex. We found that the thickness of the SV remains relatively stable throughout the levels examined in the cochlea of monkeys regardless of age or the degree of spectral impairment (largest $r = -0.47$, $p > 0.05$). This result does not support the hypothesis that the SV thickness contributes to the identified spectral impairments in monkeys.

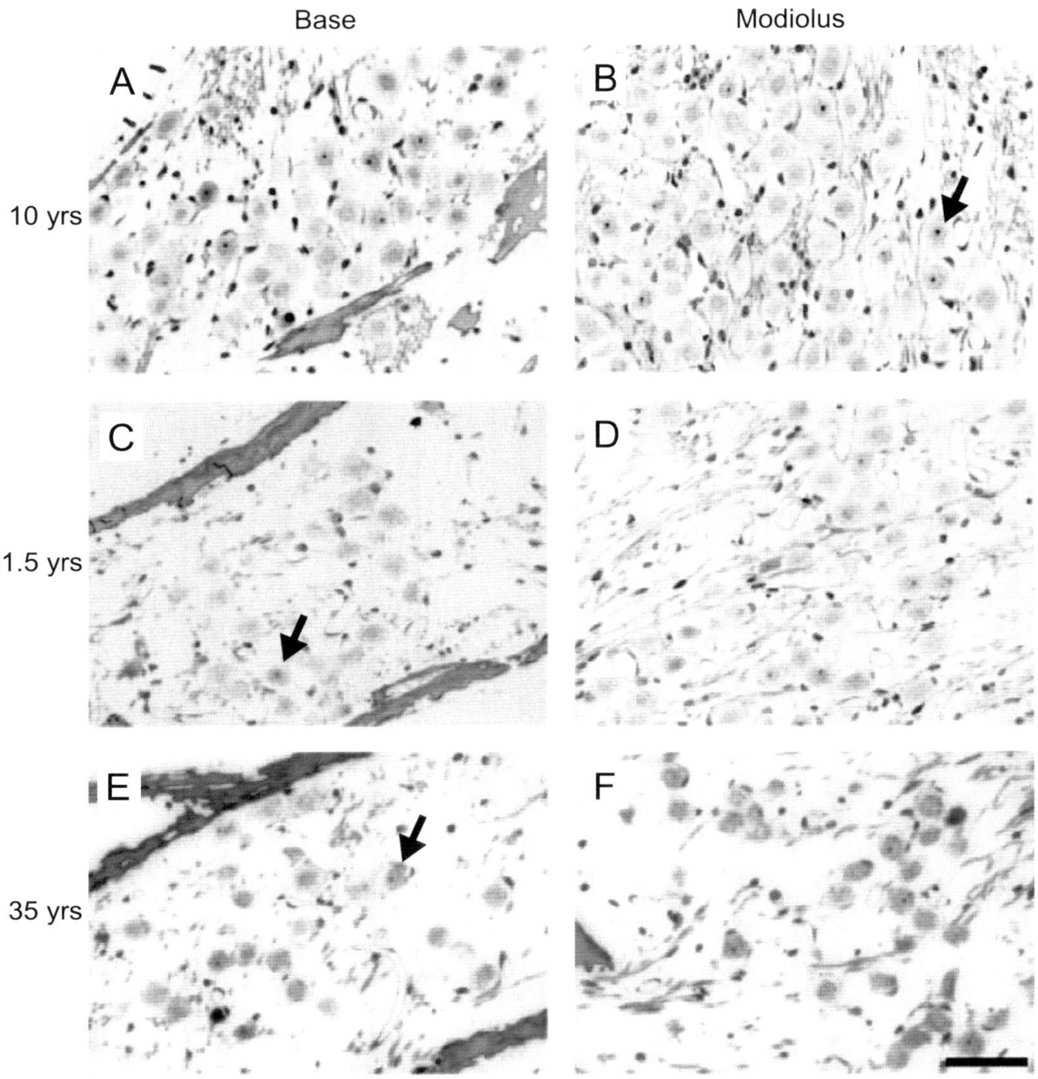

Figure 5. Spiral Ganglion Cell (SGC) loss as a function of age. Photomicrographs of SGCs in the base (left) and modiolus (right) of the 10 (A,B), 21.5 (C, D), and the 35 (E, F) year old monkeys. The packing density of SGCs decreases as a function age and region in the cochlea. Scale bar = 50 μm.

SGC Density and OHCs Contribute to the High Frequency Audiometric Hearing Impairments in Monkeys

The above results indicate that rhesus monkeys experience several age-related cochlear pathologies. We used multiple regression analysis to determine the best predictors of age-related changes in the ABR thresholds. In a step-wise manner we entered explanatory variables that could theoretically predict the ABR threshold of a specific frequency region in the cochlea. For example, we entered the cochlear features in the lower base, the upper base, and the lower middle turn as predictors of age-related change in threshold to the 16 kHz tone stimulus to determine how the highest frequency tested is influenced by these regional cochlear features. For this analysis, we found that the packing density of SGCs in the lower base ($b = -0.643$, $t(8) = -6.608$, $p<0.001$), and number of OHCs in the lower middle turn ($b = 0.596$, $t(8) = 6.123$, $p<0.001$) contributed to the age-related ABR threshold loss at 16 kHz. In the final model, the packing density of SGCs and the number of OHCs accounted for 95% of the variance in the age-related changes in ABR threshold at 16 kHz ($R^2 = 0.946$, $F(2,6) = 37.491$, $p<0.001$). Interestingly, adding the most basal turn did not improve this correlation, presumably as this region is normally processing frequencies much higher than 16 kHz in the macaque, where the hearing range extends beyond 30 kHz (see [12,19]).

The age-related decrease of SGCs contributed to a large proportion of the variance in the age-related decrease of the ABR threshold at the highest frequencies tested. It appears, however, that the age-related decrease of OHCs is the primary contributor to the age-related increase of ABR threshold to clicks, and at middle frequencies of 1, 2 and 8 kHz. IHCs and the thickness of the SV contributed a very small percentage to the variance of age-related changes in hearing thresholds. These combined results suggest that the major contributors to age-related high frequency hearing loss in monkeys are the concomitant age-related decline of SGCs and OHCs.

To build upon this analysis, we examined the number of significant age-related differences across the four features in the

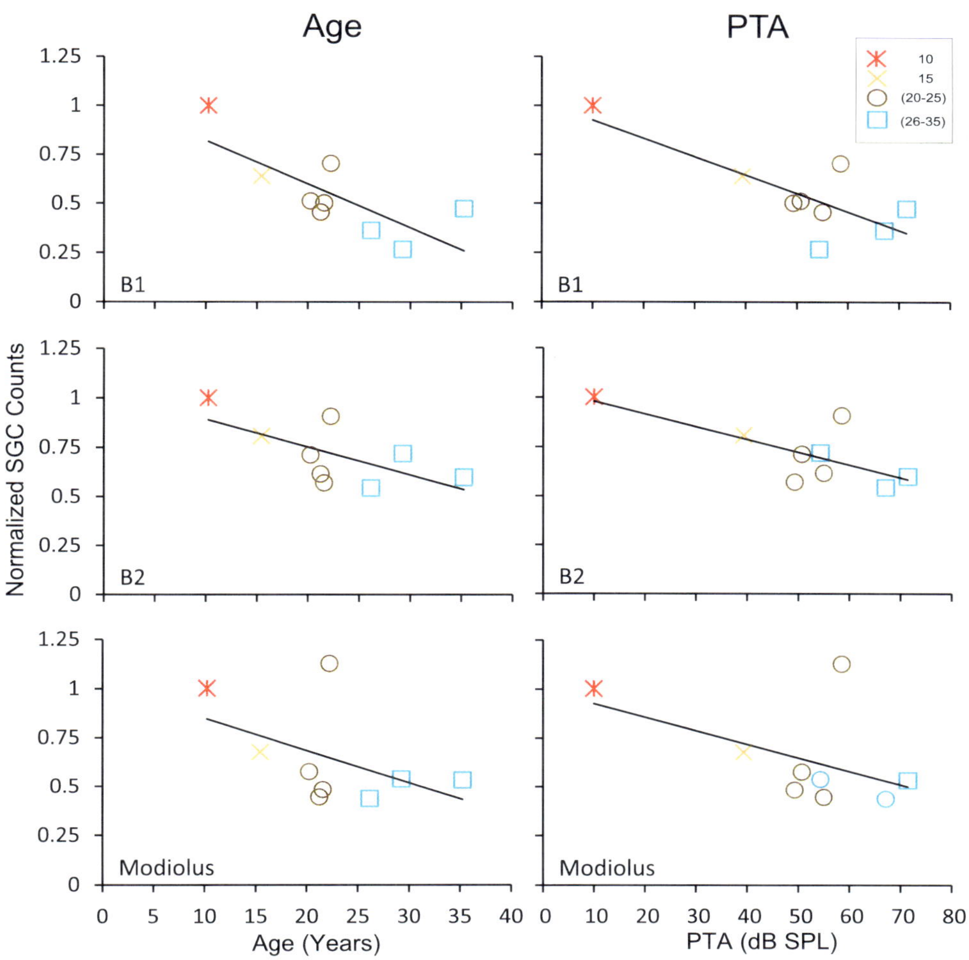

Figure 6. Effects of age and PTA on spiral ganglion cells. Age-normalized spiral ganglion cell counts as a function of age (left) and PTA (right) in the lower base (top), upper base (middle), and modiolus (bottom). There was a clear decrease in SGC as a function of both age and PTA.

cochlea that were under investigation. Significant differences were identified by making age-related comparisons after collapsing the data within a single cochlea. For example, the overall packing density was significantly lower in the 15 year old monkey compared to the 10 year old monkey (t-test, $p<0.05$) while no other differences were found. Therefore, the 15 year old monkey had only one significant age-related difference from the 10 year old monkey. On the other hand, the 35 year monkey had three features that were statistically different relative to the 10 year old monkey. The SV thickness, OHC counts and SGC counts were all significantly lower in the 35 year old monkey (t-test, $p<0.05$). The number of significant pathological differences was strongly correlated with age ($r=0.90$, $p<0.001$), and PTA ($r=0.78$, $p<0.05$). This result is shown in Figure 9 (see Figure S2 for individual data). This suggests that the number of age-related pathological features increases with both age and the severity of hearing loss. We then used multiple regression analysis to determine if age-related changes at a particular frequency could predict the number of significant pathological changes in the cochlea. For this analysis, we found that the age-related increase of ABR thresholds at 2 kHz can be used as a predictor of the age-related increase in the number of significant pathologies in the cochlea ($b=0.836$, $t(8)=4.023$, $p<0.01$). In the final model, threshold changes at 2 kHz accounted for 70% of the variance in the number of significant age-related pathological changes in the cochlea ($R^2=0.698$, $F(1,7)=16.184$, $p<0.01$). This result suggests that a frequency-specific deficit at 2 kHz is the best predictor of the extent of cochlear histopathological changes in monkeys.

Discussion

Rhesus monkeys are widely used in studies that explore system level questions in the auditory cortex (see [7,8,30,31]), and in aging [12,13]. Studies of the auditory system in aged rhesus monkeys are sparse, and the origins of the reported processing deficits are unclear. Using the auditory brainstem response to assess auditory function, this and previous studies have demonstrated increases in audiometric thresholds across the frequency spectrum with age [11,16]. In the current study this was observed as an initial age-related increase which was restricted to high frequencies and slowly progressed with age across the entire frequency spectrum. Similar patterns have been reported in humans and in animal models of presbycusis [25,32,33]. These similarities led us to examine and characterize the relationship between age-related audiometric shifts to age-related cochlear histopathological changes in rhesus monkeys.

We found several correlations between age, increases in ABR thresholds, and distinct decreases in the cochlear histopathology of

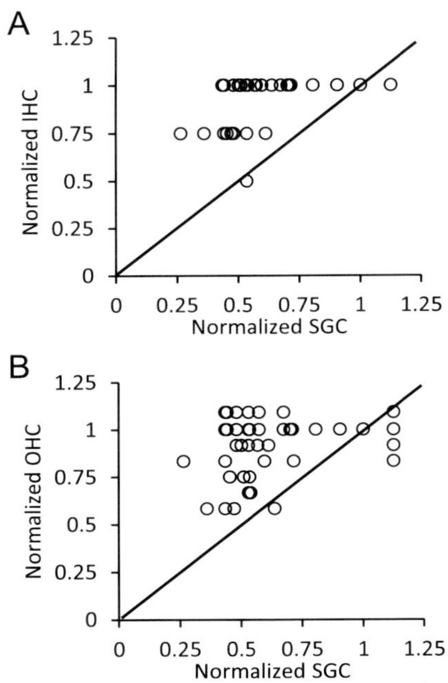

Figure 7. Relationship between the hair cells and spiral ganglion cells. Age-normalized inner (A) and outer (B) hair cell counts as a function of age-normalized packing density of SGCs. The solid diagonal line represents the unity line. Points that fall above the unity indicate a greater loss of spiral ganglion cells compared to the hair cells.

rhesus monkeys. The first important finding is that the decline in spiral ganglion cells and outer hair cells accounts for most of the decreases in high and mid frequency hearing, respectively. A second important finding is that the number of different cochlear histopathologies is very strongly correlated with age. These results suggest that rhesus monkeys experience spectral hearing impairment with mixed cochlear pathologies and indicate that a similar condition of multiple cochlear pathologies could underlie age-related audiometric deficits, as well as temporal and spatial processing deficits, in humans [34,35].

Parallels of Age-related Hearing Loss in Humans and Monkeys

Early studies of ARHL in humans indicated that specific audiometric shifts were related to a distinct cochlear histopathology [1,2,4]. Our understanding of ARHL, however, was slightly obscured by the inclusion of temporal bone specimens with potential histopathological confounds that were generated by means other than natural aging (for review see [5]), and by studies that did not find a relationship between audiometric changes and cochlear histopathology [3,36]. Recent studies of human temporal bones, however, provide a different picture due to more rigorous evaluations of patient data, and stringent inclusion criteria. Nelson and Hinojosa [5] found that the severity of the hearing loss in the aged was associated with the degeneration of IHC, OHCs, SGCs and the stria vascularis. This also applies to monkeys as this same association was found in the present study. Additionally, Nelson and Hinojosa [5] found that the extent of cochlear degeneration of the above four elements was highly associated with audiometric changes at 8 kHz in humans. In monkeys, we found that extent of cochlear degeneration of these same four elements was strongly associated with audiometric changes at 2 kHz. If these findings translate to other species, then audiometric shifts at a specific frequency can be used to identify animals with multiple cochlear pathologies. This will greatly aid in participant or specimen selection for future studies on ARHL.

Age-related Changes in the Auditory Brainstem Response of Rhesus Monkeys

We found that the ABR thresholds increased as a function of age regardless of stimulus type (Figure 1). By defining mild and moderate-to-severe hearing loss across the low, mid, and high frequencies, we found that the severity of loss in rhesus monkeys increases as a function of age. The identified patterns of hearing loss showed a transition from downward to gentle sloping ABR audiograms as a function of age, which is one of the more common conditions in humans. We did not observe elevated and flat hearing loss as has been described previously in humans [32], as well as in some instances in a larger population of monkeys [16], which is likely due to the relatively small sample of monkeys in the current study. There have been only a few studies in rhesus monkeys that probed for ARHL with ABRs. In an early study on how caloric restriction affects ARHL, ABR responses to clicks were found to only have a trend to increase with age [14], and that it increases at an approximate constant rate of 1.2 dB per year. In a follow-up study on how caloric restriction affects ARHL longitudinally, ABR thresholds increased at different rates that varied with the stimulus type and age [11]. Importantly, Fowler et al. [11] found both linear age-related increases in hearing threshold, and curvilinear age-related increases that began around 21 years of age. The results of this study indicate that the rate of hearing loss may not be constant, and that the underestimated 1.2 dB decrease may be frequency specific. Our results show age-related increases in ABR threshold to the click stimulus at an approximate rate of 1.8 dB per year. Our results also demonstrate that the rate of loss decreases at different rates across the tone frequencies tested, especially in the low and mid tone frequencies.

Age-related Histopathological Changes in the Cochlea of Rhesus Monkeys

We found several age-related histopathological changes in the cochlea of the rhesus monkey. This included an age-related decline in the packing density of SGCs, IHC loss that was primarily found in the lower base and OHC loss that extended from the lower base. For hair cells, Hawkins et al., [15] reported a similar but more extreme pattern of loss in the lower base. This difference can be accounted for by differences in our strategies to analyze the cochlear specimens. We performed our analysis on mid-modiolar cross sections that randomly sampled the tissue whereas Hawkins et al. [15] cut the Organ of Corti away from the modiolus into several millimeter sections from the apex to base, and then performed mid-modiolar cross sections on the remaining tissue. For SGCs, we found an age-related decline in the packing density that extends from the lower base into the modiolus. Although qualitative, Hawkins et al. [15] reported a similar pattern in the lower base in their sample of three aged monkeys. They also found in one middle aged animal that SGC loss throughout the modiolus was extensive, which suggests that SGC loss may be independent of hair cell loss. We found that the packing density of SGC decreased with age, but at differential rates in the lower base, upper base and the modiolus. This suggests that SGC loss may be regionally specific and then progress over the lifespan of the animal. This loss is also independent from hair cell loss, which is a pattern that has been reported in humans and in some rodents [4,37–39]. For example, Zilberstein et al. [40] highlighted this independence by showing that SGCs survive for

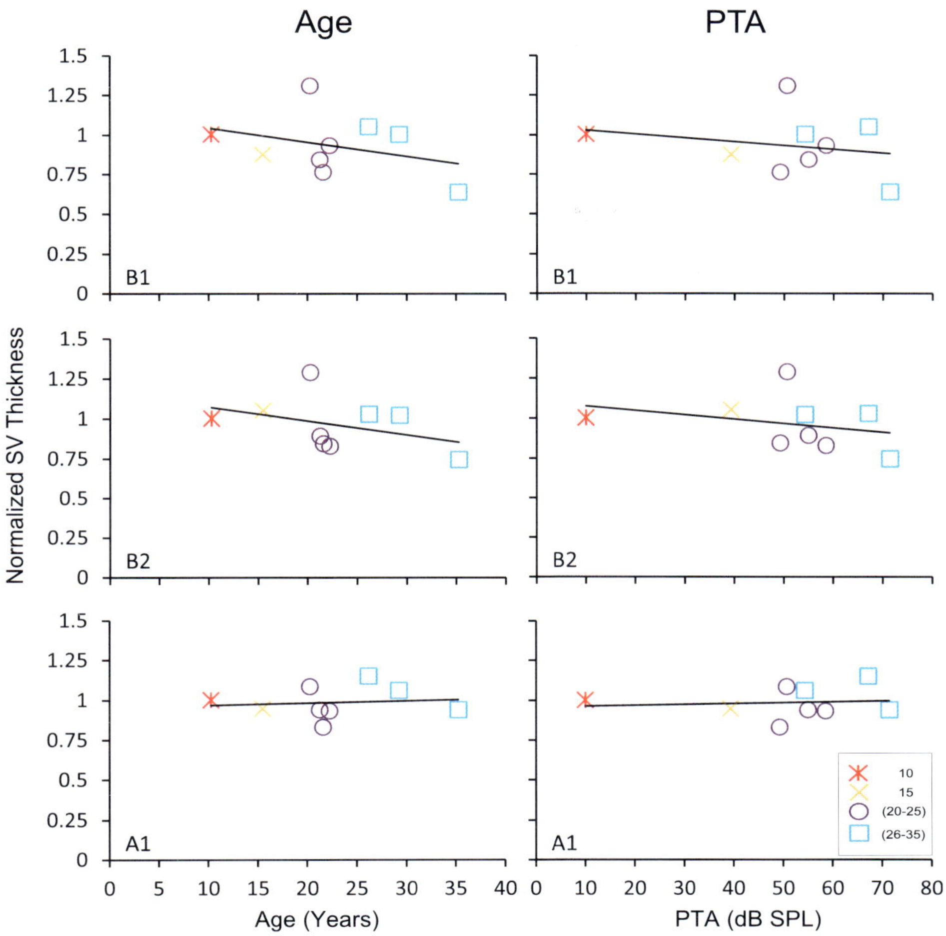

Figure 8. Effects of age and PTA on stria vascularis thickness. Age-normalized stria vascularis thickness as a function of age (left) and PTA (right) in the lower base (top), upper base (middle), and lower apex (bottom). There was no statistically significant correlation across animals.

weeks following the targeted ablation of IHCs in a mouse strain that lacks a thiamine transporter. The likely culprit behind SGC loss found in monkeys is the accumulation of mild to moderate noise overexposure over the lifespan in a similar fashion that has been shown in rodents [41]. Interestingly, we saw no difference in the spiral ganglion cell axons across age using whole-mounts of osmium stained cochleae (Figure S1). This indicates to us that this method is not sensitive enough to reveal the level of SGC loss seen in these animals, and that more sensitive anatomical techniques are required to detect a corresponding loss of SGC axons [42].

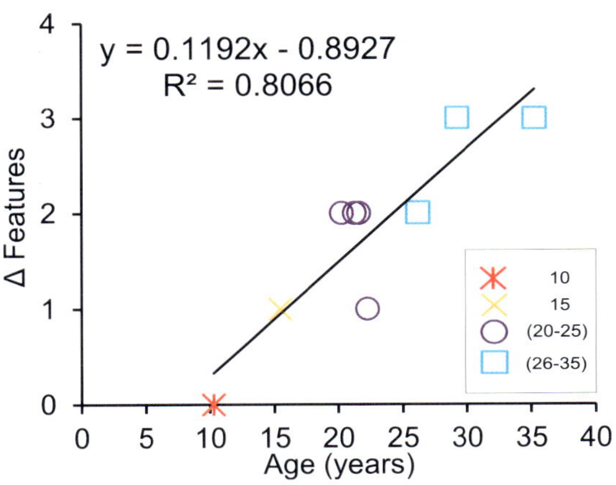

Figure 9. Age-related increase of the number of significant pathological features in the cochlea of the rhesus monkey. There was a statistically significant correlation, indicating that multiple histopathologies occur with natural aging. $r = 0.90$, $p < 0.001$.

Lastly, we found that the stria vascularis was not associated with a specific audiometric shift in hearing, which is congruent with previous observations of the stria vascularis in aged rhesus monkeys [15]. Stria vascularis thickness has been reported to be associated with the endocochlear potential, and scales with age [29]. In our hands, the thickness of the stria vascularis did not significantly change with increasing age in a similar fashion that has been reported in rodents [25]. We also found that the thickness of the stria vascularis was not significantly correlated with age-related changes in the ABR thresholds as a function of frequency. This may be due to several reasons. The lack of observing changes in strial thickness does not necessarily imply that rhesus monkeys do not experience changes to their audiogram based upon strial pathology. Our sample was fairly small and predominately female, and strial ARHL has been linked to genetic factors [43]. In addition, inspection of Figure S2 shows that there were several cases where SV thickness was reduced, but did not reach our criteria for statistical significance. An increased sample size, or inclusion of even younger monkeys may reveal differences in SV thickness with age. Future studies in rhesus monkeys could identify monkeys with flat elevated hearing loss, and then examine their relatives for similar ARHL outcomes to determine the extent of

Figure S2 Summary profile of the age-related cochlear histopathological changes. The data from each of the 8 animals is normalized by the youngest. A value of 1 indicates no difference from the youngest animal, larger values indicate a

3

Relationship between Audiometric Slope and Tinnitus Pitch in Tinnitus Patients: Insights into the Mechanisms of Tinnitus Generation

Martin Schecklmann[1,2], Veronika Vielsmeier[2,3], Thomas Steffens[3], Michael Landgrebe[1,2], Berthold Langguth[1,2], Tobias Kleinjung[2,3,4]*

1 Department of Psychiatry and Psychotherapy, University of Regensburg, Regensburg, Germany, **2** Interdisciplinary Tinnitus Clinic, University of Regensburg, Regensburg, Germany, **3** Department of Otorhinolaryngology, University of Regensburg, Regensburg, Germany, **4** Department of Otorhinolaryngology, University of Zurich, Zurich, Switzerland

Abstract

Background: Different mechanisms have been proposed to be involved in tinnitus generation, among them reduced lateral inhibition and homeostatic plasticity. On a perceptual level these different mechanisms should be reflected by the relationship between the individual audiometric slope and the perceived tinnitus pitch. Whereas some studies found the tinnitus pitch corresponding to the maximum hearing loss, others stressed the relevance of the edge frequency. This study investigates the relationship between tinnitus pitch and audiometric slope in a large sample.

Methodology: This retrospective observational study analyzed 286 patients. The matched tinnitus pitch was compared to the frequency of maximum hearing loss and the edge of the audiogram (steepest hearing loss) by t-tests and correlation coefficients. These analyses were performed for the whole group and for sub-groups (uni- vs. bilateral (117 vs. 338 ears), pure-tone vs. narrow-band (340 vs. 115 ears), and low and high audiometric slope (114 vs. 113 ears)).

Findings: For the right ear, tinnitus pitch was in the same range and correlated significantly with the frequency of maximum hearing loss, but differed from and did not correlate with the edge frequency. For the left ear, similar results were found but the correlation between tinnitus pitch and maximum hearing loss did not reach significance. Sub-group analyses (bi- and unilateral, tinnitus character, slope steepness) revealed identical results except for the sub-group with high audiometric slope which revealed a higher frequency of maximum hearing loss as compared to the tinnitus pitch.

Conclusion: The study-results confirm a relationship between tinnitus pitch and maximum hearing loss but not to the edge frequency, suggesting that tinnitus is rather a fill-in-phenomenon resulting from homeostatic mechanisms, than the result of deficient lateral inhibition. Sub-group analyses suggest that audiometric steepness and the side of affected ear affect this relationship. Future studies should control for these potential confounding factors.

Editor: Gerhard Andersson, Linkoping University, Sweden

Funding: The study was funded in part by the Tinnitus Research Initiative (TRI). No additional external funding was received for this study. The funders had no role in study design, data collection and analysis, decision to publish, or preparation of the manuscript.

Competing Interests: The authors have declared that no competing interests exist.

* E-mail: tobias.kleinjung@usz.ch

Introduction

There is a lot of evidence that tinnitus, the phantom perception of sound, is a consequence of neuroplastic alterations in the central auditory pathways [1]. These alterations are assumed to result from a dysbalance of excitatory and inhibitory mechanisms on many levels of the auditory pathways as a consequence of disturbed sensory input due to hearing loss [2]. Hearing loss can have multiple reasons within the peripheral auditory system. However, damage to cochlear structures represents the main cause of hearing loss in tinnitus subjects [3]. Defects of the cochlea can develop as a consequence of ageing, exposure to loud noise, cochlear ischemia, viral infections or ototoxic drugs [2]. In many cases middle and high frequencies are predominantly affected which leads to audiograms of characteristic shape. Different theories exist which try to explain the relationship of different types of hearing impairment and the perceived tinnitus frequency, the so-called tinnitus pitch.

One theory proposes that tinnitus results from an edge effect caused by an imbalance of lateral inhibition at the boundary of the region of normal and impaired hearing, the "edge frequency" [4]. It is assumed that a discontinuity of input along the tonotopic axis leads to a dysbalance in lateral inhibition, which in turn results in an increased firing rate and increased synchrony of the cortical representation of the edge frequency [5], finally resulting in an expansion of this area towards the deprived cortical area [6]. This theory implies that the perceived tinnitus frequency should be related to the edge frequency.

21. Hawkins JE, Jr., Johnsson LG, Stebbins WC, Moody DB, Coombs SL (1976) Hearing loss and cochlear pathology in monkeys after noise exposure. Acta oto-laryngologica 81: 337–343.
22. Tinling SP, Giberson RT, Kullar RS (2004) Microwave exposure increases bone demineralization rate independent of temperature. Journal of microscopy 215: 230–235.
23. Clark JG (1981) Uses and abuses of hearing loss classification. ASHA 23: 493–500.
24. Gundersen HJ (1977) Notes on the estimation of the numerical density of arbitrary profiles. Journal of microscopy 111: 219–223.
25. Ohlemiller KK, Gagnon PM (2004) Apical-to-basal gradients in age-related cochlear degeneration and their relationship to "primary" loss of cochlear neurons. The Journal of comparative neurology 479: 103–116.
26. Chen MA, Webster P, Yang E, Linthicum FH Jr (2006) Presbycusic neuritic degeneration within the osseous spiral lamina. Otol Neurotol 27: 316–322.
27. Moody DB, Stebbins WC, Hawkins JE, Jr., Johnsson LG (1978) Hearing loss and cochlear pathology in the monkey (Macaca) following exposure to high levels of noise. Archives of oto-rhino-laryngology 220: 47–72.
28. Kharkovets T, Dedek K, Maier H, Schweizer M, Khimich D, et al. (2006) Mice with altered KCNQ4 K+ channels implicate sensory outer hair cells in human progressive deafness. The EMBO journal 25: 642–652.
29. Ohlemiller KK, Rice ME, Gagnon PM (2008) Strial microvascular pathology and age-associated endocochlear potential decline in NOD congenic mice. Hearing research 244: 85–97.
30. Woods TM, Lopez SE, Long JH, Rahman JE, Recanzone GH (2006) Effects of stimulus azimuth and intensity on the single-neuron activity in the auditory cortex of the alert macaque monkey. Journal of neurophysiology 96: 3323–3337.
31. Miller LM, Recanzone GH (2009) Populations of auditory cortical neurons can accurately encode acoustic space across stimulus intensity. Proceedings of the National Academy of Sciences of the United States of America 106: 5931–5935.
32. Nelson EG, Hinojosa R (2003) Presbycusis: a human temporal bone study of individuals with flat audiometric patterns of hearing loss using a new method to quantify stria vascularis volume. The Laryngoscope 113: 1672–1686.
33. Bao J, Ohlemiller KK (2010) Age-related loss of spiral ganglion neurons. Hearing research 264: 93–97.
34. Frisina DR, Frisina RD (1997) Speech recognition in noise and presbycusis: relations to possible neural mechanisms. Hearing research 106: 95–104.
35. Abel SM, Giguere C, Consoli A, Papsin BC (2000) The effect of aging on horizontal plane sound localization. The Journal of the Acoustical Society of America 108: 743–752.
36. Suga F, Lindsay JR (1976) Histopathological observations of presbycusis. The Annals of otology, rhinology, and laryngology 85: 169–184.
37. Willott JF, Hunter KP, Coleman JR (1988) Aging and presbycusis: effects on 2-deoxy-D-glucose uptake in the mouse auditory brain stem in quiet. Experimental neurology 99: 615–621.
38. Linthicum FH, Jr., Fayad JN (2009) Spiral ganglion cell loss is unrelated to segmental cochlear sensory system degeneration in humans. Otology & neurotology : official publication of the American Otological Society, American Neurotology Society [and] European Academy of Otology and Neurotology 30: 418–422.
39. Suzuka Y, Schuknecht HF (1988) Retrograde cochlear neuronal degeneration in human subjects. Acta oto-laryngologica Supplementum 450: 1–20.
40. Zilberstein Y, Liberman MC, Corfas G (2012) Inner hair cells are not required for survival of spiral ganglion neurons in the adult cochlea. The Journal of neuroscience : the official journal of the Society for Neuroscience 32: 405–410.
41. Kujawa SG, Liberman MC (2009) Adding insult to injury: cochlear nerve degeneration after "temporary" noise-induced hearing loss. The Journal of neuroscience : the official journal of the Society for Neuroscience 29: 14077–14085.
42. Xing Y, Samuvel DJ, Stevens SM, Dubno JR, Schulte BA, et al. (2012) Age-related changes of myelin basic protein in mouse and human auditory nerve. PLoS One 7: e34500.
43. Gates GA, Couropmitree NN, Myers RH (1999) Genetic associations in age-related hearing thresholds. Archives of otolaryngology head & neck surgery 125: 654–659.

3

Relationship between Audiometric Slope and Tinnitus Pitch in Tinnitus Patients: Insights into the Mechanisms of Tinnitus Generation

Martin Schecklmann[1,2], Veronika Vielsmeier[2,3], Thomas Steffens[3], Michael Landgrebe[1,2], Berthold Langguth[1,2], Tobias Kleinjung[2,3,4]*

1 Department of Psychiatry and Psychotherapy, University of Regensburg, Regensburg, Germany, 2 Interdisciplinary Tinnitus Clinic, University of Regensburg, Regensburg, Germany, 3 Department of Otorhinolaryngology, University of Regensburg, Regensburg, Germany, 4 Department of Otorhinolaryngology, University of Zurich, Zurich, Switzerland

Abstract

Background: Different mechanisms have been proposed to be involved in tinnitus generation, among them reduced lateral inhibition and homeostatic plasticity. On a perceptual level these different mechanisms should be reflected by the relationship between the individual audiometric slope and the perceived tinnitus pitch. Whereas some studies found the tinnitus pitch corresponding to the maximum hearing loss, others stressed the relevance of the edge frequency. This study investigates the relationship between tinnitus pitch and audiometric slope in a large sample.

Methodology: This retrospective observational study analyzed 286 patients. The matched tinnitus pitch was compared to the frequency of maximum hearing loss and the edge of the audiogram (steepest hearing loss) by t-tests and correlation coefficients. These analyses were performed for the whole group and for sub-groups (uni- vs. bilateral (117 vs. 338 ears), pure-tone vs. narrow-band (340 vs. 115 ears), and low and high audiometric slope (114 vs. 113 ears)).

Findings: For the right ear, tinnitus pitch was in the same range and correlated significantly with the frequency of maximum hearing loss, but differed from and did not correlate with the edge frequency. For the left ear, similar results were found but the correlation between tinnitus pitch and maximum hearing loss did not reach significance. Sub-group analyses (bi- and unilateral, tinnitus character, slope steepness) revealed identical results except for the sub-group with high audiometric slope which revealed a higher frequency of maximum hearing loss as compared to the tinnitus pitch.

Conclusion: The study-results confirm a relationship between tinnitus pitch and maximum hearing loss but not to the edge frequency, suggesting that tinnitus is rather a fill-in-phenomenon resulting from homeostatic mechanisms, than the result of deficient lateral inhibition. Sub-group analyses suggest that audiometric steepness and the side of affected ear affect this relationship. Future studies should control for these potential confounding factors.

Editor: Gerhard Andersson, Linkoping University, Sweden

Funding: The study was funded in part by the Tinnitus Research Initiative (TRI). No additional external funding was received for this study. The funders had no role in study design, data collection and analysis, decision to publish, or preparation of the manuscript.

Competing Interests: The authors have declared that no competing interests exist.

* E-mail: tobias.kleinjung@usz.ch

Introduction

There is a lot of evidence that tinnitus, the phantom perception of sound, is a consequence of neuroplastic alterations in the central auditory pathways [1]. These alterations are assumed to result from a dysbalance of excitatory and inhibitory mechanisms on many levels of the auditory pathways as a consequence of disturbed sensory input due to hearing loss [2]. Hearing loss can have multiple reasons within the peripheral auditory system. However, damage to cochlear structures represents the main cause of hearing loss in tinnitus subjects [3]. Defects of the cochlea can develop as a consequence of ageing, exposure to loud noise, cochlear ischemia, viral infections or ototoxic drugs [2]. In many cases middle and high frequencies are predominantly affected which leads to audiograms of characteristic shape. Different theories exist which try to explain the relationship of different types of hearing impairment and the perceived tinnitus frequency, the so-called tinnitus pitch.

One theory proposes that tinnitus results from an edge effect caused by an imbalance of lateral inhibition at the boundary of the region of normal and impaired hearing, the "edge frequency" [4]. It is assumed that a discontinuity of input along the tonotopic axis leads to a dysbalance in lateral inhibition, which in turn results in an increased firing rate and increased synchrony of the cortical representation of the edge frequency [5], finally resulting in an expansion of this area towards the deprived cortical area [6]. This theory implies that the perceived tinnitus frequency should be related to the edge frequency.

Alternatively, it has been suggested that tinnitus is caused by homeostatic mechanisms, which aim to compensate reduced sensory input by reduction of inhibitory and/or increase of facilitatory mechanisms. This model predicts that changes in the processing of neuronal activity occur predominantly in the frequency range of reduced sensory input, which finally results in ongoing increased neuronal activity and/or synchrony in the respective central auditory pathways [7,8]. According to this theory the frequency of tinnitus perception should correspond to the frequency of hearing loss.

The relation between the individual audiometric slope and the perceived tinnitus pitch has been subject to different studies which have demonstrated somewhat inconsistent results. While some authors found a clear relationship between the tinnitus pitch and the edge frequency [9,10], others showed that the pitch corresponds to the area where hearing is impaired [11,12,13,14] and is in some specific cases congruent to the frequency of maximum hearing loss [15]. A third group could not demonstrate any correlation of audiogram shape and tinnitus pitch [16]. It has been suggested that such a relation may only exist in certain tinnitus sub-groups [14,16]. In particular perceptual characteristics of tinnitus have been proposed to be relevant [14]. Thus, the small sample sizes and the lack of sub-group analysis in most studies may provide an explanation for the conflicting results in the literature. Thus, the aim of the present study was to evaluate the relationship of hearing with tinnitus pitch in a large population of tinnitus patients and to evaluate the role of certain sub-groups. One hitherto largely neglected issue is the question whether it is of relevance if tinnitus is perceived uni- or bilaterally. Former studies only investigated patients with bilateral tinnitus [10,14]. The only study focusing on this issue did not find a clear association [16]. In relation to a recent study we were especially interested if there is an association of audiometric edge in patients with narrow-band tinnitus [14]. As former studies are highly inconsistent we additionally focused on sub-groups classified by the slope of the audiogram. Since findings from earlier studies are relatively inconsistent we resigned to formulate specific hypotheses. This study was presented in part at the Annual Meeting of the American Academy of Otolaryngology-Head and Neck Surgery, San Francisco, CA, September 10–14 2011.

Methods

Objectives

In this study we investigated in a large sample of 286 patients with tinnitus the relationship between the perceived tinnitus pitch and parameters derived from the pure tone audiogram such as the lower edge frequency and the maximum hearing loss frequency. The number of participants enabled us to perform sub-group analyses for bilateral vs. unilateral tinnitus, pure-tone vs. noise-like tinnitus, and patients with low vs. high steepness at the audiometric slope.

Ethics Statement

All participating subjects gave written informed consent for analysis of their data and inclusion of their data in the Tinnitus Research Initiative (TRI) database project. The TRI database project has been approved by the ethical committee of the University of Regensburg.

Sample

We analyzed patient data of the TRI database. The TRI database is a collaborative project of specialized tinnitus clinics following the approach to pool data in one international database [17] according to a consensus for patient assessment and outcome measurement [18]. We included only patients from the Regensburg center (Germany) in this study to ensure homogeneity of the audiometric procedures.

The flow of data selection is displayed in figure 1. The automatic data export from the database on May^{1st} 2011 included 1392 subjects. First datasets from the Regensburg center with complete data of audiometry (0.125–8 kHz) and tinnitus matching at screening/baseline visits were selected reducing the sample to 484 subjects. In the following step patients with broad-band-noise-like tinnitus and with a tinnitus pitch above 8 kHz were excluded resulting in a data set of 286 patients and 455 ears respectively (117 subjects with uni- and 169 with bilateral tinnitus). The exclusion of patients with a tinnitus pitch above 8 kHz was motivated by the fact that audiometric data were only available up to 8 kHz. Distribution of patients with uni- and bilateral and with pure-tone and narrow-band tinnitus is shown in the bottom part of figure 1.

The 286 patients which were included in the analyses were 52.9±13.7 (17.1–86.5) years old; 92 (32.4%) subjects were female. Patients suffered for 90.7±93.9 (1–456.6) months from tinnitus. Ratings and questionnaires were 48.8±22.7 (4–94) for the German version of the Tinnitus Handicap Inventory [19], 42.5±17.4 (6–79) for the German version of the Tinnitus Questionnaire [20], and 6.3±2.1 (0–10) for tinnitus loudness in a numeric rating scale.

Audiometry, pitch matching and calculation of audiogram parameters

Audiometry and tinnitus matching were done with a Madsen Itera (GN Otometrics, Germany) audiometer with Sennheiser HDA-200 supra-aural headphones (Sennheiser electronic GmbH & Co. KG, Germany). The hearing threshold for nine frequencies (0.125, 0.25, 0.5, 1, 2, 3, 4, 6, and 8 kHz) was determined by a standard Hughson-Westlake procedure (steps: 10 dB down, 5 dB up; 2 out of 3). In a second step, the frequency/pitch of the tinnitus was determined. In a first step, the pulsed tones of the audiogram where used to roughly match the tinnitus pitch and the patients were asked, whether the tinnitus sounds like a pure tone as just perceived during the audiometry, or does it sound like a broad band or a narrow band noise. To assist the comparison of the tinnitus pitch or sound quality either a pure tone or a white noise or a narrow band octave or 1/3-octave noise was presented to the ear with the tinnitus at nearly the same loudness as the tinnitus. If the pure tone threshold was too high to perceive a test signal at the side of the tinnitus, the contralateral better ear was used to present the sound. In case of a pure tone, a software sinus generator with a 1 Hz frequency resolution was then used in a bracketing procedure to match the pure tone pitch as exactly as possible. This technique is recommended for routine clinical use and seems to produce fewer octave confusions than others [21].

In case of a narrow band noise an octave or 1/3-octave filter bank with standard mid frequencies was used. The centre frequency was changed in the same way (1 Hz steps) as the bracketing procedure with pure tones until the narrow band noise matches the tinnitus pitch best. The center frequency of the matching signal was recorded as the pitch of the tinnitus.

The audiogram edge was defined as the lower frequency of two neighboring frequency pairs in the audiogram with the largest steepness, calculated as L(f2)−L(f1)/log2(f2/f1) [9]. If there were several frequency pairs with the same increase in hearing loss the lower frequency pair was used. To compute the mean audiogram edge across individuals, edge frequencies were first converted to a logarithmic scale, and then averaged, i.e. we used the geometric

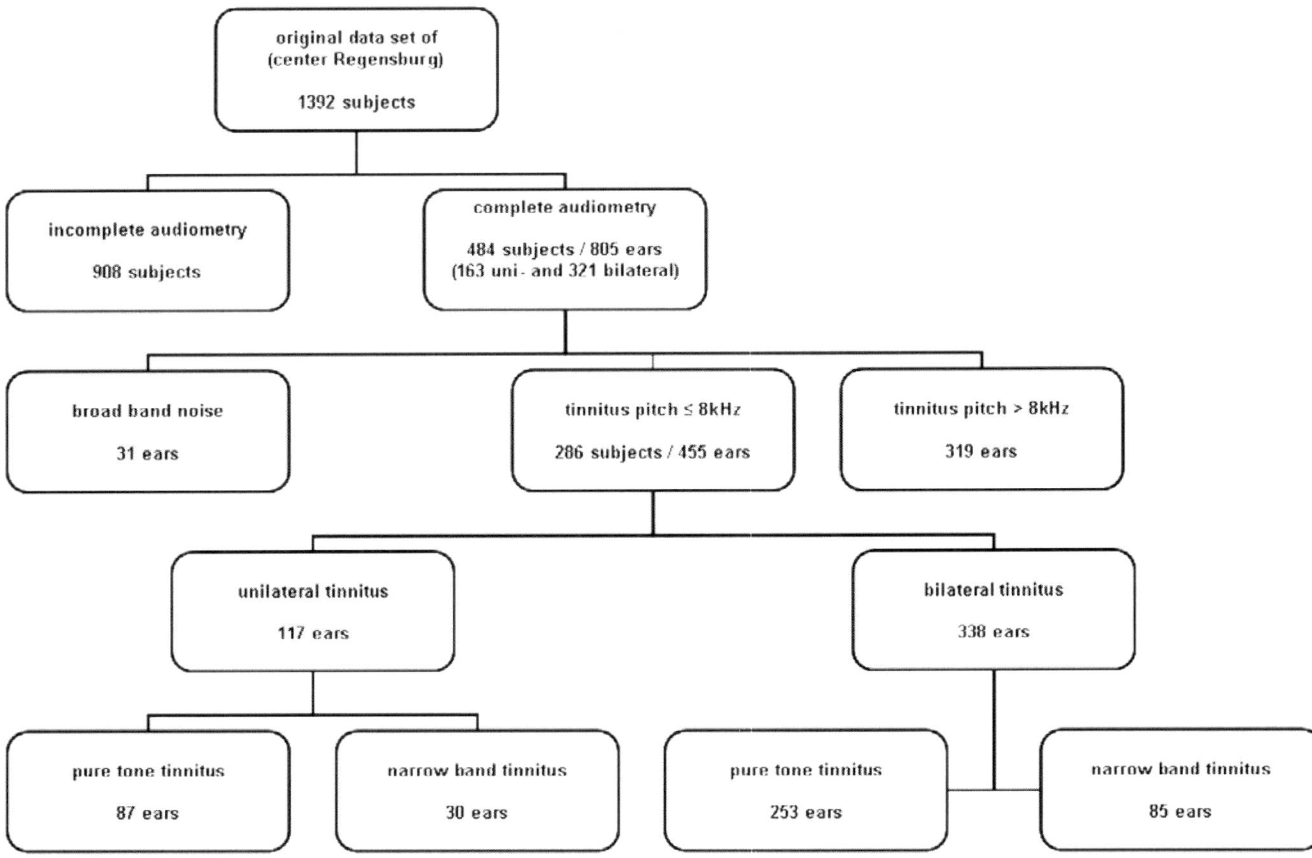

Figure 1. Study flow of inclusion of patients and ears.

mean. The slope was indicated by the hearing level difference of this frequency pair (dB/octave).

In addition, the frequency of the maximum hearing loss was evaluated for each subject. If there were several frequencies with maximum hearing loss the lowest one was used. Averaging across individuals was done accordingly to the method used for the edge. All calculations were done with MatLab® (The Mathworks Inc., USA).

Statistical analysis

The data analysis was based on data of the Tinnitus Research Initiative Database. Data management was conducted according to the Data Handling Plan (TRI-DHP V06, May 9th 2011). Data analysis was conducted according to the Standard Operating Procedure (TRI-SA V01, May 9th 2011), thereby following a study-specific Statistical Analysis Plan (SAP) that was written according to the SAP template (TRI-SAP-005, August 12th 2011) published on http://database.tinnitusresearch.org.

As all statistical tests have to fulfill the assumption that all data points have to be independent observations we separated our analyses for the right and the left ear. By this approach one subject contributed only one data point or data from only one ear respectively for each statistical test. In a first step we contrasted the tinnitus pitch with the edge frequency and with the frequency of maximum hearing loss with Student t-tests for the whole group. Thereafter, we calculated Pearson correlation coefficients between tinnitus pitch and edge, and between tinnitus pitch and frequency of maximum hearing loss. In further steps we split the samples according to tinnitus laterality (bi- vs. unilateral), tinnitus character (pure-tone vs. narrow-band tinnitus), and steepness of the slope at the audiometric edge (according to two halves of the sample as obtained by median split, i.e., low vs. high slope) and repeated the analyses in these sub-groups. Thereafter, we contrasted the sub-groups (bi- vs. unilateral, pure-tone vs. narrow-band, lower vs. higher half of the sample) for tinnitus pitch, and frequency of maximum hearing loss. As analyses were performed in logarithmic scale, we just provide back-transformed mean data of frequency space in text and abstained from presenting standard deviations.

Results

Numeric values for the frequencies/pitches for the whole group and sub-group analyses are given in table 1; statistical values for all calculations are given in table 2. Figure 2 depicts the frequency localization of the edge, the frequency of maximum hearing loss, the tinnitus pitch and the audiogram averaged for the whole group.

In the whole group analysis tinnitus pitch had a significantly higher frequency than the audiometric edge, but did not differ significantly from the frequency of maximum hearing loss for both ears. In a second analyzes of the sample with narrow band noise like tinnitus we replaced the center frequency of the narrow band noise with the lower bound frequency which is closer to the audiometric edge. This did not cause any changes of the result as there was again only significant correlation of the tinnitus pitch with the maximum hearing loss frequency but not with the edge frequency. Tinnitus pitch correlated positively with the frequency of maximum hearing loss, but not with the audiogram edge for the right ear. For the left ear no significant associations of pitch with edge and frequency of maximum hearing loss was found.

Sub-group analyses for tinnitus laterality (bi- vs. unilateral) and tinnitus character (pure-tone vs. narrow-band) showed results similar to the whole group analyses, i.e., tinnitus pitch had a significant higher frequency than the edge for both ears, frequency of maximum hearing loss did not differ from the pitch frequency for both ears, and frequency of maximum hearing loss was positively correlated with the tinnitus pitch for the right ear. Contrasts between unilateral and bilateral tinnitus did not reveal a significant difference for tinnitus pitch and frequency of maximum hearing loss. Also pure-tone and narrow-band tinnitus did not differ in these variables except for tinnitus pitch with a near-threshold p-value.

Dividing the sample in two halves by median split according to the slope at the audiometric edge showed that tinnitus pitch and frequency of maximum hearing loss was higher for the high slope in contrast to the low slope. Again the findings were comparable to the whole group analyses. In addition, frequency of maximum hearing loss was significantly higher than tinnitus pitch for the high slope group.

Discussion

We did not find an association between tinnitus pitch and audiometric edge in a sample of 286 patients (455 ears), but between pitch and frequency of maximum hearing loss, as indicated by t-tests and correlations. Frequency of maximum hearing loss and tinnitus pitch was in the same frequency range and tinnitus pitch had a higher frequency than the audiometric edge. In addition, there was a significant positive correlation between tinnitus pitch and frequency of maximum hearing loss for the right ear. For the left ear, pitch and frequency of maximum hearing loss was not correlated, although both were in the same frequency range. Edge and pitch frequency were not correlated. These findings were replicated in all analyzed sub-groups, i.e., bi- and unilateral tinnitus, pure-tone vs. narrow-band tinnitus, and tinnitus with low slope at the audiometric edge. The group with a high slope showed also a correlation between pitch and frequency of maximum hearing loss for the right ear, but in addition the frequency of maximum hearing loss was higher than tinnitus pitch which was higher than the edge frequency. Thus, our results do not support a relationship between edge frequency and tinnitus pitch, but rather confirm previous studies demonstrating that the tinnitus corresponds to the frequency region of hearing loss [11,12,13].

With respect to mechanisms involved in tinnitus generation our data favours homeostatic plasticity as the decisive mechanism of tinnitus generation [7,8]. In detail, it has been proposed that the central auditory system maintains neural homeostasis to preserve stable mean firing and neural coding efficiency. In many cases of sensory deprivation, "neural noise" might be amplified due to the overall increase of gain and result in increased neuronal activity in the deprived frequency spectrum, which is finally perceived as tinnitus [7].

Hitherto, antecedent literature indicated ambiguous results regarding the relationship of audiometric edge and tinnitus pitch (for an overview until the year 2000 see Tyler et al. [22]). A relatively large recent study ($n = 195$) could not demonstrate a significant relationship between tinnitus pitch and the low frequency edge [16]. Similar to our study, tinnitus pitch (5.0 kHz) and frequency of maximum hearing loss (5.0 kHz) were in the same frequency range in contrast to the edge (2.2 kHz) which was lower. However, in contrast to our data tinnitus pitch and the frequency of maximum hearing loss were also not correlated. In several additional analyses, they tried, but failed to find associations of edge and pitch in sub-groups based on the slope of the audiogram, tinnitus character, or tinnitus laterality. This relationship was only evident in some single cases.

In another recent study, Sereda et al. [14] studied 67 subjects with bilateral tinnitus. The complete sample failed to demonstrate an association of tinnitus pitch and edge frequency, however the tinnitus pitch was located rather within the area of hearing loss than in the area of the edge frequency in all patients. In the sub-group of subjects with narrow-band noise like tinnitus ($n = 23$) a significant positive relationship was noted for the edge frequency and tinnitus pitch, with the pitch being more than an octave above the edge frequency. In contrast to our study the audiogram involved the high frequency range up to 16 kHz and the whole perceived tinnitus frequency composition was determined. It should also be noted, that narrow-band tinnitus in this study was defined as a frequency band of 0.13–0.25 kHz bandwidth which is different from our definition of narrow-band tinnitus (<1 octave). An association of tinnitus pitch and edge within sub-groups of different slopes (shallow, moderate, and steep) could not be determined.

König and colleagues [9] also reported that tinnitus pitch was on average 1.5 ± 0.1 octaves above the edge frequency in a sub-

Table 1. Mean frequencies/pitches for the whole group and sub-groups (kHz).

	whole group		bilateral tinnitus		pure-tone tinnitus		low slope	
	right ear	left ear	right ear	left ear	right ear	left ear	right ear	left ear
tinnitus pitch	3.7	4.0	3.9	3.9	3.9	4.3	3.1	3.6
frequency of maximum hearing loss	3.9	4.3	4.1	4.2	3.9	4.3	2.5	3.3
audiometric edge	2.4	2.5	2.5	2.4	2.4	2.6	1.9	2.2
			unilateral tinnitus		narrow-band tinnitus		high slope	
			right ear	left ear	right ear	left ear	right ear	left ear
tinnitus pitch			3.2	4.3	3.4	3.2	4.6	4.5
frequency of maximum hearing loss			3.4	4.7	4.0	4.2	5.6	5.6
audiometric edge			2.1	2.8	2.3	2.3	2.9	2.8

Table 2. Contrasts and correlations of tinnitus pitch and frequency of maximum hearing loss for the whole group and sub-groups (significant or near-significant effects in bold font; T = student T; r = Pearson r).

	whole group				bilateral tinnitus				pure-tone tinnitus				low slope			
	right ear		left ear		right ear		left ear		right ear		left ear		right ear		left ear	
frequency	**T (df = 211)**	**r (n = 212)**	**T (df = 242)**	**r (n = 243)**	**T (df = 166)**	**r (n = 167)**	**T (df = 170)**	**r (n = 171)**	**T (df = 158)**	**r (n = 159)**	**T (df = 180)**	**r (n = 181)**	**T (df = 105)**	**r (n = 106)**	**T (df = 120)**	**r (n = 121)**
pitch - edge	**T = 5.324 p<0.001**	r = 0.043 p = 0.532	**T = 6.387 p<0.001**	r = −0.014 p = 0.827	**T = 4.992 p<0.001**	r = 0.029 p = 0.712	**T = 5.397 p<0.001**	r = 0.030 p = 0.692	**T = 4.881 p<0.001**	r = 0.005 p = 0.952	**T = 6.849 p<0.001**	r = 0.020 p = 0.789	**T = 2.966 p = 0.004**	r = −0.034 p = 0.732	**T = 3.943 p<0.001**	r = −0.067 p = 0.465
pitch – max. hearing loss	T = 0.489 p = 0.625	**r = 0.324 p<0.001**	T = 0.819 p = 0.413	r = 0.068 p = 0.201	T = 0.396 p = 0.693	**r = 0.236 p = 0.002**	T = 0.570 p = 0.569	r = 0.078 p = 0.312	T = 0.019 p = 0.985	**r = 0.267 p = 0.001**	T = 0.042 p = 0.966	r = 0.018 p = 0.892	T = 0.772 p = 0.442	**r = 0.240 p = 0.013**	T = 0.631 p = 0.530	r = 0.012 p = 0.897

	unilateral tinnitus				narrow-band tinnitus				high slope			
	right ear		left ear		right ear		right ear		right ear		left ear	
	T (df = 44)	**r (n = 45)**	**T (df = 71)**	**r (n = 72)**	**T (df = 52)**	**r (n = 53)**	**T (df = 61)**	**r (n = 62)**	**T (df = 105)**	**r (n = 106)**	**T (df = 121)**	**r (n = 122)**
pitch - edge	**T = 2.029 p = 0.049**	r = 0.052 p = 0.735	**T = 3.392 p = 0.001**	r = −0.185 p = 0.120	**T = 2.195 p = 0.033**	r = 0.128 p = 0.361	**T = 1.752 p = 0.085**	r = −0.090 p = 0.488	**T = 5.814 p<0.001**	r = 0.068 p = 0.489	**T = 5.621 p<0.001**	r = 0.026 p = 0.772
pitch - max. hearing loss	T = 0.303 p = 0.764	**r = 0.541 p<0.001**	T = 0.650 p = 0.518	r = 0.025 p = 0.834	T = 1.118 p = 0.269	**r = 0.487 p<0.001**	T = 1.605 p = 0.114	r = 0.188 p = 0.144	**T = 3.821 p = 0.001**	**r = 0.480 p<0.001**	**T = 2.751 p = 0.007**	r = 0.106 p = 0.246

	bi- vs. unilateral tinnitus		pure-tone vs. narrow-band tinnitus		lower vs. higher slope	
	right ear	left ear	right ear	left ear	right ear	left ear
	T (df = 210)	**T (df = 241)**	**T (df = 210)**	**T (df = 241)**	**T (df = 210)**	**T (df = 241)**
Pitch	T = 1.180 p = 0.239	T = 0.684 p = 0.495	T = 0.882 p = 0.379	**T = 2.160 p = 0.032**	**T = 2.914 p = 0.004**	**T = 1.918 p = 0.056**
Edge	T = 1.072 p = 0.285	T = 0.997 p = 0.320	T = 0.156 p = 0.876	T = 0.217 p = 0.829	**T = 5.307 p<0.001**	**T = 5.022 p<0.001**

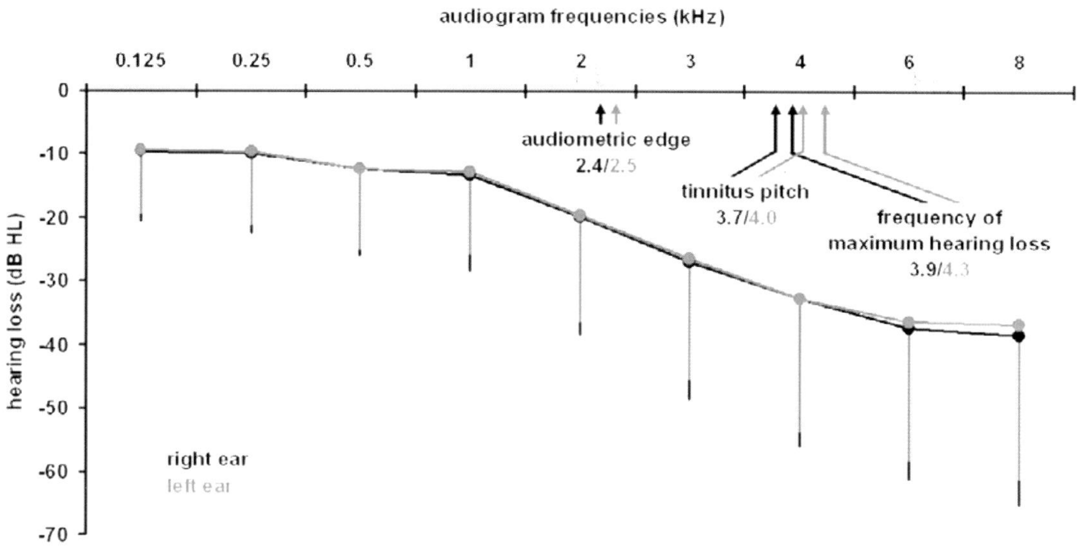

Figure 2. Relationship of audiogram and tinnitus pitch averaged for the whole sample, for the right and left ear. Please note that the averaged frequency of maximum hearing loss and the hearing loss as indicated by averaged audiogram data do not necessary result in the same values.

group of 24 patients with tonal tinnitus out of 71 patients with bilateral noise induced hearing loss. This sub-group also showed a significant correlation of pitch and edge and of pitch and frequency of the steepest slope. In contrast to our study, slope and edge were independently defined and were not necessarily related to the same frequency pair.

A recent study of Moore et al. [10] revealed a definite association between the values of the tinnitus pitch and the edge frequency with a correlation of 0.94 in 11 subjects with bilateral tonal tinnitus. This was the first study, which could show that tinnitus pitch (1.5 kHz) and audiometric edge (1.5 kHz) were in the same range. The authors remark that results depend critically on training procedures in order to avoid an octave error in tinnitus matching. Thus, patients tend to rate the frequency of their tinnitus one octave too high. In general, tinnitus pitches were one or two octaves lower after training.

The findings of König et al. [9] and Moore et al. [10] are in contrast to our results of no relationship between tinnitus pitch and audiometric edge. We rather found an association with tinnitus pitch and frequency of maximum hearing loss. Even splitting the sample in sub-groups which are considered to be specific for edge-pitch associations could not reveal such an association. Neither uni- or bilateral, nor pure-tone or narrow-band tinnitus, nor low or high sloping audiograms indicated an association of pitch and edge. This is in contrast to the findings of Sereda et al. [14] who find an association of pitch and edge in the sub-group of patients with narrow-band tinnitus. Notably the definition of narrow-band tinnitus in that study was not identical to the definition used in our study.

In our study we did not use a particular tinnitus matching training as Moore and colleagues did. Thus, we cannot exclude that some of our subjects may have an octave error at tinnitus pitch matching. However, an octave error in some patients would produce a systematic effect and could eventually explain the observed difference between the edge frequency and the tinnitus pitch, but not the lack of correlation between these two factors.

One may also argue that in the majority of patients the discontinuity in the audiogram was not very high and may not be reflected by discontinuities at the inner hair cell level which might be the necessary precondition for an edge frequency effect. However, if the edge frequency effect only explains the generation of tinnitus in patients with an extremely steep audiometric slope, then it would not provide an explanation for tinnitus generation in the vast majority of tinnitus patients with moderate hearing loss. Moreover, we did not find any differences in the relationship between edge and tinnitus pitch between the low and high slope groups. Thus, our data gives no hint that the edge frequency effect may play a major role in tinnitus generation for a relevant sub-group of tinnitus patients.

It should be noted that we excluded patients with a tinnitus pitch above 8 kHz and with broad-band tinnitus, narrowing the external validity to a certain subpopulation (see also figure 2). The prevalence of broad-band tinnitus in our sample is low maybe due to lower distress in these patients. The prevalence of high-frequency tinnitus was rather high, thus, future studies should also focus on high-frequency audiogram data. It should also be considered that definition of pure-tone or narrow-band tinnitus was done according to an audiological pitch matching procedure as there is incongruence between verbal descriptions and matching procedures. We are well aware of the fact that all pitch matching procedures have some limitations, e.g. octave error, intra-individual variation and reproducibility. An international consensus on standardized test procedures is still lacking [23]. However, with the bracketing method we chose a feasible technique which is recommended for routine clinical use in tinnitus patients [21].

In addition we found a lateralization effect. Whereas for the right ear pitch and frequency of maximum hearing loss were in the same frequency range and were correlated, for the left ear pitch and frequency of maximum hearing loss were in the same frequency range, but were not significantly correlated. Lying in the same range in a correlated manner provides a strong hint that there is a close relationship between both measures. This fits very well to the central gain hypothesis (see above). Lying in the same frequency range without correlating depicts only a coarse relationship suggesting that the neurophysiological basis of tinnitus may depend on its laterality. Further support for a lateralization effect comes from epidemiological studies showing a higher proportion of left-sided unilateral tinnitus especially in tinnitus patients with hearing loss [24] and from electrophysiological studies showing differences in laterality indices for the right and left ear [25]. However, exact mechanisms are speculative and our findings should be considered preliminary till confirmed by further studies. Nevertheless tinnitus laterality should be considered as a potential confounding factor in future studies. It is also of relevance to consider this issue methodologically, as using both ears in one analysis might introduce statistical errors as the assumption of independence of data points is not fulfilled. This was not done for most studies in this context.

Furthermore, for the high slope tinnitus group frequency of maximum hearing loss was higher than tinnitus pitch although both measures were correlated. This is in line with animal models of noise induced tinnitus which show a tinnitus pitch above the frequency of the presented noise [26]. This again might indicate another neurophysiological mechanism.

In summary, our findings are in line with most previous publications by indicating a relationship between tinnitus pitch and audiogram variables. The observed association of tinnitus pitch with the frequency of maximum hearing loss provides further support for the hypothesis of homeostatic plasticity as the relevant mechanism for tinnitus generation [7,8]. However, this model might not account completely for all subjects, especially for left-sided tinnitus and tinnitus patients with steep audiograms. This information is also relevant for illustrating the relationship of hearing loss and tinnitus in patient education and may guide the recommendation for the use of hearing aids for treating tinnitus accompanied by hearing loss [27]. We are aware that the present findings just represent a correlational, and not a causal relationship of tinnitus pitch and frequency of maximum hearing loss. Therefore the data should be complemented by further large interventional studies investigating the effect of hearing aids on the frequency composition of the tinnitus percept [28].

Acknowledgments

The authors want to thank Steven Macrum for valuable comments on the description of audiological measurements and Susanne Staudinger and Sandra Pfluegl for the collection of data in the TRI database. The authors thank Damien Sequeira MD for proofreading of the article.

Author Contributions

Conceived and designed the experiments: MS BL TK. Performed the experiments: VV TS ML TK. Analyzed the data: MS TS BL TK. Wrote the paper: MS VV TS ML BL TK.

References

1. De Ridder D, Elgoyhen AB, Romo R, Langguth B (2011) Phantom percepts: tinnitus and pain as persisting aversive memory networks. Proc Natl Acad Sci U S A 108: 8075–8080.
2. Moller AR (2003) Pathophysiology of Tinnitus. In: Sismanis A, ed. Otolaryngol Clin N Am. Amsterdam: W.B.Saunders. pp 249–266.
3. Roberts LE, Eggermont JJ, Caspary DM, Shore SE, Melcher JR, et al. (2010) Ringing ears: the neuroscience of tinnitus. J Neurosci 30: 14972–14979.
4. Kiang NY-S, Moxon EC, Levine PA (1970) Auditory-nerve activity in cats with normal and abnormal cochleas. In: Wolstenholme GEW, Knight J, eds. Sensorineural hearing loss. London: CIBA Foundation.
5. Llinas RR, Ribary U, Jeanmonod D, Kronberg E, Mitra PP (1999) Thalamocortical dysrhythmia: A neurological and neuropsychiatric syndrome characterized by magnetoencephalography. Proc Natl Acad Sci 96: 15222–15227.
6. Robertson D, Irvine DR (1989) Plasticity of frequency organization in auditory cortex of guinea pigs with partial unilateral deafness. J Comp Neurol 282: 456–471.
7. Norena AJ (2011) An integrative model of tinnitus based on a central gain controlling neural sensitivity. Neurosci Biobehav Rev 35: 1089–1109.
8. Schaette R, Kempter R (2009) Predicting tinnitus pitch from patients' audiograms with a computational model for the development of neuronal hyperactivity. J Neurophysiol 101: 3042–3052.
9. Konig O, Schaette R, Kempter R, Gross M (2006) Course of hearing loss and occurrence of tinnitus. Hear Res 221: 59–64.
10. Moore BC, Vinay, Sandhya (2010) The relationship between tinnitus pitch and the edge frequency of the audiogram in individuals with hearing impairment and tonal tinnitus. Hear Res 261: 51–56.
11. Henry JA, Meikle MB (1999) Pulsed versus continuous tones for evaluating the loudness of tinnitus. J Am Acad Audiol 10: 261–272.
12. Norena A, Micheyl C, Chery-Croze S, Collet L (2002) Psychoacoustic characterization of the tinnitus spectrum: implications for the underlying mechanisms of tinnitus. Audiol Neurootol 7: 358–369.
13. Roberts LE, Moffat G, Bosnyak DJ (2006) Residual inhibition functions in relation to tinnitus spectra and auditory threshold shift. Acta Otolaryngol Suppl. pp 27–33.
14. Sereda M, Hall DA, Bosnyak DJ, Edmondson-Jones M, Roberts LE, et al. (2011) Re-examining the relationship between audiometric profile and tinnitus pitch. Int J Audiol 50: 303–312.
15. Ochi K, Ohashi T, Kenmochi M (2003) Hearing impairment and tinnitus pitch in patients with unilateral tinnitus: comparison of sudden hearing loss and chronic tinnitus. Laryngoscope 113: 427–431.
16. Pan T, Tyler RS, Ji H, Coelho C, Gehringer AK, et al. (2009) The relationship between tinnitus pitch and the audiogram. Int J Audiol 48: 277–294.
17. Landgrebe M, Zeman F, Koller M, Eberl Y, Mohr M, et al. (2010) The Tinnitus Research Initiative (TRI) database: a new approach for delineation of tinnitus subtypes and generation of predictors for treatment outcome. BMC Med Inform Decis Mak 10: 42.
18. Langguth B, Goodey R, Azevedo A, Bjorne A, Cacace A, et al. (2007) Consensus for tinnitus patient assessment and treatment outcome measurement: Tinnitus Research Initiative meeting, Regensburg, July 2006. Prog Brain Res 166: 525–536.
19. Kleinjung T, Fischer B, Langguth B, Sand PG, Hajak G, et al. (2007) Validation of the German-version Tinnitus Handicap Inventory (THI). Psychiatrische Praxis 34: S140–S142.
20. Goebel G, Hiller W (1994) [The tinnitus questionnaire. A standard instrument for grading the degree of tinnitus. Results of a multicenter study with the tinnitus questionnaire]. HNO 42: 166–172.
21. Tyler RS, Conrad-Armes D (1983) Tinnitus pitch: a comparison of three measurement methods. Br J Audiol 17: 101–107.
22. Tyler RS (2000) Psychoacoustical measurement. In: Tyler RS, ed. Tinnitus Handbook. San Diego, CA: Singular Publishing Group. pp 149–180.
23. Henry JA, Rheinsburg B, Owens KK, Ellingson RM (2006) New instrumentation for automated tinnitus psychoacoustic assessment. Acta Otolaryngol Suppl. pp 34–38.
24. Martines F, Bentivegna D, Martines E, Sciacca V, Martinciglio G (2010) Characteristics of tinnitus with or without hearing loss: clinical observations in Sicilian tinnitus patients. Auris Nasus Larynx 37: 685–693.
25. Hine DW, Honan CA, Marks AD, Brettschneider K (2007) Development and validation of the Smoking Expectancy Scale for Adolescents. Psychol Assess 19: 347–355.
26. Kaltenbach JA (2011) Tinnitus: Models and mechanisms. Hear Res 276: 52–60.
27. Schaette R, Konig O, Hornig D, Gross M, Kempter R (2010) Acoustic stimulation treatments against tinnitus could be most effective when tinnitus pitch is within the stimulated frequency range. Hear Res 269: 95–101.
28. Moffat G, Adjout K, Gallego S, Thai-Van H, Collet L, et al. (2009) Effects of hearing aid fitting on the perceptual characteristics of tinnitus. Hear Res 254: 82–91.

4

Postlingual Hearing Loss as a Mitochondrial 3243A>G Mutation Phenotype

Katarzyna Iwanicka-Pronicka[1,2]*, Agnieszka Pollak[1,2], Agata Skórka[4], Urszula Lechowicz[1,2], Magdalena Pajdowska[5], Mariusz Furmanek[1,2], Maciej Rzeski[1,2], Lech Korniszewski[1,2], Henryk Skarżyński[1,2], Rafał Płoski[3]

1 Institute of Physiology and Pathology of Hearing, Warsaw, Poland, **2** World Hearing Center, Kajetany, Poland, **3** Department of Medical Genetics, Medical University of Warsaw, Poland, **4** Department of Paediatrics, Medical University of Warsaw, Poland, **5** Department of Biochemistry and Experimental Medicine, The Children's Memorial Health Institute, Warsaw, Poland

Abstract

Background: The prevalence of isolated hearing loss (HL) associated with the m.3243A>G mutation is unknown. The aim of this study was to assess the frequency and heteroplasmy level of the m.3243A>G mutation in a large group of Polish patients with postlingual bilateral sensorineural HL of unidentified cause.

Methodology/Principal Findings: A molecular search was undertaken in the archival blood DNA of 1482 unrelated patients with isolated HL that had begun at ages between 5 and 40 years. Maternal relatives of the probands were subsequently investigated and all carriers underwent audiological tests. The m.3243A>G mutation was found in 16 of 1482 probands (an incidence of 1.08%) and 18 family members. Of these 34 individuals, hearing impairment was detected in 29 patients and the mean onset of HL was at 26 years. Some 42% of the identified m.3243A>G carriers did not develop multisystem symptomatology over the following 10 years. Mean heteroplasmy level of m.3243A>G was lowest in blood at a level of 14% and highest in urine at 58%. These values were independent of the manifested clinical severity of the disease.

Conclusions: A single m.3243A>G carrier can usually be found among each 100 individuals who have postlingual hearing loss of unknown cause. Urine samples are best for detecting the m.3243A>G mutation and diagnosing mitochondrially inherited hearing loss.

Editor: Mathias Toft, Oslo University Hospital, Norway

Competing Interests: The authors have declared that no competing interests exist.

* E-mail: k.pronicka@ifps.org.pl

Introduction

Postlingual hearing loss (HL) occurs in 85–95% of patients with multisystem syndromes associated with an m.3243A>G mutation in the tRNA^{leu} (UUR) gene [1–4]. In the MELAS phenotype (mitochondrial encephalomyopathy lactic acidosis stroke-like episodes) [5,6], HL is the fourth most frequent of 17 symptoms [7]; in the MIDD phenotype (mitochondrially inherited diabetes-deafness syndrome), hearing impairment is usually the second most-frequent symptom [8,9]. The origin of the mitochondrial sensorineural defect may be cochlear [3,10] or retro-cochlear if there is central neurological involvement [11]. Major findings in the cochleas of subjects with the m.3243A>G mutation are degeneration and decreased cochlear neurons [12], fewer outer hair cells and endolymphatic sac cells [13], and atrophy of *stria vascularis* [12–14].

Although the prevalence of the most frequent m.3243A>G tRNA leucine (UUR) transition (MTTL1) in the general population is known [13,15–17], and the occurrence of mitochondrial disease associated with various mtDNA mutations is estimated as more than 1 in 5,000 [18], knowledge of the frequency of m.3243A>G mutation associated with isolated hearing impairment is limited [19–23] since usually, only m.1555A>G mitochondrial 12S rRNA mutation, and a few other specific mtDNA mutations associated with aminoglycoside susceptibility, are tested in patients with nonsyndromic HL [24–26].

Methods

Objectives

The aim of the study was to assess the frequency and heteroplasmy level of the m.3243A>G mutation in a large group of Polish patients with postlingual bilateral sensorineural HL of unidentified cause.

Patients

The study group was recruited from a cohort of 7000 individuals who consulted the Genetics Department of the Institute of Physiology and Pathology of Hearing (the Polish national referral centre) between the years 2000 and 2010. Only

Table 1. Characteristics of the study group: all examined patients with hearing loss (HL), and the 34 patients identified as having the m.3243A>G mutation.

	Studied patients	m.3243A>G mutation carriers
Number	1482	34*
Males	649 (44%)	13 (38%)
Females	833 (56%)	21 (62%)
Mean age at the study (years)	5–62, mean 27.0	6–61, mean 31.0
Mean age of onset of HL (years)	5–40, mean 15; SD = 10.4	8–63, mean 26[1] SD = 13.7; N = 29***
Profound degree of hearing loss**	3.8%	3.4%
Severe degree of hearing loss**	6.6%	13.8%
Moderate degree of hearing loss**	43.6%	51.8%
Mild degree of hearing loss**	46%	31%
Normal hearing	0	5
Other dysfunction of the inner ear (tinnitus/vertigo)	399/103; (27%/7%)	12/5; (35%/15%)
Progression of hearing loss during observation	ND	14
Positive family history of hearing loss	528 (35.6%)	33 (97.0%)[2]
Development of additional multi-organ 3243A>G pathology	ND	17
Number of 35delG *GJB2* heterozygotes	80 (5.5%)	1/16 (6.3%)

*16 probands and 18 relatives.
**Arithmetic mean of 0.5, 1, 2 and 4 kHz for the better-hearing ear.
***N = number of patients; 29 of 34 had HL; 5 subjects (aged 6–20) had normal hearing.
[1] $p<0.000001$ vs patients without m.3243A>G (*t*-test).
[2] $p<0.00001$.
ND = no data.

cases with bilateral HL, starting at an age between 5 and 40 years, and with available archived DNA sample, were included in the study. Patients were excluded if they had an established cause of hearing impairment, had syndromic HL of known genetic origin, or had two mutations in the connexin genes *GJB2* and *GJB6* (homozygosity or compound heterozygosity status) [27,28]. In total, 1482 archived blood DNA samples were made available for the m.3243A>G mutation search.

The data retrieved from medical reports of the recruited patients included: (1) the age of the patient, (2) gender, (3) age of HL onset (defined as the age at which the patient or his/her parents first became aware of hearing impairment), (4) the result of the first audiological examination based on pure tone audiometry (PTA), (5) the degree of HL (defined as the arithmetic mean of the frequencies 0.5, 1, 2, and 4 kHz for the better-hearing ear), (6) whether the HL was progressive or stable (determined by comparing the mean hearing threshold of each patient's initial and last audiogram), (7) the presence of additional symptoms of dysfunction of the hearing pathway like tinnitus and/or vertigo, (8) other health problems of the patient, and (9) the family history of hearing impairment, the basic health status of maternal relatives with hearing problems, and sudden deaths in the family. Characteristics of the study group are shown in Table 1.

Clinical and audiological status of the carriers of the m.3243A>G mutation were re-assessed, and they underwent genetic counselling. Maternal relatives of the m.3243A>G probands were also invited for audiological and genetic consultation. Severity of mitochondrial disease was assessed according to the Newcastle Mitochondrial Diseases Adult Scale (NMDAS) [29].

Clinical and laboratory investigations

Hearing levels were determined by pure tone audiometry. Evaluation of the degree of hearing loss was based on ANSI (American National Standards Institute) and ISO (International Standards Organization) standards. On these scales, mild hearing loss is that up to 40 dB HL, moderate is 41–70 dB HL, severe is 71–90 dB HL, and profound is more than 90 dB HL. Additional hearing tests – otoacoustic emissions, speech audiometry, tympanometry with stapedial reflexes, and brainstem evoked auditory potentials (BEAP) – were conducted to identify the character of the hearing loss (sensorineural hearing loss SNHL of cochlear origin, retro-cochlear, or conductive).

Cerebral alterations and brain lactates were assessed by magnetic resonance imaging with magnetic resonance spectroscopy (Siemens 3T). Organic acids excreted in urine were analysed using gas chromatography-mass spectroscopy (GC-MS).

Additional samples for the heteroplasmy study (urine sediment, nails, hair follicles, and buccal mucosa smear) were collected from individuals with confirmed or suspected m.3243A>G mutation and who gave signed consent.

A search for the m.3243A>G mutation was performed using TaqMan Assay on Demand from Applied Biosystems, Foster City, CA, according to the manufacturer's instructions. All positive samples were directly sequenced to confirm the presence of the mutation using primers M_F and M_R without 5′JOE modification (Table 2). The heteroplasmy level was assessed by PCR-RFLP

Table 2. The sequences of the primers M_F and M_R.

Primer	Sequence	modification
M_F	5′CCTCCCTGTACGAAAGGACA3′	none
M_R	5′AGGAGTAGGAGGTTGGCCATGG 3′	5′ JOE

Table 3. Characteristics of the patients carrying the m.3243A>G mutation patients 1–17 with multi-organ presentation (subgroup I), patients 18–29 with isolated hearing loss (subgroup II), and asymptomatic carriers 30–34 (subgroup III).

Patient number	Gender	Age (yrs)	Age of onset of HL (yrs)	HL severity	HL progression	Disease severity (NMDAS scale)	Organic acids profile in urine (GC-MS)	Increased lactates in brain (MRS)	Brain MRI	Symptoms and onset	Remarks
1	F	20	19	mild	Yes	7	NP	NP	NP	RP (20), SS	Aminogly*
2	**F**	**43**	**32**	**mild**	**No**	**15**	**MGCA**	**2**	**IMGP**	**M (40), RP (43)**	**Episode of blindness lasting 2 days**
3	**M**	**12**	**8**	**mild**	**No**	**55**	**NP**	**NP (died)**	**NP (died)**	**H (8), M (8), N (8), S (11)**	**Died at age 12**
4	F	38	35	moderate	Yes	19	MGCA LA	2	MCA IMGP	H (35), N (37), SS	Pancreatitis*
5	**F**	**41**	**10**	**moderate**	**ND**	**20 (part 2 only)**	**NP**	**NP**	**NP**	**DM (15), H (40)**	
6	M	13	9	moderate	No	81	NP	NP	NP	H (9), M (9), N (9), S (9), RP (10)	
7	**M**	**29**	**24**	**moderate**	**Yes**	**26**	**NA**	**NP (pacemaker)**	**NP**	**C (24), M (24), SS**	**Stress***
8	**M**	**27**	**20**	**moderate**	**ND**	**33 (part 2 only)**	**NP**	**NP (died)**	**NP**	**M (21), N (21), S (27), SS**	**Died at age 27**
9	**M**	**42**	**32**	**moderate**	**No**	**33**	**NA**	**1**	**MCA**	**DM (38), K (40), RP (42), I**	**Impaired spermatogenesis at biopsy, end-stage renal failure**
10	**M**	**52**	**40**	**moderate**	**No**	**77**	**MGCA**	**3**	**MCA Focal lesion after S in occ-temp-parietal area. IMGP**	**M (40), N (40), RP (45), S (45), C (45), DM (46), H (50), I, SS**	**Impaired spermatogenesis at biopsy**
11	**F**	**16**	**8**	**severe**	**Yes**	**38**	**NA**	**2**	**Diffuse bilateral lesions after S in frontal, occ-temp-parietal areas, insular cortex. IMGP MCA**	**N (8), S (8)**	**Stress***
12	F	47	37	severe	Yes	14	MGCA	2	MCA IMGP	C (40), M (45), I	Aminogly*
13	F	72	47	severe	No	74	NP	NP	NP	H (47), M (47), N (47), C (50), DM (50)	
14	M	37	19	severe	Yes	4	NA	1	MCA IMGP	SS	Noise*
15	**F**	**28**	**19**	**profound**	**Yes**	**31**	**LA**	**NP (CI)**	**NP**	**N (25), M (25)**	**Aminogly***
16	**F**	**38**	**22**	**profound**	**Yes**	**33**	**NA**	**2**	**MCA IMGP**	**H (30), DM (35), K (36), M (38), SS**	**End-stage renal failure. Stress***

Table 3. Cont.

Patient number	Gender	Age (yrs)	Age of onset of HL (yrs)	HL severity	HL progression	Disease severity (NMDAS scale)	Organic acids profile in urine (GC-MS)	Increased lactates in brain (MRS)	Brain MRI	Symptoms and onset	Remarks
17	**F**	**51**	**17**	**profound**	**Yes**	**99**	**NP**	**NP (CI)**	**NP**	**H (20), C (40), DM (40), N (40), RP (40), S (40), M (49), I, SS**	**Aminogly***
18	F	18	17	mild	No	6	NP	1	NA	-	
19	**F**	**24**	**10**	**mild**	**No**	**1**	**NP**	**NP**	**NP**	**-**	
20	F	24	23	mild	No	1	NA	1	NA	-	
21	F	35	34	mild	Yes	4	NA	1	IMGP	-	Stress*
22	F	49	48	mild	Yes	12	MGCA	0	IMGP	-	Stress*
23	**M**	**29**	**9**	**mild**	**No**	**1**	**NA**	**0**	**NA**	**-**	
24	F	78	63	moderate	No	34	NA	1	Focal spread vascuar lesions of white matter (non-specific).	-	NMDAS score probably false positive, connected with advanced age
25	**M**	**32**	**29**	**moderate**	**Yes**	**8**	**NA**	**1**		**-**	**Noise***
26	M	33	33	moderate	Yes	11	NP	NP	NP	-	Stress*
27	**M**	**51**	**20**	**moderate**	**ND**	**NP**	**NP**	**NP**	**NP**	**-**	
28	F	49	42	severe	No	25 (13 of part I - QoL)	NA	1	MCA	-	
29	**F**	**61**	**25**	**profound**	**Yes**	**7**	**NA**	**NP (CI)**	**NP**	**-**	**Pregnancy***
30	F	5	No HL	-	No HL	11	NA	NP	NP	-	Hair heteroplasmy 20.4%
31	F	10	No HL	-	No HL	24 (15 of part I - QoL)	NA	NP	NP	-	Buccal heteroplasmy 100%
32	F	10	No HL	-	No HL	0	MGCA	0	NA	-	
33	F	19	No HL	-	No HL	5	LA	1	IMGP	-	
34	M	8	No HL	-	No HL	0	NA	1	NA	-	Hair heteroplasmy 63.7%

Probands are shown in bold.

GC-MS = gas chromatography–mass spectroscopy; NMDAS = Newcastle Mitochondrial Disease Adult Scale; MGCA = 3-methylglutaconic aciduria; LA = lactic aciduria; HL = hearing loss; NP = not performed; NA = normal value; QoL = quality of life; CI = cochlear implant user; IMGP = increased mineralisation of globus pallidus; MCA = minimal cerebellar atrophy; MRS = magnetic resonance spectroscopy; MRS score: 0 = negative LA, 1 = uncertain LA, 2 = positive LA, 3 = strong LA.

C = cardiomyopathy; DM = diabetes mellitus; H = migraine; I = infertility; K = renal insufficiency; M = myopathy; N = peripheral neuropathy; RP = pigmentary degeneration of retina; S = stroke-like episodes; SS = short stature.

No HL = normal hearing.

*Stress = hearing deterioration following stressful event; Aminogly = hearing deterioration following aminoglycoside administration; Noise = hearing deterioration following noise exposure; Pancreatitis = hearing deterioration following acute pancreatitis; Pregnancy = hearing deterioration after pregnancy.

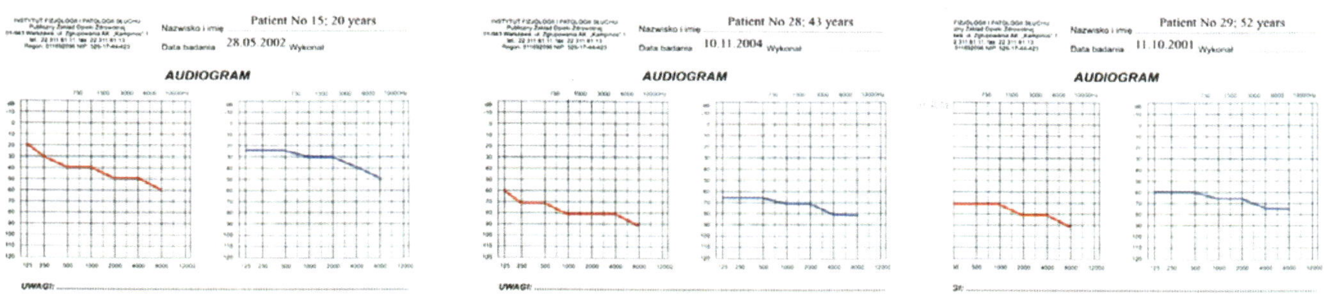

Figure 1. Audiograms of patients 15, 28, and 29 when first diagnosed with isolated hearing impairment.

using the primers and ApaI (Fermentas, Lithuania) enzyme (the m.3243A>G mutation creates a restriction site for this enzyme). Digested products were analyzed on an ABI 3130 capillary sequencer. Finally, by analysing the area under the peak the mutated/non-mutated DNA ratio was assessed.

Ethics statement

The bioethical commission of the Institute of Physiology and Pathology of Hearing approved the study and all subjects or their guardians gave signed consent.

Statistical analysis

Comparisons of mean onset of HL among m.3243A>G carriers versus other patients were done using a student *t*-test for independent samples. Comparison of heteroplasmy levels in different tissues was performed by a student *t*-test for dependent samples. Correlation between total disease score and heteroplasmy levels was performed by linear regression. All analyses were done using the Statistica software package.

Results

Prevalence of m.3243A>G

Our study of 1482 archival DNA samples of HL patients revealed m.3243A>G mutation in 16 cases (1.08%) indicating that on average the m.3243A>G mutation was found in one of 92 examined patients with isolated HL that had begun between the ages of 5 and 40 years.

In comparison with the whole studied HL group, patients with the m.3243A>G mutation had similar age, gender, degree of HL, and frequency of symptoms or other dysfunctions of the inner ear. The major features of the subgroup positive for m.3243A>G were maternal inheritance in all families (except one) and relatively later onset of HL in the m.3243A>G subgroup (Table 1).

The total of 34 identified individuals carrying the m.3243A>G mutation included 16 probands and 18 of their relatives detected at the second step by molecular investigation. Presence of the m.3243A>G mutation was not previously tested nor suspected in any of these cases.

The study group consisted of 29 patients with m.3243A>G HL (16 probands and 13 relatives). Five m.3243A>G relatives (children and young females) without hearing problems, but testing positively for the m.3243A>G mutation, were analysed separately.

Over the course of 10 years of observations, 17 of 29 HL patients developed multi-system mitochondriopathy while 12 remained oligosymptomatic. Clinical characteristics of the studied patients are shown in Table 3.

According to the clinical status, the m.3243A>G carriers were divided into three subgroups:

I. Multi-symptomatic subgroup (17 patients)
II. Isolated hearing loss subgroup (12 patients)
III. Asymptomatic subgroup (5 individuals).

Audiological assessment

Bilateral sensorineural hearing loss was the first presentation of the disease in all m.3243A>G patients (Figure 1). The mean age of onset of hearing impairment was 26 years: 18 years for men and 28 years for women (Table 4). HL started earlier in the multi-symptomatic subgroup (21 years) than in the isolated HL subgroup (32 years).

Progression of the HL was observed in 14 out of 29 (48%) patients: in 10 women and 4 men (Table 3). The proportion of patients with a progressive course of HL was similar in both multi-symptomatic and isolated HL subgroups (Table 5).

Hearing deterioration was triggered by stressful situations (6 times), medications (aminoglycosides, 4 times), noise (2 times), or other major events such as acute pancreatitis or pregnancy (Table 3) with similar frequency in both the multi-symptomatic and isolated HL subgroups.

The majority of audiograms showed a pantonal shape with high frequencies more severely affected (Figures 1, 2, and 3). BEAP did not show retro-cochlear pathology in any case and always confirmed audiometric hearing thresholds. Otoacoustic emissions were absent in all HL patients. Type A tympanograms and stapedial reflexes were registered in all ears (excluding severe and profound HL).

Heteroplasmy study

The levels of heteroplasmy in the whole m.3243A>G group decreased in the following order: urine, hair, buccal mucosa, nails, and blood (Table 4). The mean level of heteroplasmy detected in urine (57.6%) was significantly higher ($p<10^{-6}$) than in any other tested tissue, whereas blood heteroplasmy levels were significantly lower compared to other tissues ($p<0.002$, Table 4). Notably, the most pronounced mean difference (44.1%) was found in a comparison between urine and blood ($p<10^{-7}$). Analysis of heteroplasmy levels among other tissues did not reveal significant differences (data not shown). Mean heteroplasmy load was relatively higher in the multi-systemic subgroup than in the isolated HL and asymptomatic subgroups (Table 4), but the differences were relatively small. The patients from the isolated HL and the asymptomatic subgroups showed low as well as high mtDNA load in all tissues studied (Figure 4).

Table 4. Heteroplasmy levels (% of total tissue DNA) of m.3243A>G mutation in mtDNA samples isolated from: urinary sediment, hair follicles, buccal mucosa, nails and blood (put in order of heteroplasmy intensity).

No of patients in group; mean age	Females /Males	Gender-age of onset (mean age of onset in group)	No of studied samples of urinary sediment; Mean %; (Range %)	No of studied samples of hair follicles; Mean %; (Range %)	No of studied samples of buccal mucosa smear; Mean %; (Range %)	No of studied samples of nails; Mean %; (Range %)	No of studied samples of blood; Mean %; (Range %)
I group (17) 36 yrs	10/7	F–24 yrs; M–16 yrs (21 yrs)	**13**; 67%; (31.4%–96.5%)	**13**; 21.2%; (0%–77.2%)	**11**; 26.1%; (5.6%–60.2%)	**12**; 26.4%; (6.7%–65.2%)	**14**; 14,4%; (5,4%–27,8%)
II group (12) 40 yrs	8/4	F–37 yrs; M–23 yrs (32 yrs)	**11**; 51.5%; (7.6%–85.8%)	**8**; 25.8%; (1.6%–63.7%)	**10**; 21.0%; (1.2%–33.2%)	**9**; 14.2%; (1.8%–24.6%)	**12**; 9,3%; (0%–32,1%)
III group (5) 8 yrs	4/1	NA	**3**; 39.5%; (16.2%–81.3%)	**4**; 44.8%; (20.4%–66.5%)	**5**; 35.9%; (3.8%–100%)	**4**; 34.1%; (16.7%–49.6%)	**5**; 21,1%; (12,8%–32,5%)
Total 34 patients 33 yrs	22/12	F–28 yrs; M–18 yrs (26 yrs)	**27**; 57.6%; (7.6%–96.5%)	**26**; 26.5% (0%–77.2%)	**26**; 26.0%; (1.2%–100%)	**25**; 23.2%; (1.8%–65.2%)	**31**; 13,5%; (0%–32,5%)

F = female, M = male, yrs = years, NA = not applicable.
The subgroups of patients: I – multi-organ presentation, II - isolated hearing loss and III - asymptomatic are presented separately.

Table 5. Comparison of clinical status among all groups of patients (I, II and III) carrying m.3423A>G mutation: I = Multi-symptomatic subgroup, II = Isolated HL subgroup, III = Asymptomatic subgroup.

No of patients in groups	Mild degree of HL	Moderate degree of HL	Severe degree of HL	Profound degree of HL	Progression of HL	Mean value of NMDAS score (parts 1–3)	Normal value/ Examined (GC-MS)	LA/MGCA (GC-MS)	0 = no brain LA (MRS)	1 = uncertain brain LA (MRS)	2 = positive brain LA (MRS)	3 = strong brain LA (MRS)	Brain MRI alterations /Examined	Heteroplasmy level in urine (%)	Heteroplasmy level in blood (%)
I (17)	3	7	4	3	53% 9/17	39*	5/10	2/4	0	2	5	1	8/8	67	14
II (12)	5	4	2	1	42% 5/12	10**	7/8	0/1	2	6	0	0	4/8	51	9
III (5)	NA	NA	NA	NA	NA	8***	3/5	1/1	1	2	0	0	1/3	40	31
AL (34)	8	11	6	4	14/29		15/23	3/6	3	10	5	1	13/19	53	18

*2 patients had only part 2 assessed.
**11/12 patients were assessed.
***probably false positive related to high score for quality of life (part 1) of two patients.
HL = hearing loss; NMDAS = Newcastle Mitochondrial Disease Adult Scale; MRS = magnetic resonance spectroscopy,
LA = lactic acidosis, MGCA = 3-methylglutaconic aciduria, MRI = magnetic resonance imaging; NA = not applicable.
GC-MS = Gas Chromatography–Mass Spectroscopy.
Degree of HL: mild HL<40 dB; moderate 41–70 dB; severe 71–90 dB; profound >91 dB.

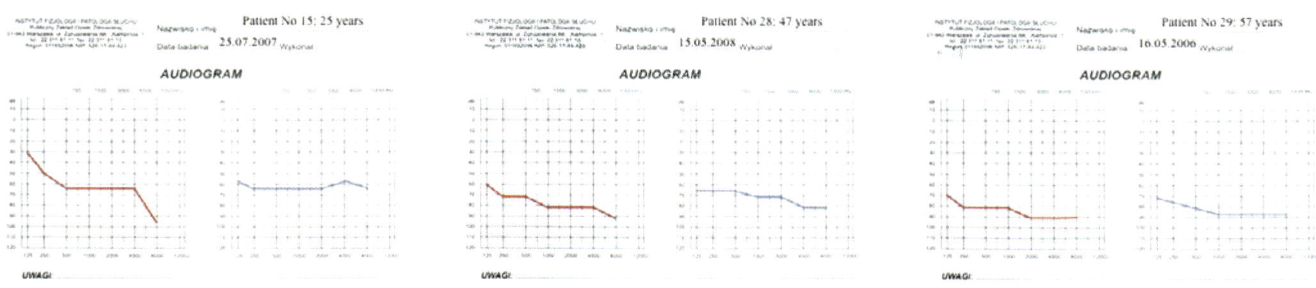

Figure 2. Subsequent audiograms of the patients presented in Fig. 1. Patient 15 has developed multisystem disorder; patients 28 and 29 have remained oligosymptomatic. Hearing loss has not progressed in patient 28.

After adjustment for age we detected a relatively weak correlation between total disease score and heteroplasmy level in urine ($p = 0.034$) or nails ($p = 0.015$), but the distribution of m.3243A>G mutation load among tissues and individuals did not allow clinically useful prediction of disease severity. There was no relation between kidney disease in the patients 9 and 16 (Table 3) and level of urine heteroplasmy [30].

Brain imaging and lactates

Magnetic resonance imaging (MRI) was abnormal in 13 of 19 examined patients (Table 5). The most frequent changes were cerebellar atrophy and increased mineralisation of the globus pallidus. Chronic and/or acute stroke-like changes were seen in two cases. Cerebral abnormalities were found in MRI, mainly in the multi-symptomatic subgroup (in all examined patients), but also in the four patients from the isolated HL and one patient from the asymptomatic subgroups. Details of the MRI findings are given in Table 3.

Magnetic resonance spectroscopy (MRS) of the brain showed increased lactate signal in 6 out of 19 examined patients (Table 5). The pathology was seen only in the multi-symptomatic subgroup. The lactate signal was absent in three MRS scans, and was uncertain in 10 patients (Table 3). Profiling of urinary organic acids revealed an increased excretion of lactic acid in three patients and/or 3-methylglutaconic acid (3-MGCA) in six patients (Table 3).

Discussion

In this hearing loss-oriented study, we found that about 1% of Polish patients presenting with isolated HL that had begun between the ages of 5 and 40 years harboured the m.3243A>G mutation in their blood DNA. This figure is lower than ~2.4% reported for Japanese HI patients [20,31,32], but similar to that reported in a diabetic Caucasian cohort [33] and 3 times less than the prevalence of m.1555A>G mutation (3.4%) reported for HL patients [34]. A similar hearing loss study was carried out by Majamaa et al. who found m.3243A>G mutation in 2.1% of 250 HL patients by applying pre-selection based on maternal inheritance [16].

The association between isolated HL and m.3243A>G is consistent with the data of Manwaring et al. who studied hair follicle mtDNA in 900 elderly individuals and found six m.3243A>G carriers, all having mild to moderate hearing impairment [35]. Uimonen et al. showed that isolated HL associated with m.3243A>G mutation resembled presbyacusis, but its progression rate was faster [22].

The m.3243A>G HL in our study was not always progressive and remained the only complaint in 42% of patients (Table 3). Mitochondrial etiology of long-standing hearing loss in a 78 year-old woman was established after development of m.3243A>G associated MELAS phenotype in her son. Molecular testing for m.3243A>G mutation was positive in at least four young adults with stable HL which had lasted more than 10 years. Data on the non-progressive course of m.3243A>G induced long-lasting HL is limited. In the key paper of Uimonen et al., the progressive pattern was the most common, with high frequencies affected first [22]. A relationship between HL progression and severity of m.3243A>G phenotype has been found [23]. This suggests that a low progression rate of hearing impairment is a good prognostic marker.

The m.3243A>G positive subgroup differed from the whole study group by having relatively later onset of HL, as well as presenting maternal inheritance of HL in all except one case. However, at the first presentation of HL in m.3243A>G carriers, the risk of developing multisystem disease cannot be predicted.

Analysis of circumstances of hearing deterioration in m.3243A>G mutation revealed various triggering factors, some of which have been suggested previously, such as exposure to aminoglycosides, valproates, noise exposure, or stress [36,37].

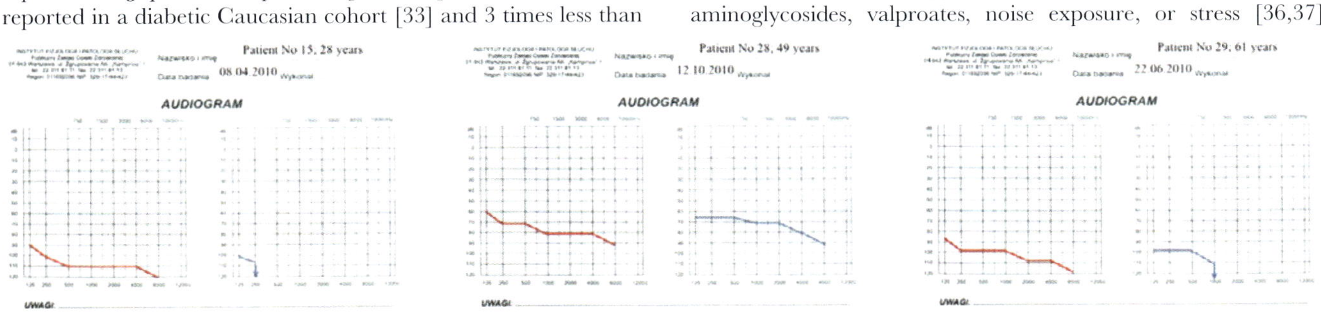

Figure 3. Latest audiograms of the three patients shown in Figs. 1 and 2. Patients 15 and 29 have become cochlear implant users. The HL threshold of patient 28 has still not changed.

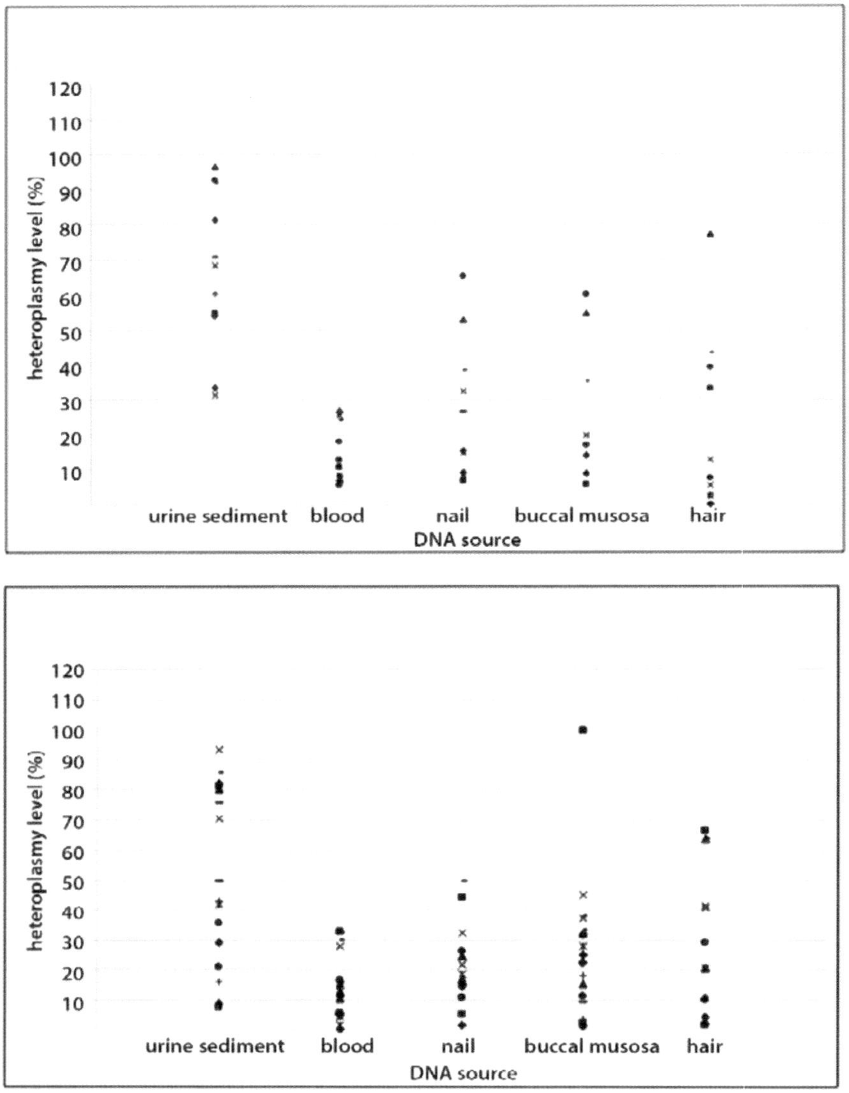

Figure 4. Heteroplasmy level of the m.3243A>G mutation in examined tissues. Above: the scores of patients with multi-symptomatic presentation (subgroup I). Below: the scores of patients with isolated hearing loss and asymptomatic carriers (subgroups II and III together).

Other triggers, such as pregnancy or pancreatitis, have not been convincingly reported in the literature.

In this study the onset of m.3243A>G associated HL was earlier in men than in women (18 and 28 years, respectively). Uimonen et al. found that being male, as well as a high heteroplasmy level of the mutation, may aggravate the severity of hearing impairment in m.3243A>G carriers [22]. More epidemiological data are needed to properly assess a sex influence on the m.3243A>G phenotype.

In our patients the m.3243A>G mutation load was lowest in the DNA derived from archived blood samples compared to other analysed tissues. It has previously been found that the mtDNA mutation load in blood decreases in older patients due to the negative selection of leukocytes carrying impaired mitochondria [38,39]; because of this, significantly better detection of m.3243A>G can be achieved by analysing urine [40], buccal mucosa, or hair [35,36,41,42].

In this study, the heteroplasmy level of m.3243A>G mutation was markedly (2–4 times) higher in DNA derived from urine compared to other tissues. Interestingly, the urinary heteroplasmy of over 30% was found not only in the classical MELAS patients, but also in the oligosymptomatic and even asymptomatic m.3243A>G persons.

Our results are consistent with those of Whittaker et al. who showed that urine is the most suitable material for detection of the m.3243A>G mutation. The authors concluded that the screening of urine for m.3243A>G mutation load is a better predictor of outcome than the gold standard of skeletal muscle [40].

Short stature [43], abnormal excretion of 3-MGCA in urine [44,45], and elevation of lactates in the brain MRS, which were seen in our oligo- and asymptomatic m.3243A>G carriers, may be helpful in identifying affected individuals, but these are not sensitive tests either.

Summarizing

People with postlingual isolated HL require testing for m.3243A>G mutation. Early detection of patients with mitochondrial isolated HL and identification of mutation-carrying healthy relatives would improve proper prophylactic management – i.e. avoidance of harmful environmental factors (noise and stress) and certain medications (aminoglicosides and valproate). New therapies may become available in the near future. Urinary sediment – not blood – is the material of choice for assessing the mtDNA mutation load in people with isolated hearing loss. The possible prognostic value of high and low levels of mtDNA heteroplasmy in urine sediment needs further study.

Author Contributions

Conceived and designed the experiments: KIP AP. Performed the experiments: KIP AP UL MP AS LK MF MR. Analyzed the data: KIP AP RP. Contributed reagents/materials/analysis tools: AP UL RP. Wrote the paper: KIP. Designed a study group: KIP AP UL. Assessment of GCMS: MP. Assessment of MRS: MF. Neurological examination: MR. Clinical genetics assessment: AS LK. Clinical assessment of the patients: KIP. Statistical analysis: RP. Support of the team: HS (Head of the Institution).

References

1. Michaelides M, Jenkins SA, Bamiou DE, Sweeney MG, Davis MB, et al. (2008) Macular dystrophy associated with the A3243G, mitochondrial DNA mutation: distinct retinal and associated features, disease variability, and characterization of asymptomatic family members. Arch Ophthalmol 126: 320–28.
2. Deschauer M, Muller T, Wieser T, Schulte-Mattler W, Kornhuber M, et al. (2001) Hearing impairment is common in various phenotypes of mitochondrial DNA A3243G mutation. Arch Neurol 58: 1885–8.
3. Damian MS, Siebel P, Reichmann H (1995) Clinical spectrum of the MELAS mutation. Acta Neurol Scand 92: 409–15.
4. Mosewich RK, Donat R, DiMauro S (1993) The syndrome of mitochondrial encephalopathy, lactic acidosis, and stroke-like episodes presenting without stroke. Arch Neurol 50: 275–8.
5. Pavlakis SG, Phillips PC, DiMauro S, De Vivo DC, Rowland LP (1984) Mitochondrial myopathy, encephalopathy, lactic acidosis, and stroke like episodes: a distinctive clinical syndrome. Ann Neurol 16: 481–8.
6. Goto Y, Nonaka I, Horai S (1990) A mutation in the tRNA leu (UUR) gene associated with the MELAS subgroup of mitochondrial encephalopaties. Nature 348: 651–3.
7. Chinnery PF, Howell N, Lightowlers RN, Turnbull DM (1997) Molecular pathology of MELAS and MERRF. The relationship between mutation load and clinical phenotypes. Brain 120: 1713–21.
8. Narbonne H, Paquis-Fluckinger V, Valero R, Heyries L, Pellissier JF, et al. (2004) Gastrointestinal tract symptoms in maternally inherited diabetes and deafness (MIDD). Diabetes Metab 30: 61–66.
9. van den Ouweland JM, Lemkes HH, Ruitenbeek W, Sandkuijl LA, de Vijlder MF, et al. (1992) Mutation in mitochondrial tRNA(Leu) (UUR) gene in a large pedigree with maternally transmitted type II diabetes mellitus and deafness. Nat Genet 1: 368–71.
10. Chinnery PF, Griffiths TS (2006) Mitochondrial otology. In: DiMauro S., Hirano M., Schon EA. Mitochondrial Medicine Informa UK Limited, pp.161–77.
11. Sawada S, Takeda T, Kakigi A, Saito H, Suehiro T, et al. (1997) Audiological findings of sensorineural deafness associated with a mutation in the mitochondrial DNA. Am J Otol 18: 332–5.
12. Nadol JB, Merchant SN (2001) Histopathology and molecular genetics of hearing loss in the human. Int J Pediatr Otorhinolaryngol 61: 1–15.
13. Uusimaa J, Moilanen JS, Vainionpaa L, Tapanainen P, Lindholm P, et al. (2007) Prevalence, segregation, and phenotype of the mitochondrial DNA 3243A>G mutation in children. Ann Neurol 62: 278–87.
14. Merchant SN (2010) Genetically determined and other developmental defects. In: Schuknecht's Pathology of the Ear, 3th Edition PMPH-USA, 209 pp.
15. Schaefer A, Taylor R, Turnbull DM, Chinnery PF (2004) The epidemiology of mitochondrial disorders - past, present and future. Bioch Biophys Acta 1659: 115–20.
16. Majamaa K, Moilanen J, Uimonen S, Remes A, Salmela P, et al. (1998) Epidemiology of A3243G, the mutation for mitochondrial encephalomyopathy, lactic acidosis, and stroke like episodes: prevalence of the mutation in an adult population. Am J Hum Genet 63: 447–54.
17. Elliot HR, Samuels DC, Eden JA, Relton CL, Chinnery PF (2008) Pathogenic mitochondrial DNA mutations are common in the general population. Am J Hum Genet 8: 254–60.
18. Chinnery PF, Wardell TM, Singh-Kler R, Hayes C, Brown DT, et al. (2000) The epidemiology of pathogenic mitochondrial DNA mutation. Ann Neurol 48: 188–93.
19. Leveque M, Marlin S, Jonard L, Procaccio V, Reynier P, et al. (2007) Whole mitochondrial genome screening in maternally inherited non-syndromic hearing impairment using a microarray resequencing mitochondrial DNA chip. Eur J Hum Genet 15: 1145–55.
20. Kato T, Nishigaki Y, Noguchi Y, Ueno H, Hosoya H, et al. (2010) Extensive and rapid screening for major mitochondrial DNA point mutations in patients with hereditary hearing loss. J Hum Genet 55: 147–54.
21. Sue CM, Quigley A, Katsabanis S, Kapsa R, Crimmins DS, et al. (1998) Detection of MELAS A3243G point mutation in muscle, blood and hair follicle. J Neurol Sci 161: 36–39.
22. Uimonen S, Moilanen JS, Sorri M, Hassinen IE, Majamaa KS (2001) Hearing impairment in patients with 3243A>G mtDNA mutation: phenotype and rate of progression Hum Genet 108: 284–9.
23. Majamaa-Voltti KA, Winqvist S, Remes AM, Tolonen U, Pyhtinen, et al. (2006) A 3-year clinical follow-up of adult patients with 3243 A>G in mitochondrial DNA Neurology 66: 1470–75.
24. Kokotas H, Petersem MB, Willems PJ (2007) Mitochondrial deafness Clin Genet 71: 379–91
25. Guan M-X (2011) Mitochondrial 12S rRNA mutations associated with aminoglycoside ototoxicity. Mitochondrion 11: 237–45.
26. Rydzanicz M, Cywińska K, Wróbel M, Pollak A, Gawęcki W, et al. (2011) The contribution of the mitochondrial COI/tRNA(Ser(UCN)) gene mutations to non-syndromic and aminoglycoside-induced hearing loss in Polish patients. Mol Genet Metab Sep–Oct;104(1–2):153–9.
27. Pollak A, Mueller-Malesinska M, Skórka A, Kostrzewa G, Ołdak M, et al. (2008) GJB2 and hearing impairment: promoter defects do not explain the excess of monoallelic mutations. J Med Genet 45(9):607–8.
28. Pollak A, Skórka A, Mueller-Malesińska M, Kostrzewa G, Kisiel B, et al. (2007) M34T and V37I mutations in GJB2 associated hearing impairment: evidence for pathogenicity and reduced penetrance. Am J Med Genet A.1;143A(21):2534–43.
29. Schaefer AM, Phoenix C, Elson JL, McFarland R, Chinnery PF, et al. (2006) Mitochondrial disease in adults: A scale to monitor progression and treatment. Neurology 66: 1932–4.
30. Dinour D, Mini S, Polak-Charcon S, Lotan D, Holtzman J (2004) Progressive nephropathy associated with mitochondrial tRNA gene mutation. Clin Nephrol 62: 149–54.
31. Oshima T, Ueda N, Ikeda K, Abe K, Takasaka T (1999) Hearing loss with a mitochondrial gene mutation is highly prevalent in Japan. Laryngoscope 109:334–8.
32. Usami Si, Abe S, Akita J, Namba A, Shinkawa H, et al. (2000) Prevalence of mitochondrial gene mutations among hearing impaired patients. J Med Genet 37:38–40.
33. Malecki M, Klupa T, Wanic K, Frey J, Cyganek K, et al. (2001) Searching for mitochondrial A3243G tRNALeu mutation in Polish patients with type 2 diabetes mellitus. Med Sci Monit 7: 249–50.
34. Rydzanicz M, Wróbel M, Pollak A, Gawecki W, Brauze D, et al. (2010) Mutation analysis of mitochondrial 12S rRNA gene in Polish patients with non-syndromic and aminoglycoside-induced hearing loss. Biochem Biophys Res Commun 395: 116–21.
35. Manwaring N, Jones MM, Wang JJ, Rochtchina E, Howard C, et al. (2007) Population prevalence of the MELAS A3243G mutation. Mitochondrion 7: 230–33.
36. Finsterer J (2007) Genetic, pathogenetic, and phenotypic implications of the mitochondrial A3243G tRNALeu (UUR) mutation. Acta Neurol Scand 116: 1–14.
37. Chinnery PF, Elliott C, Green GR, Rees A, Coulthard A, et al. (2000) The spectrum of hearing loss due to mitochondrial DNA defects. Brain 123: 82–92.
38. Sue CM, Lipsett LJ, Crimmins DS, Tsang C, Boyages SC, et al. (1998) Cochlear origin of sensorineural deafness in MELAS syndrome. Ann Neurol 43: 350–59.
39. Shanske S, Pancrudo J, Kaufmann P, Engelstad K, Jhung S, et al. (2004) Varying loads of the mitochondrial DNA A3243G mutation in different tissues: implication for diagnosis. Am J Med Genet 130: 134–7.
40. Whittaker RG, Blackwood JK, Alston CL, Blakely EL, Elson JL, et al. (2009) Urine heteroplasmy is the best predictor of clinical outcome in the m.3243A>G mtDNA mutation. Neurology 72: 568–9.
41. Manwaring N, Jones MM, Wang JJ, Rochtchina E, Howard C, et al. (2007) Mitochondrial DNA haplogroups and age-related hearing loss. Arch. Otolaryngol. Head Neck Surg 133: 929–33.
42. Narbonne H, Perucca-Lostanlen D, Desnuelle C, Vialettes B, Saunieres A, et al. (2001) Searching for A3243G mitochondrial DNA mutation in buccal mucosa in order to improve the screening of patients with mitochondrial diabetes. Eur J Endocrinol 145: 541–2.
43. Pronicki M, Sykut-Cegielska J, Mierzewska H, Tońska K, Iwanicka K, et al. (2002) Diversity of clinical symptoms in A3243G mitochondrial DNA mutation (MELAS syndrome mutation). Med Sci Monit 8: 767–73.

44. Wortmann SB, Kluijtmans LA, Engelke UF, Wevers RA, Morava E (2010) The 3-methylglutaconic acidurias: what's new? J Inherit Metab Dis on line DOI 10.1007/s10545-010-9210-7.

45. Karkucinska-Wieckowska A, Lebiedzinska M, Jurkiewicz E, Pajdowska M, Trubicka J, et al. (2011) Increased reactive oxygen species (ROS) production and low catalase level in fibroblasts of a girl with MEGDEL association (Leigh syndrome, deafness, 3-methylglutaconic aciduria). Folia Neuropathol 49: 56–63.

5

Mechanisms of Hearing Loss in Neurofibromatosis Type 2

Ashok R. Asthagiri[1]*, Raul A. Vasquez[1,2], John A. Butman[3], Tianxia Wu[4], Keaton Morgan[1], Carmen C. Brewer[5], Kelly King[5], Chris Zalewski[5], H. Jeffrey Kim[6], Russell R. Lonser[1]

1 Surgical Neurology Branch, National Institute of Neurological Disorders and Stroke, National Institutes of Health, Bethesda, Maryland, United States of America, **2** Department of Neurological Surgery, University of Florida, Gainesville, Gainesville, Florida, United States of America, **3** Radiology and Imaging Sciences, The Clinical Center at the National Institutes of Health, National Institutes of Health, Bethesda, Maryland, United States of America, **4** Clinical Neurosciences Program, National Institute of Neurological Disorders and Stroke, National Institutes of Health, Bethesda, Maryland, United States of America, **5** Audiology Unit, Otolaryngology Branch, National Institute on Deafness and Other Communication Disorders, National Institutes of Health, Bethesda, Maryland, United States of America, **6** Office of the Clinical Director, National Institute on Deafness and Other Communication Disorders, National Institutes of Health, Bethesda, Maryland, United States of America

Abstract

Introduction: Patients with neurofibromatosis type 2 (NF2) develop bilateral cochleovestibular schwannomas (CVSs) that cause binaural deafness in most individuals. Hearing loss occurs in an unpredictable manner and the underlying mechanisms are not known. To gain insight into the pathophysiologic basis for hearing loss in NF2, we performed a prospective cross-sectional study of untreated ears in NF2 patients.

Methods: One hundred consecutive NF2 patients in a prospective natural history study were included. Clinical and audiometric data were analyzed for treatment naïve ears. In addition to standard MR-imaging sequences, alterations in intralabyrinthine protein content were determined utilizing high resolution FLAIR, the presence of cochlear aperture obstruction was determined by examining 3D T2 sequences, and endolymphatic hydrops was identified on delayed post-contrast FLAIR sequences.

Results: Eighty-nine ears harboring 84 untreated CVSs in 56 consecutive NF2 patients (age 30±16 years) were analyzed. Thirty-four (38%) ears had varying degrees of hearing loss. Elevated intralabyrinthine protein was identified in 70 (75%) ears by FLAIR MR-imaging and was strongly associated with the presence of hearing loss (32/34 hearing loss ears; 94%)(Fisher's exact test; $P = .005$). Elevated intralabyrinthine protein was associated with the presence of CVS-associated cochlear aperture obstruction (64 of 67 ears with elevated protein; 96%)(Fisher's exact test; $P < 0.0001$) in both normal and hearing loss ears. Elevated intralabyrinthine protein was not identified in ears without CVS (5 ears). While larger tumor size was associated with hearing loss ($P = 0.006$), 16 hearing loss ears (47%) harbored CVSs less than 0.5 cm^3, including 14 ears (88%) with block of the cochlear aperture and elevated protein.

Discussion: These findings are consistent with a model in which hearing loss develops as a result of cochlear aperture obstruction and accumulation of intralabyrinthine protein. MRI based identification of elevated intralabyrinthine protein may help identify the ear at-risk for developing hearing loss.

Editor: Mike Chen, City of Hope, United States of America

Funding: This research was supported by the Intramural Research Program of the National Institute of Neurologic Disorders and Stroke, National Institute on Deafness and Other Communication Disorders and the Clinical Center at the National Institutes of Health. The funders had no role in study design, data collection and analysis, decision to publish, or preparation of the manuscript.

Competing Interests: The authors have declared that no competing interests exist.

* E-mail: asthagiria@ninds.nih.gov

Introduction

Neurofibromatosis type 2 (NF2) is an autosomal dominant heritable neoplasia syndrome. It results from a germline mutation of the *NF2* tumor suppressor gene located on the long arm of chromosome 22 [1]. NF2 has an incidence of 1 in 25,000 persons and a penetrance of nearly 100% by age 60 years [2,3]. While the clinical manifestations of NF2 include central and peripheral nervous system tumors (nerve sheath tumors, meningiomas and ependymomas), cutaneous lesions, ocular pathology and peripheral neuropathy [4], the hallmark of NF2 is the development of bilateral cochleovestibular schwannomas (CVSs) [5]. Bilateral CVSs are present in 90 to 95% of NF2 patients [5]. Although CVSs are benign tumors, they cause significant audiovestibular morbidity, including deafness. While binaural hearing loss occurs in nearly all NF2 patients, its course remains unpredictable and therefore management paradigms have remained inconsistent.

Despite the significant audiologic morbidity identified in patients with NF2, the mechanisms by which the CVS causes hearing loss are not understood. The most frequently cited hypothesis is the enlarging CVS causes hearing loss through direct compression and stretching of the cochlear nerve. Several phenomena, including the unpredictable onset of hearing loss, frequent association of hearing loss with small tumors and progressive hearing loss in patients with non-growing CVS specifically suggest that such a simple association between tumor size and/or growth rate with hearing loss does not exist [6,7,8,9]. Further, in addition to gradual hearing loss, progression of hearing loss may be stepwise, relapsing and remitting, or sudden. These variable patterns of hearing loss suggest that additional mechanisms of hearing loss such as intralabyrinthine hemorrhage, development of endolymphatic hydrops, disruption of cochlear vascular supply and alteration in the biochemical milieu of inner ear fluids that result in cochlear hair cell degeneration and dysfunction may play a more critical role in the pathophysiology of hearing loss in patients with NF2. Because of the incomplete understanding of the pathophysiologic mechanisms underlying onset and variable progression of hearing loss in NF2 (even between ears in the same patient), the optimal management of CVSs in NF2 has not been determined. To identify markers for hearing loss and underlying pathophysiological mechanisms, we prospectively analyzed the clinical, imaging, and audiologic findings in a large cohort of NF2 patients.

Methods

Patients

Patients enrolled in a National Institute of Neurological Disorders and Stroke (NINDS) institutional review board (IRB)-approved prospective NF2 natural history study (NIH#08-N-0044) were included. Informed written consent was obtained from all adult participants. Informed written consent from the next of kin, carers or guardians on behalf of minors participating in this study was obtained. Both written consent and assent forms were approved for the consenting procedure by the NINDS IRB. Treatment naïve ears with no evidence of conductive hearing loss were used for analysis. Patients had NF2 diagnosed by clinical and/or genetic criteria [10].

Patient Evaluation

Clinical and audiologic evaluation. Detailed histories were obtained and comprehensive otologic and neurologic examinations were conducted in all patients to exclude the presence of middle ear disease. Concurrent audiometric evaluations were performed that included air- and bone- conduction thresholds from 250–8000 Hz and 250–4000 Hz, respectively. Hearing was stratified utilizing the four frequency pure-tone average (PTA) as normal [PTA≤20 dB], mild hearing loss [PTA 21–40 dB], moderate [PTA 41–70 dB], severe [PTA 71–95 dB], or profound [PTA>95 dB] [11]. _ Ears with a conductive hearing loss component (>10 dB difference between the air and bone PTA) were excluded from the study. For statistical analysis, hearing status was simplified to a binary score based on the presence (mild, moderate, severe, profound) or absence (normal) of hearing loss.

Imaging evaluation. Patients underwent magnetic resonance (MR)-imaging with and without contrast (T1 weighted) of the craniospinal axis. A neuroradiologist, blind to the hearing status of individual patients and ears, interpreted all imaging findings. Inner ear MR-imaging was performed with less than 1 mm in plane resolution utilizing a 3T-MR-scanner (Phillips; Andover, MA). Non-contrast enhanced fluid attenuated inversion recovery (FLAIR) sequences were performed to assess for the presence of elevated protein within the inner ear. Because saline-based solutions become hyperintense relative to brain parenchyma at defined protein concentration thresholds, identification of elevated intralabyrinthine protein by pre-contrast FLAIR MR-imaging is dependable and was reported as either being "elevated" or "normal" [12]. Co-registered T2-VISTA MR-images were performed to assess for the presence of cochlear aperture obstruction, as defined by the absence of a patent cerebrospinal fluid (CSF) pathway between the posterior fossa and the cochlear aperture (cochlear nerve entry point into the osseous spiral ligament). The presence or absence of intralabyrinthine hemorrhage was assessed on precontrast T1-weighted MR-images [13]. To assess for endolymphatic hydrops, delayed FLAIR and matching T2-weighted images were obtained in a plane parallel to that of the horizontal semicircular canal 6 to 18 hours after contrast injection MR-imaging [14,15]. On the delayed FLAIR, marked distension of the scala media (normally not visible) due to the differential elimination of contrast from the endolymphatic compartment relative to the retention of contrast material within the perilymph was noted as direct visualization of endolymphatic hydrops.

Volume of the CVS was determined utilizing post-contrast T1-weighted images [16] and the following formula: volume = maximum anteroposterior dimension X maximal mediolateral dimension X maximum craniocaudal dimension / 2) [17]. Volumetric measurements for CVSs were divided into posterior fossa and canalicular components if portions of the tumor [16] were present in both anatomic areas. The multilobulated posterior fossa component of tumors was further divided into individual compartments to improve accuracy of volumetric measurement (compartmental volume determined by equation defined above). Total CVS volume was determined by summing the volumes of the individual compartments. Identification of small discrete intralabyrinthine tumors by post-contrast images was confirmed by the presence of a negative outline on T2 VISTA sequences in co-registered images.

Statistical Analysis

Statistical analyses were performed as defined in text. A P-value less than or equal to 0.05 was considered significant.

Results

Patient Characteristics

Of 100 consecutive patients (200 ears) enrolled into the NF2 natural history study, ears that underwent surgery (84 ears in 58 patients) and/or received radiation therapy (26 ears in 20 patients) for management of cochleovestibular schwannomas were excluded from this study. Additionally, 5 patients (10 ears) receiving chemotherapeutics at the time of this study and 1 patient (2 ears) unable to complete audiometric examination (English second language) were also excluded from evaluation. Three ears with mild hearing loss were also excluded from analysis due to the presence of a conductive hearing loss component by otologic and audiologic evaluation. Therefore, 89 treatment naïve ears (43 right, 46 left) in 56 consecutive patients (17 male, 39 female) were included. In 23 patients (41%), one ear met criteria for inclusion and in 33 patients (59%) both ears met inclusion criteria. MR-imaging evidence of CVS was present in 84 of the 89 ears; 5 ears had no MR-imaging evidence of CVS. Mean patient age at evaluation was 30±16 years (range, 8 to 68 years). Forty-nine patients (88%) had audiovestibular symptoms associated with a CVS (Table 1). Mean age at onset of any disease related symptom was 21.7±14.5 years (range, 0.3 to 57 years).

Audiologic Findings

Fifty-five ears (62% of all evaluated ears) had normal hearing (PTA≤20 dB), including 5 (6%) ears without a CVS. Thirty-four ears (38%) had associated hearing loss (mild, 14 ears, 16%; moderate, 12 ears, 13%; severe, 4 ears, 4%; profound, 4 ears, 4%). Mean PTA was 54±29 dB (range, 22.5 to 118.75 dB) in the ears with associated hearing loss. Hearing loss occurred gradually over

Table 1. Audiovestibular and MR-imaging findings in the 56 study patients (89 ears).

Findings	Number of patients/ears (%)*		
None	7 patients (12.5%)		
Hearing loss	34 ears (38.2%)		
Tinnitus	48 ears (53.9%)		
Vertigo	8 patients (14.2%)		
Aural fullness	9 ears (10.1%)		
MR-imaging characteristic	**Normal Hearing ears**	**Hearing Loss ears**	**Total (n = 89)**
Elevated protein	35	32	67 (75%)
Cochlear aperture block	36	31	67 (75%)
Intralabyrinthine tumor	5	8	13 (14.6%)
Discrete	*2*	*3*	*5 (5.6%)*
Direct invasion	*3*	*5*	*8 (9.0%)*
Endolymphatic hydrops	4	3	7 (7.9%)
Intralabyrinthine hemorrhage	0	0	0
Brainstem stroke	0	0	0

*Specific to the ear analyzed in the current study.

months to years (12 ears; 35% of ears with hearing loss), in a stepwise manner characterized by periodic decrements in hearing associated with intervening periods of stable hearing (10; 29%), in a relapsing-remitting pattern defined by periodic decrements in hearing coupled with partial recovery of hearing during intervening periods (4; 12%), or in a sudden and complete fashion (sudden profound sensorineural hearing loss) (5; 15%). Subjective hearing loss was not reported in 3 ears (9%) in 3 patients with audiometric evidence of mild hearing loss.

Imaging Correlates in Hearing Loss Ears

Imaging and audiologic findings. Radiographic and audiologic analysis in the 34 hearing loss ears revealed that 32 ears (94% of ears with hearing loss) had elevated intralabyrinthine protein on FLAIR MR-imaging (Figure 1). The 2 hearing loss ears without elevated intralabyrinthine protein had auditory brainstem responses that suggested central nervous system dysfunction or were associated with a large CVS (greater than 2.5 cm^3). Other imaging findings and audiovestibular symptoms in the 56 study patients (89 ears) are detailed in Table 1.

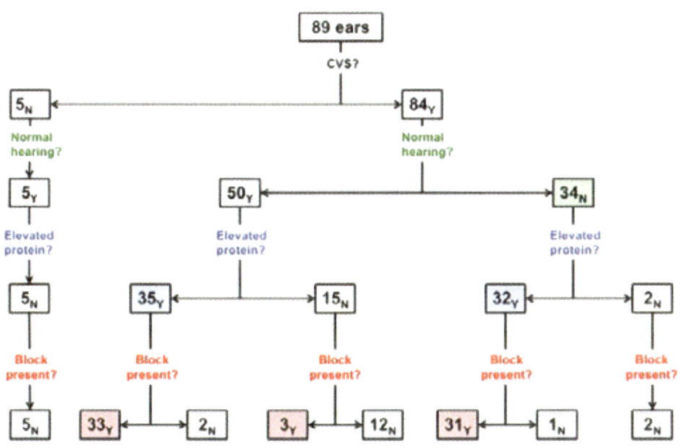

Figure 1. Features of normal hearing and hearing loss ears.

Mechanism of elevated intralabyrinthine protein. Cochlear aperture obstruction by a CVS was closely associated with identification of elevated intralabyrinthine protein in hearing loss ears (Fisher's exact test; $P = 0.005$). While 31 hearing loss ears (91%) with elevated protein in the labyrinth had cochlear aperture obstruction by a CVS, only 1 ear (3%) with elevated intralabyrinthine protein did not have evidence of cochlear aperture obstruction (Figure 1, 2). Ears with hearing loss without elevated intralabyrinthine protein (2 ears, 6%) did not demonstrate cochlear aperture obstruction.

Twenty-three ears (out of 31 hearing loss ears with elevated protein and cochlear aperture obstruction; 74%) had isolated cochlear aperture obstruction and 8 (26%) had cochlear aperture obstruction associated with either a discrete intralabyrinthine tumor (3 ears) (Figure 2) or direct invasion of the labyrinth by a CVS (5 ears). Three ears with elevated intralabyrinthine protein, cochlear aperture obstruction and discrete intralabyrinthine tumors (1 ear) or direct invasion of the labyrinth by a CVS (2 ears) also had endolymphatic hydrops based on MRI findings.

Imaging Correlates in Normal Hearing Ears

Imaging findings. Fifty normal hearing ears (91%) harbored a CVS and 5 ears (9%) did not have an associated CVS. Radiographic and audiologic analysis of the 50 normal hearing ears with a CVS demonstrated elevated intralabyrinthine protein in 35 ears (70% of all normal hearing ears with a CVS) and normal intralabyrinthine protein in 15 ears (30%) on FLAIR MR-imaging. The 5 normal hearing ears without CVS did not have evidence of elevated intralabyrinthine protein (Figure 1).

Mechanism of elevated intralabyrinthine protein. Similar to hearing loss ears, cochlear aperture obstruction by a CVS was associated with elevated intralabyrinthine protein in normal hearing ears (Fisher's exact test; $P < 0.0001$). While 33 normal hearing ears (94% of normal hearing ears with elevated intralabyrinthine protein) with elevated intralabyrinthine protein had cochlear aperture obstruction by a CVS, only 2 ears (6%) with elevated intralabyrinthine protein did not have evidence of cochlear aperture obstruction.

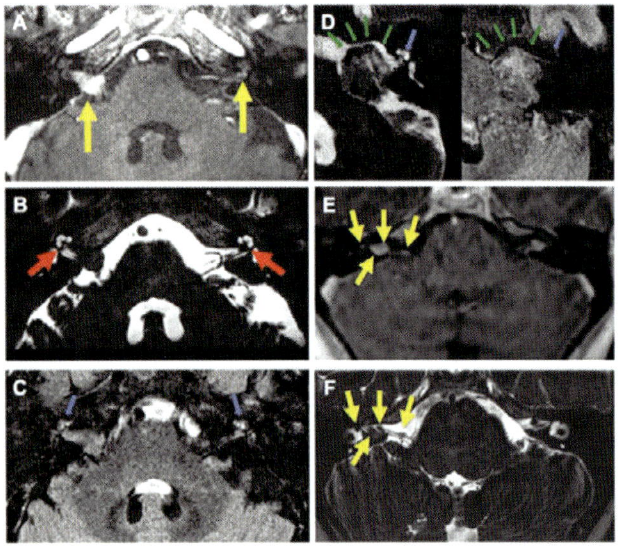

Figure 2. Magnetic resonance imaging in patients with neurofibromatosis type 2. Magnetic resonance (MR) imaging performed in a 47-year old patient with neurofibromatosis type 2 (NF2): (A) Axial, contrast enhanced, T1-weighted, magnetic resonance imaging demonstrates bilateral cochleovestibular schwannomas (CVS) (yellow arrows). (B) T2-VISTA sequence identifies the presence of a cerebrospinal fluid obstruction between the posterior fossa and the cochlear aperture (red arrows) bilaterally, independent of tumor size. (C) Pre-contrast fluid attenuated inversion recovery (FLAIR) sequence demonstrates the presence of elevated protein within the labyrinth (blue arrows). MR-imaging performed in a 48-year old patient with NF2: (D) Axial T2-VISTA and pre-contrast FLAIR sequences demonstrate the presence of normal labyrinthine protein (blue arrow) in the setting of a large CVS with an open CSF pathway (green arrows) between the posterior fossa and the cochlear aperture. MR-imaging performed in a 8-year old patient with NF2. (E) Axial, contrast enhanced, T1-weighted, magnetic resonance imaging demonstrates bilateral cochleovestibular schwannomas (CVS) with multiple tumors present on the right (yellow arrows). (F) T2-VISTA sequence identifies 4 discrete tumors, including a discrete intralabyrinthine tumor (yellow arrows).

Specific factors associated with elevated intralabyrinthine protein included isolated cochlear aperture obstruction by CVS (28 ears; 80%), cochlear aperture obstruction with direct labyrinthine invasion by CVS (3 ears; 9%), cochlear aperture obstruction with a discrete intralabyrinthine tumor (2 ears; 6%) or unknown mechanism (2 ears, 6%). Endolymphatic hydrops was also detected by MR-imaging in 3 normal hearing ears with elevated protein and block of the cochlear aperture.

Twelve normal hearing ears harboring a CVS (80% of all normal hearing ears without elevated labyrinthine protein) without elevated intralabyrinthine protein did not have block of the cochlear aperture, including 1 ear (8%) with associated hydrops. Three normal hearing ears (20%) had evidence of cochlear aperture block by CVS without elevated protein.

Tumor Volume and Hearing Loss

CVSs were identified in 84 ears (94%) and were purely intracanalicular in 38 ears (45%). Mean tumor volume (in 84 ears) was 1.8±4.0 cm^3 (approximately 1.5 cm in maximum linear dimension). While the presence of hearing loss was correlated with larger CVS volume in hearing loss ears (mean volume in normal hearing ears, 1.2±3.4 cm^3 versus hearing-loss ears, 2.5±4.6 cm^3)(Mann-Whitney; $P = 0.007$), 16 (47%) hearing loss ears had a CVS that was less than approximately 0.5 cm^3

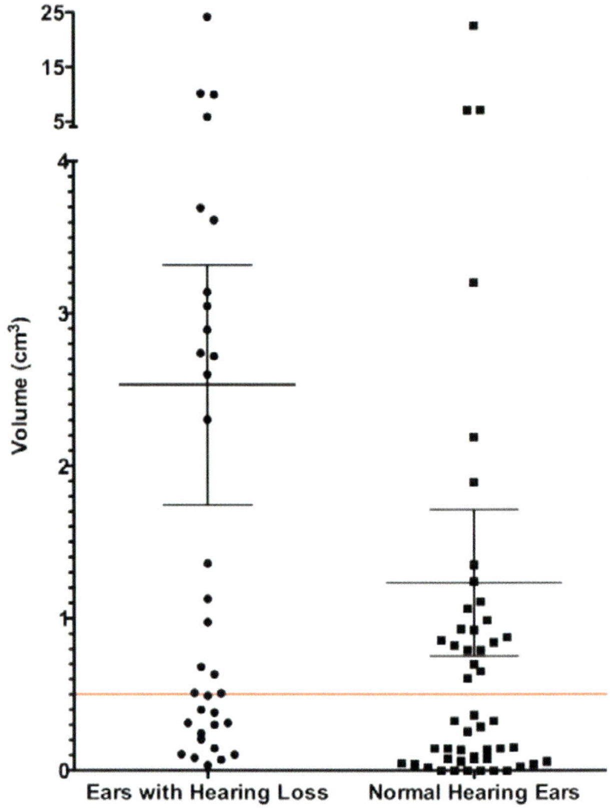

Figure 3. Graph demonstrating volume of tumors identified in ears with and without evidence of hearing loss.

(Figure 3). Among 38 ears with a purely intracanalicular CVS, hearing loss was evident in 12 ears (32%) with a mean volume of 0.2±0.2 cm^3 (range, 0.03 cm^3 to 0.7 cm^3).

Discussion

NF2-Associated Hearing Loss

Previous studies have demonstrated that CVS-associated binaural hearing loss will occur in an unpredictable manner over the lifetime of most NF2 patients [6,7,8]. Moreover, hearing loss patterns in one ear do not predict the clinical course of the contralateral ear in the same individual with NF2 [7]. Because of the uncertain clinical course associated with CVSs and because of the lack of understanding of the mechanisms that underlie hearing loss associated with CVSs in NF2, the management of these tumors has not been consistent or optimized. Here, we examined radiographic and audiometric findings associated with hearing loss in NF2 to better understand the pathophysiologic mechanisms underlying onset and progression of hearing loss in this hereditary neoplastic disorder.

Current Study

Elevated intralabyrinthine protein. The most common imaging findings identified in CVS-associated hearing loss in NF2 was the presence of elevated intralabyrinthine perilymphatic protein and the presence of cochlear aperture obstruction on MR-imaging. Elevated intralabyrinthine protein was found in 94% of hearing loss ears (32 of 34 ears) and in 70% of normal hearing ears (35 of 50 ears). Blockage of the cochlear aperture by an associated CVS was found in 96% of ears (64 of 67 ears) with elevated protein and only in 14% of ears (3 of 22 ears) without evidence of elevated intralabrynthine protein. These findings are consistent with the findings by Silverstein and colleagues [18] that demonstrated that a 2.5-fold increase in intralabyrinthine protein obtained from perilymph aspirates could accurately identify the presence of CVSs in patients in the era before MR-imaging was available for non-invasive diagnosis.

The importance that elevated intralabyrinthine protein plays in hearing loss is underscored by previous clinical-imaging studies of the inner ear in other conditions, including sporadic vestibular schwannomas and sudden sensorineural hearing loss (SNHL) [19,20]. Recent findings indicate that increased protein within the perilymph visualized on FLAIR MR-imaging can be correlated with hearing loss associated with sporadic acoustic schwannomas [20]. Elevated intralabyrinthine protein on FLAIR MR-imaging in patients with SNHL has also been correlated with hearing prognosis and extent of hearing loss that will persist [19].

Mechanisms of intralabyrinthine protein elevation. The findings of the current study indicate that cochlear aperture block underlies elevation of intralabyrinthine protein. The sensitivity and specificity of cochlear aperture obstruction in identifying elevated perilymphatic protein within the labyrinth was 96% and 87%, respectively. This indicates a pathophysiologic association between cochlear aperture obstruction and the presence of elevated intralabyrinthine protein may exist in NF2-associated CVSs. Based on the results from this study and previous studies examining elevated intralabyrinthine protein in other hearing loss syndromes, NF2-associated tumors may lead to elevated intralabyrinthine protein levels in several ways related to cochlear aperture obstruction that causes abnormal protein clearance and deposition.

Elevated intralabyrinthine protein could be the result of cochlear aperture obstruction and disruption of the blood-CSF/labyrinthine barrier caused by permeable tumor vessels [20]. CVSs cause increased protein content within the circulating cerebrospinal fluid compartment due to permeable tumor vessels, and this may be further concentrated in the lateral internal auditory canal in cases where CSF is trapped due to cochlear aperture obstruction [21,22]. Concentrated proteins can rapidly diffuse into the perilymphatic space across the porous canaliculi located within the modiolar region of the osseous spiral lamina [23]. Previous studies have shown gadolinium accumulation in the perilymphatic compartment within 10 minutes after intravenous administration in ears with CVS compared to contralateral unaffected ears, supporting the presence of a breach in the blood-CSF/labyrinthine barrier and rapid diffusion into the perilymphatic spaces in ears with CVSs [20].

Another mechanism by which protein can accumulate within the perilymph associated with cochlear aperture obstruction involves impaired clearance caused by the CVS. It has been shown that the cochlear nerve is integral in the rapid transport of proteins from the cochlea to the cochlear nucleus [24]. Although large CVSs may impact the cochlear nerve through compression within the internal auditory canal disrupting axonal transport, small tumors situated within the cochlear nerve itself may also lead to cochlear aperture obstruction and disruption of axonal transport. Therefore, when CVSs cause obstruction of the cochlear aperture, independent of size, it is likely that this results in impaired cochlear nerve axonal transport that can, in turn, underlie perilymphatic protein accumulation due to impaired clearance [25].

Elevated intralabyrinthine protein could also be the result of increased protein production or deposition. Analogous to cerebellopontine angle CVSs that are known to cause increased protein content within the circulating cerebrospinal fluid compartment [21], increased protein secretion of a plasma ultrafiltrate by permeable tumor vessels of tumors within the labyrinth (both distinct and due to CVS invasion) may permit direct extravasation of plasma proteins into the inner ear perilymph. This process could potentially underlie (in part) the protein elevation and endolymphatic hydrops seen with these tumors. Similarly, increased tumor vessel permeability with leakage of plasma ultrafiltrate and plasma proteins into the surrounding anatomic region has been described in hemangioblastomas and endolymphatic sac tumors in von Hippel-Lindau disease and may underlie peritumoral cyst formation and inner ear hydrops [26].

Mechanisms of hearing loss associated with elevated protein. Elevated intralabyrinthine protein on MR-imaging was closely associated with the presence of hearing loss. The importance of elevated intralabyrinthine protein underlying hearing loss is supported by previous studies examining unique perilymphatic proteins that are elevated in CVSs, including μ-Crystallin (CRYM) and low density lipoprotein-related protein 2 (LRP2) [27]. Mutations of these proteins are associated with genetic syndromes that present with deafness not related to tumors. Further, previous studies have utilized histopathological evaluation to indirectly support biochemical degradation of the cochlea is caused by increased protein [28,29,30,31]. Finally, multiple studies have revealed that hearing loss may progress in the absence of CVS growth [32,33], confirming that an unknown factor underlies hearing loss in these ears. Although causality cannot be directly determined by the intimate association between elevated intralabyrinthine protein and hearing loss observed in our cohort, the high sensitivity of elevated protein in identifying hearing loss ears (94%) and the high negative predictive value of normal protein content in identifying a normal hearing ear (91%) presented in this study coupled with previous studies delineating the functional and degenerative sequelae of unique perilymphatic proteins that are elevated in the setting of vestibular schwannoma indicate that the increased protein content evident by labyrinthine FLAIR MR-signal may not only be an imaging marker of hearing loss, but contribute to the pathophysiology of hearing loss and cochlear degeneration.

Tumor size and hearing loss. A simple association between tumor size and hearing loss does not explain several phenomena. For instance, hearing loss in NF2 has an unpredictable onset and variable progression, which may be gradual, stepwise, relapsing and remitting, or sudden and complete. While previous studies have attempted to link increasing tumor size with hearing loss in patients with NF2, this association has not been established because of the ubiquitous presence of small tumors within all series that are associated with hearing loss. Because hearing loss in NF2 may be caused by end organ degeneration [34] (cochlea) from accumulated protein, the functional consequences of tumor location as it relates to the cochlear aperture appears to play an important role in the pathogenesis of hearing loss. This may also explain why schwannomas of various sizes in other cranial and peripheral nerves are often not associated with neurologic deficit in patients with NF2.

Alternative mechanisms of hearing loss in NF2. Other pathophysiologic processes of the inner ear structures have been implicated with hearing loss, including the development of endolymphatic hydrops and intralabyrinthine hemorrhage [13]. Although endolymphatic hydrops was identified in 7 ears (7.6%) with CVS in this study, the MR-based identification of endolymphatic hydrops did not correlate with hearing status (Table 1). Furthermore, the infrequent identification of endolymphatic hydrops and intralabyrinthine hemorrhage (0 ears), suggests these processes are not a significant underlying mechanism of hearing loss in this patient population.

Bevacizumab induced hearing response. Bevacizumab, initially utilized in NF2 clinical trials for the treatment of growing vestibular schwannomas was associated with hearing improvement in a subset of patients (4/7 patients, 57%) [35]. While this improvement in hearing was initially thought to be due to a reduction in intraneural edema and tumor shrinkage, a subsequent larger scale follow-up study confirmed a lack of correlation between radiographic response (tumor shrinkage) and hearing response, suggesting that a stochastic mechanism underlies the rapid hearing improvement (usually within 3 months) that is observed in approximately 50% of patients [36]. Because vascular endothelial growth factor (VEGF) is a known mediator of vessel permeability, bevacizumab (a VEGF-neutralizing antibody) may be affecting hearing response through restoration of protein homeostasis within the inner ear by decreasing production of protein rich plasma ultrafiltrate from both CPA and intralabyrinthine tumors.

Identification of the at-risk ear. The appropriate stratification of benefit to risk ratio for hearing preservation attempts in NF2 requires delineation of at-risk ears for hearing loss. Because hearing loss is currently the most likely outcome in NF2 ears, it becomes imperative to avoid risk when hearing loss is unlikely to occur. Despite the variable presentation of hearing loss in NF2, most ears with normal perilymphatic protein signal had normal hearing (20/22 ears, 91%) and most ears with hearing loss had elevated perilymphatic protein (35/37 ears, 95%).

Based on the available body of evidence and the current findings that indicate elevated perilymphatic proteins may underlie the final common pathway leading to hearing loss, MR-identification of labyrinthine hyperintensity in normal hearing ears (35 of 50 ears in this study) may serve as a potent imaging biomarker of ears at-risk for developing hearing loss.

Author Contributions

Conceived and designed the experiments: ARA JAB RRL. Performed the experiments: ARA RAV JAB KM CCB KK CZ HJK. Analyzed the data: ARA RAV JAB TW CCB KK CZ HJK RRL. Contributed reagents/materials/analysis tools: ARA JAB TW CCB HJK RRL. Wrote the paper: ARA RAV RRL.

References

1. Trofatter JA, MacCollin MM, Rutter JL, Murrell JR, Duyao MP, et al. (1993) A novel moesin-, ezrin-, radixin-like gene is a candidate for the neurofibromatosis 2 tumor suppressor. Cell 75: 826.
2. Evans DG, Huson SM, Donnai D, Neary W, Blair V, et al. (1992) A genetic study of type 2 neurofibromatosis in the United Kingdom. I. Prevalence, mutation rate, fitness, and confirmation of maternal transmission effect on severity. J Med Genet 29: 841–846.
3. Evans DG, Moran A, King A, Saeed S, Gurusinghe N, et al. (2005) Incidence of vestibular schwannoma and neurofibromatosis 2 in the North West of England over a 10-year period: higher incidence than previously thought. Otol Neurotol 26: 93–97.
4. Asthagiri AR, Parry DM, Butman JA, Kim HJ, Tsilou ET, et al. (2009) Neurofibromatosis type 2. Lancet 373: 1974–1986.
5. Evans DG, Huson SM, Donnai D, Neary W, Blair V, et al. (1992) A clinical study of type 2 neurofibromatosis. Q J Med 84: 603–618.
6. Abaza MM, Makariou E, Armstrong M, Lalwani AK (1996) Growth rate characteristics of acoustic neuromas associated with neurofibromatosis type 2. The Laryngoscope 106: 694–699.
7. Fisher LM, Doherty JK, Lev MH, Slattery WH (2009) Concordance of bilateral vestibular schwannoma growth and hearing changes in neurofibromatosis 2: neurofibromatosis 2 natural history consortium. Otol Neurotol 30: 835–841.
8. Masuda A, Fisher LM, Oppenheimer ML, Iqbal Z, Slattery WH (2004) Hearing changes after diagnosis in neurofibromatosis type 2. Otol Neurotol 25: 150–154.
9. Graamans K, Van Dijk JE, Janssen LW (2003) Hearing deterioration in patients with a non-growing vestibular schwannoma. Acta oto-laryngologica 123: 51–54.
10. Baser ME, Friedman JM, Wallace AJ, Ramsden RT, Joe H, et al. (2002) Evaluation of clinical diagnostic criteria for neurofibromatosis 2. Neurology 59: 1759–1765.
11. King KA, Makishima T, Zalewski CK, Bakalov VK, Griffith AJ, et al. (2007) Analysis of auditory phenotype and karyotype in 200 females with Turner syndrome. Ear and hearing 28: 831–841.
12. Melhem ER, Jara H, Eustace S (1997) Fluid-attenuated inversion recovery MR imaging: identification of protein concentration thresholds for CSF hyperintensity. AJR Am J Roentgenol 169: 859–862.
13. Butman JA, Kim HJ, Baggenstos M, Ammerman JM, Dambrosia J, et al. (2007) Mechanisms of morbid hearing loss associated with tumors of the endolymphatic sac in von Hippel-Lindau disease. JAMA 298: 41–48.
14. Tagaya M, Yamazaki M, Teranishi M, Naganawa S, Yoshida T, et al. (2011) Endolymphatic hydrops and blood-labyrinth barrier in Meniere's disease. Acta Otolaryngol 131: 474–479.
15. Nakashima T, Naganawa S, Teranishi M, Tagaya M, Nakata S, et al. (2010) Endolymphatic hydrops revealed by intravenous gadolinium injection in patients with Meniere's disease. Acta Otolaryngol 130: 338–343.
16. Slattery WH, Lev MH, Fisher LM, Connell SS, Iqbal Z, et al. (2005) MRI evaluation of neurofibromatosis 2 patients: a standardized approach for accuracy in interpretation. Otol Neurotol 26: 733–740.
17. Lundin P, Pedersen F (1992) Volume of pituitary macroadenomas: assessment by MRI. J Comput Assist Tomogr 16: 519–528.
18. Silverstein H (1973) Labyrinthine tap as a diagnostic test for acoustic neurinoma. OTOLARYNGCLINNAMER 6: 229–244.
19. Yoshida T, Sugiura M, Naganawa S, Teranishi M, Nakata S, et al. (2008) Three-dimensional fluid-attenuated inversion recovery magnetic resonance imaging findings and prognosis in sudden sensorineural hearing loss. The Laryngoscope 118: 1433–1437.
20. Yamazaki M, Naganawa S, Kawai H, Nihashi T, Fukatsu H, et al. (2009) Increased signal intensity of the cochlea on pre- and post-contrast enhanced 3D-FLAIR in patients with vestibular schwannoma. Neuroradiology 51: 855–863.
21. Gardner WJ, Spitler DK, Whitten C (1954) Increased intracranial pressure caused by increased protein content in the cerebrospinal fluid; an explanation of papilledema in certain cases of small intracranial and intraspinal tumors, and in the Guillain-Barre syndrome. The New England journal of medicine 250: 932–936.
22. Froin G (1903) Inflammations méningées avec reaction chromatique, fibrineuse et cytologique du liquide céphalo-rachidien. Gaz d hop 76.
23. Shepherd RK, Colreavy MP (2004) Surface microstructure of the perilymphatic space: implications for cochlear implants and cell- or drug-based therapies. Archives of otolaryngology–head & neck surgery 130: 518–523.
24. Wenthold RJ, McGarvey ML (1982) Changes in rapidly transported proteins in the auditory nerve after hair cell loss. Brain research 253: 263–269.
25. Thomsen J, Saxtrup O, Tos M (1982) Quantitated determination of proteins in perilymph in patients with acoustic neuromas. ORL; journal for oto-rhino-laryngology and its related specialties 44: 61–65.
26. Butman JA, Linehan WM, Lonser RR (2008) Neurologic manifestations of von Hippel-Lindau disease. JAMA : the journal of the American Medical Association 300: 1334–1342.
27. Lysaght AC, Kao SY, Paulo JA, Merchant SN, Steen H, et al. (2011) Proteome of human perilymph. Journal of proteome research 10: 3845–3851.
28. Eckermeier L, Pirsig W, Mueller D (1979) Histopathology of 30 non-operated acoustic schwannomas. Archives of oto-rhino-laryngology 222: 1–9.
29. Schuknecht HF, Ishii T (1966) Hearing loss caused by atrophy of the stria vascularis. Nihon Jibiinkoka Gakkai kaiho 69: 1825–1833.
30. Silverstein H, Schuknecht HF (1966) Biochemical studies of inner ear fluid in man. Changes in otosclerosis, Meniere's disease, and acoustic neuroma. Archives of otolaryngology 84: 395–402.
31. Dix MR, Hallpike CS (1950) Observations on the pathological mechanism of conductive deafness in certain cases of neuroma of the VIIIth nerve. The Journal of laryngology and otology 64: 658–666.
32. Graamans K, Van Dijk JE, Janssen LW (2003) Hearing deterioration in patients with a non-growing vestibular schwannoma. Acta oto-laryngologica 123: 51–54.
33. Pennings RJE, Morris DP, Clarke L, Allen S, Walling S, et al. (2011) Natural history of hearing deterioration in intracanalicular vestibular schwannoma. Neurosurgery 68: 68–77.
34. Roosli C, Linthicum FH, Jr., Cureoglu S, Merchant SN (2012) Dysfunction of the cochlea contributing to hearing loss in acoustic neuromas: an underappreciated entity. Otology & neurotology : official publication of the American Otological Society, American Neurotology Society [and] European Academy of Otology and Neurotology 33: 473–480.
35. Plotkin SR, Stemmer-Rachamimov AO, Barker FG, 2nd, Halpin C, Padera TP, et al. (2009) Hearing improvement after bevacizumab in patients with neurofibromatosis type 2. The New England journal of medicine 361: 358–367.
36. Plotkin SR, Merker VL, Halpin C, Jennings D, McKenna MJ, et al. (2012) Bevacizumab for progressive vestibular schwannoma in neurofibromatosis type 2: a retrospective review of 31 patients. Otology & neurotology : official publication of the American Otological Society, American Neurotology Society [and] European Academy of Otology and Neurotology 33: 1046–1052.

6

Age-Related Hearing Impairment (ARHI) Associated with *GJB2* Single Mutation IVS1+1G>A in the Yakut Population Isolate in Eastern Siberia

Nikolay A. Barashkov[1,2*¶], Fedor M. Teryutin[1,2¶], Vera G. Pshennikova[1], Aisen V. Solovyev[2], Leonid A. Klarov[3], Natalya A. Solovyeva[1], Andrei A. Kozhevnikov[4], Lena M. Vasilyeva[5], Elvira E. Fedotova[5], Maria V. Pak[6], Sargylana N. Lekhanova[7], Elena V. Zakharova[8], Kyunney E. Savvinova[2,9], Nyurgun N. Gotovtsev[2,9], Adyum M. Rafailo[9], Nikolay V. Luginov[3], Anatoliy N. Alexeev[10], Olga L. Posukh[11,12], Lilya U. Dzhemileva[13], Elza K. Khusnutdinova[13,14], Sardana A. Fedorova[1,2]

1 Department of Molecular Genetics, Yakut Scientific Centre of Complex Medical Problems, Siberian Branch of the Russian Academy of Medical Sciences, Yakutsk, Russian Federation, **2** Laboratory of Molecular Biology, Institute of Natural Sciences, M.K. Ammosov North-Eastern Federal University, Yakutsk, Russian Federation, **3** Department of Radiology, Republican Hospital #2– Center of Emergency Medicine, Ministry of Public Health of the Sakha Republic, Yakutsk, Russian Federation, **4** Republican Centre of Professional Pathology, Republican Hospital #2– Center of Emergency Medicine, Ministry of Public Health of the Sakha Republic, Yakutsk, Russian Federation, **5** Audiology-Logopaedic Center, Republican Hospital #1– National Medical Centre, Ministry of Public Health of the Sakha Republic, Yakutsk, Russian Federation, **6** Department of Pediatric, Medical Institute, M.K. Ammosov North-Eastern Federal University, Yakutsk, Russian Federation, **7** Department of Normal and Abnormal Anatomy, Operative Surgery with Topographic Anatomy and Forensic Medicine, Medical Institute, M.K. Ammosov North-Eastern Federal University, Yakutsk, Russian Federation, **8** Institute of Foreign Philology and Regional Studies, M.K. Ammosov North-Eastern Federal University, Yakutsk, Russian Federation, **9** Institute of Natural Sciences, M.K. Ammosov North-Eastern Federal University, Yakutsk, Russian Federation, **10** Institute of Humanitarian Research and Indigenous Peoples of the North, Siberian Branch of the Russian Academy of Sciences, Yakutsk, Russian Federation, **11** Institute of Cytology and Genetics, Siberian Branch of the Russian Academy of Sciences, Novosibirsk, Russian Federation, **12** Novosibirsk State University, Novosibirsk, Russian Federation, **13** Department of Genomics, Institute of Biochemistry and Genetics, Ufa Scientific Centre, Russian Academy of Sciences, Ufa, Russian Federation, **14** Department of Genetics and Fundamental Medicine, Bashkir State University, Ufa, Russian Federation

Abstract

Age-Related Hearing Impairment (ARHI) is one of the frequent sensory disorders registered in 50% of individuals over 80 years. ARHI is a multifactorial disorder due to environmental and poor-known genetic components. In this study, we present the data on age-related hearing impairment of 48 heterozygous carriers of mutation IVS1+1G>A (*GJB2* gene) and 97 subjects with *GJB2* genotype wt/wt in the Republic of Sakha/Yakutia (Eastern Siberia, Russia). This subarctic territory was found as the region with the most extensive accumulation of mutation IVS1+1G>A in the world as a result of founder effect in the unique Yakut population isolate. The *GJB2* gene resequencing and detailed audiological analysis in the frequency range 0.25, 0.5, 1.0, 2.0, 4.0, 8.0 kHz were performed in all examined subjects that allowed to investigate genotype-phenotype correlations between the presence of single mutation IVS1+1G>A and hearing of subjects from examined groups. We revealed the linear correlation between increase of average hearing thresholds at speech frequencies ($PTA_{0.5,1.0,2.0,4.0\ kHz}$) and age of individuals with *GJB2* genotype IVS1+1G>A/wt ($r_s = 0.499$, $p = 0.006860$ for males and $r_s = 0.427$, $p = 0.000277$ for females). Moreover, the average hearing thresholds on high frequency (8.0 kHz) in individuals with genotype IVS1+1G>A/wt (both sexes) were significantly worse than in individuals with genotype wt/wt ($p < 0.05$). Age of hearing loss manifestation in individuals with genotype IVS1+1G>A/wt was estimated to be ~40 years ($r_s = 0.504$, $p = 0.003$). These findings demonstrate that the single IVS1+1G>A mutation (*GJB2*) is associated with age-related hearing impairment (ARHI) of the IVS1+1G>A carriers in the Yakuts.

Editor: Francesc Palau, Instituto de Ciencia de Materiales de Madrid – Instituto de Biomedicina de Valencia, Spain

Funding: The authors thank all patients and blood sample donors who have contributed to this study. This study was supported by the Russian Foundation for Basic Research (12-04-00342_a, 12-04-98520_r_vostok_a, 12-04-97004_r_povolzhye_a, 12-04-31230_mol_a, 14-04-01741_A), Federal Program «Scientific and educational staff for innovative Russia» (#16.740.11.0190, #16.740.11.0346), Integration project of SB RAS #92 «Ethnogeny of indigenous peoples in Siberia and North Asia: comparative, historical, ethno-social and genomic analysis», the Sakha Republic President Grant#80 for Young Researchers for 2014 year, Scientific and Educational Foundation for Young Scientists of Republic of Sakha (Yakutia) for 2014 year, Project #656 of Ministry of Education and Science of Russia, by grant #30 (2013–2015) of RAS Program «Fundamental Sciences for Medicine». The funders had no role in study design, data collection and analysis, decision to publish, or preparation of the manuscript.

Competing Interests: The authors have declared that no competing interests exist.

* Email: barashkov2004@mail.ru

¶ These authors contributed equally to this work.

Introduction

Age-related hearing impairment (ARHI), or presbyacusis, is a common sensory disorder characterized by bilateral sensorineural hearing loss more evident at high frequencies [1], [2]. According to some data, hearing acuity decrease occurs in one out of 25 persons at age older than 45 [3], and about 50% of population over 80 years has a significant hearing impairment [4]. ARHI is a multifactorial disease [1], [5], but the age of disease onset has not been determined. Recently, using a genomewide analysis two loci 8q24.13-q24.22 (ARHI 1, OMIM 612448) [1], [6], 3p26.1-p.25.1 (ARHI 2, OMIM 612976) [1], [7], [8] were linked with this disease.

Genes already known to be associated with hearing impairment are not investigated enough for the presence of genetic associations with ARHI. Mutations in *GJB2* gene coding protein connexin 26 (Cx26) in homozygous and compound-heterozygous states are responsible for a significant part of inherited autosomal recessive forms of hearing loss in different populations [9]. However, several studies suggest that even single mutations in *GJB2* gene (in heterozygous state) have influence on hearing function [10–16]. These studies of hearing thresholds in carriers of recessive mutations in *GJB2* gene – c.35delG, p.Met34Thr, c.167delT (most frequently registered in Europe), and c.235delC single mutation (the study was carried out in China) – had controversial results [10–13], [15], [16].

Splice site mutation IVS1+1G>A in *GJB2* gene is relatively rare, and audiological analysis of hearing threshold in carriers of this single mutation has not been performed previously. High rates of IVS1+1G>A mutation (2–11.7%) were found among some indigenous populations of Eastern Siberia, Russia (Yakuts, Dolgans, Evenks and Evens), with the highest carrier frequency (11.7%) in isolated Yakut population [17]. The genetic data revealed a relatively small size of Yakut ancestor population and the strong bottleneck effect in the Yakut paternal line (80% of Y chromosomes of Yakuts belong to one haplogroup – N1c) [18–21]. Extremely high rate of IVS1+1G>A mutation in relatively genetic homogenous Yakut population gives a unique opportunity to investigate hearing status in individuals heterozygous for this *GJB2* gene mutation.

The purpose of this study is to analyze age-related hearing alteration in *GJB2* mutation IVS1+1G>A carriers versus individuals with normal *GJB2* genotype in Yakut population.

Material and Methods

Sampling design

To form the total sample we invited random volunteers without any complaints on hearing (both in the Yakut Scientific Centre of Complex Medical Problems and during field trips in regions of inhabitance of the Yakutia indigenous population) and informed the potential participants about the aims of upcoming study. We also invited the parents and siblings of deaf children homozygous for the IVS1+1G>A mutation, as they could be the carriers of this mutation. All the volunteers (214 individuals in total) passed otologic-audiological evaluation and genotyping for the *GJB2* gene mutations (spectrum of *GJB2* genotypes is given in Table 1). For the further analysis we selected 145 individuals that matched the following criteria: had *GJB2* genotypes wt/wt or IVS1+1G>A/wt; were older than 20 years old; belonged to Yakut ethnicity (predominantly to the third generation); had no recent history of fever, otitis media, tinnitus; and had no obvious contacts with occupational noise. From those 145 individuals based on genotyping data we formed two groups: Cx26-H – the group included the carriers of single mutation IVS1+1G>A (*GJB2* genotype IVS1+1G>A/wt, 48 individuals or 96 ears); and Cx26-Wt – the group of non-carriers of the IVS1+1G>A mutation (*GJB2* genotype wt/wt, 97 individuals or 194 ears). Subsequently, we stratified these two groups according to age and sex for the purpose of correct comparison (Figure 1).

Audiological examination

Audiological examination was conducted on all 214 individuals (n = 428 ears). Otologic examination was performed with the «Basic-Diagnostik-Set» (KaWe, Germany), tuning fork standard set. Acoustic impedance was measured with impedance meter (Interacoustics AS, Denmark). Air conduction thresholds were measured on frequencies 0.25, 0.5, 1.0, 2.0, 4.0, 8.0 kHz and bone conduction thresholds – on frequencies 0.25, 0.5, 1.0, 2.0, 4.0 kHz with audiometer «MAICO ST20» (MAICO, Germany) in the same conditions for all participants. The results were assessed separately for each ear on air conduction thresholds as on all measured frequencies, and speech range of frequencies – $PTA_{0.5,1.0,2.0,4.0\ kHz}$ separately.

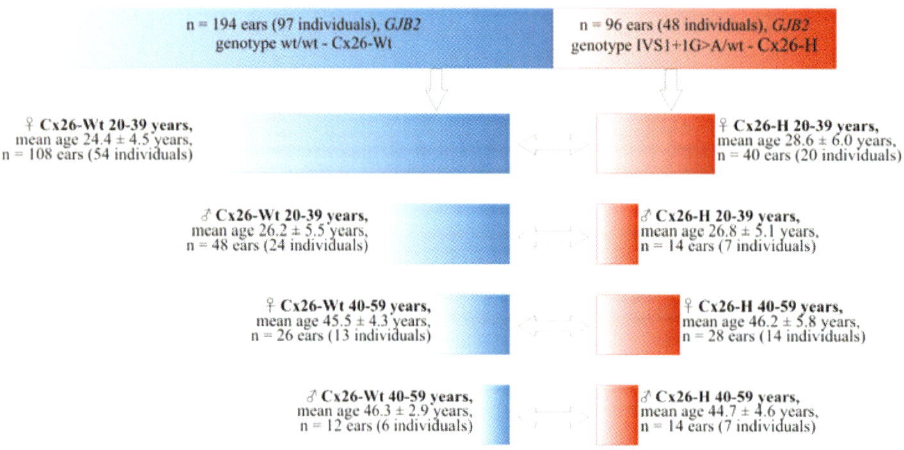

Figure 1. Design of Cx26-H and Cx26-Wt groups. Note: Cx26-Wt (IVS1+1G>A non-carriers) is shown in blue, Cx26-H (IVS1+1G>A carriers) is shown in red; bilateral arrows show the compared subgroups; ♀ – female, ♂ – male.

Table 1. Mutation analysis of *GJB2* gene.

№	*GJB2* **genotype**	**Relatives of the deaf children with mutations in** *GJB2* **gene**	**Random sample from Yakut population**	**Frequency of** *GJB2* **genotypes*, %**
1	**wt/wt**	**4**	**113**	**66.47**
2	**IVS1+1G>A/wt**	**35**	**17**	**10.00**
3	IVS1+1G>A/p.Val27Ile	2	2	1.18
4	p.Val27Ile/wt	1	21	12.35
5	p.Val27Ile/p.Val27Ile+p.Thr123Asn	-	1	0.59
6	p.Val27Ile+p.Glu114Gly/wt	-	6	3.53
7	p.Val27Ile+p.Thr123Asn/wt	-	5	2.94
8	p.Met34Thr/wt	-	1	0.59
9	p.Val37Ile/wt	-	3	1.76
10	c.35delG/wt	2	-	-
11	c.360_362delGAG/wt	-	1	0.59
Total number and percentage of *GJB2*-mutations and polymorphisms		40	57	33.53
Total number of individuals		44	170	-
Total number and percentage		214		100

Note: * The frequency of *GJB2* genotypes was calculated in random sample; in bold are *GJB2* genotypes selected for comparative analysis of hearing thresholds.

Mutation analysis of GJB2 gene

A total of 214 genomic DNA samples, which were extracted from leukocytes of peripheral blood, were used for *GJB2* gene mutation analysis. Amplification of the coding (exon 2) and noncoding (exon 1) and flanking intronic regions of *GJB2* gene was conducted with PCR on thermocycler «MJ Mini» (Bio-Rad) using appropriate primers [22–25]. The PCR products were subjected to direct sequencing using the same primers on ABI PRISM 3130XL (Applied Biosystems, USA) («Genomics» Core Facility; Institute of Chemical Biology and Fundamental Medicine, Siberian Branch of the Russian Academy of Sciences, Novosibirsk, Russia). The results of mutation analysis of *GJB2* gene are shown in the Table 1.

Statistical analysis

The results of audiological examination and mutation analysis of *GJB2* gene were summarized in the unified database. Regression and correlation analysis of «age-hearing threshold» association were assessed with Spearman's rank correlation coefficient r_s. Significance of hearing thresholds on measured frequencies was statistically evaluated with the Mann-Whitney U test using software STATISTICA version 8.0. (StatSoft Inc, USA) and Biostatd (McGraw-Hill, Inc.Version 3.03). Differences were statistically significant when $p<0.05$.

Ethical approval

Written informed consent was obtained from all individuals. This study was approved by the local Committee on Biomedical Ethics of Yakut Scientific Center of Complex Medical Problems,

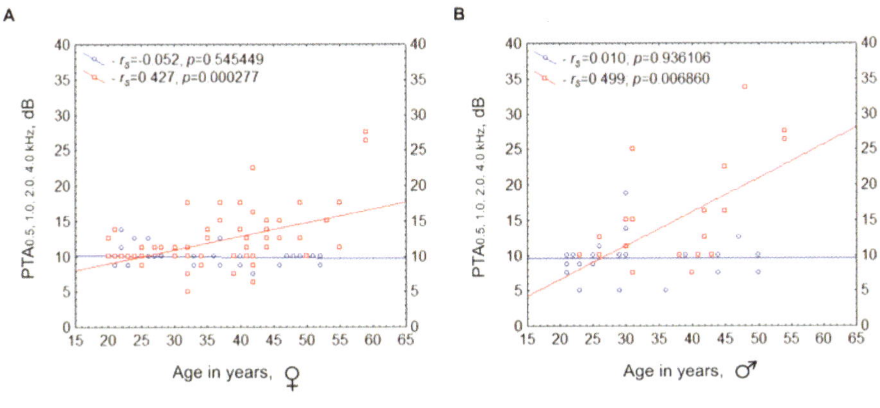

Figure 2. The correlation of increase of hearing thresholds according to age in individuals with genotype IVS1+1G>A/wt. Note: Y-axis – hearing thresholds (dB), X-axis – age in years; r_s – the Spearman's rank correlation coefficient, p – statistical significance of Spearman's rank correlation; blue circles – individuals with *GJB2* genotype wt/wt, red squares – individuals heterozygous for mutation (genotype IVS1+1G>A/wt); blue line shows the absence of hearing thresholds correlation with age in individuals with *GJB2* genotype wt/wt, red line – the linear regression of increase in hearing thresholds according to age in individuals with *GJB2* genotype IVS1+1G>A/wt; A – ♀ female, B – ♂ male.

Table 2. Correlation of increase of hearing thresholds in $PTA_{0.5,1.0,2.0,4.0\ kHz}$ according to age in individuals with *GJB2* genotype wt/wt and IVS1+1G>A/wt.

GJB2 genotype	Parameters	20–29 years	30–39 years	40–49 years	50–59 years
wt/wt	n= ears	128	28	28	10
	r_s	0.036	−0.245	0.159	0.272
	p	0.682	0.208	0.417	0.445
IVS1+1G>A/wt	n= ears	28	26	32	10
	r_s	0.228	−0.125	**0.504**	**0.697**
	p	0.243	0.542	**0.003**	**0.024**

Note: r_s – the Spearman's rank correlation coefficient; values with statistically significant correlation ($p<0.05$) of increase of hearing thresholds with age are shown in bold.

Siberian Branch of the Russian Academy of Medical Sciences, Yakutsk, Russia (Yakutsk, Protocol No 16, April 16, 2009).

Results

Correlation analysis of hearing thresholds in $PTA_{0.5,1.0,2.0,4.0\ kHz}$ according to age

We conducted correlation analysis of «age-hearing thresholds at $PTA_{0.5,1.0,2.0,4.0\ kHz}$» in IVS1+1G>A single mutation carriers (group Cx26-H) and non-carriers (group Cx26-Wt), for females and males separately. Statistically significant ($p<0.05$) correlation of increase in hearing threshold according to age was detected in IVS1+1G>A carriers (group Cx26-H: $r_s=0.427$, $p=0.000277$ in females, $r_s=0.499$, $p=0.006860$ in males) and not observed in non-carriers (group Cx26-Wt: $r_s=-0.052$, $p=0.545449$ in females, $r_s=0.010$, $p=0.936106$ in males) (Figure 2 A, B).

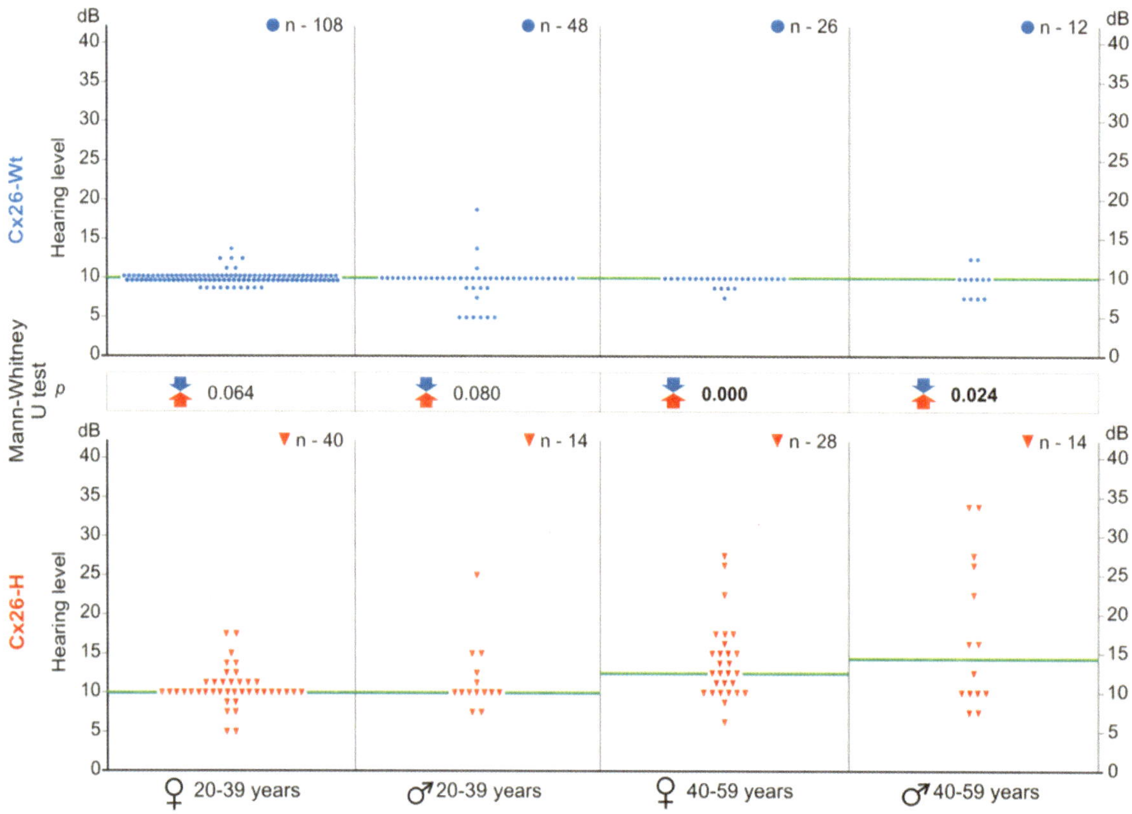

Figure 3. Scatter plots of the hearing thresholds at $PTA_{0.5,\ 1.0,\ 2.0,\ 4.0\ kHz}$ of individuals from compared Cx26-Wt and Cx26-H subgroups according to sex and age. Note: Y-axis – hearing level (hearing threshold, dB). X-axis – audiometric parameters of individuals according to sex and age. Blue circle denotes an individual with *GJB2* genotype wt/wt, red delta denotes an individual with *GJB2* genotype IVS1+1G>A/wt; n – number of ears; statistically significant differences ($p<0.05$) by the Mann-Whitney U test between the compared subgroups are shown in bold; median hearing thresholds are shown by green line. ♀ – female; ♂ – male.

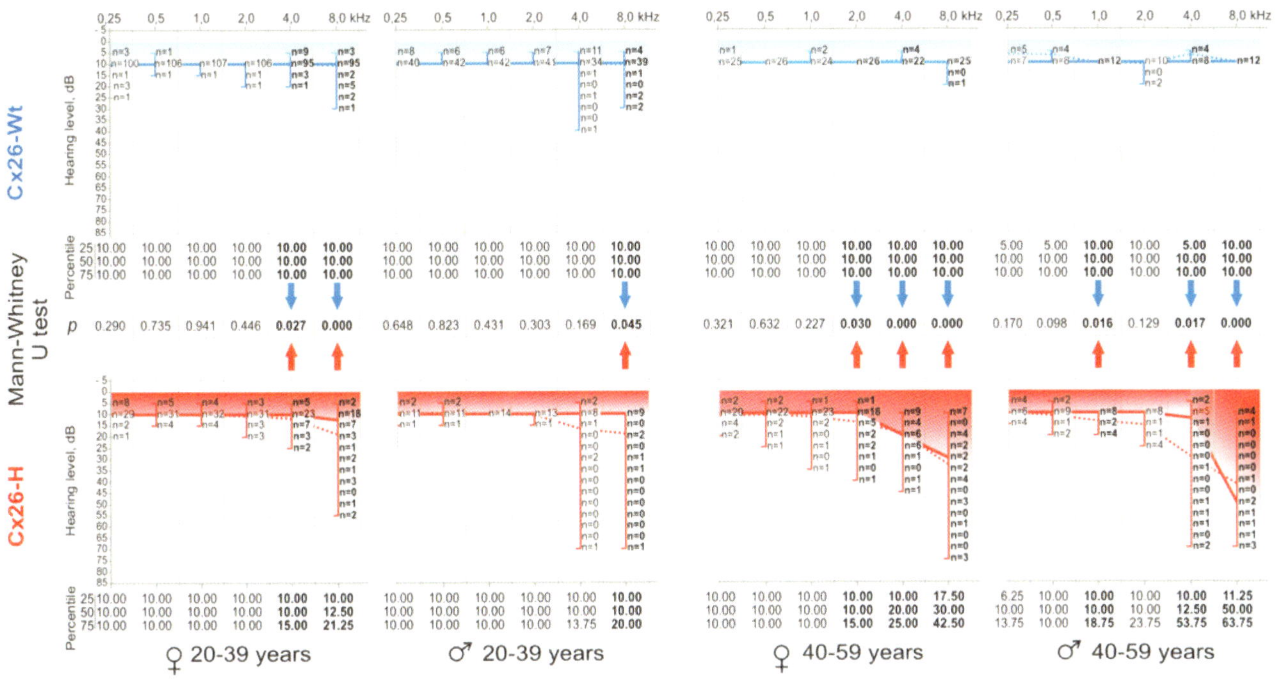

Figure 4. Audiometric parameters at all measured frequencies (0.25, 0.5, 1.0, 2.0, 4.0, 8.0 kHz) of individuals from compared subgroups Cx26-Wt and Cx26-H according to sex and age. Note: Y-axis – hearing thresholds (dB), X-axis – measured frequency (kHz), the audiometric parameters of individuals with *GJB2* genotype wt/wt are shown in blue and of individuals with *GJB2* genotype IVS1+1G>A/wt – in red; n – the number of ears; the frequencies (%) with statistically significant differences ($p<0.05$) by the Mann-Whitney U test are shown in bold; the arrows show statistically significant differences ($p<0.05$) by the Mann-Whitney U test; median hearing thresholds are shown by solid line, average hearing thresholds – by dotted line. ♀ – female; ♂ – male.

The age of onset of hearing impairment in single mutation IVS1+1G>A carriers

To determine onset of presbyacusis manifestation, both studied groups Cx26-H and Cx26-Wt were divided into age cohorts 20–29, 30–39, 40–49, and 50–59 years. Correlation analysis of association «age-hearing threshold in $PTA_{0.5,1.0,2.0,4.0\ kHz}$» was performed in these age cohorts (Table 2). Correlation was not observed in individuals of all age cohorts from group Cx26-Wt and in individuals at ages 20–29 and 30–39 years from group Cx26-H. Statistically significant ($p<0.05$) correlation was observed in hearing thresholds of individuals from group Cx26-H at ages 40–49 years ($r_s=0.504$, $p=0.003$), and 50–59 years ($r_s=0.697$, $p=0.024$) (Table 2). Thus, hearing impairment onset was identified as approximately 40 years, and further analysis was conducted in two age subgroups: 20–39 and 40–59 years (for females and males, separately).

Detailed audiometric analysis of hearing thresholds in IVS1+1G>A carriers and non-carriers

Comparative analysis of hearing thresholds at frequencies of significant speech range ($PTA_{0.5,1.0,2.0,4.0\ kHz}$) did not identify differences between groups Cx26-Wt and Cx26-H at age 20–39 years (females $p=0.064$, males $p=0.080$). However, statistically significant differences in hearing thresholds were observed at age 40–59 years in both groups Cx26-Wt and Cx26-H (females $p=0.000$, males $p=0.024$) (Figure 3).

Following analysis at all measured frequencies (0.25, 0.5, 1.0, 2.0, 4.0, 8.0 kHz) revealed that in group Cx26-Wt averaged audiological profile of females and males aged 20–39 and 40–59 years had a shape of flat curve. Averaged audiological profile of females and males aged 20–39 years in group Cx26-H had a shape of sloping curve, aged 40–59 years – steep-sloping curve in high-frequent range (4.0–8.0 kHz) (Figure 4).

Hearing threshold median at all measured frequencies did not reach 20.0 dB in males and females aged 20–39 years from both groups (Cx26-Wt and Cx26-H) (Figure 4). However, statistically significant ($p<0.05$) differences were observed at frequency 8.0 kHz in both sexes and at frequency 4.0 kHz – in females (Figure 4).

Statistically significant differences ($p<0.05$) in hearing thresholds at frequencies 4.0–8.0 kHz between groups Cx26-Wt and Cx26-H were observed in females and males aged 40–59 years (differences for females were observed starting from frequency 2.0 kHz, for males – from 1.0 kHz). Moreover, median value of hearing threshold was ≥20.0 dB in single mutation IVS1+1G>A carriers at 4.0–8.0 kHz for females, and at 8.0 kHz – for males (Figure 4).

Discussions

ARHI is multifactorial disorder due to environmental and poor-known genetic components. Studying the contribution of single mutations in *GJB2* gene to ARHI had somewhat controversial results.

Engel-Yeger et al. did not detect difference in mean hearing thresholds between c.35delG mutation – carriers (n = 40 persons) and individuals with normal *GJB2* genotype [11]. However, they found proved differences in otoacoustic emission amplitude between the compared groups [26]. Also, associations between c.35delG heterozygous carrier state and age-related hearing alterations with influence of occupational noise were not shown even on more representative sample (2311 individuals) [13]. It is possible that in these studies the difference in hearing thresholds between carriers and non-carriers was not detected due to the inadequate sample size or due to specific features of the chosen method of analysis.

Moreover, there is a study that detected statistically significant differences in mean hearing thresholds on high frequencies (6.0 and 8.0 kHz) between mutation c.35delG carriers (n = 31) and individuals with normal *GJB2* genotype (n = 29) in Italy, however, this study failed to find a correlation of hearing threshold increase with age [12]. Hearing loss predominantly on high and extra-high frequencies (8.0–16.0 kHz) was found to be significantly more severe in *GJB2* c.35delG heterozygous females in comparison with controls [15]. The recent study of hearing status in carriers of *GJB2* single mutations, c.35delG and p.Met34Thr (c.101T>C), conducted in a UK population from 1991 to 2011 with three-step audiological test of children aged 3, 7 and 11 years (9202 children) showed that hearing thresholds on extra-high frequency (16.0 kHz) in c.35delG and p.Met34Thr (c.101T>C) carriers was significantly worse than in children without *GJB2* gene mutation and tend to increase with age [14].

A recently published study provides the data comparable to our results. The study carried out in China (2011) showed that in c.235delC heterozygous carriers hearing for high-frequency (4.0 and 8.0 kHz) increases at the age of 30–59 years and hearing thresholds in the intermediate frequencies may deteriorate over the age of 40 [16].

Our study provides the first evidence that in a relatively isolated Yakut population the average hearing thresholds at the speech frequencies ($PTA_{0.5,1.0,2.0,4.0\ kHz}$) linearly increase ($p<0.05$) with age in the heterozygous carriers of single site splicing mutation IVS1+1G>A (*GJB2* gene) of both sexes. This correlation is more expressed in males, which probably associated with physiological features and environmental factors. Moreover, audiometric analysis showed that hearing thresholds at high frequency (8.0 kHz) in heterozygous for IVS1+1G>A females and males aged 20–39 years were definitely worse ($p<0.05$) than in non-carriers. We also found that hearing on lower frequencies (1.0–2.0 kHz) was affected in both heterozygous for IVS1+1G>A females and males aged 40–59 years (Figure 4). At the same time, these parameters in non-carriers do not cause concerns about hearing impairment regardless of age and sex. We determined onset of hearing worsening in individuals with genotype IVS1+1G>A/wt as ~40 years ($r_s = 0.504$, $p = 0.003$). Thus, we identified that hearing acuity of single mutation IVS1+1G>A carriers on particular frequencies was decreased compared to non-carriers, regardless of sex and age. Splice site mutation IVS1+1G>A, probably leads to a deficiency of normal Cx26 molecules that form intercellular gap junction channels, and this results in impaired recycling of potassium ions in the cochlea with a local organ of Corti intoxication [27]. Thus, carrying the single mutation IVS1+1G>A may cause hearing worsening with ageing.

Conclusion

Despite the controversial results of previous audiological analysis of the c.35delG mutation in heterozygous carriers from Caucasian populations [10–15], the results of this study demonstrate that the single IVS1+1G>A mutation (*GJB2*) is associated with age-related hearing impairment (ARHI) of the IVS1+1G>A carriers among the Yakuts.

Acknowledgments

We thank all patients and blood sample donors who have contributed to this study. This study was supported by the Russian Foundation for Basic Research (12-04-00342_a, 12-04-98520_r_vostok_a, 12-04-97004_r_povolzhye_a, 12-04-31230_mol_a, 14-04-01741_A), Federal Program «Scientific and educational staff for innovative Russia» (#16.740.11.0190, #16.740.11.0346), Integration project of SB RAS #92 «Ethnogeny of indigenous peoples in Siberia and North Asia: comparative, historical, ethno -social and genomic analysis», the Sakha Republic President Grant #80 for Young Researchers for 2014 year, Scientific and Educational Foundation for Young Scientists of Republic of Sakha (Yakutia) for 2014 year, Project #656 of Ministry of Education and Science of Russia, by grant #30 (2013–2015) of RAS Program «Fundamental Sciences for Medicine».

Author Contributions

Conceived and designed the experiments: NB FT SF. Performed the experiments: NB FT VP AS LK NS AK LV EF NL. Analyzed the data: NB FT MP SL EZ KS NG OP LD. Contributed reagents/materials/analysis tools: AR AA OP LD EK SF. Wrote the paper: NB FT OP LD.

References

1. Huyghe JR, Van Laer L, Hendrickx JJ, Fransen E, Demeester K, et al. (2008) Genome-wide SNP-based linkage scan dentifies a locus on 8q24 for an age-related hearing impairment trait. Am. J. Hum. Genet. 83: 401–407.
2. Yamasoba T, Lin FR, Someya S, Kashio A, Sakamoto T, et al. (2013) Current concepts in age-related hearing loss: Epidemiology and mechanistic pathways. Hear. Res. 303: 30–8.
3. Smith RJ, Bale JF Jr, White KR (2005) Sensorineural hearing loss in children. Lancet 365: 879–890.
4. Morton NE, Ann NY (1991) Genetic epidemiology of hearing impairment. Acad. Sci. 630: 16–31.
5. Fransen E, Topsakal V, Hendrickx JJ, Van Laer L, Huyghe JR, et al. (2008) Occupational noise, smoking, and a high body mass index are risk factors for age-related hearing impairment and moderate alcohol consumption is protective: a European population-based multicenter study. J. Assoc. Res. Otolaryngol. 9(3): 264–76.
6. Van Laer L, Van Eyken E, Fransen E, Huyghe JR, Topsakal V, et al. (2008) The grainyhead like 2 gene (GRHL2), alias TFCP2L3, is associated with age-related hearing impairment. Hum. Mol. Genet. 17: 159–169.
7. Friedman RA, Van Laer L, Huentelman MJ, Sheth SS, Van Eyken E, et al. (2009) GRM7 variants confer susceptibility to age-related hearing impairment. Hum. Mol. Genet. 18: 785–796.
8. Van Laer L, Huyghe JR, Hannula S, Van Eyken E, Stephan DA, et al. (2010) A genome-wide association study for age-related hearing impairment in the Saami. European Journal of Human Genetics 18: 685–693.
9. Ballana E, Ventayol M, Rabionet R, Gasparini P, Estivill X Connexins and deafness Homepage. Available: http://www.crg.es/deafness.
10. Morell RJ, Kim HJ, Hood LJ, Goforth L, Friderici K, et al. (1998) Mutations in the connexin 26 gene (GJB2) among Ashkenazi Jews with nonsyndromic recessive deafness. N. Engl. J. Med. 339: 1500–1505.
11. Engel-Yeger B, Zaaroura S, Zlotogora J, Shalev S, Hujeirat Y, et al. (2002) The effects of a connexin 26 mutation 35delG on oto-acoustic emissions and brainstem evoked potentials: homozygotes and carriers. Hearing Research 163: 93–100.
12. Franzé A, Caravelli A, Di Leva F, Marciano E, Auletta G, et al. (2005) Audiometric evaluation of carriers of the connexin 26 mutation 35delG. Eur. Arch. Otorhinolaryngol. 262: 921–924.
13. Van Eyken E, Van Laer L, Fransen E, Topsakal V, Hendrickx JJ, et al. (2007) The contribution of GJB2 (Connexin 26) 35delG to age-related hearing impairment and noise-induced hearing loss. Otol. Neurotol. 28: 970–975.
14. Hall A, Pembrey M, Lutman M, Steer C, Bitner-Glindzicz M (2012) Prevalence and audiological features in carriers of GJB2 mutations, c.35delG and c.101T>C (p.M34T), in a UK population study. BMJ Open 31 2(4): 3–8.
15. Groh D, Seeman P, Jilek M, Popelář J, Kabelka Z, et al. (2013) Hearing function in heterozygous carriers of a pathogenic GJB2 mutation. Phisiol. Res. 62(3): 323–30.
16. Li Q, Fang RP, Wang GJ, Liu F, Dai P (2011) Tonal audiometry of GJB2 235delC single heterozygous mutation carriers. Zhonghua Er Bi Yan Hou Tou Jing Wai Ke Za Zhi 46(7): 543–6. (Article in Chinese).
17. Barashkov NA, Dzhemileva LU, Fedorova SA, Teruytin FM, Posukh OL, et al. (2011) Autosomal recessive deafness 1A (DFNB1A) in Yakut population isolate in Eastern Siberia: extensive accumulation of the splice site mutation IVS1+1G>A in GJB2 gene as a result of founder effect. Journal of Human Genetics 9: 631–639.

18. Zerjal T, Dashnyam B, Pandya A, Kayser M, Roewer L, et al. (1997) Genetic relationships in Asians and Nothern Europeans, revalated by Y-chromosomal analysis. Am. J. Hum. Genet. 60: 1174–1183.
19. Pakendorf B, Novgorodov IN, Osakovskij VL, Danilova AP, Protod'jakonov AP, et al. (2006) Investigating the effects of prehistoric migrations in Siberia: genetic variations and the origins of Yakuts. Hum. Genet. 120: 334–353.
20. Khar'kov VN, Stepanov VA, Medvedev OF, Spiridonova MG, Maksimova NR, et al. (2008) The origin of Yakuts: analysis of Y-chromosome haplotypes. Mol. biol. (Mosk.) 42: 226–237.
21. Fedorova SA, Reidla M, Metspalu E, Metspalu M, Rootsi S, et al. (2013) Autosomal and uniparental portraits of the native populations of Sakha (Yakutia): implications for the peopling of Northeast Eurasia. BMC Evolutionary Biology 13: 127.
22. Kelsell DP, Dunlop J, Stevens HP, Lench NJ, Liang JN, et al. (1997) Connexin 26 mutations in hereditary non-syndromic sensorineural deafness. Nature 387: 80–83.
23. Zelante L, Gasparini P, Estivill X, Melchionda S, D'Agruma L, et al. (1997) Connexin 26 mutations associated with the most common form of non-syndromic neurosensory autosomal recessive deafness (DFNB1) in Mediterraneans. Hum. Mol. Genet. 6: 1605–1609.
24. Kelley PM, Harris DJ, Comer BC, Askew JW, Fowler T, et al. (1998) Novel mutations in the connexin 26 gene (GJB2) that cause autosomal recessive (DFNB1) hearing loss. Am. J. Hum. Genet. 62: 792–799.
25. Sirmaci A, Akcayoz-Duman D, Tekin M (2006) The c.IVS1+1G>A mutation in the GJB2 gene is prevalent and large deletions involving the GJB6 gene are not present in the Turkish population. J. Genet. 85: 213–216.
26. Engel-Yeger B, Zaaroura S, Zlotogora J, Shalev S, Hujeirat Y, et al. (2003) Otoacoustic emissions and brainstem evoked potentials in compound carriers of connexin 26 mutations. Hearing Research 175 (1–2): 140–51.
27. Lefebvre PP, Van De Water TR (2000) Connexins, hearing and deafness: clinical aspects of mutations in the connexin 26 gene. Brain Res. Brain Res. Rev. 32: 159–162.

7

Application of Massively Parallel Sequencing to Genetic Diagnosis in Multiplex Families with Idiopathic Sensorineural Hearing Impairment

Chen-Chi Wu[1,2], Yin-Hung Lin[1,3], Ying-Chang Lu[1], Pei-Jer Chen[4,5], Wei-Shiung Yang[2,4,5,6], Chuan-Jen Hsu[1]*, Pei-Lung Chen[2,5,6,7]*

1 Department of Otolaryngology, National Taiwan University Hospital, Taipei, Taiwan, **2** Department of Medical Genetics, National Taiwan University Hospital, Taipei, Taiwan, **3** Graduate Institute of Molecular Medicine, National Taiwan University College of Medicine, Taipei, Taiwan, **4** Graduate Institute of Clinical Medicine, National Taiwan University College of Medicine, Taipei, Taiwan, **5** Department of Internal Medicine, National Taiwan University Hospital, Taipei, Taiwan, **6** Research Center for Developmental Biology and Regenerative Medicine, National Taiwan University, Taipei, Taiwan, **7** Graduate Institute of Medical Genomics and Proteomics, National Taiwan University College of Medicine, Taipei, Taiwan

Abstract

Despite the clinical utility of genetic diagnosis to address idiopathic sensorineural hearing impairment (SNHI), the current strategy for screening mutations via Sanger sequencing suffers from the limitation that only a limited number of DNA fragments associated with common deafness mutations can be genotyped. Consequently, a definitive genetic diagnosis cannot be achieved in many families with discernible family history. To investigate the diagnostic utility of massively parallel sequencing (MPS), we applied the MPS technique to 12 multiplex families with idiopathic SNHI in which common deafness mutations had previously been ruled out. NimbleGen sequence capture array was designed to target all protein coding sequences (CDSs) and 100 bp of the flanking sequence of 80 common deafness genes. We performed MPS on the Illumina HiSeq2000, and applied BWA, SAMtools, Picard, GATK, Variant Tools, ANNOVAR, and IGV for bioinformatics analyses. Initial data filtering with allele frequencies (<5% in the 1000 Genomes Project and 5400 NHLBI exomes) and PolyPhen2/SIFT scores (>0.95) prioritized 5 indels (insertions/deletions) and 36 missense variants in the 12 multiplex families. After further validation by Sanger sequencing, segregation pattern, and evolutionary conservation of amino acid residues, we identified 4 variants in 4 different genes, which might lead to SNHI in 4 families compatible with autosomal dominant inheritance. These included *GJB2* p.R75Q, *MYO7A* p.T381M, *KCNQ4* p.S680F, and *MYH9* p.E1256K. Among them, *KCNQ4* p.S680F and *MYH9* p.E1256K were novel. In conclusion, MPS allows genetic diagnosis in multiplex families with idiopathic SNHI by detecting mutations in relatively uncommon deafness genes.

Editor: Andreas R. Janecke, Innsbruck Medical University, Austria

Funding: This study was supported by research grants from the National Health Research Institute (NHRI-EX101-10147PI), National Science Council of the Executive Yuan of the Republic of China (NSC 100-2314-B-002-031-MY3), and National Taiwan University (UN1UN101-013). The funders had no role in study design, data collection and analysis, decision to publish, or preparation of the manuscript.

Competing Interests: The authors have declared that no competing interests exist.

* E-mail: cjhsu@ntu.edu.tw (CJH); paylong@ntu.edu.tw (PLC)

Introduction

Hearing loss is a common sensory disorder. Approximately 1 in 500 newborns are affected with bilateral moderate or more severe sensorineural hearing impairment (SNHI). Before the age of 5, the prevalence increases to 2.7 per 1,000, and during adolescence, to 3.5 per 1,000 [1]. It has been revealed that more than 50% of children with SNHI have attributable genetic factors [2]. As such, genetic testing is a powerful tool for a precise genetic diagnosis in hearing-impaired children. In addition, this diagnostic approach provides clues concerning the pathogenesis of hearing impairment, and allows for an accurate prognosis [3,4], facilitates genetic counseling [5], prevents further hearing loss [6], and might help to design novel strategies for future treatment.

However, the genetic heterogeneity of hereditary hearing impairment remains a major obstacle to obtaining molecular diagnoses in the majority of cases. To date, more than 100 genes are associated with deafness, and approximately 50 genes have been identified to cause nonsyndromic hereditary hearing impairment (The Hereditary Hearing Loss Homepage, http://hereditaryhearingloss.org/) [7]. For example, in Taiwan, although mutations in certain genes such as *GJB2* (or *Cx26*) (Gene ID: 2706), *SLC26A4* (or *PDS*) (Gene ID: 5172), and the mitochondrial 12SrRNA gene (*MTRNR1*) (Gene ID: 4549) have been shown to be much more prevalent than other genes, a definitive diagnosis by direct sequencing of these coding regions could only be established in approximately 1/3 patients with idiopathic SNHI [8] and 1/4 patients with cochlear implantation [4], respectively. It is likely that there are other, relatively uncommon, genetic mutations that contribute to SNHI in some of the remaining families, especially those with many affected members (i.e., multiplex families). Recently, the development of massively parallel sequencing (MPS), also known as next-generation sequencing (NGS), which generates millions of DNA sequence reads in parallel during a single experimental run, offers a potential solution to approach

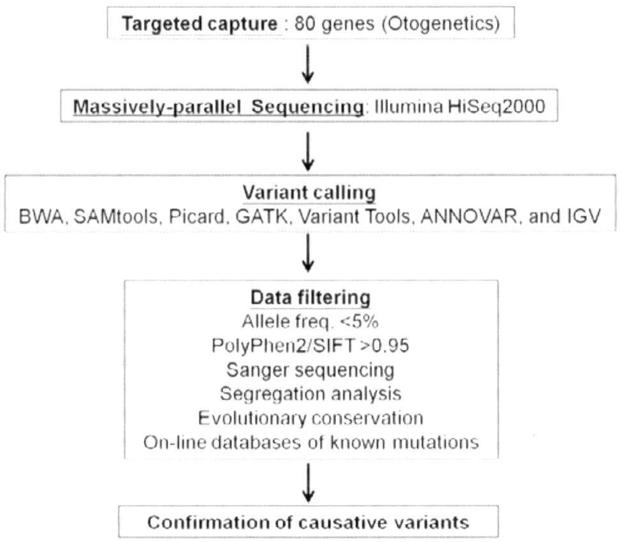

Figure 1. Pipeline to identify causative variants in the present study. Causative variants in the 12 families were confirmed through the steps of targeted capture of 80 known deafness genes; massively parallel sequencing with the Illumina platform; variant calling using the BWA, SAMtools, Picard, GATK, and IGV software packages; and data filtering with various criteria, including allele frequencies <5% in both the 1000 Genomes Project and NHLBI-ESP 5400 exome project, both PolyPhen2 and SIFT scores >0.95, Sanger sequencing, segregation pattern, evolutionary conservation of amino acid residues, and on-line databases of known deafness mutations.

hereditary disorders with genetic heterogeneity such as retinitis pigmentosa [9], breast cancer [10], cardiomyopathy [11], and hereditary hearing impairment [12,13]. To investigate the diagnostic utility of MPS, we applied the MPS technique to a cohort composed of 12 families with idiopathic SNHI in which common deafness mutations had been ruled out as the cause.

Materials and Methods

Family Recruitment and Phenotype Characterization

Twelve multiplex families with idiopathic nonsyndromic SNHI, including 10 families compatible with autosomal dominant inheritance and 2 families compatible with autosomal recessive inheritance (Figure S1), were enrolled in the present study. All 12 families were Han Chinese from Taiwan in ethnicity. Prior mutation screening using the SNaPshot multiplex assays, which targeted 20 common deafness-associated mutations in the Han Chinese population of Taiwan [14], did not detect mutations in these 12 families. For the proband and affected family members, comprehensive family history and past medical records were obtained, and physical examination, neurological examination, audiological results, and temporal bone imaging results were obtained and analyzed. Audiological results were assessed and characterized in terms of 2 parameters: hearing levels and audiogram shapes [15]. The hearing level of the better ear, calculated by a 4-tone average (0.5, 1, 2, and 4 kHz), was labeled as mild (20~40 dBHL), moderate (41~70 dBHL), severe (71~95 dBHL), or profound (>95 dBHL) hearing loss (GEN-DEAF: http://audiology.unife.it/www.gendeaf.org/index.html). Temporal bone imaging results were obtained using high-resolution computed tomography and/or magnetic resonance imaging, and inner ear malformations (IEMs) were identified and determined according to the criteria in the literature [15]. Written informed consent for participation in the project was obtained from the subjects, and all procedures were approved by the Research Ethics Committee of the National Taiwan University Hospital.

Target Enrichment, Massively Parallel Sequencing and Variant Calling

Figure 1 depicts the major criteria for identification of causative variants in the affected families, including target enrichment, massively parallel sequencing, variant calling, and data filtering. Genomic DNA (gDNA) was extracted from the probands of the 12 families and submitted to Otogenetics Corporation (Norcross, GA, USA) for exome capture and sequencing. Briefly, gDNA was

Table 1. Number of Variants Detected in the Probands of the 12 Families.

Proband	Inheritance	Variants (freq. <5%)			Potentially functional variants				
		SNP	Private indels	Total	Nonsense	Missense	Splice junctions	Frameshift	Total
DE2087	ADNSHL	296	4	300	1	3	1	0	5
DE2180	ADNSHL	284	4	288	2	5	1	0	8
DE2548	ADNSHL	298	4	302	1	4	1	0	6
DE2616	ADNSHL	278	4	282	1	3	0	1	5
DE2624	ADNSHL	98	3	101	1	2	1	0	4
DE2675	ADNSHL	138	4	142	1	7	2	0	10
DE2721	ADNSHL	182	4	186	2	10	0	0	12
DE2737	ARNSHL	284	4	288	2	3	0	0	5
DE2827	ADNSHL	109	3	112	1	4	0	0	5
DE2939	ARNSHL	367	8	375	2	0	1	0	3
DE3050	ADNSHL	171	3	174	1	10	0	1	12
DE3281	ADNSHL	148	2	150	1	6	0	0	7

SNP, single nucleotide polymorphism; ADNSHL, autosomal dominant nonsyndromic hearing loss; ARNSHL, autosomal recessive nonsyndromic hearing loss.

subjected to agarose gel and O.D. ratio tests to confirm its purity and concentration prior to Covaris fragmentation (Covaris, Inc., Woburn, MA, USA). Fragmented gDNAs were tested for size distribution and concentration using the Agilent Bioanalyzer 2100 (Agilent Technologies, Inc., Santa Clara, CA, USA) and NanoDrop (Thermo Fisher Scientific, Inc., Wilmington, DE, USA). Illumina libraries were generated from fragmented gDNA (only after the gDNA passed the quality control checks) using NEBNext reagents (New England Biolabs, Ipswich, MA, USA; catalog# E6040), and the resulting libraries were subjected to target enrichment using custom probes targeting the Human Deafness Gene DA1 panel (Otogenetics Corporation) following the manufacturer's instructions. The libraries were first tested for enrichment by qPCR and for size distribution and concentration using the Agilent Bioanalyzer 2100. The samples were then sequenced on an Illumina HiSeq2000 that generated paired-end reads of 100 nucleotides.

We aligned the raw sequencing data to the latest reference human genome (Feb. 2009, GRCh37/hg19) using the BWA software (version 0.5.9) [16]. We used SAMtools (version 0.1.18) [17] and Picard (version 1.54) (http://picard.sourceforge.net) to perform the necessary data conversion, sorting, and indexing. The main variant calling process, for both indels (insertion/deletions) and single nucleotide variants, was operated by using the GATK software package (version 1.2-59-gd74367c1) [18,19]. We applied Variant Tools (version 1.0.2) to select and analyze the variants [20]. ANNOVAR (version 2012-03-08) was used to appropriately annotate the genetic variants [21]. This included gene annotation, amino acid change annotation, SIFT scores [22], PolyPhen2 scores [23], dbSNP identifiers, 1000 Genomes Project allele frequencies, and NHLBI-ESP 5400 exome project allele frequencies. We then used IGV (version 2.1.16) to view the mapping and annotation of sequences on a graphic interface [24,25].

Data Filtering

After variant calling, we used ANNOVAR to annotate genetic variants, identify variants that are reported in dbSNP135, and check if variants have already been reported in the 1000 Genomes Project (Feb. 2012) or NHLBI-ESP 5400 exome project (all ethnicity). Only variants with allele frequencies <5% in both the 1000 Genomes Project and NHLBI-ESP 5400 exome project were selected. Among these variants, all frameshift and non-frameshift indel variants, nonsense variants, and splice site variants were included for further analysis. In contrast, for missense variants, PolyPhen2 and SIFT (http://sift.jcvi.org/) were used to assess the effect on the protein. SIFT prediction is based on the degree of conservation of amino acid residues in multiple alignment information. The amino acid substitution is predicted damaging if the score is >0.95, and tolerated if the score is <0.95. Accordingly, missense variants with a score <0.95 in PolyPhen2 or SIFT were excluded. Variants meeting the aforementioned criteria were then subjected to Sanger sequencing to confirm the nucleotide change; segregation pattern were obtained to determine if the variant co-segregated with the hearing impairment phenotype in the pedigrees, and the evolutionary conservation of amino acid residues was assessed. Known variants present in databases (http://deafnessvariationdatabase.org/) and published in the literature as disease-causing were regarded as pathogenic mutations. The mutated gene identified in each family was classified as autosomal dominant or autosomal recessive according to the Hereditary Hearing Loss Homepage (http://hereditaryhearingloss.org), and was then correlated to the inheritance pattern in each family. Allele frequencies of the

Table 2. The Variants Identified in the 6 Families Compatible with Autosomal Dominant Inheritance.

Proband	Inheritance	Genomic Coordinates	Reference reads	Variant reads	Total reads	Gene	cDNA (RefSeq ID)	Protein (RefSeq ID)	SIFT	PolyPhen2	5400 NHLBI exomes	1000 Genomes
DE2624	ADNSHL	Chr13:20763497 C>T	130	120	251	*GJB2*	c.224G>A (NM_004004.5)	p.R75Q (NP_003995.2)	1	1	0	0
DE2675	ADNSHL	Chr1:41304146 C>T	156	97	253	*KCNQ4*	c.1877C>T (NM_004700.3)	p.S680F (NP_004691.2)	0.98	0.999	0	0
DE2721	ADNSHL	Chr22:36690209 C>T	122	78	201	*MYH9*	c.3766G>A (NM_002473.4)	p.E1256K (NP_002464.1)	1	1	0	0
DE2827	ADNSHL	Chr1:35227362 C>G	120	102	222	*GJB4*	c.507C>G (NM_153212.2)	p.C169W (NP_694944.1)	1	1	0.028	0.03
DE3050	ADNSHL	Chr11:76871270 C>T	32	41	73	*MYO7A*	c.1142C>T (NM_000260.3)	p.T381M (NP_000251.3)	0.98	0.996	0	0
DE3281	ADNSHL	Chr1:35227362 C>G	155	150	305	*GJB4*	c.507C>G (NM_153212.2)	p.C169W (NP_694944.1)	1	1	0.028	0.03

ADNSHL, autosomal dominant nonsyndromic hearing loss.

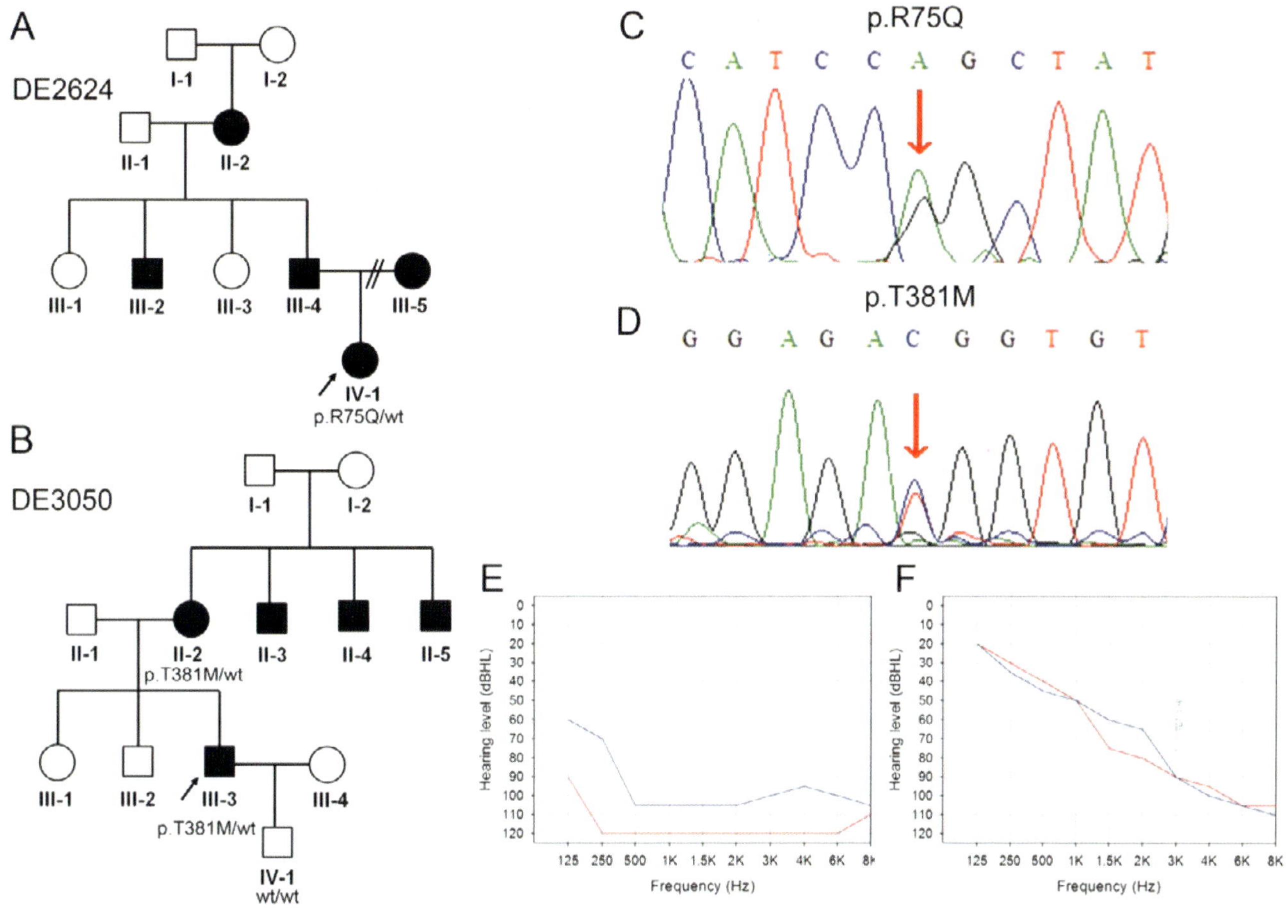

Figure 2. The *GJB2* p.R75Q mutation in Family DE2624 and the *MYO7A* p.T381M mutation in Family DE3050. (A) Pedigree and segregation pattern in Family DE2624. (B) Pedigree and segregation pattern in Family DE3050. (C) Sanger sequence of the *GJB2* p.R75Q mutation. Arrow: nucleotide change c.224G>A (p.R75Q) variant. (D) Sanger sequence of the *MYO7A* p.T381M mutation. Arrow: nucleotide change c.1142C>T (p.T381M) variant. (E) Audiogram of the proband of Family DE2624. (F) Audiogram of the proband of Family DE3050. Hearing levels of the right ear and left ear are marked with red and blue lines, respectively.

variants detected were also verified in a panel of 100 controls with normal hearing of the same ethnicity.

Results

Target Enrichment and Massively Parallel Sequencing

DNA libraries were created from the probands of the 12 multiplex families with SNHI (Table 1). As shown in Supplementary Material, Table S1, the Human Deafness DA1 Panel was designed to enrich for all coding sequences (CDSs) and splicing sites of 80 confirmed human deafness genes. This covered 1,253 exons with a total coding region of 193,634 bp. The enriched targets then were submitted to MPS using the Illumina HiSeq2000 and the paired-end protocol with a length of 100 bp. The average coverage was 490 folds. 99.3% of sequences had coverage greater than 30 folds, 99% greater than 50 folds, and 95.3% greater than 100 folds.

Data Filtering and Identification of Causative Variants

Initial data filtering with allele frequencies and PolyPhen2/SIFT scores prioritized 5 indels and 36 missense variants in the 12 multiplex families. After further validation by Sanger sequencing, segregation pattern, and assessment of evolutionary conservation of amino acid residues, we identified 5 variants in 5 different genes, which might have led to SNHI in 6 of the families compatible with autosomal dominant inheritance. These included *GJB2* p.R75Q, *MYO7A* (GeneID 4647) p.T381M, *KCNQ4* (GeneID 9132) p.S680F, *MYH9* (GeneID 4627) p.E1256K, and *GJB4* (GeneID 127534) p.C169W (Table 2).

Known Causative Variants: *GJB2* p.R75Q and *MYO7A* p.T381M

We identified 2 known causative variants, *GJB2* p.R75Q (c.224G>A) and *MYO7A* p.T381M (c.1142C>T), in Family DE2624 and Family DE3050, respectively (Figure 2). Variant reads of *GJB2* p.R75Q were 48% (120/251) of total reads in the proband of Family DE2624, suggesting heterozygosity of the allele (Table 2). p.R75Q has been associated to both autosomal dominant nonsyndromic hearing loss (ADNSHL) [26] and autosomal dominant SNHI with palmoplantar keratoderma [27]. The proband of Family DE2624 was a 5-year-old girl with profound hearing loss (Figure 2E) and normal temporal bone imaging results. Palmoplantar keratoderma was not observed in the affected members of Family DE2624, thus indicating that the phenotype associated with *GJB2* p.R75Q in this family was nonsyndromic hearing loss.

In the proband of Family DE3050, variant reads of *MYO7A* p.T381M were 56% (41/73) of the total reads, suggesting

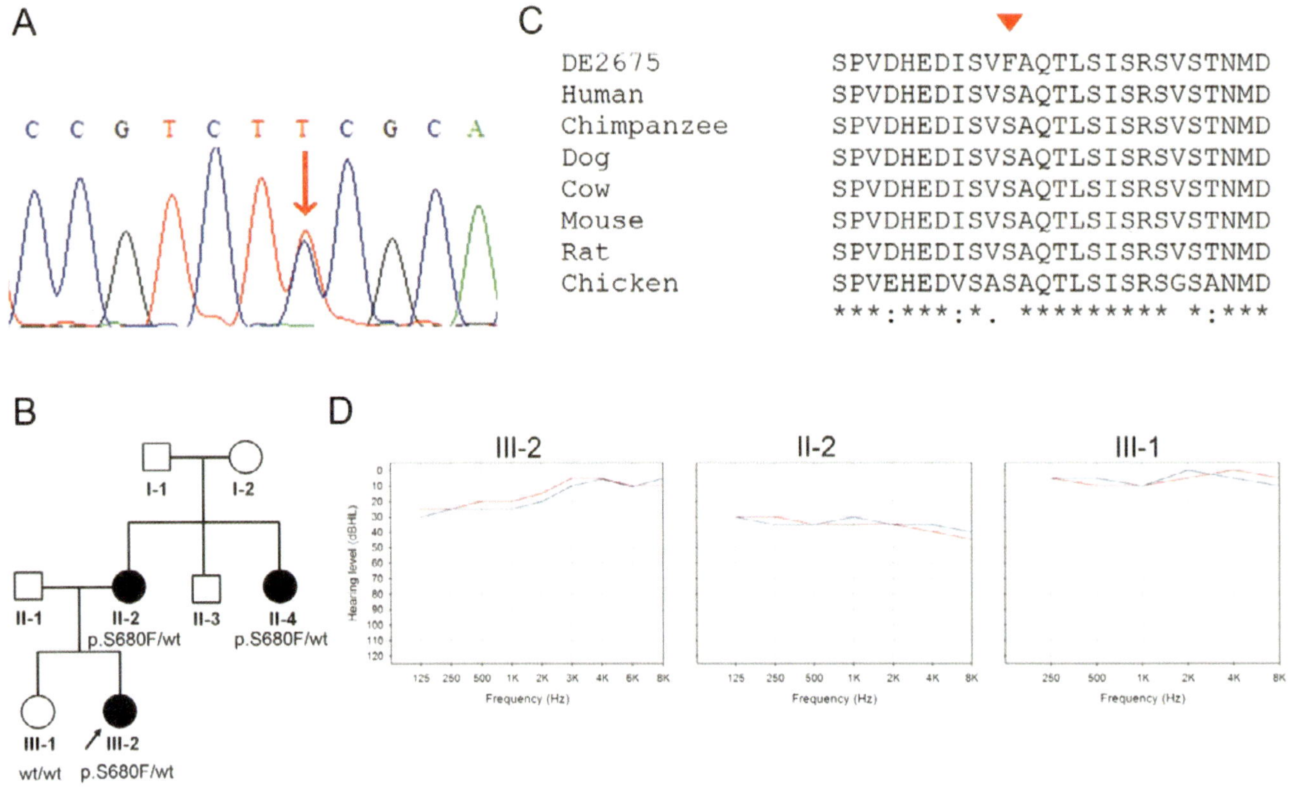

Figure 3. The *KCNQ4* p.S680F variant identified in Family DE2675. (A) Sanger sequence of the *KCNQ4* p.S680F variant. Arrow: nucleotide change c.1877C>T (p.S680F) variant. (B) Pedigree and segregation pattern in Family DE2675. (C) Evolutionary conservation of the p.S680 residue. Arrowhead: variant site. (D) Audiograms of the affected family members (II-2 & III-2) and an unaffected member (III-1) of Family DE2675. Hearing levels of the right ear and left ear are marked with red and blue lines, respectively.

heterozygosity of the allele (Table 2). Heterozygosity for *MYO7A* p.T381M has been documented in 3 unrelated patients with nonsyndromic SNHI from Taiwan [28], and co-segregated with the phenotype of hearing impairment in the pedigree of Family DE3050 (Figure 2B). The proband of Family DE3050 was a 31-year-old man with progressive, moderate SNHI (Figure 2F) and no inner ear malformations (IEM) on temporal bone imaging studies. None of the affected members in Family DE3050 exhibited retinitis pigmentosa.

Novel Causative Variants: *KCNQ4* p.S680F and *MYH9* p.E1256K

In Family DE2675, we identified the p.S680F (c.1877C>T) variant in the *KCNQ4* gene, which has not been reported previously (Figure 3A). The pathogenicity of *KCNQ4* p.S680F was supported by its high SIFT (0.98) and PolyPhen2 (0.99) scores, as well as its absence in the 5400 NHLBI exomes, 1000 Genomes, and the 100 normal hearing controls of the present study (Table 2). Furthermore, heterozygosity for p.S680F co-segregated with the phenotype of hearing impairment in the pedigree (Figure 3B), and the amino acid residue p.S680 was evolutionarily conserved (Figure 3C). The proband (III-2) of Family DE2675 was a 7-year-old girl with mild low-tone hearing loss, and her mother's (II-2) hearing loss began at adolescence and gradually deteriorated to mild SNHI until her current age (Figure 3D). Both exhibited normal temporal bone imaging results. By contrast, the elder sister (III-1) of the proband who did not segregate the p.S680F variant demonstrated a normal audiogram.

In Family DE2721, we identified the p.E1256K (c.3766G>A) variant in the *MYH9* gene, which has not been reported previously (Figure 4A). The pathogenicity of *MYH9* p.E1256K was supported by its high SIFT (1.00) and PolyPhen2 (1.00) scores, as well as its absence in 5400 NHLBI exomes, 1000 Genomes, and the 100 normal hearing controls (Table 2). In addition, heterozygosity for p.E1256K co-segregated with the phenotype of hearing impairment in the pedigree (Figure 4B), and the amino acid residue p.E1256 was evolutionarily conserved (Figure 4C). The proband of Family DE2721 was a 57-year-old woman with profound SNHI that had progressed since 10 years of age (Figure 4D). One of her sons had segregated the *MYH9* p.E1256K variant and also exhibited progressive SNHI of moderate severity. The result of the temporal imaging study performed in the proband was normal. Comprehensive renal, hematological, and ophthalmological studies in the proband revealed normal results, and her affected son (III-2) also showed normal laboratory findings on complete blood count and serum renal profiles. Hematologic and renal disorders were ruled out in other affected members of Family DE2721 by history.

Probable Non-causative Variant: *GJB4* p.C169W

In Family DE2827 and Family DE3281, we identified the p.C169W (c.507C>G) variant in the *GJB4* gene (Figure 5A). In both Family DE2827 and Family DE3281, heterozygosity for *GJB4* p.C169W co-segregated with the hearing impairment phenotype in the pedigree (Figure 5B and 5C), except for case I-1 of Family DE2827, which exhibited normal hearing that corresponded to his age. The proband of Family DE2827 was a

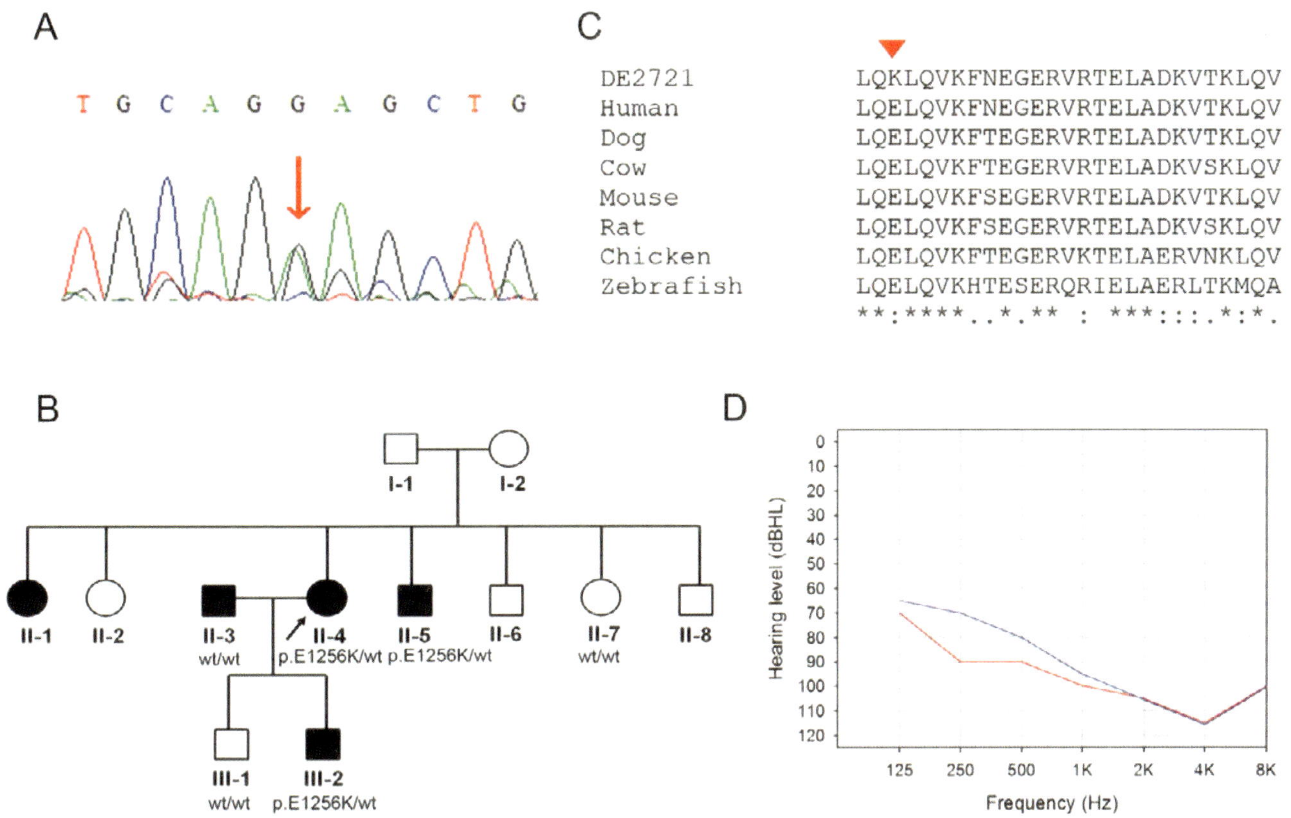

Figure 4. The *MYH9* p.E1256K variant identified in Family DE2721. (A) Sanger sequence of the *MYH9* p.E1256K variant. Arrow: nucleotide change c.3766G>A (p.E1256K) variant. (B) Pedigree and segregation pattern of Family DE2721. (C) Evolutionary conservation of the p.E1256 residue. Arrowhead: variant site. (D) Audiogram of the proband of Family DE2721. Hearing levels of the right ear and left ear are marked with red and blue lines, respectively.

44-year-old woman with progressive severe SNHI (Figure 5E, upper panel), whereas the proband of Family DE3281 was a 50-year-old woman with progressive SNHI of moderate severity (Figure 5E, lower panel). Both probands exhibited normal temporal bone imaging results. The SIFT and PolyPhen2 scores of *GJB4* p.C169W were 1.00 (Table 2). The amino acid residue p.C169 was evolutionarily conserved (Figure 5D), and heterozygosity for the nonsense mutation at this amino acid residue (i.e., p.C169X) has been related to nonsyndromic SNHI in a Han Chinese family from Taiwan [29]. However, the allele frequencies of *GJB4* p.C169W were as high as 2.8% and 3.0% in 5400 NHLBI exomes and 1000 Genomes, respectively. Among the 100 normal hearing controls, we also identified 6 carriers with *GJB4* p.C169W, revealing an allele frequency of 3.0% (6/200 chromosomes). Therefore, probably *GJB4* p.C169W is a non-pathogenic variant.

Discussion

In the present study, we applied MPS to 12 multiplex families with idiopathic SNHI. We identified 5 variants in 5 different genes, which might have led to SNHI in 6 families compatible with autosomal dominant inheritance, including *GJB2* p.R75Q, *MYO7A* p.T381M, *KCNQ4* p.S680F, *MYH9* p.E1256K, and *GJB4* p.C169W (Figure 6). Four variants were classified as pathogenic variants, including 2 known variants (*GJB2* p.R75Q and *MYO7A* p.T381M) and 2 novel variants (*KCNQ4* p.S680F and *MYH9* p.E1256K). The remaining variant, *GJB4* p.C169W, was classified as a probable non-causative variant, as its allele frequency was as high as ~3% in the general population.

Among the deafness-associated genes identified thus far, mutations in *GJB2* are the most common cause of monogenic hearing impairment worldwide. *GJB2* encodes a gap junction protein, connexin 26, and the major function of connexin 26 in the inner ear is to regulate potassium recycling [30]. To date, 2 mutations at the p.R75 amino acid residue of connexin 26 have been related to autosomal dominant SNHI with or without palmoplantar keratoderma: p.R75W [31,32] and p.R75Q [26,27]. *GJB2* p.R75Q was identified in 1 Turkish and 2 French families, with the severity of hearing loss ranging from mild to profound SNHI in the affected individuals [26,27]. We failed to detect p.R75Q in our first pass of mutation screening using the SNaPshot multiplex assays, as p.R75Q was not included in the screening panels because it had never been detected in our previous genetic epidemiological survey [8].

Another known causative variant identified in the present study is *MYO7A* p.T381M. The human *MYO7A* gene consists of 48 coding exons, and encodes the unconventional myosin MYO7A with 2,215 amino acids [33]. Different *MYO7A* mutations might lead to a wide variety of phenotypes with different inheritance patterns, ranging from Usher syndrome type 1B [34], autosomal recessive nonsyndromic hearing loss (ARNSHL) (DFNB2) [33,35], to ADNSHL (DFNA11) [36]. *MYO7A* p.T381M is located in the MYO7A motor head domain, and the previously reported 3 unrelated Han Chinese patients who segregated 1 allele of *MYO7A* p.T381M revealed nonsyndromic severe-to-profound SNHI [28].

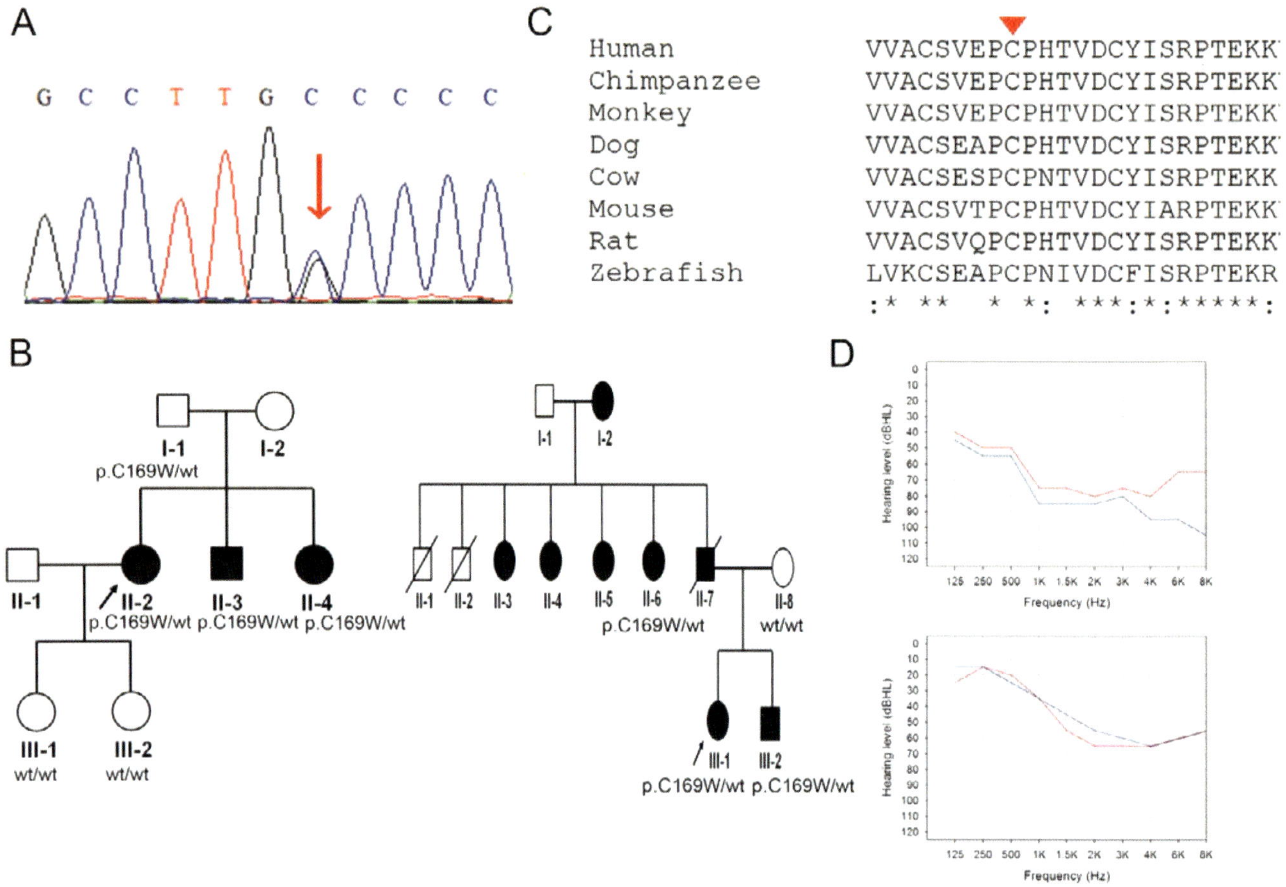

Figure 5. Probable non-causative *GJB4* p.C169W variant identified in Family DE2827 and Family DE3281. (A) Sanger sequence of the *GJB4* p.C169W variant. Arrow: nucleotide change c.507C>G (p.C169W) variant. (B) Pedigree and segregation patterns of Family DE2827 and Family DE3281. (C) Evolutionary conservation of the p.C169 residue. Arrowhead: variant site. (D) Audiograms of the probands of Family DE2827 (upper panel) and Family DE3281 (lower panel). Hearing levels of the right ear and left ear are marked with red and blue lines, respectively.

Together with the results of this study, it is likely that *MYO7A* p.T381M is associated with ADNSHL.

In addition to the 2 known causative variants, we identified 2 novel variants, i.e., *KCNQ4* p.S680F and *MYH9* p.E1256K, in 2 families, respectively. The *KCNQ4* gene, which encodes the voltage-gated potassium channel KCNQ4 in outer hair cells, has been identified at the ADNSHL DFNA2 locus on the human chromosome 1p34 [37]. To date, 11 missense mutations, 1 nonsense mutation, and 2 deletion mutations of the *KCNQ4* gene have been documented in DFNA2 patients with various clinical phenotypes (The Deafness Variation Database: http://deafnessvariationdatabase.org) [38]. *KCNQ4* p.S680F is located at the cytoplasmic C terminus and contributes to progressive SNHI in the affected members of Family DE2675. The *MYH9* gene encodes myosin IIA heavy chain, which is involved in actomyosin-microtubule crosstalk, cell motility, and maintenance of cell shape [39]. Defects in *MYH9* have been associated with ADNSHL DFNA17 [40], as well as a plethora of autosomal dominant syndromes with hematologic and/or renal manifestations in addition to progressive SNHI [41]. As none of the affected members in Family DE2721 demonstrated symptoms other than SNHI, the p.E1256K variant might lead to nonsyndromic SNHI only.

The *GJB4* p.C169W variant was detected in 2 other autosomal dominant families. *GJB4* p.C169W fulfilled most criteria used for data filtering in the present study, including allele frequency <5% in the general population, high PolyPhen2 and SIFT scores, and evolutionary conservation of p.C169 amino acid residues. It is important to note, that the allele frequency of *GJB4* p.C169W is approximately 3% in the general population, which is, to some extent, higher than the convention definition of a mutation, i.e., the allele frequency of a mutation should be less than 1% [42]. It has been demonstrated that the allele frequencies of several common deafness mutations are higher than 1% in the general population, e.g., *GJB2* p.V37I (~10% in some East Asian general populations) [43,44], c.235delC (~1.5% in the Chinese general population) [45], and c.35delG (~1.3% in the European general population) [46]. However, all these mutations are recessive. As such, it is unlikely that *GJB4* p.C169W leads to ADNSHL given its high allele frequency in the population. However, there might be hypothetical possibility that this variant indeed contributes to SNHI through "autosomal dominant but low penetrance" or "oligogenic" inheritance pattern; we therefore still presented the results in this paper for the sake of completeness.

In addition to the 2 families with *GJB4* p.C169W, we were not able to obtain a genetic diagnosis in the other 4 ADNSHL families and the 2 ARNSHL families using the current MPS panel (Figure 6), although many affected members strongly suggest a genetic cause of deafness in these families. As the MPS diagnostic panel of the present study only targeted the coding sequences and

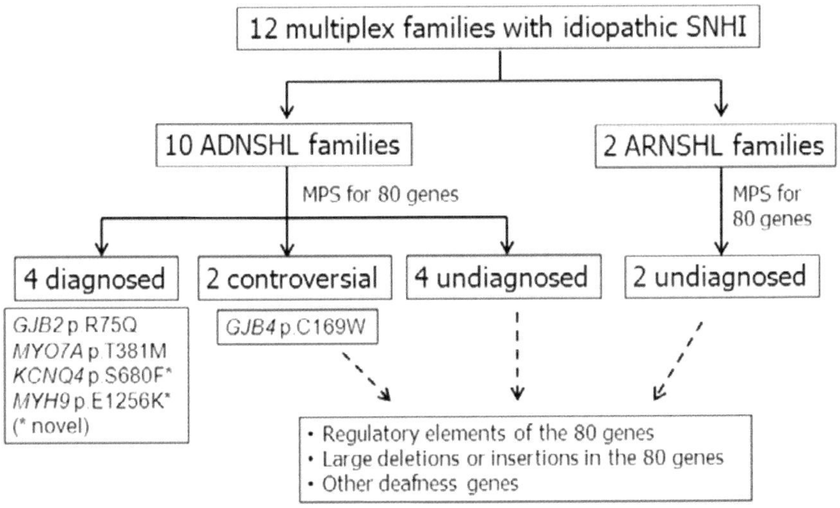

Figure 6. Summary of the genetic diagnostic results obtained in the present study. Twelve multiplex families with idiopathic SNHI, including 10 ADNSHL and 2 ARNSHL families, were subjected to MPS for 80 known human deafness genes. Four out of 10 ADNSHL families were diagnosed to segregate causative variants, including *GJB2* p.R75Q, *MYO7A* p.T381M, *KCNQ4* p.S680F, and *MYH9* p.E1256K. The *GJB4* p.C169W variant of controversial pathogenicity was identified in another two ADNSHL families. In addition to the 2 families with *GJB4* p.C169W, we were unable to achieve a genetic diagnosis in the other 4 ADNSHL families and the 2 ARNSHL families. The cause of SNHI in these undiagnosed families might be attributed to genetic defects in the regulatory elements of the 80 genes, large deletions or insertions of >100 bp in the 80 genes, or even other deafness genes. SNHI, sensorineural hearing impairment; ADNSHL, autosomal dominant nonsyndromic hearing loss; ARNSHL, autosomal recessive nonsyndromic hearing loss; MPS, massively parallel sequencing.

splicing sites of known deafness genes, genetic defects in regulatory elements, e.g., un-translated regions (UTRs), enhancers, promoters, and intronic splicing regulatory elements, could not be examined. Large deletions or insertions of >100 bp, as well as inversions, might also be missed because of the short average read length of the Illumina platform used in our MPS diagnostic panel. Another possibility is that deafness in these families might be caused by mutations in genes other than the 80 known deafness genes targeted in the present study. For the latter possibility, whole exome sequencing might be helpful in identifying novel deafness genes in the future.

The MPS technology, via targeted sequencing of whole exomes [47] or specific chromosomal regions confined by linkage analysis and homozygosity mapping [48], has been proven to be a powerful tool for discovering novel deafness genes (for a detailed review, please refer to [49]). In addition to gene discovery, the

Table 3. Summary of the 5 Series Investigating the Diagnostic Utility of MPS.

Reference	Targeted regions	Subjects enrolled for MPS	Main results
Shearer *et al.*	54 known deafness genes in humans; exons and 50 bp flanking introns	3 positive controls with mutations detected previously by Sanger sequencing and 6 patients with idiopathic SNHI. The 6 idiopathic SNHI patients included 4 with ADNSHL and 2 with ARNSHL. [ethnicity: NA]	Causative mutations were confirmed in the 3 positive controls. Pathogenic mutations were identified in 5 of the 6 idiopathic SNHI patients, including 3 novel mutations. Genetic diagnosis remained elusive in an ADNSHL patient.
Brownstein *et al.*	246 genes responsible for deafness in humans (85 genes) and mice (161 genes); exons and 40 bp flanking introns	11 unrelated families with idiopathic SNHI, including 2 with ADNSHL and 9 with ARNSHL. [ethnicity: 5 Israeli Jewish and 6 Palestinian Arab]	Pathogenic mutations were identified in 2 ADNSHL and 4 ARNSHL families, including 4 novel mutations. Genetic diagnosis could be achieved in all 5 Jewish families, but in only 1 Palestinian family.
Tang *et al.*	5 selected known deafness genes in humans; exons and 50 bp flanking introns	10 positive controls previously detected to have mutations in *GJB2* by Sanger sequencing. [ethnicity: NA]	Causative *GJB2* mutations were confirmed in the positive controls, and additional variants in other selected targeted genes were identified.
De Keulenaer *et al.*	15 ARNSHL genes in humans; exons and most of the UTRs	1 positive control and 3 ARNSHL families (4 individuals). [ethnicity: the 3 ARNSHL families included 2 Iranian and 1 Turkish]	The causative mutation was confirmed in the positive control. Pathogenic mutations were identified in 2 ARNSHL families, including 2 novel mutations.
This study	80 known deafness genes in humans; exons and 100 bp flanking introns	12 multiplex families with idiopathic SNHI, including 10 with ADNSHL and 2 with ARNSHL. [ethnicity: all Han Chinese]	Causative variants were identified in 4 ADNSHL families, including 2 novel variants.

MPS, massively parallel sequencing; SNHI, sensorineural hearing impairment; ADNSHL, autosomal dominant nonsyndromic hearing loss; ARNSHL, autosomal recessive nonsyndromic hearing loss; NA, not available; UTR, untranslated region.

diagnostic utility of MPS in addressing genetically heterogeneous nonsyndromic hearing loss has also been examined in several studies (Table 3). Shearer *et al.* performed targeted capture of 54 known deafness genes in 9 individuals, including 3 positive controls with mutations detected previously and 6 patients with idiopathic SNHI. Causative mutations were confirmed in all 3 positive controls, and genetic diagnosis was achieved in 5 of the 6 idiopathic SNHI patients [12]. Brownstein *et al.* developed a targeted capture pool composed of 246 deafness genes (85 human and 161 mouse genes), and applied it to 11 unrelated families with idiopathic SNHI, including 2 with ADNSHL and 9 with ARNSHL. They established genetic diagnosis in 2 ADNSHL and 4 ARNSHL families, and identified 4 novel mutations. Interestingly, a genetic diagnosis was made in all 5 Jewish families, but in only 1 of the 6 Palestinian families. A possible explanation for the difference in the diagnostic yield between populations, as proposed by the authors, is that inherited hearing loss in the Palestinian population is more heterogeneous than in the Israeli population because of historical marriage patterns [13]. Tang *et al.* selected 5 known deafness genes to test the diagnostic efficacy of MPS in 10 positive controls previously identified to have *GJB2* mutations by Sanger sequencing. They successfully confirmed the causative mutations in all positive controls and detected additional variants in the other selected genes [50]. De Keulenaer *et al.* screened 15 ARNSHL genes in 1 positive control and 3 ARNSHL families with MPS and identified a pathogenic mutation in 2 ARNSHL families of Iranian ancestry [51]. In the present study, we performed targeted capture of 80 known deafness genes in 10 ADNSHL and 2 ARNSHL families and identified causative variants in 4 ADNSHL families. In summary, MPS accurately detected causative mutations in the positive controls in these series and facilitated the genetic diagnosis in a certain proportion of idiopathic SNHI families. However, the diagnostic yield of MPS may depend on several factors, including the number of targeted genes, the MPS platform used, the inheritance pattern, and the ethnic background of the families tested.

In conclusion, by applying the MPS diagnostic panel targeting 80 deafness genes to 12 multiplex Han Chinese families with idiopathic nonsyndromic SNHI, we identified 4 variants in 4 different genes, which might have led to SNHI in 4 families compatible with autosomal dominant inheritance, including *GJB2* p.R75Q, *MYO7A* p.T381M, *KCNQ4* p.S680F, and *MYH9* p.E1256K. Among them, *KCNQ4* p.S680F and *MYH9* p.E1256K are novel variants. Thus, MPS enables genetic diagnosis in multiplex families with idiopathic SNHI by detecting mutations in relatively uncommon deafness genes.

Supporting Information

Figure S1 The pedigrees of the 12 multiplex families recruited in the present study. Families compatible with autosomal dominant inheritance and autosomal recessive inheritance are marked with AD and AR, respectively. Arrows indicate the probands.

Table S1 The 80 known human deafness genes included in DA1.

Author Contributions

Conceived and designed the experiments: CCW CJH PJC PLC. Performed the experiments: YHL YCL. Analyzed the data: PLC YHL. Contributed reagents/materials/analysis tools: YHL YCL. Wrote the paper: CCW WSY PJC PLC.

References

1. Morton CC, Nance WE (2006) Newborn hearing screening a silent revolution. N Engl J Med 354: 2151–2164.
2. Smith RJ, Bale JF Jr, White KR (2005) Sensorineural hearing loss in children. Lancet 365: 879–890.
3. Wu CC, Lee YC, Chen PJ, Hsu CJ (2008) Predominance of genetic diagnosis and imaging results as predictors in determining the speech perception performance outcome after cochlear implantation in children. Arch Pediatr Adolesc Med 162: 269–276.
4. Wu CC, Liu TC, Wang SH, Hsu CJ, Wu CM (2011) Genetic characteristics in children with cochlear implants and the corresponding auditory performance. Laryngoscope 121: 1287–1293.
5. Wu CC, Lin SY, Su YN, Fang MY, Chen SU, et al. (2010) Preimplantation genetic diagnosis (embryo screening) for enlarged vestibular aqueduct due to SLC26A4 mutation. Audiol Neurootol 15: 311–317.
6. Hamasaki K, Rando RR (1997) Specific binding of aminoglycosides to a human rRNA construct based on a DNA polymorphism which causes aminoglycoside-induced deafness. Biochemistry 36: 12323–12328.
7. Hilgert N, Smith RJ, Van Camp G (2009) Forty-six genes causing nonsyndromic hearing impairment: which ones should be analyzed in DNA diagnostics? Mutat Res 681: 189–196.
8. Wu CC, Chen PJ, Chiu YH, Lu YC, Wu MC, et al. (2008) Prospective mutation screening of three common deafness genes in a large Taiwanese Cohort with idiopathic bilateral sensorineural hearing impairment reveals a difference in the results between families from hospitals and those from rehabilitation facilities. Audiol Neurootol 13: 172–181.
9. Simpson DA, Clark GR, Alexander S, Silvestri G, Willoughby CE (2011) Molecular diagnosis for heterogeneous genetic diseases with targeted high-throughput DNA sequencing applied to retinitis pigmentosa. J Med Genet 48: 145–151.
10. Morgan JE, Carr IM, Sheridan E, Chu CE, Hayward B, et al. (2010) Genetic diagnosis of familial breast cancer using clonal sequencing. Hum Mutat 31: 484–491.
11. Meder B, Haas J, Keller A, Heid C, Just S, et al. (2011) Targeted next-generation sequencing for the molecular genetic diagnostics of cardiomyopathies. Circ Cardiovasc Genet 4: 110–122.
12. Shearer AE, Deluca AP, Hildebrand MS, Taylor KR, Gurrola J Jr, et al. (2010) Comprehensive genetic testing for hereditary hearing loss using massively parallel sequencing. Proc Natl Acad Sci U S A 107: 21104–21109.
13. Brownstein Z, Friedman LM, Shahin H, Oron-Karni V, Kol N, et al. (2011) Targeted genomic capture and massively parallel sequencing to identify genes for hereditary hearing loss in middle eastern families. Genome Biol 12: R89.
14. Wu CC, Lu YC, Chen PJ, Liu AY, Hwu WL, et al. (2009) Application of SNaPshot multiplex assays for simultaneous multigene mutation screening in patients with idiopathic sensorineural hearing impairment. Laryngoscope 119: 2411–2416.
15. Wu CC, Chen YS, Chen PJ, Hsu CJ (2005) Common clinical features of children with enlarged vestibular aqueduct and Mondini dysplasia. Laryngoscope 115: 132–137.
16. Li H, Durbin R (2009) Fast and accurate short read alignment with Burrows-Wheeler transform. Bioinformatics 25: 1754–1760.
17. Li H, Handsaker B, Wysoker A, Fennell T, Ruan J, et al. (2009) The Sequence Alignment/Map format and SAMtools. Bioinformatics 25: 2078–2079.
18. McKenna A, Hanna M, Banks E, Sivachenko A, Cibulskis K, et al. (2010) The Genome Analysis Toolkit: a MapReduce framework for analyzing next-generation DNA sequencing data. Genome Res 20: 1297–1303.
19. DePristo MA, Banks E, Poplin R, Garimella KV, Maguire JR, et al. (2011) A framework for variation discovery and genotyping using next-generation DNA sequencing data. Nat Genet 43: 491–498.
20. San Lucas FA, Wang G, Scheet P, Peng B (2012) Integrated annotation and analysis of genetic variants from next-generation sequencing studies with variant tools. Bioinformatics 28: 421–422.
21. Wang K, Li M, Hakonarson H (2010) ANNOVAR: functional annotation of genetic variants from high-throughput sequencing data. Nucleic Acids Res 38: e164.
22. Kumar P, Henikoff S, Ng PC (2009) Predicting the effects of coding non-synonymous variants on protein function using the SIFT algorithm. Nat Protoc 4: 1073–1081.
23. Adzhubei IA, Schmidt S, Peshkin L, Ramensky VE, Gerasimova A, et al. (2010) A method and server for predicting damaging missense mutations. Nat Methods 7: 248–249.
24. Robinson JT, Thorvaldsdottir H, Winckler W, Guttman M, Lander ES, et al. (2011) Integrative genomics viewer. Nat Biotechnol 29: 24–26.

25. Thorvaldsdottir H, Robinson JT, Mesirov JP (2012) Integrative Genomics Viewer (IGV): high-performance genomics data visualization and exploration. Brief Bioinform.
26. Feldmann D, Denoyelle F, Blons H, Lyonnet S, Loundon N, et al. (2005) The GJB2 mutation R75Q can cause nonsyndromic hearing loss DFNA3 or hereditary palmoplantar keratoderma with deafness. Am J Med Genet A 137: 225-227.
27. Uyguner O, Tukel T, Baykal C, Eris H, Emiroglu M, et al. (2002) The novel R75Q mutation in the GJB2 gene causes autosomal dominant hearing loss and palmoplantar keratoderma in a Turkish family. Clin Genet 62: 306-309.
28. Su MC, Yang JJ, Su CC, Hsin CH, Li SY (2009) Identification of novel variants in the Myosin VIIA gene of patients with nonsyndromic hearing loss from Taiwan. Int J Pediatr Otorhinolaryngol 73: 811-815.
29. Yang JJ, Wang WH, Lin YC, Weng HH, Yang JT, et al. (2010) Prospective variants screening of connexin genes in children with hearing impairment: genotype/phenotype correlation. Hum Genet 128: 303-313.
30. Kikuchi T, Kimura RS, Paul DL, Takasaka T, Adams JC (2000) Gap junction systems in the mammalian cochlea. Brain Res Brain Res Rev 32: 163-166.
31. Richard G, White TW, Smith LE, Bailey RA, Compton JG, et al. (1998) Functional defects of Cx26 resulting from a heterozygous missense mutation in a family with dominant deaf-mutism and palmoplantar keratoderma. Hum Genet 103: 393-399.
32. Janecke AR, Nekahm D, Loffler J, Hirst-Stadlmann A, Muller T, et al. (2001) De novo mutation of the connexin 26 gene associated with dominant non-syndromic sensorineural hearing loss. Hum Genet 108: 269-270.
33. Weil D, Kussel P, Blanchard S, Levy G, Levi-Acobas F, et al. (1997) The autosomal recessive isolated deafness, DFNB2, and the Usher 1B syndrome are allelic defects of the myosin-VIIA gene. Nat Genet 16: 191-193.
34. Weil D, Blanchard S, Kaplan J, Guilford P, Gibson F, et al. (1995) Defective myosin VIIA gene responsible for Usher syndrome type 1B. Nature 374: 60-61.
35. Liu XZ, Walsh J, Mburu P, Kendrick-Jones J, Cope MJ, et al. (1997) Mutations in the myosin VIIA gene cause non-syndromic recessive deafness. Nat Genet 16: 188-190.
36. Liu XZ, Walsh J, Tamagawa Y, Kitamura K, Nishizawa M, et al. (1997) Autosomal dominant non-syndromic deafness caused by a mutation in the myosin VIIA gene. Nat Genet 17: 268-269.
37. Kubisch C, Schroeder BC, Friedrich T, Lutjohann B, El-Amraoui A, et al. (1999) KCNQ4, a novel potassium channel expressed in sensory outer hair cells, is mutated in dominant deafness. Cell 96: 437-446.
38. Nie L (2008) KCNQ4 mutations associated with nonsyndromic progressive sensorineural hearing loss. Curr Opin Otolaryngol Head Neck Surg 16: 441-444.
39. Even-Ram S, Yamada KM (2007) Of Mice and Men: Relevance of Cellular and Molecular Characterizations of Myosin IIA to MYH9-Related Human Disease. Cell Adhesion & Migration 1: 152-155.
40. Lalwani AK, Goldstein JA, Kelley MJ, Luxford W, Castelein CM, et al. (2000) Human nonsyndromic hereditary deafness DFNA17 is due to a mutation in nonmuscle myosin MYH9. Am J Hum Genet 67: 1121-1128.
41. Seri M, Pecci A, Di Bari F, Cusano R, Savino M, et al. (2003) MYH9-related disease: May-Hegglin anomaly, Sebastian syndrome, Fechtner syndrome, and Epstein syndrome are not distinct entities but represent a variable expression of a single illness. Medicine (Baltimore) 82: 203-215.
42. Harris H, Hopkinson DA, Luffman J (1968) Enzyme diversity in human populations. Ann N Y Acad Sci 151: 232-242.
43. Hwa HL, Ko TM, Hsu CJ, Huang CH, Chiang YL, et al. (2003) Mutation spectrum of the connexin 26 (GJB2) gene in Taiwanese patients with prelingual deafness. Genet Med 5: 161-165.
44. Wattanasirichaigoon D, Limwongse C, Jariengprasert C, Yenchitsomanus PT, Tocharoenthanaphol C, et al. (2004) High prevalence of V37I genetic variant in the connexin-26 (GJB2) gene among non-syndromic hearing-impaired and control Thai individuals. Clin Genet 66: 452-460.
45. Dai P, Yu F, Han B, Liu X, Wang G, et al. (2009) GJB2 mutation spectrum in 2,063 Chinese patients with nonsyndromic hearing impairment. J Transl Med 7: 26.
46. Van Eyken E, Van Laer L, Fransen E, Topsakal V, Hendrickx JJ, et al. (2007) The contribution of GJB2 (Connexin 26) 35delG to age-related hearing impairment and noise-induced hearing loss. Otol Neurotol 28: 970-975.
47. Rehman AU, Morell RJ, Belyantseva IA, Khan SY, Boger ET, et al. (2010) Targeted capture and next-generation sequencing identifies C9orf75, encoding taperin, as the mutated gene in nonsyndromic deafness DFNB79. Am J Hum Genet 86: 378-388.
48. Walsh T, Shahin H, Elkan-Miller T, Lee MK, Thornton AM, et al. (2010) Whole exome sequencing and homozygosity mapping identify mutation in the cell polarity protein GPSM2 as the cause of nonsyndromic hearing loss DFNB82. Am J Hum Genet 87: 90-94.
49. Brownstein Z, Bhonker Y, Avraham KB (2012) High-throughput sequencing to decipher the genetic heterogeneity of deafness. Genome Biol 13: 245.
50. Tang W, Qian D, Ahmad S, Mattox D, Todd NW, et al. (2012) A low-cost exon capture method suitable for large-scale screening of genetic deafness by the massively-parallel sequencing approach. Genet Test Mol Biomarkers 16: 536-542.
51. De Keulenaer S, Hellemans J, Lefever S, Renard JP, De Schrijver J, et al. (2012) Molecular diagnostics for congenital hearing loss including 15 deafness genes using a next generation sequencing platform. BMC Med Genomics 5: 17.

8

Trauma-Associated Tinnitus: Audiological, Demographic and Clinical Characteristics

Peter M. Kreuzer[1]*, Michael Landgrebe[1,2], Martin Schecklmann[1], Susanne Staudinger[1], Berthold Langguth[1], The TRI Database Study Group[¶]

1 Department of Psychiatry and Psychotherapy, University of Regensburg, Regensburg, Germany, 2 Department of Psychiatry, Psychosomatic Medicine and Psychotherapy, Sozialstiftung Bamberg, Bamberg, Germany

Abstract

Background: Tinnitus can result from different etiologies. Frequently, patients report the development of tinnitus after traumatic injuries. However, to which extent this specific etiologic factor plays a role for the phenomenology of tinnitus is still incompletely understood. Additionally, it remains a matter of debate whether the etiology of tinnitus constitutes a relevant criterion for defining tinnitus subtypes.

Objective: By investigating a worldwide sample of tinnitus patients derived from the Tinnitus Research Initiative (TRI) Database, we aimed to identify differences in demographic, clinical and audiological characteristics between tinnitus patients with and without preceding trauma.

Materials: A total of 1,604 patients were investigated. Assessment included demographic data, tinnitus related clinical data, audiological data, the Tinnitus Handicap Inventory, the Tinnitus Questionnaire, the Beck Depression Inventory, various numeric tinnitus rating scales, and the World Health Organisation Quality of Life Scale (WHOQoL).

Results: Our data clearly indicate differences between tinnitus patients with and without trauma at tinnitus onset. Patients suffering from trauma-associated tinnitus suffer from a higher mental burden than tinnitus patients presenting with phantom perceptions based on other or unknown etiologic factors. This is especially the case for patients with whiplash and head trauma. Patients with posttraumatic noise-related tinnitus experience more frequently hyperacousis, were younger, had longer tinnitus duration, and were more frequently of male gender.

Conclusions: Trauma before tinnitus onset seems to represent a relevant criterion for subtypization of tinnitus. Patients with posttraumatic tinnitus may require specific diagnostic and therapeutic management. A more systematic and – at best - standardized assessment for hearing related sequelae of trauma is needed for a better understanding of the underlying pathophysiology and for developing more tailored treatment approaches as well.

Editor: Xi (Erick) Lin, Emory Univ. School of Medicine, United States of America

Funding: The study was supported by the Tinnitus Research Initiative/TRI (www.tinnitusresearch.org). All authors confirm no conflicts of interest in regard to the manuscript. The funders had no role in study design, data collection and analysis, decision to publish, or preparation of the manuscript.

Competing Interests: The authors have declared that no competing interests exist.

* E-mail: peter.kreuzer@medbo.de

¶ Membership of The TRI Database Study Group is provided in the Acknowledgments

Introduction

Each year, approximately 1–2 million people experience a traumatic brain injury (= TBI) in the United States [1,2]. Apart from that, TBI is found among the most common war related injuries due to blast and concussion [3]. Recent studies revealed that 15.8% of service members in the Iraq war experienced traumatic brain injury [4,5], in combat team samples an even higher prevalence ranging up to 22.8% was reported [6].

Trauma to the head – especially to the ear – is often associated with tinnitus [7], defined as an intermittent or constant sound sensation which cannot be attributed to an external sound source. In military personnel with TBI up to 38% reported comorbid tinnitus complaints [8]. A random sample of the Iraq war records revealed that 71% of soldiers experienced loud noises and that 15.6% had tinnitus [9,10]. According to the American Tinnitus Association 3 to 4 million veterans suffer from tinnitus and compensation payments for combat related hearing loss [10] and tinnitus account for approximately US$ 1.2 billion per year [11]. But also in civil populations acoustic trauma is among the most frequently reported triggers for the development of chronic tinnitus [12,13].

Notably, many different types of trauma can precede tinnitus onset. Noise trauma typically causes damage to the inner ear, and as a consequence leads to tinnitus [14]. Brain injuries can cause a variety of auditory symptoms such as hearing loss, tinnitus, and central deficits indicating the vulnerability of the auditory pathways to traumatic injury [15]. Moreover, also neck [16] injuries and emotional trauma [17,18] are well known triggers of tinnitus [19,20]. Therefore, we investigated the categories "noise trauma", "whiplash", and "head trauma", and its combinations with regard to a large sample of tinnitus patients presenting in specialized tinnitus centers worldwide. The term "post-traumatic" or "trauma-associated" as mentioned in the present manuscript does not refer to the psychological aspects of trauma in the sense of "posttraumatic stress (disorder)". It is rather applied to subsume the trauma categories "noise trauma", "whiplash", and "head trauma" (without further specification of its extent).

Tinnitus can vary in its phenomenological characteristics and in the amount of the related distress. It can cause severe distress on individuals and it has been shown to be correlated with sleeping disorders [21], depression [18,22] and anxiety [23,24,25,26,27,28,29,30]. It may affect the individual's concentration and ability for attentional focusing and working memory [31,32]. Development of tinnitus may even end up in suicidal attempts [33,34,35,36]. Perceptual characteristics such as tinnitus loudness [37] or tinnitus frequency [38] only explain to a small extent the amount of tinnitus suffering. Other relevant factors include age at onset [39], personality factors [40] and coping behavior [41]. It has also been proposed that etiologic factors such as head and neck injuries related to tinnitus onset may exert an influence on the amount of tinnitus complaints [16].

In order to find out whether trauma and especially the different types of trauma at tinnitus onset are of relevance for perceptual, demographic and clinical characteristics of tinnitus a large worldwide sample of patients presenting at specialized tinnitus clinics has been investigated. The main objectives were to 1) to determine the percentage of cases of chronic tinnitus related to different types of trauma; 2) to describe the characteristics of these population and 3) to compare these characteristics with tinnitus patients whose tinnitus onset was not associated with trauma.

Materials and Methods

The data presented in this study derive from the Tinnitus Research Initiative Database [42]. Data management was conducted according to the Data Handling Plan (TRI-DHP V07, May 9th, 2011). Data analysis was conducted according to the Standard Operating Procedure (TRI-SA V01, May 9th, 2011), thereby following a study-specific Statistical Analysis Plan (SAP-008, 20/12/2011) that was written according to the SAP template (TRI-SAP V01, May 9th, 2011). All documents can be accessed under http://database.tinnitusresearch.org/. Analysis details can found at the end of this section.

The default dataset import (November 1st, 2011) from the Tinnitus Research Initiative (TRI) Database consisted of 2,184 patients (see figure 1). Patients presented between 2005 and 2011 at different tinnitus centres worldwide (mainly from Brasil and Europe; center specific analysis could not be done due to irregular frequencies for the single trauma types with respect to centres; more detailed information about contributing tinnitus centres can be found at http://database.tinnitusresearch.org/en/map/map_en.php). Patients gave written informed consent to record their data in the database and to perform analyses with the data. The project has been approved by the local ethics committee of the Medical Faculty of the University of Regensburg. The database project is coordinated by the department of psychiatry and psychotherapy of the University of Regensburg, Germany, and the database server is located at the ManaTheam GmbH in Regensburg.

The variable "onset related event" was deduced from the question of the Tinnitus Sample Case History Questionnaire (TSCHQ; 45) "Was the initial onset of your tinnitus related to:" with the pre-formulated answers "loud blast of sound", "whiplash", "change in hearing", "stress", "head trauma", and "other". Patients who did not answer the TSCHQ were excluded from analysis resulting in a sample of 1,604 patients (see figure 1). Patients were grouped according to their self-reported onset related events (see figure 1).

We built the five categories "no trauma", "noise trauma", "whiplash", and "head trauma", and "other tinnitus related onset". If one patient reported multiple events including one single trauma this patient was subsumed to the group of this trauma. Patients with multiple traumata were excluded from primary analysis (n = 23; 1.4%) (see figure 1).

Assessment was performed before the first consultation in the tinnitus clinics and included the Tinnitus Sample Case History Questionnaire (TSCHQ), the Tinnitus Handicap Inventory (THI) [43], the Tinnitus Questionnaire (TQ) [44], the Beck Depression Inventory (BDI) [45], and four domains of the World Health Organisation Quality of Life Scale (WHOQoL). The different domains of the WHOQOL measure 1st "physical health", in particular activities of daily living, dependence on medicinal substances and medical aids, energy and fatigue, mobility, pain and discomfort, sleep and rest, work capacity; 2nd "psychological health", in particular bodily image and appearance, negative/positive feelings, self-esteem, spirituality/religion/personal beliefs, thinking, learning, memory and concentration; 3rd "social relationships", in particular personal relationships, social support, sexual activity; and 4th "environmental factors", in particular financial resources, freedom, physical safety and security, health and social care, home environment, opportunities for acquiring new information and skills, opportunities for recreation, physical environment, and transport [46].

Subjectively perceived loudness, discomfort, annoyance, ignorability, and unpleasantness were assessed by numeric rating scales (range: 0–10).

In addition to these variables, we were interested in the demographic characteristics age, gender and age at tinnitus onset. Furthermore, we investigated the tinnitus duration until presentation at our clinic, the way of onset (gradual/abrupt), number of preceding treatments until presentation, tinnitus characteristics such as pulsatile or non-pulsatile sound perception, tonal or noise-like tinnitus, the possibility of masking the tinnitus by music or sounds and the ability of modulating the tinnitus by somatic manoeuvres. Comorbid symptoms of tinnitus such as headaches, vertigo/dizziness, temporomandibular disorders, neck pain or other pain symptoms were asked for. Hyperacousis was checked by the following TSCHQ-items (number 28 and 29): a) "Do you have a problem tolerating sounds because they often seem much too loud? That is, do you often find too loud or hurtful sounds which other people around you find quite comfortable?" with the predetermined response possibilities "never/rarely/sometimes/usually/always" and b) "Do sounds cause you pain or physical discomfort? "yes/no/I don't know".

In addition, current psychiatric treatment was assessed. The mean hearing level (dB hearing level (pure tone audiogram) over eight frequencies (0.125/0.250/0.500/1/2/4/6/8 kHz) of both ears was documented and averaged."

If no data were available at the screening visit (first consultation), we used data from the baseline visit of a clinical intervention. If both screening and baseline data were available we used the mean of both time points. For statistical analyses we used analyses of variance (ANOVAs) for continuous variables (e.g., age) and chi-square-tests for categorical variables (e.g., gender) with the variable onset (no trauma/noise/whiplash/head/other) as group variable (table 1). Significance threshold was set to a Bonferroni corrected

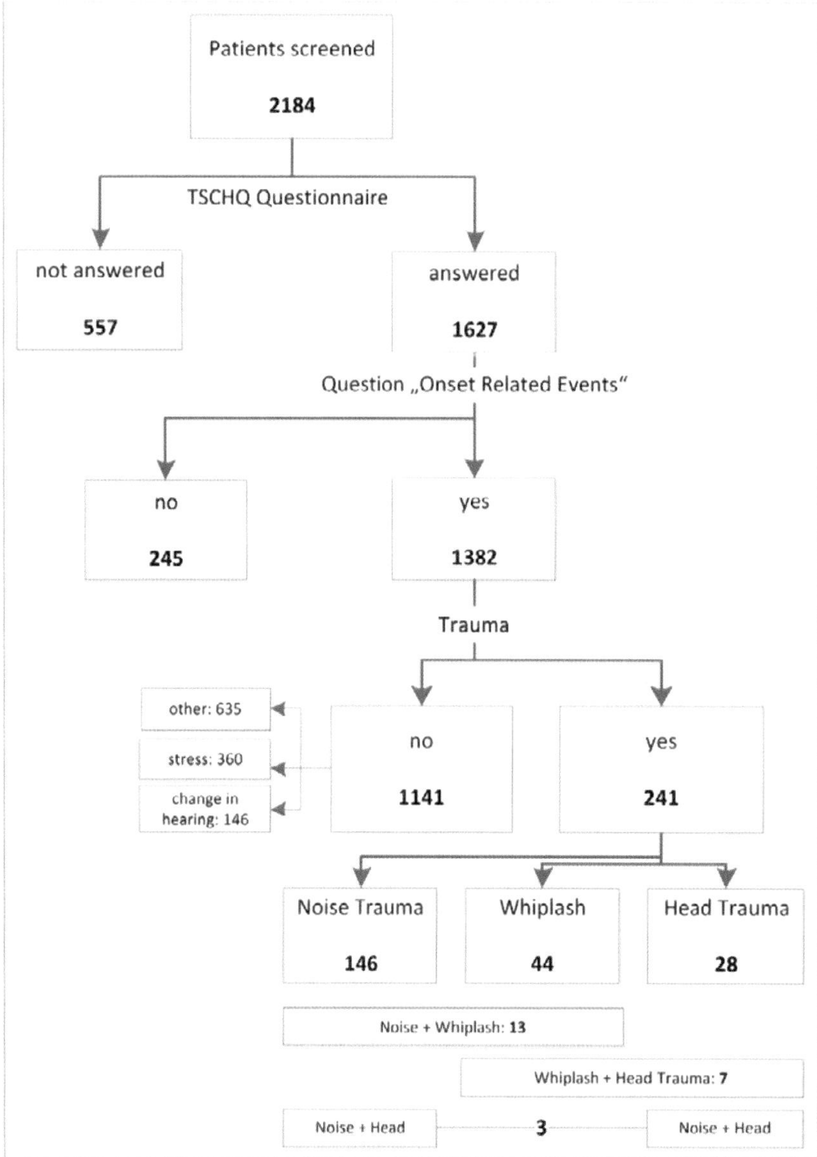

Figure 1. Patients' flowchart, data provided in absolute numbers.

level of 0.0016 (0.0016 = 0.05/31 included variables). In case of significant results in the ANOVA, post-hoc tests were performed by using t-tests for continuous variables and using z-standardized residuals of the frequencies of the single cells of the chi-square-tests for categorical variables. These post-hoc tests are displayed graphically (figure 2 to 5). For post-hoc tests significance threshold was set to an uncorrected level of 0.05.

Results

A total of 1,604 patients answered the TSCHQ-Question concerning onset-related events thus providing a self-report of possible triggering factors of the phantom perception. 241 individuals reported a trauma-associated tinnitus onset. 146 reported a history of noise trauma, 44 a history of whiplash, and 28 a history of head trauma as an *isolated* trigger for their tinnitus. Detailed information is given in figure 1.

We found significant group effects for the variables age at presentation, age at onset, gender, tinnitus duration, vertigo/dizziness, neck pain, other pain symptoms, current psychiatric treatment, TQ, THI, BDI, WHOQOL domain 1 and 4, and both hyperacousis-questions regarding "sound toleration" and "sounds causing pain and physical discomfort".

Groups did not differ for the variables "number of preceding treatments", "pulsatile vs. non-pulsatile tinnitus character", "tonal/noise-like/cricket-like tinnitus", "maskability", "somatic modulation", "headache", "temporomandibular joint disorders (TMJD)", "hearing level", WHOQOL domains 2 and 3, and the five numeric tinnitus rating scales regarding the aspects "loudness", "discomfort", "annoyance", "ignorability", and "unpleasantness".

As patients with multiple trauma history (n = 23; see figure 1) have been excluded from analysis as described in the methods section of this manuscript, we additionally calculated thirty (as shown in table 1) group contrasts of single trauma cases vs.

Table 1. Sample characteristics and clinical assessment scales (given as mean±standard deviation); significant results after Bonferroni correction for multiple testing are highlighted in bold letters.

	no trauma	noise	whiplash	head	other	F/χ^2	df	p
sample characteristics								
age at presentation	**54.3±13.8**	**49.3±15.1**	**54.4±8.1**	**47.6±14.6**	**52.9±12.8**	**4.589**	**4**	**.001**
age at tinnitus onset	**45.3±15.2**	**36.2±15.3**	**47.4±8.5**	**41.2±16.5**	**44.3±13.6**	**11.820**	**4**	**<.000**
gender (female/male)	**94/151**	**32/114**	**12/32**	**10/18**	**447/693**	**18.606**	**4**	**.001**
tinnitus and audiologic characteristics								
duration in months	**103.7±108.7**	**144.5±135.5**	**75.1±82.7**	**75.6±69.0**	**95.6±104.0**	**7.096**	**4**	**<.000**
preceding treatments	2.61±1.040	2.77±1.159	3.05±1.011	2.54±1.170	2.78±1.052	2.806	4	.042
pulsatile (no/yes with heartbeat/yes other than heartbeat)	196/22/19	115/11/18	32/4/6	22/3/1	899/123/106	5.861	8	.663
tone/noise/crickets/other	120/46/54/19	85/30/18/11	19/8/6/10	14/8/3/3	616/204/210/97	21.432	12	.044
maskable (no/yes)	55/161	22/104	5/30	7/13	244/734	6.750	4	.150
somatic modulation (no/yes)	169/71	97/48	19/23	15/12	751/377	11.626	4	.020
headache (no/yes)	155/81	82/60	21/22	8/17	686/426	14.544	4	.006
vertigo/dizziness (no/yes)	**179/57**	**86/53**	**19/23**	**11/15**	**732/369**	**25.953**	**4**	**<.000**
temporomandibular disorder (no/yes)	196/42	108/34	26/17	15/8	874/237	13.173	4	.010
neck pain (no/yes)	**123/119**	**61/82**	**5/38**	**10/17**	**482/630**	**23.573**	**4**	**<.000**
other pain (no/yes)	**169/70**	**87/57**	**19/22**	**12/16**	**632/465**	**20.258**	**4**	**<.000**
current psychiatric treatment (no/ yes)	**226/17**	**125/20**	**35/8**	**17/10**	**945/180**	**24.156**	**4**	**<.000**
sound tolerance (low/high)	**178/63**	**73/73**	**28/15**	**16/11**	**732/398**	**23.025**	**4**	**<.000**
painful sounds (no/yes)	**133/85**	**49/87**	**11/23**	**9/18**	**441/569**	**31.384**	**4**	**<.000**
hearing level (median HL)	23.2±20.31	21.4±13.38	18.8±11.83	18.7±9.92	20.7±13.51	1.395	4	.233
tinnitus questionnaires								
TQ	**36.2±18.53**	**42.5±18.14**	**49.2±14.74**	**51.8±20.81**	**40.6±17.37**	**7.090**	**4**	**<.000**
THI	**42.8±24.82**	**51.5±23.44**	**55.3±23.70**	**60.7±24.44**	**48.0±22.55**	**6.770**	**4**	**<.000**
BDI	**9.8±8.72**	**11.6±8.07**	**15.4±10.20**	**15.6±9.19**	**11.1±8.56**	**5.733**	**4**	**<.000**
WHOQOL domain 1	**14.7±3.27**	**13.9±3.22**	**12.7±3.51**	**12.5±3.63**	**14.4±2.98**	**4.735**	**4**	**.001**
WHOQOL domain 2	14.2±2.98	13.9±2.52	12.6±2.66	12.6±2.78	14.0±2.74	3.154	4	.014
WHOQOL domain 3	15.0±3.22	13.9±3.03	13.3±3.27	13.5±2.38	14.5±3.17	3.094	4	.015
WHOQOL domain 4	**15.7±2.80**	**15.0±2.56**	**14.7±2.90**	**13.5±3.06**	**15.8±2.37**	**6.487**	**4**	**<.000**
numeric rating scales								
loudness	6.2±2.34	6.4±2.34	6.9±2.16	6.9±2.29	6.4±2.13	1.472	4	.208
discomfort	6.9±2.55	7.0±2.29	7.7±1.94	7.4±2.15	7.0±2.26	1.359	4	.246
annoyance	6.4±2.62	6.5±2.36	7.4±2.05	7.3±2.23	6.6±2.34	2.009	4	.091
ignorability	6.6±2.90	6.6±2.71	7.7±2.03	7.2±2.87	6.7±2.57	1.774	4	.131
unpleasantness	6.5±2.61	6.6±2.45	7.5±1.81	7.2±2.29	6.6±2.37	2.046	4	.086

multiple trauma cases (n = 218; subsuming all patients with noise or head trauma or whiplash) resulting in no significant results (lowest p-values = .017 and.028 (uncorrected for multiple comparisons) for the items "preceding treatment approaches" and tinnitus questionnaire total score, respectively.

Comprehensive information about clinical characteristics, questionnaire ratings and audiological data is given in table 1.

Discussion

Occurrence of Tinnitus Onset Related Traumata

With a percentage of 4.9% (=(44+28+7)/1604; see figure 1) patients suffering from a tinnitus induced by whiplash or head trauma (or a combination) represent only a small subsample in our database derived from several tinnitus centers worldwide participating in the Tinnitus Research Initiative (TRI). In an earlier study, Folmer and Griest reported a prevalence of a history of head and neck trauma in more than 10 percent of the patients presenting in the specialized tinnitus clinic in Portland, Oregon [16]. Vice versa, in the literature there is evidence that tinnitus is found to be highly prevalent in patients with a history of trauma. Flint *et al.* investigated the incidence of persisting auditory and vestibular sequelae in a group of 30 young adults (aged 21–45 years) recovering from traumatic brain injury, that had taken place previously (range 19 months to 27 years). A variety of sequelae to TBI were reported including tinnitus (53%), vestibular dysfunction (83%), abnormal facial sensory symptoms (27%) and intolerance to loud/sudden noises (87%) [19]. Ten (33%) participants demon-

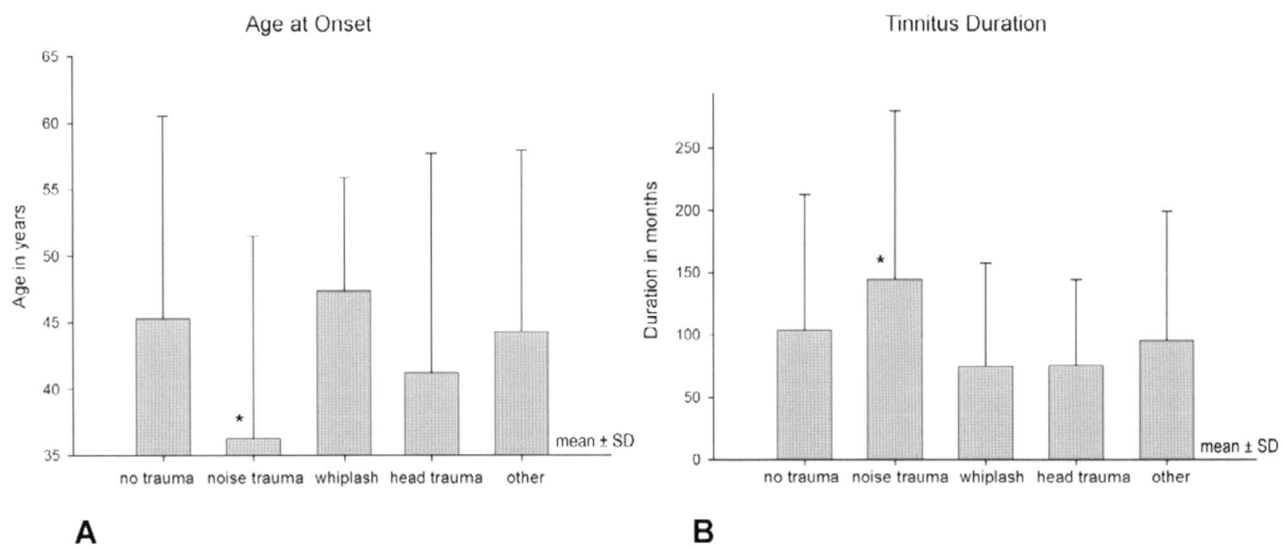

Figure 2. Age at Tinnitus Onset and Tinnitus Duration (mean ± SD). A * Statistically significant between-groups contrasts ($p<0.001$) to groups "no trauma", "whiplash", and "other". **B** * Statistically significant between-groups contrasts ($p<0.005$) to groups "no trauma", "whiplash", "head trauma" and "other".

strated significant sensorineural hearing impairment in addition to speech recognition performance significantly worse than would have been predicted from their hearing impairment [19].

But also in total, given the high prevalence of head, neck and noise trauma and the frequent occurrence of tinnitus after these traumas the rate of reported trauma at tinnitus onset in our sample is very low. Different explanations may account for this finding: a) trauma at tinnitus onset may be underreported by patients especially when there was a delay between trauma and tinnitus onset; b) patients with posttraumatic tinnitus may be preferentially encountered in specific settings such as military medicine or occupational medicine; c) posttraumatic tinnitus might be underestimated by treating physicians with respect to other trauma-related symptoms and therefore these patients might not be referred to tinnitus clinics and be underrepresented in this study population; d) Patients with trauma-associated tinnitus experience tinnitus frequently but rarely present themselves to specialized tinnitus centres because they do not suffer a lot from it compared to other trauma-related impairments; The last explanation is rather unlikely as in our study sample patients with trauma-associated tinnitus showed greater symptom-related burden (see figure 4).

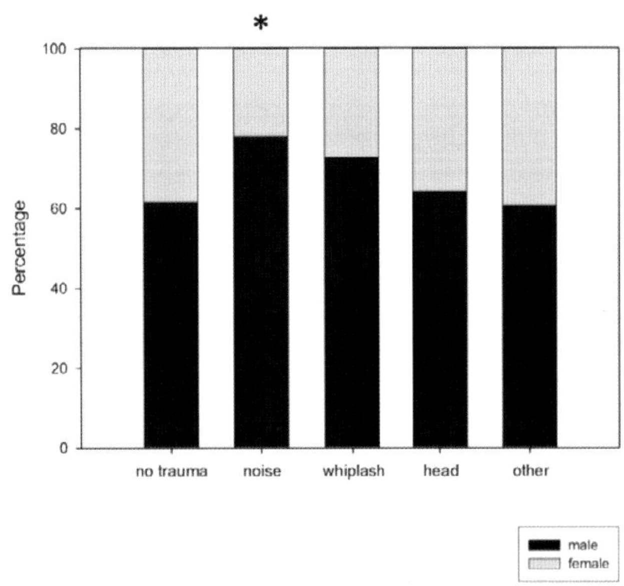

Figure 3. Gender distribution shown in percentage of male/female patients. * Proportion of male patients higher than statistically expected.

We are aware that our study can only provide a vague estimation of the prevalence of trauma preceding tinnitus onset. First, our analyses rely entirely on patients' self reports; secondly even if our sample is large and derives from many centers world-wide it is biased since it reflects the patient population in specialized tinnitus clinics. Therefore, further prospective and population based studies are needed for a more precise estimation of the prevalence of trauma before tinnitus onset.

Summary of the TRI Database Findings

Posttraumatic tinnitus was associated with higher distress levels reflected by higher scores in TQ, THI, BDI, and WHOQoL subscores 1 and 4 as compared to tinnitus patients without trauma at tinnitus onset. These findings reached statistical significance for whiplash and head trauma (TQ, THI, BDI, WHOQOL Dom1 and Dom4) (see figures 4 and 5). This is in line with the findings of the study of Folmer and Griest, who reported both higher Tinnitus Severity Index Scores. However, these authors found also more pronounced tinnitus loudness (measured by 1-to-10 scales and tinnitus matching) in patients suffering from trauma-associated tinnitus [16]. Whereas, our data did not show any effects in tinnitus ratings as elicited by numeric rating scales. In addition, these patients reported greater difficulties with concentration, memory, and clear thinking [16]. Possibly, trauma-associated tinnitus might constitute a subtype connected with higher symptom-related distress levels. Another explanation would be that the higher impairment of posttraumatic tinnitus is not directly associated with a specific trauma associated pathophysiology but rather reflects dysfunctional coping strategies. A "fateful" tinnitus

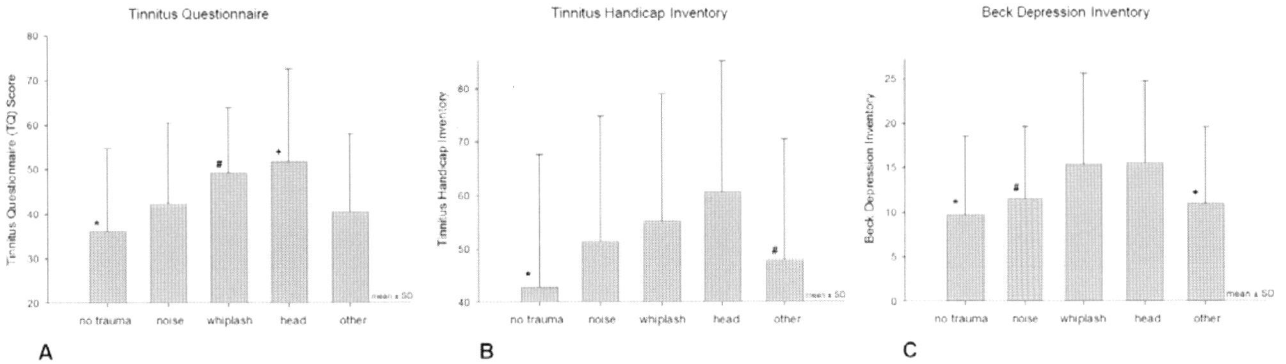

Figure 4. Clinical Questionnaire Assessment Scales at Presentation (mean ± SD). A * Statistically significant between-groups contrasts to all other groups ($p<0.005$). # Statistically significant between-groups contrasts to groups "no trauma", "noise", and "other" ($p<0.05$). + Statistically significant between-groups contrasts to groups "no trauma" and "other" ($p<0.05$). **B** * Statistically significant between-groups contrasts to all other groups ($p<0.005$). # Statistically significant between-groups contrasts to groups "no trauma", "whiplash", and "head" ($p<0.05$). **C** * Statistically significant between-groups contrasts to all other groups ($p<0.05$). # Statistically significant between-groups contrasts to groups "no trauma", "whiplash", and "head" ($p<0.05$). + Statistically significant between-groups contrasts to groups "no trauma", "whiplash", and "head" ($p<0.05$).

onset without any triggering factors might be tolerable, habituable and integrable more easily than a trauma-associated onset which is often accompanied by strong emotions such as surprise, helplessness, pain, and fear, especially when the trauma has not been caused by the patient but by a second party. In many of these cases, patients suffer not only from a bodily damage but tend to regard themselves as "victims" and spend much time with ruminating thoughts about the traumatic event and its preventability such as "If I hadn't gone there and wouldn't have done that… I would not have met this…". Similarly, the expectation for compensation payments may influence habituation. These dysfunctional coping strategies may particularly explain the elevated depression scores in the BDI after head and whiplash trauma. The participation rate in psychiatric treatment reflects this situation, indicating that trauma patients in our sample underwent current psychiatric treatment more frequently than patients without trauma-related onset (see table 1). However, this finding might be biased by psychiatric trauma consequences unrelated to tinnitus. Also, the WHOQOL Quality of Life Questionnaires showed similar patterns like the THI, TQ, and BDI. Apparently, trauma patients as a whole suffered from a more pronounced impairment of their quality of life than tinnitus patients of other etiologies. This pattern was similar for all of the four WHOQOL domains (see Figure 5).

Patients without tinnitus related onset events (including trauma and non-trauma events) reported less frequently that sounds can cause them pain or physical discomfort (see figure 6). Furthermore, the tolerance to loud or hurtful sounds is reduced especially in the subgroup of noise trauma patients (see figure 6). As patient groups did not differ in their hearing levels, recruitment phenomena are considered unlikely to account for these symptoms. In particular, there was no significant between-groups contrast of hearing loss levels at 4 kHz ($F=0.906$; $df=4$; $p=0.460$) and no at the remaining frequencies either ($F=1.414$; $df=4$; $p=0.227$) suggesting that no typical c5-dip [47] was present in noise trauma patients. Rather, the impairment assessed by both questionnaire items suggests a more frequent occurrence of hyperacousis in patients with noise related posttraumatic tinnitus, thus indicating differences in central auditory processing [48]. In this regard our findings of an increased rate of hyperacousis in posttraumatic tinnitus correspond well with earlier studies demonstrating high rates of intolerance to loud sounds after TBI [19]. These findings indicate that in TBI in addition to potential cochlear damage the direct impact on the central auditory pathways is relevant for the etiology of posttraumatic tinnitus. As also mentioned above, no difference in cumulative hearing loss between patients with trauma and non-trauma-groups was observed in our study (see table 1). On a descriptive level, patients without a history of trauma showed higher levels of cumulative hearing loss than patients affected by noise trauma but this difference did not reach significance. This is surprising because it has been reported that acoustic trauma and blast injuries result typically in high-frequency hearing loss [15,47]. However, Nicolas-Puel *et al.* reported similar findings in a sample of 555 patients attending the specialized Tinnitus Clinic in Montpellier, France. Patients with a reported history of noise trauma (17% of the total sample) showed symmetrical hearing loss without differences in lateralization of the tinnitus percept. As in our study, this subset of patients was mainly male and on average 10 years younger than other tinnitus patients. Possibly, young men tend to live an active life and execute risky behavior more frequently thus undergoing an increased risk for accidents. In this French study hearing loss of patients with noise trauma was significantly less pronounced than that measured in the other patients [49]. The observed less pronounced hearing loss in tinnitus patients with noise trauma may be a hint for the relevance of the temporal dynamics of hearing loss for tinnitus generation. As compared with slowly progressing hearing loss in presbyacousis, noise trauma causes a sudden hearing impairment which might trigger specific neuroplastic mechanisms in the brain which in turn induce tinnitus. The induced tinnitus may then persist, even if hearing function recovers in many patients.

Further studies in humans and experimental studies in animals demonstrate that the extent of permanent threshold shift after trauma is variable and may depend on the type of trauma. Nölle *et al.* reported in a sample of 31 patients (24–56 years) after a history of blunt head trauma that initial sensorineural hearing loss (as a result of the inner ear fluid concussion) was transiently perceived only. Auditory brainstem responses (ABR) were normal in all patients, but 76% experienced lowered loudness discomfort levels. The authors stated that blunt trauma of the head can lead to auditory dysfunction, probably as a result of diffuse axonal injury of the central auditory pathway [50]. In contrast, Nageris *et al.* reported in a sample of 73 patients exposed to physical trauma in case of explosion, that 78% experienced high-frequency accentuated sensorineural hearing loss with only 7% improving over time [51]. Apparently, the correlation of head and acoustic

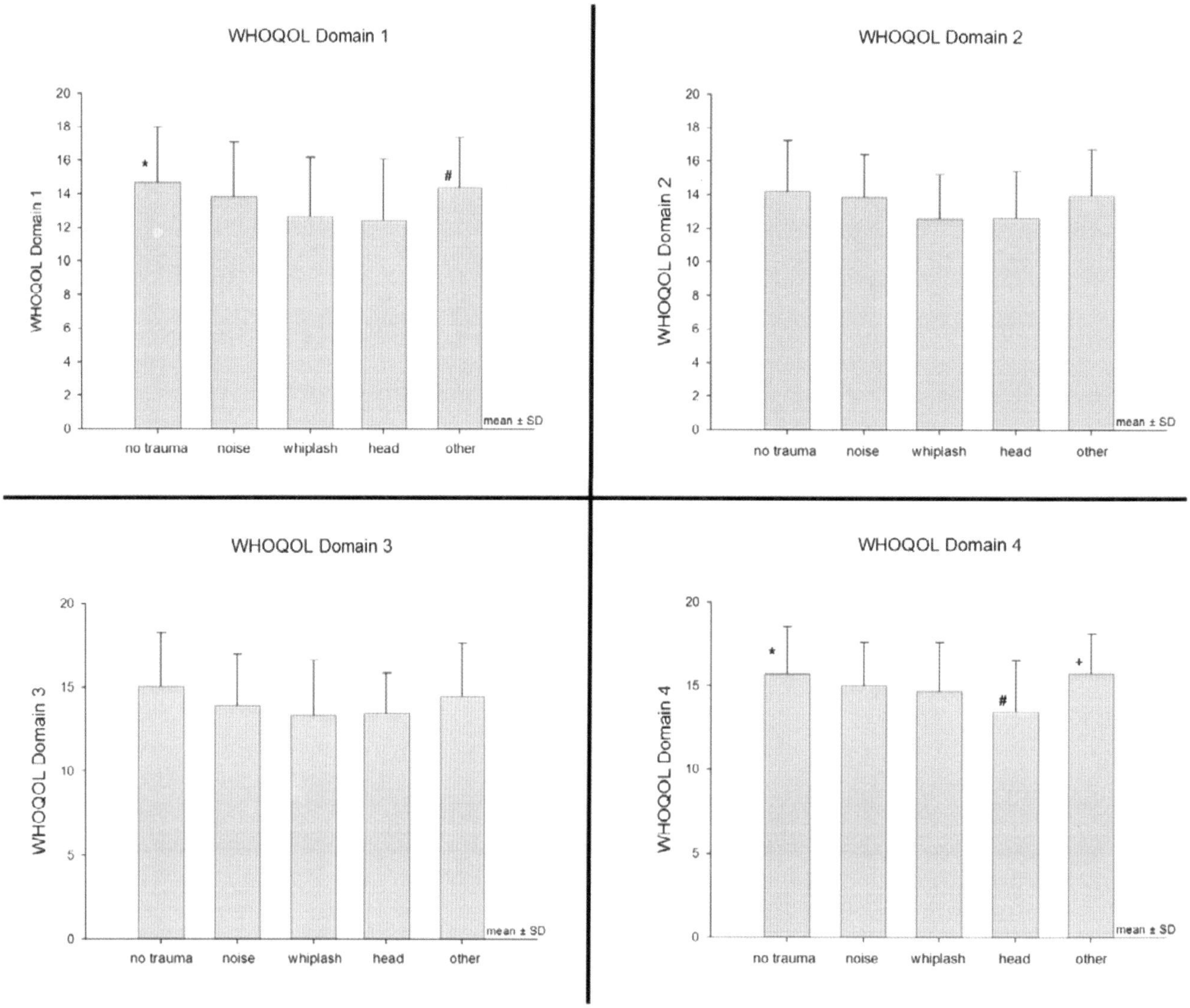

Figure 5. WHOQOL Questionnaire. Domain 1 * Statistically significant between-groups contrasts($p<0.05$) to groups "noise", "whiplash", and "head". # Statistically significant between-groups contrasts ($p<0.05$) to groups "whiplash" and "head". **Domain 4** * Statistically significant between-groups contrasts ($p<0.05$) to groups "noise" and "head". # Statistically significant between-groups contrasts ($p<0.05$) to groups "noise", "whiplash", and "head". + Statistically significant between-groups contrast ($p<0.05$) to group "noise".

trauma with hearing loss strongly depends on the specific form of trauma and its *extent*, so a more detailed, structured and - at best - standardized assessment of trauma-related information is considered vital for the drawing of outlines both in post-trauma research and the definition of therapeutic needs and the prediction of clinical outcomes.

In view of the findings described above patients with noise trauma are more frequently of male gender. Those with a history of noise trauma are younger and describe an earlier onset and longer tinnitus duration at first consultation in a contributing tinnitus center of the TRI consortium. This is well in line with the findings of Nicolas-Puel *et al.*, from a sample presenting at the tinnitus clinic in Montpellier. The patients presenting with noise-induced tinnitus were reported to be mainly male and on average were 10 years younger than other tinnitus patients. In contrast to our results, these patients were reported to differ also in their perceptional characteristics mainly suffering from bilateral high-pitched "whistling" tinnitus in correlation with their high-frequency hearing loss [52]. Especially in young people relevant noise exposure from recreational activities is expected. Between 50 and 70% of young people who expose themselves to loud recreational noise have temporarily experienced tinnitus [53]. Up to 75% of Disc jockeys develop tinnitus, They develop hearing loss both at high frequencies and at low frequencies and have tinnitus of the same sound spectra [54].

A further clinical observation was the fact that patients suffering from trauma-associated tinnitus reported pain symptoms more frequently than other non-trauma-patients. Whiplash patients indicated coincidence of neck pain at a significantly higher rate than all other groups (see figure 6). Vertigo and dizziness were more prevalent in patients suffering from tinnitus associated with whiplash and head trauma as already reported in the literature [55]. These findings support the notion of a generally strong correlation of tinnitus and pain syndromes [56] which might be even more pronounced in patients with trauma-associated tinnitus and merits careful prospective observational studies in the future.

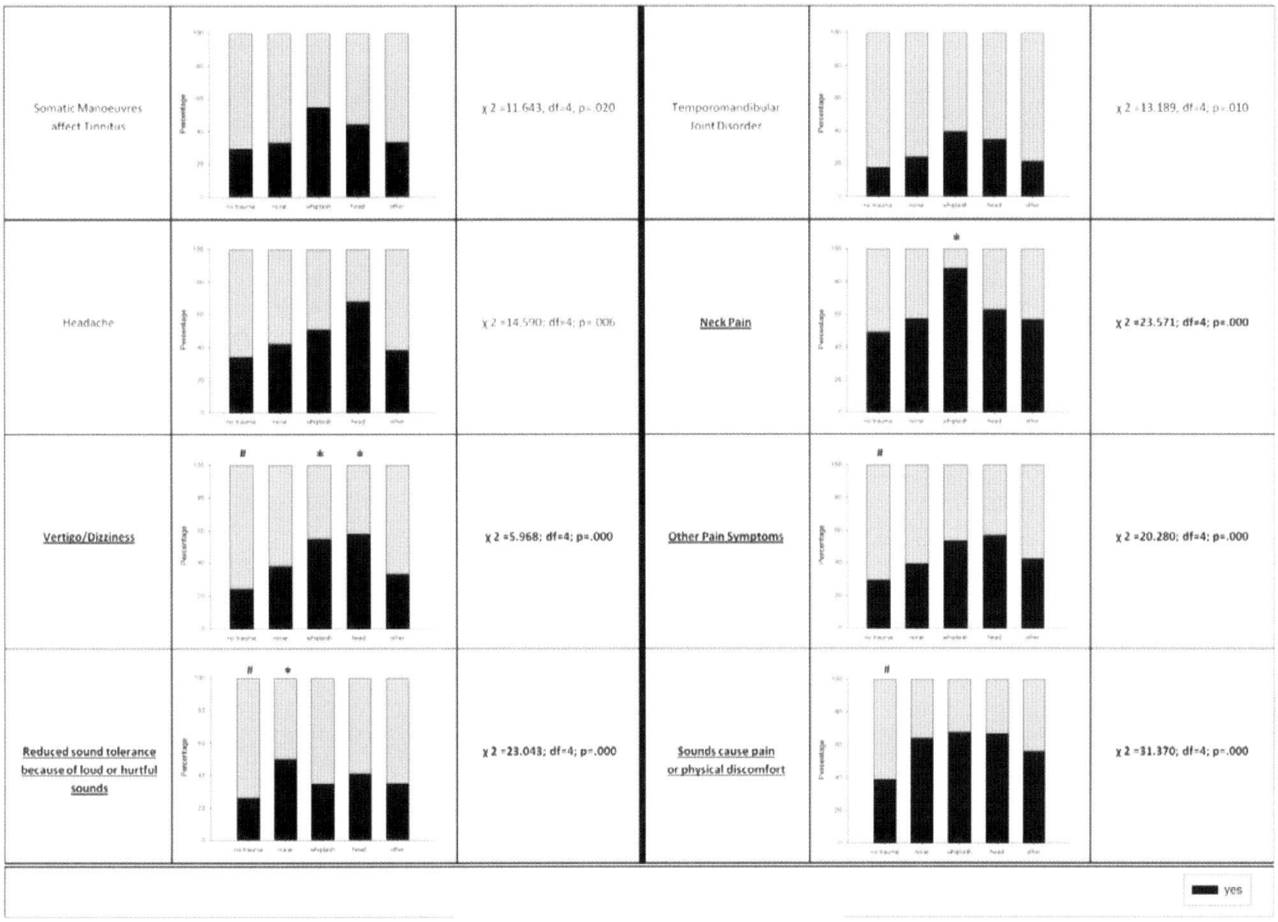

Figure 6. Percentage of accompanying factors of tinnitus with respect to different trauma-associated and non-trauma-associated tinnitus patients' groups. Significant results (after Bonferroni correction for multiple testing) are highlighted in bold and underlined letters; * higher proportion of patients with yes-answer than expected; # lower proportion of patients with yes-answer than expected.

Conclusion and Outlook

Our data clearly indicate differences between tinnitus patients with and without trauma at tinnitus onset. Patients suffering from trauma-associated tinnitus suffer from a higher mental burden than tinnitus patients presenting with phantom perceptions based on other or unknown etiologic factors. This is especially the case for patients with whiplash and head trauma. Patients with posttraumatic noise-related tinnitus experience more frequently hyperacousis, were younger, had longer tinnitus duration, and more frequently male.

Thus, trauma before tinnitus onset seems to represent a relevant criterion for subtypization of tinnitus. Patients with posttraumatic tinnitus may require specific diagnostic and therapeutic management. A more systematic and – at best - standardized assessment for hearing related sequelae of trauma is needed for a better understanding of the underlying pathophysiology and for developing more tailored treatment approaches as well.

Acknowledgments

We want to thank Sandra Pfluegl, Helene Niebling, Jarmila Gerxhaliu-Holan and Constantin Martin for their help and effort in collecting and handling data. The members of The TRI Database Study Group are: Veronika Vielsmeier, Tobias Kleinjung, Astrid Lehner, Timm B. Poeppl, Ricardo Figueiredo, Andréia Azevedo, Ana Carolina Binetti, Ana Belén Elgoyhen, Marcelo Rates, Claudia Coelho, Sven Vanneste, Dirk de Ridder, Paul van de Heyning, Florian Zeman, Markus Mohr, Michael Koller.

Author Contributions

Conceived and designed the experiments: PMK ML BL. Performed the experiments: PMK ML BL. Analyzed the data: MS SS. Wrote the paper: PMK ML MS BL. The data analysed in this study derive from the Tinnitus Research Iniative (TRI) Database. All members of the TRI Database Study Group contributed data.

References

1. Thurman D, Guerrero J (1999) Trends in hospitalization associated with traumatic brain injury. JAMA 282: 954–957.
2. Thurman DJ, Alverson C, Dunn KA, Guerrero J, Sniezek JE (1999) Traumatic brain injury in the United States: A public health perspective. J Head Trauma Rehabil 14: 602–615.
3. Warden D (2006) Military TBI during the Iraq and Afghanistan wars. J Head Trauma Rehabil 21: 398–402.
4. MacGregor AJ, Dougherty AL, Galarneau MR (2011) Injury-specific correlates of combat-related traumatic brain injury in Operation Iraqi Freedom. J Head Trauma Rehabil 26: 312–318.
5. MacGregor AJ, Shaffer RA, Dougherty AL, Galarneau MR, Raman R, et al. (2010) Prevalence and psychological correlates of traumatic brain injury in operation iraqi freedom. J Head Trauma Rehabil 25: 1–8.

6. Terrio H, Brenner LA, Ivins BJ, Cho JM, Helmick K, et al. (2009) Traumatic brain injury screening: preliminary findings in a US Army Brigade Combat Team. J Head Trauma Rehabil 24: 14–23.
7. Sindhusake D, Golding M, Wigney D, Newall P, Jakobsen K, et al. (2004) Factors predicting severity of tinnitus: a population-based assessment. J Am Acad Audiol 15: 269–280.
8. Lew HL, Jerger JF, Guillory SB, Henry JA (2007) Auditory dysfunction in traumatic brain injury. J Rehabil Res Dev 44: 921–928.
9. Geckle L, Lee R (2004) Soldier perceptions of deployment environmental exposures. Albuquerque: NM: Force Health Protection Conference.
10. Mao JC, Pace E, Pierozynski P, Kou Z, Shen Y, et al. (2011) Blast-Induced Tinnitus and Hearing Loss in Rats: Behavioral and Imaging Assays. J Neurotrauma.
11. Yankaskas K (2012) Prelude: Noise-induced tinnitus and hearing loss in the military. Hear Res.
12. Axelsson A, Sandh A (1985) Tinnitus in noise-induced hearing loss. Br J Audiol 19: 271–276.
13. Leske MC (1981) Prevalence estimates of communicative disorders in the U.S. Language, hearing and vestibular disorders. ASHA 23: 229–237.
14. Bauer CA, Brozoski TJ (2001) Assessing tinnitus and prospective tinnitus therapeutics using a psychophysical animal model. J Assoc Res Otolaryngol 2: 54–64.
15. Fausti SA, Wilmington DJ, Gallun FJ, Myers PJ, Henry JA (2009) Auditory and vestibular dysfunction associated with blast-related traumatic brain injury. J Rehabil Res Dev 46: 797–810.
16. Folmer RL, Griest SE (2003) Chronic tinnitus resulting from head or neck injuries. Laryngoscope 113: 821–827.
17. Hinton DE, Chhean D, Pich V, Hofmann SG, Barlow DH (2006) Tinnitus among Cambodian refugees: relationship to PTSD severity. J Trauma Stress 19: 541–546.
18. Langguth B, Landgrebe M, Kleinjung T, Sand GP, Hajak G (2011) Tinnitus and depression. World J Biol Psychiatry 12: 489–500.
19. Jury MA, Flynn MC (2001) Auditory and vestibular sequelae to traumatic brain injury: a pilot study. N Z Med J 114: 286–288.
20. Moller A, Langguth B, de Ridder D, Kleinjung T (2011) Textbook of Tinnitus.: Springer.
21. Cronlein T, Langguth B, Geisler P, Hajak G (2007) Tinnitus and insomnia. Prog Brain Res 166: 227–233.
22. Dobie RA (2003) Depression and tinnitus. Otolaryngol Clin North Am 36: 383–388.
23. Belli S, Belli H, Bahcebasi T, Ozcetin A, Alpay E, et al. (2008) Assessment of psychopathological aspects and psychiatric comorbidities in patients affected by tinnitus. Eur Arch Otorhinolaryngol 265: 279–285.
24. Folmer RL, Griest SE, Meikle MB, Martin WH (1999) Tinnitus severity, loudness, and depression. Otolaryngol Head Neck Surg 121: 48–51.
25. Malouff JM, Schutte NS, Zucker LA (2011) Tinnitus-related distress: A review of recent findings. Curr Psychiatry Rep 13: 31–36.
26. Marciano E, Carrabba L, Giannini P, Sementina C, Verde P, et al. (2003) Psychiatric comorbidity in a population of outpatients affected by tinnitus. Int J Audiol 42: 4–9.
27. Andersson G, Freijd A, Baguley DM, Idrizbegovic E (2009) Tinnitus distress, anxiety, depression, and hearing problems among cochlear implant patients with tinnitus. J Am Acad Audiol 20: 315–319.
28. Crocetti A, Forti S, Ambrosetti U, Bo LD (2009) Questionnaires to evaluate anxiety and depressive levels in tinnitus patients. Otolaryngol Head Neck Surg 140: 403–405.
29. Halford JB, Anderson SD (1991) Anxiety and depression in tinnitus sufferers. J Psychosom Res 35: 383–390.
30. Hesser H, Andersson G (2009) The role of anxiety sensitivity and behavioral avoidance in tinnitus disability. Int J Audiol 48: 295–299.
31. Rossiter S, Stevens C, Walker G (2006) Tinnitus and its effect on working memory and attention. J Speech Lang Hear Res 49: 150–160.
32. Stevens C, Walker G, Boyer M, Gallagher M (2007) Severe tinnitus and its effect on selective and divided attention. Int J Audiol 46: 208–216.
33. Jacobson GP, McCaslin DL (2001) A search for evidence of a direct relationship between tinnitus and suicide. J Am Acad Audiol 12: 493–496.
34. Lewis JE (2002) Tinnitus and suicide. J Am Acad Audiol 13: 339; author reply 339–341.
35. Lewis JE, Stephens SD, McKenna L (1994) Tinnitus and suicide. Clin Otolaryngol Allied Sci 19: 50–54.
36. Turner O, Windfuhr K, Kapur N (2007) Suicide in deaf populations: a literature review. Ann Gen Psychiatry 6: 26.
37. Hiller W, Goebel G (2006) Factors influencing tinnitus loudness and annoyance. Arch Otolaryngol Head Neck Surg 132: 1323–1330.
38. Adamchic I, Hauptmann C, Tass PA (2012) Changes of oscillatory activity in pitch processing network and related tinnitus relief induced by acoustic CR neuromodulation. Front Syst Neurosci 6: 18.
39. Schlee W, Kleinjung T, Hiller W, Goebel G, Kolassa IT, et al. (2011) Does tinnitus distress depend on age of onset? PLoS One 6: e27379.
40. Langguth B, Kleinjung T, Fischer B, Hajak G, Eichhammer P, et al. (2007) Tinnitus severity, depression, and the big five personality traits. Prog Brain Res 166: 221–225.
41. Budd RJ, Pugh R (1996) Tinnitus coping style and its relationship to tinnitus severity and emotional distress. J Psychosom Res 41: 327–335.
42. Landgrebe M, Zeman F, Koller M, Eberl Y, Mohr M, et al. (2010) The Tinnitus Research Initiative (TRI) database: a new approach for delineation of tinnitus subtypes and generation of predictors for treatment outcome. BMC Med Inform Decis Mak 10: 42.
43. Newman CW, Jacobson GP, Spitzer JB (1996) Development of the Tinnitus Handicap Inventory. Arch Otolaryngol Head Neck Surg 122: 143–148.
44. Hallam RS, Jakes SC, Hinchcliffe R (1988) Cognitive variables in tinnitus annoyance. Br J Clin Psychol 27 (Pt 3): 213–222.
45. Steer RA, Beck AT, Riskind JH, Brown G (1986) Differentiation of depressive disorders from generalized anxiety by the Beck Depression Inventory. J Clin Psychol 42: 475–478.
46. WHOQOL-BREF: Introduction, Administration, Scoring. (1996) World's Health Organization. Geneva, Switzerland.
47. Shida S, Yoshida M (1990) [Clinical observation on the dip location of industrial deafness and physiological consideration on the dip origin]. Nihon Jibiinkoka Gakkai Kaiho 93: 1823–1831.
48. Gu JW, Halpin CF, Nam EC, Levine RA, Melcher JR (2010) Tinnitus, diminished sound-level tolerance, and elevated auditory activity in humans with clinically normal hearing sensitivity. J Neurophysiol 104: 3361–3370.
49. Nicolas-Puel C, Akbaraly T, Lloyd R, Berr C, Uziel A, et al. (2006) Characteristics of tinnitus in a population of 555 patients: specificities of tinnitus induced by noise trauma. Int Tinnitus J 12: 64–70.
50. Nolle C, Todt I, Seidl RO, Ernst A (2004) Pathophysiological changes of the central auditory pathway after blunt trauma of the head. J Neurotrauma 21: 251–258.
51. Nageris BI, Attias J, Shemesh R (2008) Otologic and audiologic lesions due to blast injury. J Basic Clin Physiol Pharmacol 19: 185–191.
52. Nicolas-Puel C, Akbaraly T, Lloyd R, Berr C, Uziel A, et al. (2006) Characteristics of tinnitus in a population of 555 patients: specificities of tinnitus induced by noise trauma. Int Tinnitus J 12: 64–70.
53. Quintanilla-Dieck Mde L, Artunduaga MA, Eavey RD (2009) Intentional exposure to loud music: the second MTV.com survey reveals an opportunity to educate. J Pediatr 155: 550–555.
54. Potier M, Hoquet C, Lloyd R, Nicolas-Puel C, Uziel A, et al. (2009) The risks of amplified music for disc-jockeys working in nightclubs. Ear Hear 30: 291–293.
55. Boniver R (2002) Temporomandibular joint dysfunction in whiplash injuries: association with tinnitus and vertigo. Int Tinnitus J 8: 129–131.
56. De Ridder D, Elgoyhen AB, Romo R, Langguth B (2011) Phantom percepts: Tinnitus and pain as persisting aversive memory networks. Proc Natl Acad Sci U S A 108: 8075–8080.

Etiology and Audiological Outcomes at 3 Years for 364 Children in Australia

Hans-Henrik M. Dahl[1,2], Teresa Y.C. Ching[3,4]*, Wendy Hutchison[1], Sanna Hou[3,4], Mark Seeto[3,4], Jessica Sjahalam-King[3,4]

1 Murdoch Childrens Research Institute, Royal Children's Hospital, Melbourne, Australia, **2** Department of Pediatrics, University of Melbourne, Melbourne, Australia, **3** National Acoustic Laboratories, Sydney, Australia, **4** HEARing Cooperative Research Centre, Melbourne, Australia

Abstract

Hearing loss is an etiologically heterogeneous trait with differences in the age of onset, severity and site of lesion. It is caused by a combination of genetic and/or environmental factors. A longitudinal study to examine the efficacy of early intervention for improving child outcomes is ongoing in Australia. To determine the cause of hearing loss in these children we undertook molecular testing of perinatal "Guthrie" blood spots of children whose hearing loss was either detected via newborn hearing screening or detected later in infancy. We analyzed the *GJB2* and *SLC26A4* genes for the presence of mutations, screened for the mitochondrial DNA (mtDNA) *A1555G* mutation, and screened for congenital CMV infection in DNA isolated from dried newborn blood spots. Results were obtained from 364 children. We established etiology for 60% of children. One or two known *GJB2* mutations were present in 82 children. Twenty-four children had one or two known *SLC26A4* mutations. *GJB2* or *SLC26A4* changes with unknown consequences on hearing were found in 32 children. The *A1555G* mutation was found in one child, and CMV infection was detected in 28 children. Auditory neuropathy spectrum disorder was confirmed in 26 children whose DNA evaluations were negative. A secondary objective was to investigate the relationship between etiology and audiological outcomes over the first 3 years of life. Regression analysis was used to investigate the relationship between hearing levels and etiology. Data analysis does not support the existence of differential effects of etiology on degree of hearing loss or on progressiveness of hearing loss.

Editor: Andreas R. Janecke, Innsbruck Medical University, Austria

Funding: The project described was partly supported by Award Number R01DC008080 from the National Institute on Deafness and Other Communication Disorders. The content is solely the responsibility of the authors and does not necessarily represent the official views of the National Institute on Deafness and Other Communication Disorders or the National Institutes of Health. The authors acknowledge the financial support of the Commonwealth of Australia through the establishment of the HEARing CRC and the Cooperative Research Centres Program. The authors also acknowledge the financial support of the Victorian Government's Operational Infrastructure Support Program in Australia. The funders had no role in study design, data collection and analysis, decision to publish, or preparation of the manuscript.

Competing Interests: The authors have declared that no competing interests exist.

* E-mail: Teresa.Ching@nal.gov.au

Introduction

Permanent childhood hearing loss, which occurs in 1–2 per 1000 live births [1], is associated with significant under-achievement in education and lifetime costs of care and lost productivity [2]. Universal newborn hearing screening (UNHS) has been adopted in many regions as a means to speed diagnosis and intervention. Despite its widespread implementation, the available evidence on whether earlier intervention improves long-term speech and language outcomes is flawed in important ways, including cohort composition and potential for systematic bias (reliance on parent-report measures only, non-blinded assessment, and selective follow up) [3]. To address the question of whether, at a population level, UNHS is effective in reducing the gap in speech and language skills between hearing-impaired children and their normal-hearing peers, we conducted the Longitudinal Outcomes of Children with Hearing Impairment (LOCHI) study to directly compare outcomes of children with or without access to UNHS in a prospective manner. The existence of uniform auditory intervention for all hearing-impaired children in Australia, within the government-funded national service provision system (Australian Hearing), serves to minimize variables that might affect outcomes.

Childhood hearing loss is an etiologically heterogeneous condition, caused by environmental factors and/or genetic factors. Despite this heterogeneity, mutations in the *GJB2* (connexin 26, Cx26) gene, the *SLC26A4* (pendred) gene and in the mitochondrial DNA at position 1555 (*A1555G* mutation) and congenital cytomegalovirus (CMV) infection have been considered as the major causes of congenital hearing loss in developed countries [4]. No previous population-based longitudinal studies on child outcomes have examined etiologies and related these to audiological outcomes in the same cohort. We have performed molecular testing for the four common causes to determine the frequency of occurrence in a community sample, and examined the relationship between etiology and audiological outcomes of children over their first 3 years of life. We hypothesized that there will be no difference in hearing level between children with known etiologies and children with none of the etiologies (Hypothesis 1). We also hypothesized that there will be no difference in progression of hearing loss over the first 3 years of life between children with known etiologies and children with none of the tested etiologies (Hypothesis 2).

Subjects and Methods

Ethics Statement

The study was approved by institutional ethics review boards (Royal Children's Hospital HREC 28055 and Australian Hearing HREC 2008-3).

Subjects

The LOCHI study commenced in 2005, with recruitment completed in 2007. All families with children born in Australia between 2002 and 2007 and who presented for hearing services below 3 years of age at Australian Hearing (AH) were invited to participate. Parents of children enrolled in the LOCHI study provided written, informed consent to participate. All participants were invited to give additional informed consent for molecular testing. Of the 451 eligible children, written consent was obtained for 387 children for molecular testing. There was no significant difference in hearing loss (average of 0.5, 1, 2 kHz) between the consent group and the non-consent group ($p = 0.605$). A total of 364 Guthrie card samples were obtained from the custodian authorities of health records. The sample comprised 280 whose hearing loss was detected via UNHS, 64 who did not have access to UNHS and 20 whose screening status was unknown.

Audiologic Assessments

In Australia, the hearing of newborns is screened using automated auditory brainstem response (AABR). Infants who do not pass hearing screening are referred for diagnostic audiological assessment. These include tympanometry, middle ear muscle reflexes, otoacoustic emissions (OAEs), click-evoked auditory brainstem response (ABR) testing, and ABR or auditory steady-state responses (ASSR) testing using frequency-specific stimuli. Following diagnosis, children are referred to AH for assessment of hearing and provision of amplification, at no cost to families. Electrophysiological tests results are converted to estimated behavioral thresholds for fitting of hearing aids [5,6]. Behavioral hearing thresholds are obtained using visual reinforcement audiometry or conditioned play audiometry, depending on the child's age and ability. According to national protocols, hearing levels are monitored at regular intervals by experienced AH pediatric audiologists.

Characteristics of Hearing Loss

The hearing thresholds of participants from inception to 44 months of age were retrieved from clinical records held at the AH national database, with written permission from parents. Hearing thresholds at 0.25, 0.5, 1, 2, and 4 kHz for each ear were obtained. These audiometric thresholds were used to characterize evolution of children's hearing loss over the first 3 years of life as fluctuating, progressive, or stable. In accordance with the audiological protocol of AH, fluctuating hearing loss is defined as a change in hearing threshold of 15 dB or greater at any octave frequency between 0.5 and 4 kHz, but subsequently recover over the period of investigation. Progressive hearing loss is defined as a decrease in 10 dB or greater at two or more adjacent frequencies between 0.5 and 4 kHz or a decrease in 15 dB at one octave frequency in the same frequency range over the period of investigation. Longitudinal audiograms that do not demonstrate the changes specified above are labeled as stable.

ANSD is characterized by a dysfunction in neural/brainstem transmission of auditory stimuli in the presence of normal cochlear outer hair cell function. The clinical presentation is an absent or abnormal ABR responses and the presence of otoacoustic emissions or cochlear microphonics.

Information about enlarged vestibular aqueduct (EVA) was obtained from clinical records held at the AH national database. The diagnosis of EVA was based on CT scan. Radiographic imaging was not part of routine clinical service offered to children identified with hearing loss.

Etiologic Evaluation

Lysates for molecular screening were prepared from Guthrie blood spots, using a modification of the method described by Barbi *et al.* [7]. Briefly, 3 mm diameter disks were punched from the Guthrie blood spot and soaked in 100 µl lysis buffer (50 mM Tris-HCl (pH 8.5); 50 mM NaCl; 2.5 mM $MgCl_2$; 1 mg/ml Proteinase K; 1% Tween-20) at 56°C for 1 hour. Following incubation at 100°C for 7 mins. the samples were rapidly cooled on ice. The samples were centrifuged (10 minutes at 10,000 rpm) and the supernatants frozen for >4 hours at −80°C.

Lysates were screened for mutations in the coding region of *GJB2* (exon 2) and the splice site mutation in intron 1 (IVS1+1 G>A). Exon 2 PCR products were sequenced in both directions. The IVS1+1 G>A mutation was screened for by Hph1 digestion of a PCR product which spans the splice site. If a single mutation in *GJB2* was found, connexin-30 deletions del(GJB6-D13S1830) and del(GJB6d13s1854) were screened for as described by Castillo *et al.* [8].

Each of the *SLC26A4* gene exons was PCR amplified. Following nested PCR, the products were analyzed by High Resolution Melt (HRM) on the Corbett Rotorgene 6000 (Corbett Life Science, Australia). Primary PCR products were sequenced when HRM variants were identified.

We used *in silico* approaches to assess if unreported changes in the *GJB2* and *SLC26A4* genes are likely to affect protein function: PolyPhen-2 [9], SIFT BLink and SIFT Sequence [10].

The mitochondrial 12S rRNA *A1555G* mutation introduces a *HaeIII* restriction enzyme site. PCR products were digested with *Hae*III and analyzed by agarose gel electrophoresis.

The presence of CMV DNA was determined in a multiplex, quantitative, real-time PCR assay, using the CMV and CPOL probes published in Sanchez *et al.* [11] with the probes labelled as described in Scanga *et al.* [12]. Fifteen µl DNA lysate isolated from a disk was used in the PCR reaction, allowing two real-time PCR reactions to be analyzed from each 3 mm disk. The CMV tests were replicated on a second disk.

Analysis

The results are summarized as means and percentages. To investigate the relationship between etiology and hearing thresholds at 3 years of age (Hypothesis 1), multiple regression analysis was carried out using the four-frequency average hearing loss (4FAHL, average of hearing threshold levels at 0.5, 1, 2, and 4 kHz in the better ear at 3 years of age) as dependent variable and etiology as a predictor variable. To determine the evolution of hearing loss, children were grouped according to the AH national protocols into those with fluctuating, progressive, or stable hearing loss. To consider the relation between progression of hearing loss and etiology (Hypothesis 2), a mixed-effects model was fitted using the longitudinal 4FA HL (four frequency average (average of 0.5, 1, 2, and 4 kHz) hearing level) data as dependent variable, the fixed effects were age (continuous variable), the seven etiologies (one mutation for *GJB2*, two mutations for *GJB2*, one mutation for *SLC26A4* gene, two mutations for *SLC26A4* gene, CMV infection, enlarged vestibular aqueduct (EVA), conductive loss) as two-category predictors, and the interactions between etiologies and age. We used two-tailed tests for all analyses and set statistical significance at $p<0.05$. The statistical analysis was performed using Statistica (Statsoft Inc, 2005) and R [13] with the additional packages ggplot2 [14] and nlme [15].

Results

We use the wording "reported mutations" for DNA and protein changes classified as causative mutations in *Cx26* and *SLC26A4* mutation databases [16,17,18]. DNA changes with uncertain consequence on hearing are referred to as "ambiguous changes".

Figure 1 shows the distribution of predicted diagnoses. Reported mutations or congenital CMV infection were identified in 135 (37%) children, and ambiguous changes in the *GJB2* or *SLC26A4* gene were detected in 31 (9%) children. We did not detect mutations or ambiguous changes or evidence of congenital CMV infection in 198 (54%) children. These findings were supplemented by information retrieved from clinical records and parental reports. The cause of hearing loss remained unknown for 146 children (40%).

Reported mutations of *GJB2* were present in 82 children. Of these, 48 (58.5%) had two known mutations and 35 (41.5%) children had one mutation. The inheritance is in all cases compatible with a recessive inheritance pattern. Details of mutations and the evolution of hearing loss for individual children are shown in Table S1. Stable, fluctuating and progressive hearing losses are associated with GJB2 mutations, but specific genotypes do not appear to be exclusively associated with a phenotype. We assume that the hearing loss in children with two known mutations is attributable to *GJB2*. Of the children with two mutations of Cx26, one child passed hearing screening at birth, but was diagnosed with moderate hearing loss at 19.4 months of age. Another child was diagnosed with auditory neuropathy spectrum disorder (ANSD), and two children had EVA. Ambiguous changes in the *GJB2* gene were detected in 24 children, 22 of whom have one mutation and the remaining 2 have two mutations.

Reported mutations of *SLC26A4* [17,18] were found in 24 children. Of these, seven (29.2%) had two known mutations, one of whom was also positive for CMV infection. Seventeen (70.8%) children carried one known *SLC26A4* mutation, two of whom also carried one uncertain mutation and four others also carried *GJB2* mutations. For 8 other children, one ambiguous change of the *SLC26A4* gene was detected. Details of mutations and evolution of hearing thresholds are shown in Table S2.

Mutations in the *SLC26A4* gene are associated with Pendred syndrome (PS, MIM 274600) and non-syndromic enlarged vestibular aqueduct (EVA, MIM 600791). Three children who carried one mutation of *SLC26A4* also had EVA, and one child who carried two mutations of *SLC26A4* also had EVA. EVA was also found for 4 children who had *Cx26* mutations, 1 who had CMV infection, and 8 who had normal results for the four causes tested. The number of children who had EVA could not be

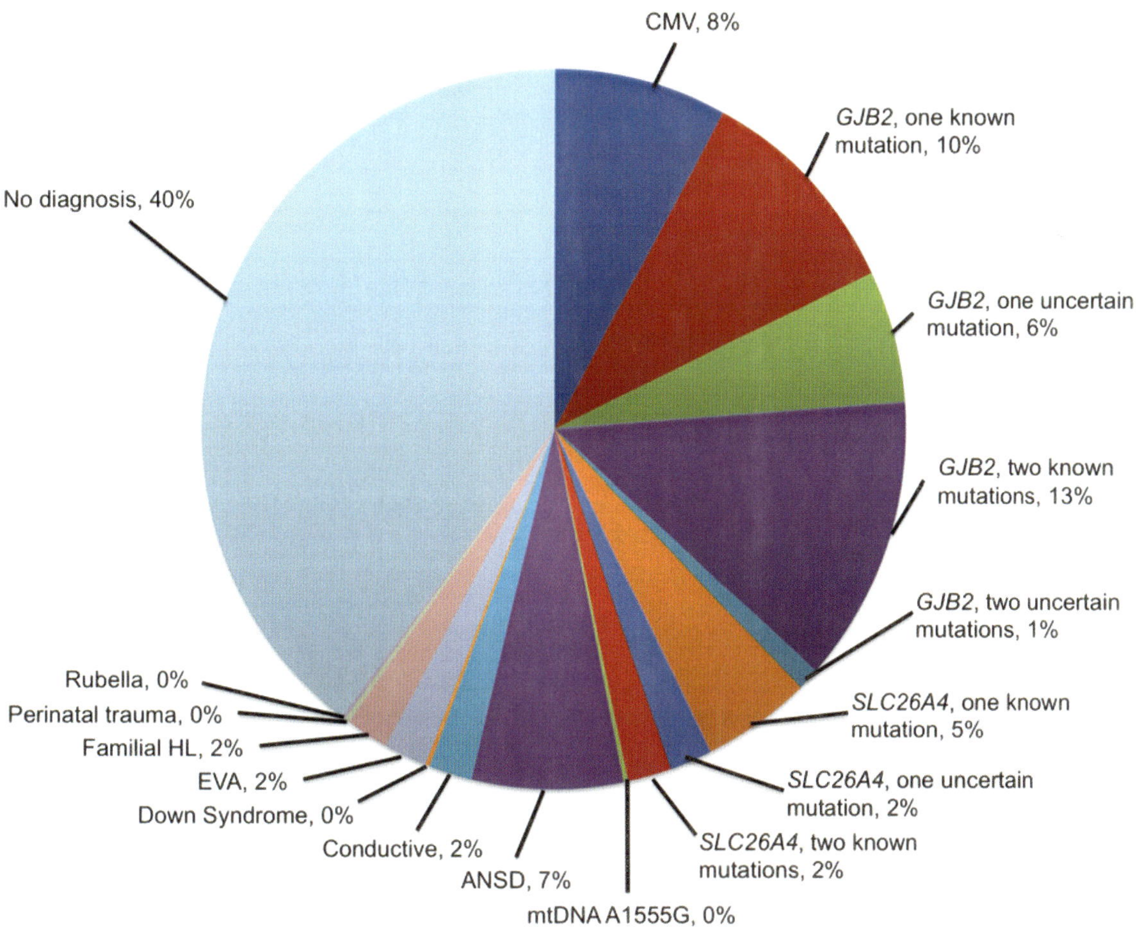

Figure 1. Results of the search for hearing loss etiology in 364 Australian children.

ascertained because information was available only for those with imaging results recorded in their clinical files.

The mtDNA *A1555G* mutation was detected in one child. The mutation appeared homoplasmic on agarose gel electrophoresis. The child has bilateral ANSD with profound hearing loss. It is not known whether the child had been exposed to aminoglycosides.

Cytomegalovirus infection was detected in 28 children. Of these, one child passed UNHS but was diagnosed with meningitis and hearing loss at 5.1 months of age. A second child with congenital CMV infection also had one mutation of Cx26, and was referred for unilateral hearing loss after screening. One CMV positive child also carried two mutations of the *SLC26A4* gene. Details of the evolution of hearing loss for children who are CMV positive are presented in Table S3.

In the regression analysis examining the relation between etiology and hearing threshold levels at 3 years of age, the overall p-level for the regression model was 0.27. Table 1 shows the estimate and 95% confidence interval for the regression coefficients. For each of the etiologies tested, there was insufficient evidence at the 5% significance level to reject the null hypothesis that the average hearing loss (4FA HL) for children with that etiology is the same as children without the etiology.

Table 2 shows the estimates of the effect of etiology on progression of hearing loss over the first 3 years of life. For each of the seven etiologies investigated, there was insufficient evidence at the 5% significance level to reject the null hypothesis that the average rate of change of 4FA HL in the better ear for children with that etiology is the same as children without the etiology.

Table 2. Progression of hearing loss over the first 3 years of life, expressed in terms of slope in dB/year, with respect to predictors.

Predictor	Estimate	95% CI	p-value
Age	1.99	(−0.42, 4.41)	0.11
Cx26, one mutation × Age	−2.22	(−6.31, 1.87)	0.29
Cx26, two mutations × Age	1.12	(−2.38, 4.61)	0.53
SLC26A4, one mutation × Age	2.52	(−1.80, 6.84)	0.25
SLC26A4, two mutations × Age	0.18	(−8.11, 8.47)	0.97
CMV × Age	2.57	(−2.01, 7.15)	0.27
EVA × Age	3.97	(−0.64, 8.58)	0.09
Conductive × Age	−3.71	(−9.53, 2.11)	0.21

The estimated effect size, 95% confidence interval (CI), and the probability level (p-value) for each predictor term are shown.

Discussion

The incidence of permanent childhood hearing loss is 1 to 1.2 per 1000 at birth increasing to about 1.5 by 3 years of age [19] in Australia where compliance with confirmatory testing after hearing screening is excellent and loss to follow-up for intervention is below 1%. As a sub-component of the LOCHI study, the present study conducted molecular testing of dried newborn blood spots for *GJB2*, *SLC26A4*, *A1555G* and CMV infection, and established a likely etiologic diagnosis for 166 (45.6%) of the 364 cases tested. Of the causes identified, a genetic cause was present in 138 children (83.1%) and an environmental cause in 28 children (16.9%).

It has previously been suggested that hearing loss attributable to congenital CMV may be progressive in >50% of cases [20]. However, we did not find this trend when examining hearing level data of children from diagnosis to 3 years of age. Whether the progression extends beyond this young age will be revealed in future follow-ups within the context of the LOCHI study. It is possible that some children with progressive hearing loss had congenital CMV infection that was not detected, as the use of Guthrie blood spot DNA in CMV testing may result in false negatives [21]. Dilution studies suggest that our CMV assay will detect the presence of a few copies of CMV DNA present in the 15 μl lysate used in the PCR reaction. Even with such sensitivity, CMV levels might be too low to be detected in Guthrie blood cards. More sensitive is the detection of CMV virus in the newborn's blood, saliva urine or other tissues or body fluids within 2–3 weeks of birth. However, such tissues or fluids were not available in this cohort. Our finding that 8% of blood spots were positive for CMV is likely to be an underestimation of the true number of newborn Australian children with a congenital CMV infection. This frequency of infection is indeed lower than the 18.8% (9 of 48 infants with hearing loss) at a tertiary center of UNHS in Flanders [22]. In that study, CMV was detected through PCR assays with the blood spots on Guthrie cards, viral cultures, or blood serological tests. The present findings are nonetheless consistent with those reported by Stehel *et al* for infants at a hospital in the US showing that 6% (16 of 256 infants with hearing loss) were CMV positive through urine cultures [23]. Even though hearing loss in children with congenital CMV infection is likely to have been caused by the infection, we cannot conclude that this is the case in all children because most children with congenital CMV infection do not develop hearing loss [20].

Table 1. Multiple regression analysis of hearing loss at 3 years of age with respect to etiology.

Predictor	Estimate	95% CI	p-value
Cx26, one mutation	−7.8	(−20.8, 5.1)	0.23
Cx26, two mutations	7.4	(−3.3, 18.1)	0.17
SLC26A4, one mutation	−7.0	(−21.0, 7.0)	0.32
SLC26A4, two mutations	−3.4	(−34.8, 27.9)	0.83
CMV	9.9	(−3.9, 23.8)	0.16
EVA	0.2	(−14.9, 15.3)	0.98
Conductive	−7.2	(−29.8, 15.3)	0.53

The estimated effect size, 95% confidence interval (CI), and the probability level (p-value) for each predictor term are shown.

Looking specifically at the genetic causes of hearing loss in our population (n = 138), mutations in the *GJB2* gene accounted for 76.1% of the genetic cases. This frequency of occurrence is higher than the 50% previously reported for congenital, autosomal recessive, nonsyndromic, sensorineural hearing loss in the white population [24]. Consistent with previous studies on children of northern European ancestry [22,25], the c35delG (35delG mutation) variant was the most common allele variant of GJB2, with 60 of 135 mutant alleles (44%) being 35delG. As shown in Table S1, there was a variable genotype-phenotype correlation even among children homozygous for 35delG. Our finding that progressiveness of hearing loss in children with *GJB2* mutations was not significantly different from those without the mutations is consistent with previous reports [26,27]. Unlike previous reports that revealed an association of biallelic truncating mutations (such as 35delG) with more severe loss than those with biallelic non-truncating mutations [28], our study did not reveal such a relation between mutations and hearing level.

One known mutation in the *GJB2* gene was detected in 35 children. The pathogenic effect of these single mutations are uncertain, but we have attributed the hearing losses to thise *GJB2* gene changes, because the proportion of children with hearing loss and one detectable recessive *GJB2* mutation is significantly higher than that of the general population (approximately 1%) [29]. The pathogenic effects of a number of other changes in the *GJB2* gene of 24 children are also ambiguous. We have classified the V27I and E114G changes, when together, as a mutation in accordance with the *Connexins and Deafness Homepage* [16]. However, recent data suggest that the V27I+E114G changes might not be pathogenic [30]. Although sometimes classified as polymorphisms [16], it is likely that M34T [28,31,32,33,34], R127H [35,36,37], M195V [38,39], and I203T [40,41] contribute to hearing loss. The V153I change is usually considered to be a polymorphism, although it has been suggested that the mutant *GJB2* protein is unable to form functional gap junction channels [42]. We have previously reported the T186A change [43], but the pathogenicity of this change has not been established. The T186A change was seen in two affected siblings together with the 35delG mutation. PolyPhen-2, SIFT BLink and SIFT Sequence analyses all predict this change to affect protein function (Table S4). The K108N change has not been reported before, but the *in silico* analysis suggests that is unlikely to cause hearing loss. Although SIFT Sequence analysis predicts that it is "likely to affect protein function", PolyPhen-2 and SIFT BLink predict it is benign (Table S4).

Previous studies have shown the presence of two *SLC26A4* mutations in many patients with Pendred syndrome, whereas one mutation is common in patients with EVA [44,45] *SLC26A4* mutations [17,18] were found in 32 children. Of these, 7 (21.9%) had two known mutations, 17 (53.1%) had one known mutation and 8 (25.0%) had one uncertain mutation. As shown in Table S2, there was a complex genotype-phenotype correlation. The c.919_936delinsCCCCA change has not been described before, but the exon 8 mutation results in a frameshift and premature termination of the protein. As with the *GJB2* mutations, the pathogenic effects of some of the *SLC26A4* changes haven't been fully established and are controversial. This is the case for L597S [45,46,47,48,49,50,51,52], IVS1-2A>G [51], and F335L [45]. PolyPhen-2 and SIFT Sequence predict the L597S and F335L changes are "probably damaging", while SIFT BLink suggests they affect protein function (Table S4). Only 4 of the cases identified with one or two mutations in the SLC26A4 also had EVA. The status for the remaining cases could not be ascertained from clinical records. Therefore, the pathogenicity of detected mutations in those with one mutation is uncertain.

We detected 3 previously unreported missense changes: R43H, R79Q and S780F. A mutation, R43S, has been reported in R43 suggesting that this amino acid might be important for protein function [17]. R43 and R79 are both highly conserved amino acids suggesting that the R43H and R79Q changes might affect SLC26A4 function. However, PolyPhen-2, SIFT BLink and SIFT Sequence analyses predict the R43H change to be benign. PolyPhen-2 predicts the R79Q change to be "probably damaging" to protein function, while the two SIFT programs predict that the change is "tolerated" (Table S4). Despite being the C-terminal amino acid, S780 is conserved in most species. However, in the Common Shrew (Sorex araneus) the corresponding amino acid is a phenylalanine. This suggests that the S780F change might be a polymorphism. PolyPhen-2 predicts this change to be benign, while SIFT BLink and SIFT Sequence predict that the change affects protein function (Table S4). However, the *in silico* predictions at the C-terminal amino acid are with low confidence because only short sequence regions can be compared.

To assess the contribution of single mutations in the *GJB2* or *SLC2A4* gene to a hearing loss is challenging. The study by Wang et al [53] in which 14,913 newborn Chinese children had both a newborn hearing test and a genetic screen for *GJB2* and *SLC2A4* mutations showed significantly increased risks of hearing loss in *GJB2* and *SLC2A4* heterozygous carrier children.

The *A1555G* mtDNA mutation increases susceptibility to aminoglycoside induced hearing loss. Because many newborns and young children are exposed to aminoglycoside antibiotics, its potential presence is often of concern to health professionals and families. The *A1555G* mtDNA mutation was found in only one of the 364 hearing-impaired children. Our result is consistent with previous observations that this mutation is not a common cause of hearing loss in children less than 3 years of age in the general Australian population. [43].

A diagnosis of ANSD was established for 39 children. Of the children diagnosed with ANSD, four had one *SLC26A4* mutation also; six had one GJB2 mutation and one child had two GJB2 mutations. Twenty-six of the children with ANSD did not have detectable mutations or evidence of CMV infection. The presence of ANSD results in degraded oral language development.

The limitations of this study include its reliance on newborn blood spots for CMV testing. Supplementing UNHS with molecular testing would enable pre-symptomatic detection of preventable hearing loss for some children. Despite testing for four common causes of childhood hearing loss, the etiology for 54% of the cohort remains unknown. Future molecular testing for etiology of hearing loss will need to include mutations in other genes, such as *OTOF*, encoding otoferlin, in which mutations are commonly found in children with ANSD. It was not possible to do a comprehensive audiological and genetic study of parents, siblings and other relatives of affected children. Such study could be helpful in assessing the inheritance and consequence of a *GJB2* or *SLC26A4* change. Future follow-up of the present cohort as part of the longitudinal study will examine the relation between an identified genetic/viral cause and the type and degree of hearing loss as the children grow.

The strengths of the LOCHI study include its longitudinal, community-based design, with prospective, repeated measurements of hearing and developmental outcomes. The longer term audiological outcomes of children with different etiologies will be evaluated.

Conclusion

This study presents the first comprehensive evaluation of four common causes of childhood hearing loss in a community cohort. After etiologic evaluation of 364 children identified with hearing loss below 3 years of age, a genetic diagnosis could be made in 46% of those children. Approximately another 14% of children had clinical abnormalities or syndromes without identified *GJB2* or *SLC26A4* mutations. Our findings provide a basis for future studies to determine the impact of mutations of the *GJB2* and *SLC26A4* genes and congenital CMV infection on speech and language outcomes in children with hearing loss. Establishing the etiology of an identified hearing loss provides answers to parents, facilitates planning of hearing loss management and provides information that is relevant to the prognosis for the child.

Supporting Information

Table S1 Genotype-phenotype correlation in children with GJB2 mutations and evolution of hearing loss.

Table S2 Genotype-phenotype correlation in children with *SLC26A4* mutations and evolution of hearing loss. Children with *SLC26A4* mutations with additional diagnostic information regarding enlarged vestibular aqueduct (EVA), auditory neuropathy spectrum disorder (ANSD) and congenital cytomegalovirus infection (CMV) are also indicated.

Table S3 Hearing thresholds at time of diagnosis and evolution in children with hearing loss attributable to congenital CMV infection.

Table S4 PolyPhen-2, SIFT BLink and SIFT Sequence predictions of novel or controversial amino acid changes on *GJB2* and *SLC26A4* gene product functions.

Acknowledgments

We gratefully thank all the families for their participation. We thank the many persons who served as clinicians for the study participants or assisted in other administrative capacities at Australian Hearing. We also thank the Genetic Service Laboratories in Victoria, NSW and Queensland who retrieved Guthrie Blood Cards as well as Marit Wiersma for her assistance in genetic analyses.

Author Contributions

Assessed audiological profiles: TC SH MS JS-K. Conceived and designed the experiments: HD TC. Performed the experiments: HD WH SH MS JS-K. Analyzed the data: HD TC WH JS-K. Contributed reagents/materials/analysis tools: HD TC WH SH MS JS-K. Wrote the paper: HD TC.

References

1. Davis A, Davis KAS (2011) Chapter 5. Descriptive epidemiology of childhood hearing impairment. In: , editor. Comprehensive Handbook of Pediatric Audiology: Plural Publishing, Abingdon, UK. pp. 85–111.
2. Access Economics (2006) Listen Hear. The Economic Impact and Cost of Hearing Loss in Australia.
3. Thompson DC, McPhillips H, Davis RL, Lieu TL, Homer CJ, et al. (2001) Universal newborn hearing screening: summary of evidence. JAMA 286: 2000–2010.
4. Morton CC, Nance WE (2006) Newborn hearing screening–a silent revolution. N Engl J Med 354: 2151–2164.
5. King AC, Parkinson KN, Adamson AJ, Murray L, Besson H, et al. (2011) Correlates of objectively measured physical activity and sedentary behaviour in English children. Eur J Public Health 21: 424–431.
6. Vander Werff KR, Prieve BA, Georgantas LM (2009) Infant air and bone conduction tone burst auditory brain stem responses for classification of hearing loss and the relationship to behavioral thresholds. Ear Hear 30: 350–368.
7. Barbi M, Binda S, Primache V, Caroppo S, Dido P, et al. (2000) Cytomegalovirus DNA detection in Guthrie cards: a powerful tool for diagnosing congenital infection. J Clin Virol 17: 159–165.
8. del Castillo FJ, Rodriguez-Ballesteros M, Alvarez A, Hutchin T, Leonardi E, et al. (2005) A novel deletion involving the connexin-30 gene, del(GJB6-d13s1854), found in trans with mutations in the GJB2 gene (connexin-26) in subjects with DFNB1 non-syndromic hearing impairment. J Med Genet 42: 588–594.
9. Adzhubei IA, Schmidt S, Peshkin L, Ramensky VE, Gerasimova A, et al. (2010) A method and server for predicting damaging missense mutations. Nature methods 7: 248–249.
10. Kumar P, Henikoff S, Ng PC (2009) Predicting the effects of coding non-synonymous variants on protein function using the SIFT algorithm. Nature protocols 4: 1073–1081.
11. Sanchez JL, Storch GA (2002) Multiplex, quantitative, real-time PCR assay for cytomegalovirus and human DNA. J Clin Microbiol 40: 2381–2386.
12. Scanga L, Chaing S, Powell C, Aylsworth AS, Harrell LJ, et al. (2006) Diagnosis of human congenital cytomegalovirus infection by amplification of viral DNA from dried blood spots on perinatal cards. J Mol Diagn 8: 240–245.
13. The "R Project for Statistical Computing" website. R Development Core Team. A language and environment for statistical computing (Version 2.13.1). Available: http://www.r-project.org/. Accessed 2012 May 8.
14. The "ggplot2: An implementation of the Grammar of Graphics" website. Wickham H and Chang W. Available: http://cran.r-project.org/package=ggplot2. Accessed 2012 May 8.
15. The "nlme: Linear and Nonlinear Mixed Effects Models" website. Pinheiro J, Bates, D., DebRoy, S., Sarkar, D. & R Development Core Team. Available: http://cran.r-project.org/package=nlme. Accessed 2012 May 8.
16. Connexin-deafness Homepage website. Ballana E, Ventayol M, Rabionet R, Gasparini P, Estivill X. Available: http://davinci.crg.es/deafness/. Accessed 2012 Aug 26.
17. Pendred/BOR Homepage website. Chang E, Kölln KA, Nishimura CJ, Fischer S, Smith RJH. Available: http://www.healthcare.uiowa.edu/labs/pendredandbor/. Accessed 2012 Aug 26.
18. Deafness Gene Mutation Database website. Harvard Medical School Center for Hereditary Deafness (2012). Available: http://hearing.harvard.edu/genepages/pdsdream.htm. Accessed 2012 Aug 26.
19. Australian Hearing website Demographic Details of Persons under the age of 21 years with a Hearing Impairment who are fitted with a Hearing Aid - 2011. Available: http://www.hearing.com.au/digitalAssets/13809_1352761241226_Demographics%20of%20Persons%20under%20the%20age%20of%2021%20years%20with%20Hearing%20Aids.pdf. Accessed 2012 May 8.
20. Fowler KB, Boppana SB (2006) Congenital cytomegalovirus (CMV) infection and hearing deficit. J Clin Virol 35: 226–231.
21. Boppana SB, Ross SA, Novak Z, Shimamura M, Tolan RW Jr, et al. (2010) Dried blood spot real-time polymerase chain reaction assays to screen newborns for congenital cytomegalovirus infection. Jama 303: 1375–1382.
22. Declau F, Boudewyns A, Van den Ende J, Peeters A, van den Heyning P (2008) Etiologic and audiologic evaluations after universal neonatal hearing screening: analysis of 170 referred neonates. Pediatrics 121: 1119–1126.
23. Stehel EK, Shoup AG, Owen KE, Jackson GL, Sendelbach DM, et al. (2008) Newborn hearing screening and detection of congenital cytomegalovirus infection. Pediatrics 121: 970–975.
24. Smith RJ, Bale JF Jr, White KR (2005) Sensorineural hearing loss in children. Lancet 365: 879–890.
25. Denoyelle F, Weil D, Maw MA, Wilcox SA, Lench NJ, et al. (1997) Prelingual deafness: high prevalence of a 30delG mutation in the connexin 26 gene. Hum Mol Genet 6: 2173–2177.
26. Denoyelle F, Marlin S, Weil D, Moatti L, Chauvin P, et al. (1999) Clinical features of the prevalent form of childhood deafness, DFNB1, due to a connexin-26 gene defect: implications for genetic counselling. Lancet 353: 1298–1303.
27. Murgia A, Orzan E, Polli R, Martella M, Vinanzi C, et al. (1999) Cx26 deafness: mutation analysis and clinical variability. J Med Genet 36: 829–832.
28. Snoeckx RL, Huygen PL, Feldmann D, Marlin S, Denoyelle F, et al. (2005) GJB2 mutations and degree of hearing loss: a multicenter study. Am J Hum Genet 77: 945–957.
29. Dahl HH, Saunders K, Kelly TM, Osborn AH, Wilcox S, et al. (2001) Prevalence and nature of connexin 26 mutations in children with non-syndromic deafness. Med J Aust 175: 191–194.
30. Tekin M, Xia XJ, Erdenetungalag R, Cengiz FB, White TW, et al. (2010) GJB2 mutations in Mongolia: complex alleles, low frequency, and reduced fitness of the deaf. Ann Hum Genet 74: 155–164.
31. Cucci RA, Prasad S, Kelley PM, Green GE, Storm K, et al. (2000) The M34T allele variant of connexin 26. Genet Test 4: 335–344.
32. Houseman MJ, Ellis LA, Pagnamenta A, Di WL, Rickard S, et al. (2001) Genetic analysis of the connexin-26 M34T variant: identification of genotype M34T/M34T segregating with mild-moderate non-syndromic sensorineural hearing loss. J Med Genet 38: 20–25.
33. Kenna MA, Feldman HA, Neault MW, Frangulov A, Wu BL, et al. (2010) Audiologic phenotype and progression in GJB2 (Connexin 26) hearing loss. Arch Otolaryngol Head Neck Surg 136: 81–87.
34. Teek R, Kruustuk K, Zordania R, Joost K, Reimand T, et al. (2010) Prevalence of c.35delG and p.M34T mutations in the GJB2 gene in Estonia. Int J Pediatr Otorhinolaryngol 74: 1007–1012.
35. Dahl HH, Tobin SE, Poulakis Z, Rickards FW, Xu X, et al. (2006) The contribution of GJB2 mutations to slight or mild hearing loss in Australian elementary school children. J Med Genet 43: 850–855.
36. Palmada M, Schmalisch K, Bohmer C, Schug N, Pfister M, et al. (2006) Loss of function mutations of the GJB2 gene detected in patients with DFNB1-associated hearing impairment. Neurobiol Dis 22: 112–118.
37. Thonnissen E, Rabionet R, Arbones ML, Estivill X, Willecke K, et al. (2002) Human connexin26 (GJB2) deafness mutations affect the function of gap junction channels at different levels of protein expression. Hum Genet 111: 190–197.
38. Dai P, Yu F, Han B, Liu X, Wang G, et al. (2009) GJB2 mutation spectrum in 2,063 Chinese patients with nonsyndromic hearing impairment. J Transl Med 7: 26.
39. Tsukada K, Nishio S, Usami S (2010) A large cohort study of GJB2 mutations in Japanese hearing loss patients. Clin Genet 78: 464–470.
40. Han SH, Park HJ, Kang EJ, Ryu JS, Lee A, et al. (2008) Carrier frequency of GJB2 (connexin-26) mutations causing inherited deafness in the Korean population. J Hum Genet 53: 1022–1028.
41. Kim HJ, Park CH, Lee KO, Won HH, Ko MH, et al. (2010) Sequence Variations and Haplotypes of the GJB2 Gene Revealed by Resequencing of 192

Chromosomes from the General Population in Korea. Clin Exp Otorhinolaryngol 3: 65–69.

42. Mese G, Londin E, Mui R, Brink PR, White TW (2004) Altered gating properties of functional Cx26 mutants associated with recessive non-syndromic hearing loss. Hum Genet 115: 191–199.
43. Siemering K, Manji SS, Hutchison WM, Du Sart D, Phelan D, et al. (2006) Detection of mutations in genes associated with hearing loss using a microarray-based approach. J Mol Diagn 8: 483–489; quiz 528.
44. Azaiez H, Yang T, Prasad S, Sorensen JL, Nishimura CJ, et al. (2007) Genotype-phenotype correlations for SLC26A4-related deafness. Hum Genet 122: 451–457.
45. Choi BY, Stewart AK, Madeo AC, Pryor SP, Lenhard S, et al. (2009) Hypo-functional SLC26A4 variants associated with nonsyndromic hearing loss and enlargement of the vestibular aqueduct: genotype-phenotype correlation or coincidental polymorphisms? Hum Mutat 30: 599–608.
46. Albert S, Blons H, Jonard L, Feldmann D, Chauvin P, et al. (2006) SLC26A4 gene is frequently involved in nonsyndromic hearing impairment with enlarged vestibular aqueduct in Caucasian populations. Eur J Hum Genet 14: 773–779.
47. Blons H, Feldmann D, Duval V, Messaz O, Denoyelle F, et al. (2004) Screening of SLC26A4 (PDS) gene in Pendred's syndrome: a large spectrum of mutations in France and phenotypic heterogeneity. Clin Genet 66: 333–340.
48. Campbell C, Cucci RA, Prasad S, Green GE, Edeal JB, et al. (2001) Pendred syndrome, DFNB4, and PDS/SLC26A4 identification of eight novel mutations and possible genotype-phenotype correlations. Hum Mutat 17: 403–411.
49. Fugazzola L, Cerutti N, Mannavola D, Crino A, Cassio A, et al. (2002) Differential diagnosis between Pendred and pseudo-Pendred syndromes: clinical, radiologic, and molecular studies. Pediatr Res 51: 479–484.
50. Pera A, Dossena S, Rodighiero S, Gandia M, Botta G, et al. (2008) Functional assessment of allelic variants in the SLC26A4 gene involved in Pendred syndrome and nonsyndromic EVA. Proc Natl Acad Sci U S A 105: 18608–18613.
51. Pryor SP, Madeo AC, Reynolds JC, Sarlis NJ, Arnos KS, et al. (2005) SLC26A4/PDS genotype-phenotype correlation in hearing loss with enlargement of the vestibular aqueduct (EVA): evidence that Pendred syndrome and non-syndromic EVA are distinct clinical and genetic entities. J Med Genet 42: 159–165.
52. Yang T, Vidarsson H, Rodrigo-Blomqvist S, Rosengren SS, Enerback S, et al. (2007) Transcriptional Control of SLC26A4 Is Involved in Pendred Syndrome and Nonsyndromic Enlargement of Vestibular Aqueduct (DFNB4). Am J Hum Genet 80: 1055–1063.
53. Wang QJ, Zhao YL, Rao SQ, Guo YF, He Y, et al. (2011) Newborn hearing concurrent gene screening can improve care for hearing loss: a study on 14,913 Chinese newborns. Int J Pediatr Otorhinolaryngol 75: 535–542.

10

Hearing Ability with Age in Northern European Women: A New Web-Based Approach to Genetic Studies

Lisa E. Wolber*, Claire J. Steves, Tim D. Spector, Frances M. K. Williams

Department of Twin Research & Genetic Epidemiology, King's College London, London, United Kingdom

Abstract

Age-related hearing impairment (ARHI) affects 25–40% of individuals over the age of 65. Despite the high prevalence of this complex trait, ARHI is still poorly understood. We hypothesized that variance in hearing ability with age is largely determined by genetic factors. We collected audiologic data on females of Northern European ancestry and compared different audiogram representations. A web-based speech-to-noise ratio (SNR) hearing test was compared with pure-tone thresholds to see if we could determine accurately hearing ability on people at home and the genetic contribution to each trait compared. Volunteers were recruited from the TwinsUK cohort. Hearing ability was determined using pure-tone audiometry and a web-based hearing test. Different audiogram presentations were compared for age-correlation and reflection of audiogram shape. Using structural equation modelling based on the classical twin model the heritability of ARHI, as measured by the different phenotypes, was estimated and shared variance between the web-based SNR test and pure-tone audiometry determined using bivariate modelling. Pure-tone audiometric data was collected on 1033 older females (age: 41–86). 1970 volunteers (males and females, age: 18–85) participated in the SNR. In the comparison between different ARHI phenotypes the difference between the first two principle components (PC1–PC2) best represented ARHI. The SNR test showed a sensitivity and specificity of 89% and 80%, respectively, in comparison with pure-tone audiogram data. Univariate heritability estimates ranged from 0.70 (95% CI: 0.63–0.76) for (PC1–PC2) to 0.56 (95% CI: 0.48–0.63) for PC2. The genetic correlation of PC1–PC2 and SNR was −0.67 showing that the 2 traits share variances attributed to additive genetic factors. Hearing ability showed considerable heritability in our sample. We have shown that the SNR test provides a useful surrogate marker of hearing. This will enable a much larger sample to be collected at a fraction of the cost, facilitating future genetic association studies.

Editor: Julian Little, University of Ottawa, Canada

Funding: The authors would like to acknowledge Action on Hearing Loss and Research into Ageing for the financial support of this work. The funders had no role in study design, data collection and analysis, decision to publish, or preparation of the manuscript.

Competing Interests: The authors have declared that no competing interests exist.

* E-mail: lisa.wolber@kcl.ac.uk

Introduction

ARHI, also referred to as presbycusis, is a complex age-related disorder affecting 25–40% of all individuals older than 65 years. Hearing loss can cause severe communication disability, leading to social isolation [1] and incapacity to work. ARHI is a common complex trait with few risk factors reliably identified. The presentation of presbycusis is diverse, showing high variance in age of onset and severity. In most cases, both ears are affected equally by sensori-neural hearing loss. Loss of hearing sensitivity with age generally starts in the higher frequencies and progresses to the lower frequencies, leading to a characteristic down-slope in the pure-tone audiogram starting at the higher frequencies and increasing in steepness.

Complex traits may be attributed to a combination of environmental and genetic factors. Several environmental factors have been implicated in the development of ARHI. Significant environmental risk factors include noise exposure ($p = 1.0\times10^{-17}$) [2], smoking ($p = 0.0009$) [2], alcohol consumption (OR = 0.59 95% CI: 0.43–0.80) [3], as well as cardiovascular disease (OR = 2.0, 95% CI:1.15–3.46) [4] and diabetes mellitus ($p<0.05$) [5].

Heritability is defined as the proportion of phenotypic variance caused by genetic factors. Heritability is a population measure and thus depends on the variance of the trait seen in the respective population. Several heritability studies have been conducted for presbycusis resulting in heritability estimates ranging from 25%–42% for strial presbycusis (atrophy of the stria vascularis, causing a flat slightly descending audiogram [6]) in families of the Framingham cohort [7] to 75% (95% CI: 0.76–0.81) for the better ear hearing threshold level (BEHL) (0.5–4 kHz) in Finnish female twins (age range: 63–76 years) [8]. Heritability was shown to decrease with increasing age and increasing environmental risk factor exposure in a cohort of male twins [9]. In general, prevalence of ARHI is higher in men, presumably due to higher occupational noise exposure, and heritability estimates for presbycusis are higher in females [7].

Several linkage, candidate gene and genome-wide association (GWA) studies have attempted to elucidate the genetic background of ARHI. Linkage studies revealed 6 loci linked to presbycusis on Chromosomes 11, 10, 14 and 18 (LOD>1.5) [10], for the *DFNA18* locus (LOD = 2.5) [11] and a locus on chromosome 8q (LOD = 4.23) [12]. Candidate gene studies focused on loci implicated in congenital deafness and reactive oxygen species removal. Associations have been suggested for the *NAT2*6A* polymorphism (G590A, $p = 0.013$) [13], polymorphisms in *GSTT1* and *GSTM1* ($p = 0.035$ and $p = 0.027$, respectively) [14], as well as for a polymorphism in *GRHL2* ($p = 8.38 \times 10^{-5}$) [15]. Only the association with *NAT2*6A* could be replicated in an independent European cohort ($p = 0.013$) [14]. Variable phenotype definitions, different age ranges, sample sizes and types of study populations used for hearing ability with age in various studies impairs the comparison of results and conclusions that can be reached.

Two GWA studies have been conducted for ARHI, showing suggested associations with polymorphisms in the *GRM7* gene ($p = 9 \times 10^{-5}$) in a European mixed gender case-control cohort ($n = 1692$, age range: 53–67 years) [16] and the *IQGAP2* gene ($p = 3.55 \times 10^{-7}$) in the Finnish Saami ($n = 347$, age range: 50–75 years) [17]. Both studies initially failed to reach genome-wide significance levels, which most likely reflects low sample size [18]. The association with GRM7 has been replicated in a group of 120 subjects after 23 single nucleotide polymorphisms (SNPs) were selected and tested for association [16].

This study aimed to determine genetic causal factors of differences in hearing ability with age in middle aged female twins of Northern European ancestry using two different objective measures of hearing ability: the standard pure-tone audiogram administered in controlled conditions to twins visiting the department and a web-based speech-to-noise ratio test which twins were invited by email, to perform online from home [19]. We aimed to identify the phenotype that best reflects the characteristics of hearing loss with age in particular and to establish its heritability based on the classical twin model. The novel speech-to-noise ratio (SNR) hearing test was validated against pure-tone audiometry and shared causal factors determined using bivariate structural equation modeling.

Methods

Pure-tone Audiogram Data Collection

Twin subjects were recruited from the TwinsUK registry at St. Thomas' Hospital, King's College London (www.twins.ac.uk). This twin registry comprises mainly female, adult volunteer twins recruited previously via UK media campaigns [20]. Participants were recruited from the TwinsUK registry over the age of 40. All participants underwent a detailed questionnaire on medical and environmental risk factors relevant for hearing, including auditory diseases, self reported hearing ability, hearing aid usage, occupation and noise exposure (see File S1). An otoscopic examination followed by an air-conduction pure-tone audiogram was conducted by trained personnel under standard conditions. Audiometric measures were performed using a Madsen XETA audiometer including TDH39 headphones. Audiologic equipment was calibrated on a regular basis. All research was conducted according to the ethical standards as defined by the Helsinki declaration. Ethical approval for this study was obtained from the National Research Ethics service London-Westminster (REC reference number: 07/H0802/84). Written informed consent was obtained from all participants prior to study conduction.

Phenotype Definition

There is no gold standard method for defining ARHI and different groups have used pure tone averages (PTAs) for different frequency ranges, standardized Z-scores [21], a better ear hearing level threshold (BEHL) [8] or principal component (PC) scores calculated in a principal component analysis [12].

The PTA and BEHL are averages calculated from pure-tone thresholds of all frequencies or 0.5 kHz–4.0 kHz for the better ear, respectively. Principal component analysis is a statistical procedure based on correlations between variables. Underlying correlations between the pure-tone thresholds are determined and summarised in new variables, referred to as PCs. In case of pure-tone audiogram data, three PCs have been reported that account for size and shape of the audiogram, respectively [12]. Log transformed pure-tone thresholds (0.125–8.0 kHz) were used in this analysis. A variable combining PC1 and PC2 was generated by subtracting PC2 from PC1.

Two criteria were applied to define a good phenotypic representation for hearing loss with age: high correlation with age and the characteristic downslope of the pure-tone audiogram. As PC2 has been shown previously to capture the slope of the audiogram [22], shared variance with PC2 was determined in a linear regression on PC2, adjusted for age and twin relatedness. Each phenotype was ranked based on these two criteria. Correlation with age was determined for PTA, PC1, PC2, (PC1–PC2) and BEHL (Table 1). Mean age, mean PTA, PC scores, (PC1–PC2) scores and BEHL were compared for MZ twins, DZ twins and unpaired twins (singletons) using Kruskal-Wallis test.

Speech-to-noise Ratio Test Data Collection

The SNR test measures the ability to understand words against increasing background noise. Difficulty in following a conversation in a noisy environment is one of the main symptoms of hearing loss due to advanced age. The test used in this study was originally developed for use on a telephone [23]. The SNR test was converted for web based usage by Action on Hearing loss (previously RNID). In the test, combinations of digit-triplets (i.e. 3–4–6 spoken as three-four-six) were presented at a constant sound intensity against a variable background noise [23]. The starting speech sound intensity was adapted individually by asking the subject to increase or decrease the sound intensity until a comfortable intensity was reached at which the digit triplets could be identified correctly. The initial speech sound intensity was kept constant, while the background noise increased or decreased in steps of 2 dB, depending on whether the complete triplet was understood correctly or not, respectively. The measured speech-to-noise ratio gives the ratio of speech to noise sound intensity at which half of the presentations were understood correctly.

Validation of Speech-to-noise Ratio Test

To determine the reproducibility of the SNR test we selected 17 individuals (age range 20–83) to perform the test twice under similar conditions (same environment and same personal computer). We compared the test results using a Bland-Altman comparison [24] and Pitman's test of difference in variance.

The results of the web based SNR test were validated against the pure-tone audiogram data. Subjects for the validation experiment ($n = 351$) were selected from the TwinsUK cohort if they participated both in the pure-tone audiogram and the SNR. The validation experiment included only female participants. The SNR validation cohort showed a similar age and hearing ability distribution as the pure-tone audiogram cohort (mean age: 59.8 ± 8.5; mean PTA: 21.4 ± 10.2; mean SNR: -10.1 ± 2.2; all values given with $\pm$standard deviation). The correlation of the SNR test results were determined for different pure-tone audiogram presentations (PTA, BEHL, PC1,PC2 and PC1–PC2). Sensitivity and specificity of the SNR test was compared to a PTA>40 dB and a (PC1–PC2) score of 3.4 as thresholds for good hearing ability. Receiver operating curves were calculated. To determine shared causal factors between both hearing tests, bivariate structural equation modelling based on a correlated factors model was performed for PTA and SNR as well as (PC1–

Table 1. Demographic and phenotypic profile of study sample with pure-tone audiogram data.

zygosity	n	age range	mean age (SD)	mean PTA (SD)	mean PC1 (SD)	mean PC2 (SD)	mean PC1–PC2 (SD)	mean BEHL (SD)
MZ	464	44–83	62.37 (7.93)	23.2 (10.10)	−0.01 (2.02)	0.01 (1.32)	−0.02 (2.33)	19.53 (9.91)
DZ	528	41–86	62.14 (8.10)	23.8 (11.58)	0.07 (2.16)	−0.06 (1.23)	0.14 (2.51)	20.26 (11.25)
singletons	41	41–83	62.46 (10.24)	25.3 (15.63)	0.24 (2.89)	0.32 (1.31)	−0.08 (3.13)	20.52 (15.24)
total	1033	41–86	62.23 (8.12)	23.5 (11.13)	0.04 (2.13)	−0.01 (1.27)	0.05 (2.46)	19.93 (10.85)

The study sample was separated into monozygotic twins (MZ), dizygotic twins (DZ) and singletons. Each group was further described by its sample size (n), age-range, mean age, pure-tone average (PTA), principal component 1 (PC1), principal component 2 (PC2) as well as their difference (PC1–PC2) and better ear hearing level threshold (BEHL) values. Measurements for the mean age, pure-tone average and principle components are given as mean with standard deviation (SD).

PC2) and SNR. For the bivariate analysis, SNR data was normalized using a cubic transformation.

Univariate Heritability of Different Phenotypes

Heritability estimates for hearing ability with age as a quantitative trait were calculated using structural equation modelling in Mx [25] on the basis of the classical twin model. The model assumes that phenotypic variance is determined by additive genetic (A), unique environmental (E) and common environmental (C) factors. MZ twins share all of their additive genetic factors, whereas DZ twins share on average half of their additive genetics. Common environmental factors are fully shared within MZ and DZ twin pairs, while unique environmental factors are unshared within twin pairs. In the structural equation modelling A is modelled as twice the difference between phenotypic covariance in MZ and DZ twin pairs. E is modelled as phenotypic variation not explained by shared additive genetics [1-cov(MZ)]. As phenotypic similarity in dizygotic twins is caused by shared genetic and common environmental factors, C is calculated as the phenotypic correlation in dizygotic twins minus half the heritability. Mx compares reduced models (AE, CE and E) to the saturated ACE model using a −2 log likelihood statistic. Heritability was estimated for PTA, PC1, PC2 and BEHL and (PC1–PC2).

Results

Description of Study Sample with Pure-tone Audiogram Data

Pure-tone audiograms and hearing questionnaire data were collected from 1033 female participants, including 264 DZ and 232 MZ pairs and 41 singletons. The mean age was 62.23 years (± 8.12 years of standard deviation), range 41–86 years. There was no significant age-difference ($p = 0.97$) for MZs, DZs and singletons (Table 1). PCA was conducted and the first two principal components, PC1 and PC2, gave eigenvalues >1 and were therefore considered important components. Together, PC1 and PC2 captured 78% of the variation in the pure tone audiogram data. While the loadings for PC1 were stable across all frequencies, loadings for PC2 were high for the low frequencies (0.125–1.0 kHz) and decreased for the higher frequencies (2.0–8.0 kHz).

Pure-tone audiogram data as measured by PTA, PC1, PC2, (PC1–PC2) and BEHL did not differ significantly between MZs, DZs and singletons (PTA: $p = 0.88$; PC1: $p = 0.86$; PC2: $p = 0.06$; PC1–PC2: $p = 0.52$; BEHL: $p = 0.48$). PC1 values increased with raised hearing thresholds whereas PC2 values decreased with increasing downslope in the audiogram (high frequency hearing loss, increasing with steepness of slope and affection of lower frequencies). We concluded that a low PC1–PC2 value (i.e. low PC1-high PC2) would reflect good hearing ability, whereas a high PC1–PC2 value (i.e. high PC1-low PC2) would represent hearing loss with age. The highest correlation with age was determined for the combined variable of PC1–PC2 ($r = 0.61$) (Table 2). This combined variable also explained the highest proportion of variance in PC2 ($R^2 = 0.26$) and thus resulted in the lowest rank (Table 2).

Speech-to-noise Ratio Test

1970 subjects responded to the web-based SNR test within the first 3 months. This first sample set included 348 MZ and 179 DZ twin pairs, as well as 916 unpaired twins. SNR scores did not differ significantly between both sexes (Kruskal-Wallis test, $p = 0.09$). SNR scores ranged from 6 dB −13.5 dB (Table 3).

Validation of Speech-to-noise Ratio Test in Comparison to Pure-tone Audiometry

The results of the SNR test were reproducible with a mean difference between repeat measurements of −0.43 (95% CI: (−0.956) – 0.095). Pitman's test for difference in variance showed no significant difference ($p = 0.879$).

The highest correlation with the SNR was found with PTA ($r = 0.62$). We decided to validate the SNR test results against PTA and PC1–PC2, which gave the best ranking in the comparison of pure-tone audiogram phenotypes. Moderate hearing impairment is defined as a PTA> 40 dB [26]. We used this criterion as the reference measurement to determine the sensitivity and specificity of the SNR test in subjects having completed both pure-tone audiogram and SNR ($n = 351$), although the PTA> 40 dB might not be the best criterion for hearing loss due to age. A PTA of 40 dB corresponded to a (PC1–PC2) score of 3.4. Receiver operating curves were calculated that plot 1-specficity versus sensitivity of the SNR test against a PTA threshold of 40 dB (Figure 1) and a (PC1–PC2) threshold of 3.4 (Figure 2). For a threshold of −9.25 dB SNR, a sensitivity of 89% and a specificity of 80% were obtained in comparison to the PTA (Figure 1). For a threshold of −9 dB SNR, a sensitivity of 87% and a specificity of 82% were determined when compared to (PC1–PC2) (Figure 2).

Tests measuring the same trait might also reflect a high proportion of shared genetic factors. We investigated bivariate heritability between the two best pure-tone audiometry measures ((PC1–PC2) and PTA) and SNR results. For all bivariate analyses, the AE model gave the better model fit compared to the saturated ACE model (Table S1). Correlations between the additive genetic estimates for both tests ranged from −0.61 for age-adjusted PTA & SNR scores to −0.67 for age-adjusted (PC1–PC2) & SNR values (Figure 3, Table S1). This corresponded to 65% and 88% of

Table 2. Ranking of pure-tone audiogram phenotypes.

phenotype	r(age) [rank]	proportion of variance shared with PC2 [rank]
PC1–PC2	0.61 [1]	0.26 [1]
PTA	0.55 [2]	0.08 [3]
PC1	0.53 [3]	0.12 [2]
BEHL	0.49 [4]	0.08 [3]
PC2	−0.29 [5]	1.00 [N.A.]

Pure-tone audiogram phenotypes were ranked according to their correlation with age (Pearson's correlation coefficient) and representation of audiogram shape (measured as proportion of variance shared with PC2). Ranks are given in square brackets.

phenotypic correlation due to genetic effects for PTA & SNR and PC1–PC2 & SNR, respectively.

Univariate Heritability Study for Pure-tone Audiogram Phenotypes

Univariate structural equation modelling was used to determine the variance in phenotype explained by additive genetic factors (heritability), common environmental and unique environmental factors for different ARHI phenotype presentations. There was a high correlation with age, so age-adjusted residuals were calculated. Results of the univariate heritability study are given in Table 4. Model fit was determined using a −2 log Likelihood (−2 log L) statistic. Different nested models (AE, CE, E) were compared to the saturated ACE model based on a −2 log L difference test [27]. The Akaike information criterion (AIC) gives a measure of model fit, taking into consideration the balance of the χ^2 statistic and the number of degrees of freedom. For each phenotype the saturated ACE model as well as nested models with better model fits are reported (Table 4). The AE model gave the best model fit for all phenotype representations. Heritability estimates ranged from 0.70 (95% CI: 0.64–0.76) for PC1–PC2 to 0.57 (95% CI: 0.49–0.63) for PC2 (Table 4).

Discussion

For this study, we collected pure-tone audiogram data and SNR data of 1033 and 1970 mainly female participants, respectively. (PC1–PC2) was suggested as new phenotype definition for hearing ability with age, which showed a high correlation with age and best captured high frequency hearing loss. We have shown that the SNR is a valid tool when compared with the standard test and will allow us to increase our sample size for future GWAs on hearing ability with age as a quantitative trait. The moderate univariate heritability determined for pure-tone audiogram phenotypes suggests causal genetic factors involved in the etiology of hearing ability with age.

The TwinsUK cohort has been shown to be widely representative of the general singleton North European population [28] and their involvement in numerous genome wide association study meta-analyses attests to their comparability with other populations [29].

For the pure-tone audiogram representations, the values of the better ear were chosen for analysis, as it is considered to be less representative of environmental factors affecting hearing ability. Exposure to such factors would not represent natural age-related hearing and therefore bias the search for an ageing phenotype. We decided not to adjust for noise exposure in this study, due to minimal self reported exposure in the presented cohort (less than 8% of participants reported to have been exposed to occupational noise for more than one year). In addition, noise exposure was not significantly associated with hearing ability ($p = 0.92$) in our cohort.

Several phenotypes have been used to represent hearing ability with age in previous studies, however, no gold standard could be decided on. Moderate hearing impairment (PTA>40 dB), as defined by the WHO [26] is a very stringent criteria. In addition, averaging hearing ability over all frequencies (i.e. PTA) might not be suitable to measure hearing ability with age as it neglects the characteristic downslope of the audiogram. We therefore compared different phenotypes as measured by pure-tone audiometry including PTAs, BEHL, scores for PC1 and PC2. Two criteria important for hearing impairment with age were defined: the correlation with age (for an age-related trait) and capture of the characteristic down-slope seen for high frequency hearing loss, the most common variant of ARHI. As PC1 and PC2 alone captured only fractions of the variance in pure-tone

Table 3. Demographic and phenotypic profile of study sample with speech-to-noise ratio data.

zygosity	n	sex (M/F)	mean age (SD)	age range	mean SNR	min SNR	max SNR
MZ	696	70/627	53.3 (2.08)	20–85	−10.26	−13.25	4.38
DZ	358	28/330	57.2 (2.17)	28–78	−10.19	−13.5	6.00
singletons	916	143/772	53.63 (2.18)	18–84	−13.25	−13.25	6.00
total	1970	241/1729	54.18 (2.14)	18–85	−10.21	−13.5	4.38

Test participants for the SNR test were described by zygosity (MZ, DZ, singletons), sample size (n), sex (male (M), female (F)) of participants, mean age with standard deviation (SD) and the age range. Mean speech-to-noise ratios (SNR) are given with minimal (min SNR) and maximal (max SNR) values.

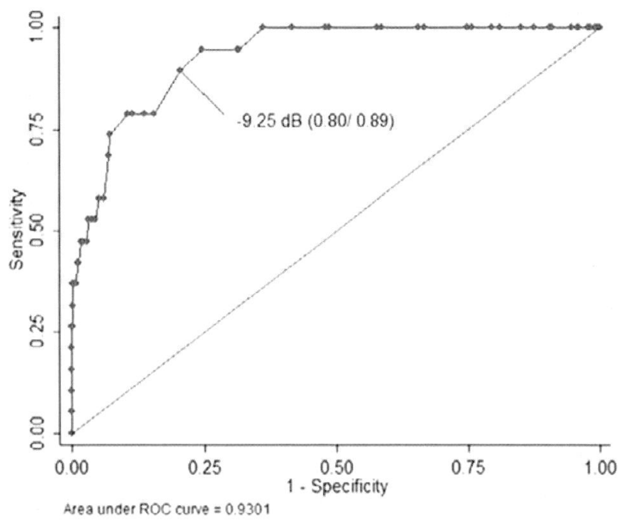

Figure 1. Receiver operating curve for SNR in comparison to PTA>40 dB. The receiver operating curve plots the specificity versus the sensitivity of the Speech-to-noise ratio in comparison to hearing ability measured by the pure-tone average >40 dB.

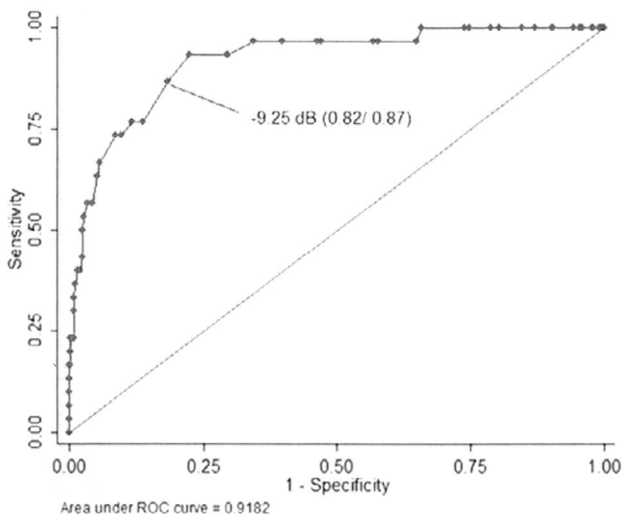

Figure 2. Receiver operating curve of SNR in comparison to PC1–PC2>3.4. The receiver operating curve plots the specificity versus the sensitivity of the Speech-to-noise ratio in comparison to hearing ability measured by a (PC1–PC2) >3.4.

audiograms, we decided to combine both variables by taking their difference (PC1–PC2). In the ranking according to the above criteria, (PC1–PC2) gave the best rank. We therefore propose (PC1–PC2) as a new phenotype to measure ARHI from pure-tone audiogram data. We acknowledge that principal component loadings are dependent on the study population and more complicated to adapt than PTAs but their advantage is that they capture magnitude and shape of the audiogram, whereas average variables (PTA, BEHL) mainly represent the magnitude alone. Nevertheless, this problem could be targeted by deciding on equal PC loadings in replication studies or meta analyses.

In this study, we validated a measure of hearing ability obtained via the web, the SNR test. This test has previously been validated for telephone usage [23] producing a sensitivity of 79% and specificity of 100% of the BEHL as measured by pure-tone audiometry versus the telephone based SNR [23]. A new method should always be validated against the existing standard measure: we therefore determined the sensitivity and specificity of the web based SNR against the PTA and (PC1–PC2) as obtained by the pure-tone audiogram. Sensitivity and specificity was high in comparison to the PTA (89% and 80%, respectively), but decreased slightly when the SNR was validated against (PC1–PC2) (87% and 82%, respectively). This could be expected considering that PC1 and PC2 together account for 78% of the variances in pure-tone thresholds while the PTA reflects 100%.

These sensitivity and specificity values might be too low for a diagnostic test, but appropriate for a screening test, as used here. Word recognition and hearing sensitivity at different frequencies represent different aspects of ARHI and might be explained by different causal factors. To reduce the effect of cognitive ability on word recognition digit combinations were used as speech material rather than complete sentences. We hypothesized that variances in both measurements could be explained by shared causal genetic factors and our bivariate heritability results underline this notion. Genetic correlations between pure-tone audiogram measurements (PTA and (PC1-PC2)) and SNR determined in the bivariate analyses ranged from $r = -0.61$ to $r = -0.67$. According to the sensitivity and specificity as well as the high bivariate heritability correlations determined, we conclude that the SNR represents a satisfactory surrogate to the pure-tone audiogram and that both tests could serve as complements to each other.

The heritability estimates from the univariate analysis ranged from 70% (95% CI: 0.64–0.76) for (PC1–PC2) to 57% (95% CI: 0.49–0.63) for PC2. This is comparable to a heritability of 75% for pure-tone thresholds reported for female Finnish twins [8] and a heritability of 66.3% for PC1 achieved in a population of singletons [12]. Our twin sample was composed exclusively of females with relatively minor exposure to environmental risk factors, high occupational status and a broader age range and

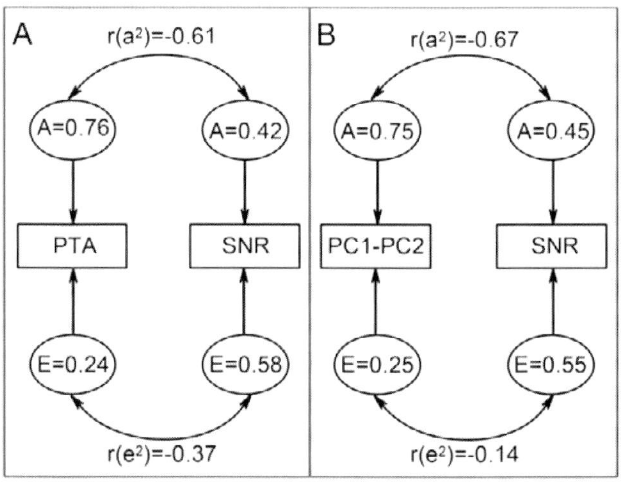

Figure 3. Results of bivariate variance component modelling. Graphical presentation of bivariate variance modelling results for PC1–PC2 &SNR (Panel A) and PTA & SNR (Panel B). Univariate heritability (A) and unique environmental factor (E) estimates are given separately for each trait. Correlation between these factors are given by $r(a^2)$ and $r(e^2)$, respectively.

Table 4. Results of univariate variance modelling for age-adjusted pure-tone audiogram phenotypes.

phenotype	model fit			model comparison				estimates % (95%CI)		
	Model	−2 log L	df	Δ −2 log L	Δ df	p-value	AIC	A	C	E
PTA age-adjusted	ACE	7386.954	1025	–	–	–	–	67 (52–73)	0.0(0.0–12)	33 (27–41)
	AE	7386.954	1026	0.000	1	1.000	−2.000	67(59–73)	–	33 (27–41)
PC1 age-adjusted	ACE	4006.850	1025	–	–	–	–	59 (35–69)	3 (0.0–23)	38 (31–46)
	AE	4006.919	1026	0.069	1	0.792	−1.931	63 (55–69)	–	37 (31–45)
PC2 age-adjusted	ACE	3235.682	1025	–	–	–	–	40 (14–62)	16 (0.0–37)	45 (37–53)
	AE	3237.390	1026	1.709	1	0.191	−0.291	57 (49–63)	–	43 (37–51)
(PC1–PC2) age-adjusted	ACE	4167.301	1025	–	–	–	–	70 (58–76)	0.0 (0.0–11)	30 (24–36)
	AE	4167.301	1026	0.000	1	1.000	−2.000	70 (64–76)	–	30(24–36)
BEHL age-adjusted	ACE	7421.538	1025	–	–	–	–	65 (54–72)	0.0 (0.0–8.0)	35 (28–42)
	AE	7421.538	1026	0.000	1	1.000	−2.000	65 (58–72)	–	35 (28–42)

Three nested models were compared to the saturated ACE model, taking into account different causal factors: AE (additive genetics and unshared environmental factors), CE (shared and unshared environmental factors) and E (unshared environmental factors). For each phenotype the saturated model and nested models with a better model fit (minus 2 log likelihood(−2 logL), degrees of freedom (df)) are shown. Model comparison is only given for nested models as they are compared to the full (ACE) model. Estimated variances explained by the specific causal factors (A = additive genetics, C = shared environment and E = unshared environment) are given with 95% confidence intervals for each model.

lower mean age than previously conducted heritability studies on ARHI. Therefore, a lower phenotypic variance could be expected for this population due to decreased heterogeneity.

The moderate to high heritability estimates confirm the involvement of genetic factors in the etiology of ARHI as well as the reliability of the phenotype measure.

We accept that there were limitations to our data collection. Conductive hearing loss, commonly diagnosed as an air-bone gap of >20 dB, could not be fully excluded, due to a lack of bone conduction measurements. However, auditory diseases leading to conductive hearing loss (i.e. Otosclerosis, cholesteatoma and chronic otitis media) were covered in the questionnaire and subjects were excluded upon these pathologies. In addition, hearing loss generally refers to a longitudinal process, whereas the data we presented here was cross-sectional. The percentage of subjects with moderate hearing loss as defined by the WHO (PTA>40 dB) [26] was relatively low for the TwinsUK cohort. This might be explained by better hearing ability than average for this cohort. Considering that ARHI affects predominantly the higher frequencies, elderly subjects with a PTA<40 dB might still be affected by ARHI. For the validation of the SNR test, the number of subjects having performed both tests was limited (n = 351, only females) compared to the overall sample size. However, the audiometric profile of the SNR validation cohort resembled that of the complete pure-tone audiogram and SNR cohort. We also acknowledge that the web-based test attracted slightly younger subjects and was not limited to female participants like the pure-tone audiogram. We will address this by a correction for age and gender in the future analysis of this data set.

Supporting Information

File S1 Copy of hearing questionnaire. The Hearing questionnaire was developed to test for self reported hearing loss and exposure to environmental risk factors for hearing ability.

Table S1 Results of bivariate variance modelling for PTA & SNR and PC1–PC2 & SNR. Results of bivariate structural equation modelling are given for unadjusted and age-adjusted pure-tone audiogram phenotypes. The nested AE models were compared to the saturated ACE model. Model fit is given as minus 2 log likelihood (−2 log L), degrees of freedom (df) and difference in −2 log L and df between the nested and saturated model (Δ −2 log L, Δ df) are shown. Estimated variances explained by the specific causal factors (A = additive genetics, C = shared environment and E = unshared environment) are given with 95% confidence intervals for each model. For each model, univariate estimates for each phenotype separately and the correlation ($r(a^2)$, $r(e^2)$ and $r(c^2)$) between these estimates are reported.

Acknowledgments

We would like to acknowledge Action on Hearing Loss and in particular Thomas Fiddian, for his collaboration and help in the establishment of the SNR test. The authors would particularly like to thank Dr Sally Dawson for her advice and comments on the questionnaire and conduction of the project.

Author Contributions

Conceived and designed the experiments: LW CS FW. Performed the experiments: LW CS. Analyzed the data: LW FW. Contributed reagents/materials/analysis tools: TS. Wrote the paper: LW.

References

1. Dalton DS, Cruickshanks KJ, Klein BE, Klein R, Wiley TL, et al. (2003) The impact of hearing loss on quality of life in older adults. Gerontologist 43: 661–668.
2. Fransen E, Topsakal V, Hendrickx JJ, Van Laer L, Huyghe JR, et al. (2008) Occupational noise, smoking, and a high body mass index are risk factors for age-related hearing impairment and moderate alcohol consumption is

protective: a European population-based multicenter study. J Assoc Res Otolaryngol 9: 264–276; discussion 261–263.
3. Itoh A, Nakashima T, Arao H, Wakai K, Tamakoshi A, et al. (2001) Smoking and drinking habits as risk factors for hearing loss in the elderly: epidemiological study of subjects undergoing routine health checks in Aichi, Japan. Public Health 115: 192–196.
4. Torre P III, Cruickshanks KJ, Klein BEK, Klein R, Nondahl DM (2005) The Association Between Cardiovascular Disease and Cochlear Function in Older Adults. J Speech Lang Hear Res 48: 473–481.
5. Kakarlapudi V, Sawyer R, Staecker H (2003) The effect of diabetes on sensorineural hearing loss. Otol Neurotol 24: 382–386.
6. Schuknecht HF, Gacek MR (1993) Cochlear pathology in presbycusis. Ann Otol Rhinol Laryngol 102: 1–16.
7. Gates GA, Couropmitree NN, Myers RH (1999) Genetic associations in age-related hearing thresholds. Arch Otolaryngol Head Neck Surg 125: 654–659.
8. Viljanen A, Era P, Kaprio J, Pyykkö I, Koskenvuo M, et al. (2007) Genetic and Environmental Influences on Hearing in Older Women. The Journals of Gerontology Series A: Biological Sciences and Medical Sciences 62: 447–452.
9. Karlsson KK, Harris JR, Svartengren M (1997) Description and primary results from an audiometric study of male twins. Ear Hear 18: 114–120.
10. DeStefano AL, Gates GA, Heard-Costa N, Myers RH, Baldwin CT (2003) Genomewide linkage analysis to presbycusis in the Framingham Heart Study. Arch Otolaryngol Head Neck Surg 129: 285–289.
11. Garringer HJ, Pankratz ND, Nichols WC, Reed T (2006) Hearing Impairment Susceptibility in Elderly Men and the DFNA18 Locus. Arch Otolaryngol Head Neck Surg 132: 506–510.
12. Huyghe JR, Van Laer L, Hendrickx JJ, Fransen E, Demeester K, et al. (2008) Genome-wide SNP-based linkage scan identifies a locus on 8q24 for an age-related hearing impairment trait. Am J Hum Genet 83: 401–407.
13. Unal M, Tamer L, Dogruer ZN, Yildirim H, Vayisoglu Y, et al. (2005) N-acetyltransferase 2 gene polymorphism and presbycusis. Laryngoscope 115: 2238–2241.
14. Van Eyken E, Van Camp G, Fransen E, Topsakal V, Hendrickx JJ, et al. (2007) Contribution of the N-acetyltransferase 2 polymorphism NAT2*6A to age-related hearing impairment. J Med Genet 44: 570–578.
15. Van Laer L, Van Eyken E, Fransen E, Huyghe JR, Topsakal V, et al. (2008) The grainyhead like 2 gene (GRHL2), alias TFCP2L3, is associated with age-related hearing impairment. Hum Mol Genet 17: 159–169.
16. Friedman RA, Van Laer L, Huentelman MJ, Sheth SS, Van Eyken E, et al. (2009) GRM7 variants confer susceptibility to age-related hearing impairment. Hum Mol Genet 18: 785–796.
17. Van Laer L, Huyghe JR, Hannula S, Van Eyken E, Stephan DA, et al. (2010) A genome-wide association study for age-related hearing impairment in the Saami. European Journal of Human Genetics 18: 685–693.
18. Manolio TA, Collins FS, Cox NJ, Goldstein DB, Hindorff LA, et al. (2009) Finding the missing heritability of complex diseases. Nature 461: 747–753.
19. ActionOnHearingLoss (2011) Check your Hearing- online hearing test. London: Action on Hearing Loss.
20. Spector TD, Williams FM (2006) The UK Adult Twin Registry (TwinsUK). Twin Res Hum Genet 9: 899–906.
21. Fransen E, Van Laer L, Lemkens N, Caethoven G, Flothmann K, et al. (2004) A novel Z-score-based method to analyze candidate genes for age-related hearing impairment. Ear Hear 25: 133–141.
22. Van Laer L, Huyghe JR, Hannula S, Van Eyken E, Stephan DA, et al. (2010) A genome-wide association study for age-related hearing impairment in the Saami. Eur J Hum Genet 18: 685–693.
23. Smits C, Kapteyn TS, Houtgast T (2004) Development and validation of an automatic speech-in-noise screening test by telephone. International Journal of Audiology 43: 15–28.
24. Martin Bland J, Altman D (1986) Statistical methods for assessing agreement between two methods of clinical measurement. The Lancet 327: 307–310.
25. Neale MC, Boker SM, Xie G, Maes HH (2006) Mx: Statistical Modeling. 7th Edition.
26. WHO (2011) Grades of hearing impairment. In: Organization WH, ed. Prevention of Blindness and Deafness Geneva: World Health Organization.
27. Neale MC, Walters EE, Eaves LJ, Maes HH, Kendler KS (1994) Multivariate genetic analysis of twin-family data on fears: Mx models. Behav Genet 24: 119–139.
28. Andrew T, Hart DJ, Snieder H, de Lange M, Spector TD, et al. (2001) Are twins and singletons comparable? A study of disease-related and lifestyle characteristics in adult women. Twin Res 4: 464–477.
29. Perry JRB, Stolk L, Franceschini N, Lunetta KL, Zhai G, et al. (2009) Meta-analysis of genome-wide association data identifies two loci influencing age at menarche. Nat Genet 41: 648–650.

11

An Eye-Tracking Paradigm for Analyzing the Processing Time of Sentences with Different Linguistic Complexities

Dorothea Wendt*, **Thomas Brand**, **Birger Kollmeier**

Medizinische Physik and Cluster of Excellence Hearing4all, Universität Oldenburg, Oldenburg, Germany

Abstract

An eye-tracking paradigm was developed for use in audiology in order to enable online analysis of the speech comprehension process. This paradigm should be useful in assessing impediments in speech processing. In this paradigm, two scenes, a target picture and a competitor picture, were presented simultaneously with an aurally presented sentence that corresponded to the target picture. At the same time, eye fixations were recorded using an eye-tracking device. The effect of linguistic complexity on language processing time was assessed from eye fixation information by systematically varying linguistic complexity. This was achieved with a sentence corpus containing seven German sentence structures. A novel data analysis method computed the average tendency to fixate the target picture as a function of time during sentence processing. This allowed identification of the point in time at which the participant understood the sentence, referred to as the decision moment. Systematic differences in processing time were observed as a function of linguistic complexity. These differences in processing time may be used to assess the efficiency of cognitive processes involved in resolving linguistic complexity. Thus, the proposed method enables a temporal analysis of the speech comprehension process and has potential applications in speech audiology and psychoacoustics.

Editor: Joseph Najbauer, University of Pécs Medical School, Hungary

Funding: This study was supported by the Deutsche Forschungsgemeinschaft (DFG) within the AULIN Project (grant numbers KO 942/20-1 and BR 3668/1-2). The funders had no role in study design, data collection and analysis, decision to publish, or preparation of the manuscript.

Competing Interests: The authors have declared that no competing interests exist.

* Email: wendt@elektro.dtu.dk

Introduction

Speech intelligibility tests are an indispensable tool in clinical audiology. They can evaluate the consequence of sensory hearing loss (characterized by a frequency dependent hearing impairment) for the patient's communication abilities [1–4]. Beyond diagnostic applications, speech intelligibility tests are also often used to quantify the benefit of hearing aids or cochlear implants for individual patients. Typically, speech intelligibility tests measure the proportion of correctly repeated speech items, usually single words or single sentences [5–8]. However, research has shown that additional performance information about the ease of speech comprehension or cognitive effort during speech processing can complement traditional speech intelligibility measures. Increased cognitive effort is indicated by poorer task performance and processing time and can be measured in terms of recognition accuracy or reaction time, for instance [9,10]. The current study focuses on developing a method for assessing the speech comprehension process and processing speed as indicators of the cognitive effort required at levels of high intelligibility. The proposed method is characterized by two main aspects: Firstly, a special speech corpus is applied that is optimized for both speech intelligibility measurements and controlled variation of linguistic complexity. Secondly, eye movements are tracked to provide an online assessment of speech processing during sentence comprehension. This study aims to determine whether this combination of speech intelligibility testing and eye tracking can detect a systematic deceleration in speech processing due to an increase in cognitive processing effort that is sufficiently large and robust to be used in audiology. A further question is whether the deceleration effect is detected by either recognition scores or reaction times alone.

A. Speech intelligibility and linguistic complexity

Several studies reported that speech intelligibility is influenced by linguistic aspects of the speech material, such as context information, sentence structure, or level of complexity [11–13]. However, the role of linguistic aspects in speech comprehension, in particular in connection with hearing loss, has been largely neglected in standard audiological testing. In addition, speech intelligibility measurements provide little information about linguistic aspects in language comprehension, such as processing costs arising from different levels of cognitive load and/or linguistic complexity [13]. Recently, Uslar et al. [14] developed the Oldenburg Linguistically and Audiologically Controlled Sentences (OLACS) material to differentiate between acoustical and linguistic factors and their respective contributions to speech intelligibility measurement. Using the OLACS corpus, Uslar et al. measured speech reception thresholds (SRT) and reported a small effect of complexity on speech intelligibility (about 1–2 dB). However, studies in which participants were asked a comprehension question following sentence presentation revealed a stronger effect of linguistic complexity on sentence processing. For instance, Tun and colleagues [10] measured reaction times for sentences with different sentence structures presented at a clearly audible level. They observed reduced speech processing speeds for structures with higher linguistic complexity. It was argued that the reduced comprehension speed was caused by the increased cognitive processing demands of the more complex sentence structures. Hence, sentence complexity can lead to slower sentence processing. This suggests that sentence processing speed may be a more sensitive measure for detecting difficulties during sentence understanding than standard methods used in audiology, such as speech intelligibility tests. Reaction time, as reported by Tun et al. [10], and speech intelligibility measures are taken after the speech is presented. These offline measures do not provide any time-resolved information about the process of sentence comprehension, but instead reflect the end point of this process. On the other hand, an online analysis of processing time occurring *during* the presentation of the sentence is expected to provide a more direct measure of any temporal changes in speech processing that are not reflected by offline measures.

Another advantage of using response measures based on eye movements is their relative robustness against age effects [15]; latency and reaction times using a button press exhibit age-related differences [16]. This is an important issue when testing listeners with hearing impairment because hearing loss typically increases with age. For this reason, this study recorded both eye fixation and reaction time derived from pressing buttons.

B. Analysis of eye movements with respect to speech processing

Eye movements are frequently used in psycholinguistic research in order to better understand how people process spoken sentences and to investigate linguistic aspects during sentence processing. A temporal relationship between speech processing and eye movements was shown in the pioneering study by Cooper [17], and confirmed in more recent studies (see [18] for a review). The visual world paradigm [19–21] was introduced in psycholinguistics to reveal the interaction between language and vision. In that paradigm, eye movements were recorded while simultaneously presenting spoken language and a visual scene that typically included the objects mentioned in the presented speech. Participants spontaneously fixated on the object that corresponded to the acoustical input. Several subsequent studies have investigated how and when the linguistic and visual information are integrated [22–29]. These recorded data were often used to investigate how linguistic processes determine the participants' sentence processing and understanding.

The method of analyzing the recorded eye-tracking data in the visual world paradigm, however, depends on the research question [18] and has not been adapted for use in audiology or made available to answer the research questions of the current study. For these reasons, an approach was adapted which combined several techniques from other (visual world) studies. The new approach was designed to meet the following requirements: a) the eye-tracking data must have a high temporal resolution; b) the test design must be symmetric, averaging out any systematic eye movement strategies, such as a preference for analyzing the pictures from left to right; c) the eye-tracking data analysis should shed light on speech comprehension and the decision process. Since the combination of these processing techniques is novel, the motivation behind each step is outlined in the following.

To investigate the effect of linguistic aspects on the comprehension process, the speech stimuli (words or sentences) were subdivided into separate time windows, as in previous studies [22,26]. Due to the nature of speech, these segments varied slightly in duration. For this reason, a time alignment was applied. This allowed temporal averaging across segments and a high temporal resolution on a sub-segment basis.

As in previous visual world studies, the visual stimulus was subdivided into regions of interest (ROIs): one for the target picture and one for the competitor picture. Previous studies have analyzed whether these ROIs differ in their likelihoods of being fixated during each time segment [30,31], or whether a ROI is looked at earlier in an experimental condition than in a control condition [22,23]. Accordingly, the current study analyzed fixation rate as a function of time for different ROIs. Previous studies found that one region of interest was more likely to be fixated even before stimulus presentation, and emphasized that these baseline effects should be taken into account when analyzing the eye-tracking data [32]. However, methods that account for baseline effects have not often been applied in visual world studies. Therefore, the current study proposes a method that calculates the rates of fixations towards a target picture (in the current study a picture that matches the spoken sentence) in relation to the rate of fixation towards a competitor picture. As this is done both for target pictures on the left and on the right side, any systematic eye movement strategy that the participant uses, such as gazing preferably from left to right, is averaged out from the data. This is referred to as *symmetrizing* in the following. The applicability of assessing differences between fixations towards a target and a competitor was previously shown by other studies [33,34]. A post-processing step is proposed that includes a bootstrap method to calculate the 95% confidence interval of the estimated probability that the participant fixates the target picture. Bootstrapping is an appropriate method for analyzing measurement statistics in situations where observed values violate normality or are unknown [35,36]. In order to obtain a defined measure of processing speed and to detect the point in time when the target is recognized by the participant, a fixed threshold criterion is used, as described by McMurray and colleagues [37,38].

The underlying hypothesis of this study is that the proposed eye-tracking paradigm can detect significant and robust reductions in sentence processing speed for sentence structures with increased linguistic complexity. This would qualify the proposed method for use in audiology. An increase in processing time, indicated by eye fixations as well as by reaction times, is then interpreted as evidence for a greater cognitive processing effort during sentence comprehension. This study had three main goals:

- Introduction of an eye-tracking paradigm that is adapted to the OLACS speech intelligibility test and enables online analysis of the time course of the sentence comprehension process for use in audiology.
- Introduction of a time-resolved statistical analysis technique for eye-tracking data that derives the decision moment (DM), defined as the point in time when the target is recognized by the participant. The analysis should take into account any systematic eye movement strategy employed by the participants.
- Evaluation of this paradigm and provision of normative data testing listeners with normal hearing in quiet.
- Identification of those sentence structures that show the most significant effects of linguistic complexity. As a prerequisite for a time-efficient clinical application, a reduced subset of test sentences will be needed for testing speech processing in listeners with hearing impairment in quiet and in noise.

Material and Methods

A. Participants

Seventeen volunteer participants (ten male and seven female) with normal hearing took part in the experiment. Hearing thresholds were measured at octave frequencies from 125 Hz to 8000 Hz. All participants had hearing thresholds less than 15 dB above normal threshold according to DIN EN ISO 8253-1 for all frequencies. All participants were native German speakers between 18 and 30 years of age (average age: 26 years) and either had uncorrected vision or wore corrective eyewear (glasses or contact lenses) when necessary.

B. Ethics statement

Written consent was obtained from each participant prior to the experiments. The experiments were approved by the local ethics committee of the University of Oldenburg.

C. Stimuli

Speech material. A total of 148 sentences from the OLACS corpus were used ([14]; a subset of the OLACS corpus can be obtained at http://www.aulin.uni-oldenburg.de/49349.html). Each sentence corresponded to one of seven different syntactic structures; there were approximately 21 sentences of each structure. The seven syntactic sentence structures fall into two major groups: verb-second structures and relative-clause structures (Table 1). Both groups contain sentences with canonical (subject-before-object) and non-canonical (object-before-subject) word orders.

The group of verb-second structures includes three sentence structures: subject-verb-object (SVO), object-verb-subject (OVS), and ambiguous object-verb-subject (ambOVS). The SVO structure has the canonical word order for simple main clauses in German and is considered syntactically simple and easy to process [39]. The OVS structure is more complex because of its non-canonical word order [40]. The SVO and OVS structures are unambiguous with respect to their meaning and to the grammatical role of the sentence components (see Table 1). For example, the grammatical function of the first noun phrase is clearly marked for both the SVO structure (*Der kleine Junge*$_{PTD}$, 'The $_{nom}$ little$_{nom}$ boy$_{nom}$' *nom* indicates the nominative case marking) and the OVS structure (*Den lieben Vater*$_{PTD}$, 'The$_{acc}$ nice$_{acc}$ father' *acc* indicates the accusative case marking). In both of these sentence structures, the disambiguating word, which is the word that clarifies the agent/object role assignment, is the first noun. For instance, the noun, *Junge*$_{PTD}$ 'boy$_{nom}$' in the SVO sentence disambiguates the sentence in such a way that participants are theoretically able to relate the spoken sentence to the target picture as soon as the noun is spoken. In all cases, the onset of the word that disambiguates subject and object is termed the point of target disambiguation (PTD). Thus,

Table 1. The Oldenburg Linguistically and Audiologically Controlled Sentences (OLACS).

Verb-second structures							
SVO	Der	kleine	Junge$_{PTD}$	grüßt	den	lieben	Vater.
	The$_{nom}$	little$_{nom}$	boy$_{nom}$	greets$_{3sg}$	the$_{acc}$	nice$_{acc}$	father.
	The little boy greets the nice father.						
OVS	Den	lieben	Vater$_{PTD}$	grüßt	der	kleine	Junge.
	The$_{acc}$	nice$_{acc}$	father	greets$_{3sg}$	the$_{nom}$	little$_{nom}$	boy$_{nom}$.
	It is the nice father that the little boy is greeting.						
ambOVS	Die	liebe	Königin	grüßt	der$_{PTD}$	kleine	Junge.
	The$_{amb}$	nice$_{amb}$	queen$_{fem,amb}$	greets$_{3sg}$	the$_{nom}$	little$_{nom}$	boy$_{nom}$.
	It is the nice queen that the little boy is greeting.						
Relative-clause structures							
SR	Der	Bauer,	der $_{PTD}$	die	Ärztinnen	fängt,	lacht.
	The$_{nom,sg}$	farmer$_{nom,sg}$	who$_{nom,sg}$	the$_{nom}$	doctors$_{amb,pl,fem}$	catches$_{3sg}$	laughs$_{3sg}$.
	The farmer who is catching the doctors is laughing.						
OR	Der	Bauer,	den $_{PTD}$	die	Ärztinnen	fangen,	lacht.
	The$_{nom,sg}$	farmer$_{nom,sg}$	who$_{acc,\ sg}$	the	doctors$_{amb,pl,fem}$	catch$_{3pl}$	laugh$_{3sg}$.
	The farmer whom the doctors are catching is laughing.						
ambSR	Die	Bäuerinnen,	die	die	Ärztin	fangen$_{PTD}$,	lachen.
	The$_{amb}$	farmers$_{amb,pl,fem}$	who$_{amb}$	the$_{amb}$	doctor$_{sg,fem}$	catch$_{3pl}$	laugh$_{3pl}$.
	The farmers who are catching the doctor are laughing.						
ambOR	Die	Bäuerinnen,	die	die	Ärztin	fängt$_{PTD}$,	lachen.
	The$_{amb}$	farmers$_{amb,pl,fem}$	who$_{amb}$	the$_{amb}$	doctor$_{amb,sg,\ fem}$	catches$_{3sg}$	laugh$_{3pl}$.
	The farmers whom the doctor is catching are laughing.						

Example sentences for the seven sentence structures of the OLACS corpus. The disambiguating word from which the target picture could theoretically first be identified by the participant is indicated with *PTD* (point of target disambiguation). *Nom* (nominative), *acc* (accusative), and *amb* (ambiguous case) indicate the relevant case markings. *Sg* indicates singular forms and *pl* indicates plural forms. Verbs are either in their third person singular (*3sg*) or third person plural (*3pl*) form. *fem* indicates feminine nouns. *SVO, OVS,* and *ambOVS* sentence structures belong to the verb-second structures since they have either a subject-verb-object or an object-verb-subject sentence structure. *SR, OR, ambSR,* and *ambOR* sentence structures belong to the relative-clause structures. An English translation of the meaning of each example sentence is given in italics.

the PTD was defined as the onset of the word that first enabled correct recognition of the target picture. Note that we chose the onset of the word even though in some sentence structures the recognition of the target was only made possible by the suffix of the disambiguating word. This was necessary because it was not possible to determine the exact point in time at which the disambiguation occurs during the spoken word.

The third verb-second structure, ambOVS, has an object-before-subject structure with a later point of disambiguation. In these sentences, the first article is ambiguously marked for case: the first article, *Die* ('The$_{amb}$' *amb* indicates the ambiguous case marking; see Table 1) could indicate either subject or object function (and subsequently agent or object role) and only the article of the second noun, *der*$_{PTD}$ ('the$_{nom}$' *nom* indicates the nominative case marking; see Table 1) is unambiguously case-marked.

The second group of sentence structures, which have relative-clause structures, includes four different structures of embedded relative clauses (Table 1): subject-relative (SR) clauses and object-relative (OR) clauses, with a PTD at the first relative pronoun *der*$_{PTD}$ ('who$_{nom,sg}$') or *den*$_{PTD}$ ('who$_{acc,sg}$' *sg* indicates singular form; see Table 1); and ambiguous subject-relative clauses (ambSR) and ambiguous object-relative clauses (ambOR) with a late PTD. The ambSR and ambOR sentence structures are disambiguated by the verb, *fangen*$_{PTD}$ ('catch$_{3pl}$' *3pl* indicates the third person plural form) or *fängt*$_{PTD}$ ('catches$_{3sg}$'), of the embedded clause (Table 1).

The speech material provides different levels of linguistic complexity by varying three different structural factors of the sentence material: word order, embedding, and ambiguity. The preferred, canonical word order in German, like many other languages, is subject-before-object [41,42]. The non-canonical object-before-subject word order is considered syntactically more complex [43] and has been shown to increase processing costs in the form of reduced accuracy and longer reaction times [9,10,44]. Another factor leading to increased processing costs is embedded relative-clauses [45,46]. Within the relative-clause structures, processing costs can be further increased by word order [41,46] (SR and OR structures in Table 1). The OLACS corpus further includes temporally ambiguous sentence structures, in which disambiguation occurs later. The ambiguity of these sentence structures (ambOVS, ambSR, ambOR) can lead to temporary uncertainty with regard to the grammatical role of the sentence components [14,47]. Because of this ambiguity, the participant has to reanalyze the initial subject after the point of disambiguation. Hence, the ambiguity can lead to both increased processing cost and temporary misinterpretation of the sentence.

Visual stimuli. In total, picture sets for 150 sentences of the OLACS corpus were created. Each picture set consisted of two pictures (Figure 1). One of the two pictures, the target picture, illustrated the situation described by the sentence. In the competitor picture, the roles of agent (the active character) and object (the passive character) were interchanged. In each picture, the agent was always shown on the left side in order to facilitate fast comprehension of the depicted scene. Presenting both pictures at the same time ensured that participants did not assign agent and object roles using only visual information. All of the figures illustrated in the picture sets had the same size in order to avoid effects of contrast between the figures. Care was taken in selecting actions, agents, and objects that were non-stereotypical, such that the action was not characteristic for the agent (for example, baking is a typical action of a baker). This constraint was employed to make sure that participants did not make premature role assignments based on any anticipation of an agent's characteristic action. The picture set was divided into three regions of interest (ROI): ROI1 defined the target picture, ROI2 the competitor picture, and ROI3 defined the background. The target picture was shown randomly either on the left or right side of the computer screen. Consequently, the positions of ROI1 and ROI2 were not fixed, but changed randomly from trial to trial.

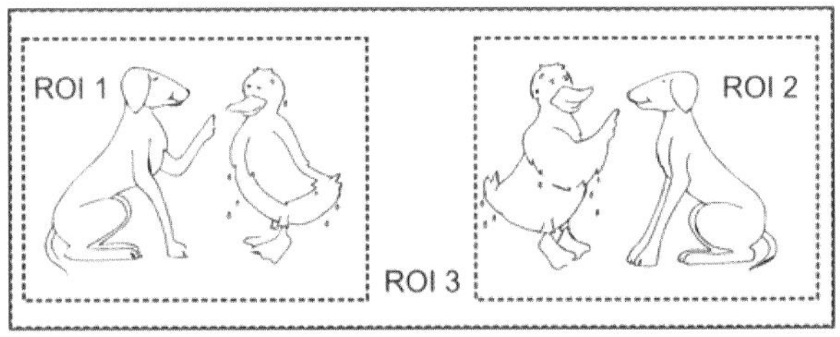

Figure 1. The visual stimulus. Example picture set for a sentence of the ambOVS sentence structure: *Die nasse Ente tadelt der treue Hund.* (The wet duck (acc.) reprimands the loyal dog (nom.), which means, "It is the wet duck that is reprimanded by the loyal dog"). A picture set consists of two single pictures. The dashed lines indicate the three regions of interest (ROI) and are not visible for the participants. ROI1 is the target picture and can be located on the left or right side of the picture set. ROI2 is the competitor picture. ROI3 is the background.

Validation of the visual stimuli. To ensure that both pictures in a particular picture set could be parsed and interpreted equally well, a subset of the graphical material was tested by measuring the reaction times of 20 participants. For 106 picture sets, the reaction time for each picture was measured (212 single pictures). For that purpose, each sentence was presented visually in written form on a computer screen for 1500 ms. Afterward one picture, either the target or the competitor picture, was shown on the computer screen, and the participants had to decide whether the presented picture matched the previously displayed sentence. Participants were instructed to respond as quickly as possible and reaction times were measured. Note that the sentences were simplified for the validation of the visual stimuli: the modified sentences all had a subject-verb-object structure, and the adjectives of the verb-second structures and the matrix verbs of the relative-clause structures were omitted in this pre-test. For instance, Figure 1 shows the picture corresponding to the example sentence, "The dog reprimands the duck." By modifying the sentences to have the same syntactical structure, any effects of linguistic complexity on reaction times were avoided. The statistical significance of the differences in reaction times for the two pictures of one set was calculated for all participants using a paired t-test with a 5% significance level. If a significant difference was found, the picture set was excluded from the eye-tracking study. Of the 106 picture sets tested, two sets were excluded. Because so few picture sets had to be excluded, no formal reaction time validation was performed for the additional 44 picture sets that were produced later and added to the experimental set. Thus, in total, 148 different picture sets were used for the eye-tracking experiment.

D. Procedure

For the experiments, an OLACS picture set was presented visually on a computer screen while the recorded sentence was presented via headphones. First, the participants performed one training block, which contained all 148 picture sets. After training, six test blocks, containing 110 sentences each, were performed. In total, each participant listened to 660 sentences. 148 sentences were presented in quiet at a level of 65 dB SPL. Two conditions with different background noises were employed for a different study: 444 sentences were presented in different noise conditions.

Table 2. Time segments used for time alignment across sentences.

	Segment 1	Segment 2	Segment 3	Segment 4	Segment 5	Segment 6
Segment borders/sample	0–100	100–200	200–300	300–400	400–500	500–end
Verb-second structure	*no acoustic stimulus*	Der kleine	Junge	grüβt den	lieben Vater.	*response time*
		The little	boy	greets the	nice father.	
Mean segment borders/ ms	0–1000	1000–1745 (±130)	1745–2340 (±135)	2340–2995 (±130)	2995–4140 (±151)	4140–end (±114)
Relative-clause structure	*no acoustic stimulus*	Der Bauer,	der die Ärtzinnen	fängt,	lacht.	*response time*
		The farmer	who the doctors	catches	smiles.	
Mean segment borders/ ms	0–1000	1000–1885 (±200)	1885–2755 (±136)	2755–3430 (±131)	3430–4450 (±143)	4450–end (±238)

Time segments for the verb-second and relative-clause structures used for time alignment across sentences. The first row gives the borders of each segment in time samples. Segment 1 describes the time from the onset of the measurement until the onset of the acoustical stimulus. The spoken sentence was presented during segments 2 through 5. Segment 6 corresponds to the time between the end of the spoken sentence and the participant's response. An example sentence is given for each group. The mean segment borders (in milliseconds) were calculated over all sentences in the group after the resampling procedure (± standard deviation).

These 592 sentences were randomly distributed across the six test blocks. In order to avoid retrieval strategies, 68 filler trials were presented across all test blocks (11–12 filler trials per test block). During a filler trial, either the target or the competitor picture was depicted on both sides of the screen, with the positions of the agent and object reversed in one of the two pictures. Therefore, either both of the pictures matched the spoken sentence or neither did. These trials forced the participants to fixate on both pictures.

The visual stimulus was presented 1000 ms before the onset of the acoustic stimulus. Participants were instructed to identify the picture that matched the acoustic stimulus by pressing one of three keys as quickly as possible: The "A" indicated that participants assigned the target to the left picture, and "L" indicated assignment to the right picture; participants were instructed to press the space bar if they were not able to clearly assign one target picture to the spoken sentence. The position of the selected keys enabled the participants to leave their hands on the keyboard during the experiment so they did not have to look at the keyboard to search for the right key. After each trial, participants were asked to look at a marker at the center of the screen so that a drift correction could be performed. At the beginning of each test block a calibration was done using a nine-point fixation stimulus. The completion of one test block of trials took about 20 min. After each block, participants had a ten-minute break. The entire measurement took about three hours per participant, which was divided into two sessions.

E. Apparatus

An eye-tracker system (EyeLink 1000 desktop system including the EyeLink CL high-speed camera, SR Research Ltd.) was used to monitor participants' eye fixations with a sampling rate of 1000 Hz. The pictures were presented on a 22″ multi-scan color computer screen with a resolution of 1680×1050 pixels. Participants were seated 60 cm from the computer screen. A chin rest was used to stabilize the participant's head. Although, viewing was binocular, the eye-tracker sampled only from the dominant eye. Auditory signals were presented via closed headphones (Sennheiser HDA 200) that were free-field compensated according to DIN EN ISO 389-8 (2004). For the calibration of the speech signals, a Brüel & Kjær (B&K) 4153 artificial ear, a B&K 4134 1/2 inch microphone, a B&K 2669 preamplifier, and a B&K 2610 measuring amplifier were used. All experiments took place in a sound-insulated booth.

Data Analysis

A. Time alignment

Since the sentences differed in length, a time alignment was employed to allow comparisons across sentences. This was realized by dividing each trial into six segments, as shown in Table 2. Note that the choice of segment borders and the evaluation of eye-tracking data during these segments were selected to best fit the employed OLACS speech material. Knoeferle and colleagues [26] showed that for German sentences with an initially ambiguous structure, sentence interpretation happens immediately after the point in time at which the combination of visual and linguistic information disambiguates the sentence. Therefore, segment borders were defined according to the word that first enabled correct recognition of the target picture. Segment 1 corresponds to the time from the onset of the visual stimulus until the onset of the acoustical stimulus. The spoken sentence was presented during segments 2 through 5. The time from the end of the spoken sentence until the participant responded by pressing the response key was denoted as segment 6. The segment borders and the corresponding points in time (in ms) during the eye-tracking recordings were determined for each sentence and averaged over all sentences of a single sentence structure (see Table 2).

B. Calculation of the target detection amplitude (TDA)

The eye-tracking data were used to calculate the target detection amplitude (TDA). The TDA quantifies the tendency of the participant to fixate on the target picture in the presence of the competitor picture. The data analysis for the TDA was divided into three stages (Figures 2 and 3). In the first stage, the calculation was sentence based (left panel in Figure 2). The recorded eye-tracking data were analyzed and the fixations on the target (ROI1), the competitor (ROI2), and the background (ROI3) were calculated as functions of time. Trials in which the target was presented on the left side were considered separately from those in which the target was on the right. A time alignment and a resampling stage were employed to associate the observed fixations of the ROIs with the appropriate sentence segment (see Table 2). To synchronize the segment borders across sentences, the first five segments were individually rescaled to a fixed length of 100

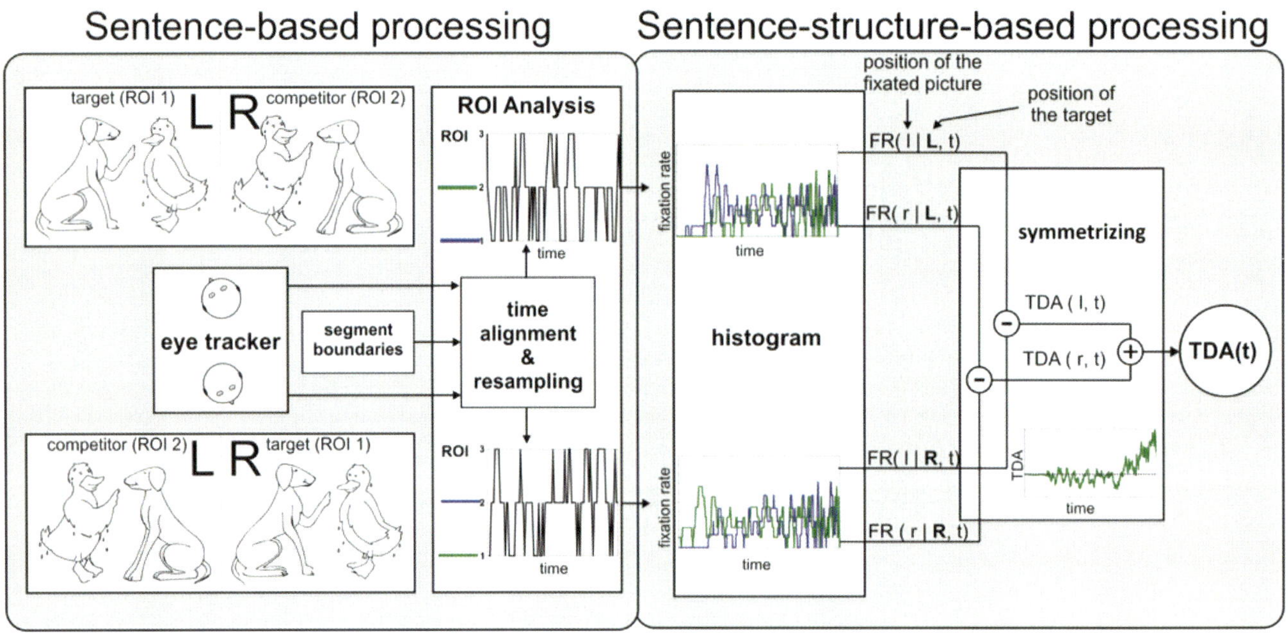

Figure 2. Schematic diagram for the analysis of the recorded eye fixation data. The first two stages of the calculation of the target detection amplitude (TDA) are depicted, namely the sentence-based processing and the sentence-structure-based processing stages.

samples using an interpolation algorithm. The length of segment 6 depended on the mean reaction time of the participant, with a maximal length of 200 samples (see Table 2). For instance, if the reaction time was 1500 ms, the last segment was rescaled to a length of 150 samples. For reaction times longer than 2000 ms, the signal was cut to a length of 200 samples. This was done because 1000 ms after the offset of the sentence, on average, participants fixated less frequently on the target picture (as can be seen in segment 6 in Figure 4 and Figure 5). This may have been because no more information could be gained after this time. The segment-based resampling used a fixed number of samples per segment (except for the last segment), which resulted in a segment-dependent sampling rate depending on the individual length of each segment. This resampling not only allowed comparison

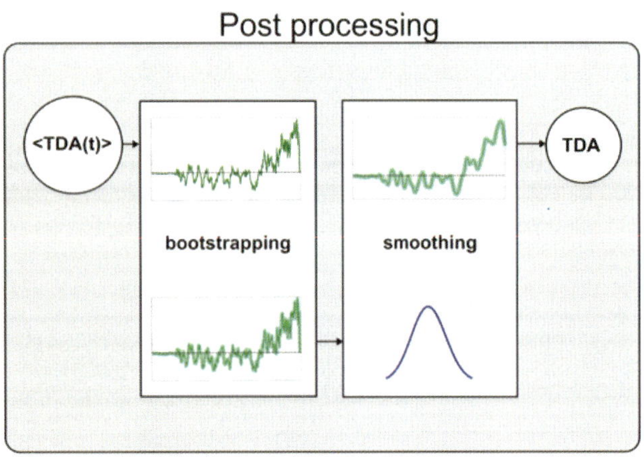

Figure 3. Post-processing stage of the analysis of the recorded eye-fixation data. Post processing of the target detection amplitude (TDA), including the bootstrap method and Gaussian smoothing.

across sentences of one structure, but also across different sentence structures.

The second stage of the TDA calculation was sentence-structure based (Figure 2). For a given (interpolated) time sample, the fixated ROIs were averaged across all sentences of a given sentence structure, resulting in an average fixation rate (right panel in Figure 2). Further analysis of the data showed that the fixation rates of the background (ROI3) did not differ significantly between sentence structures. Since this study examines the differences in the time courses of the TDAs for different sentence structures, the fixation rates of the background (ROI3) were not considered in the calculation of the TDA. Thus, the fixation rates of target (ROI1) and competitor (ROI2) did not add up to 100%. Only trials in which the participants selected the correct picture were used for further analysis. This selection was done in order to analyze time patterns of eye fixations that reflected the dynamics of the recognition process for correctly identified sentences only.

Symmetrizing. In general, participants tended to fixate more frequently on the left picture. This effect was independent of the position of the target picture and was most noticeable in segment 1, before the acoustical stimulus was presented. This tendency towards the left picture probably arose from the usual reading direction and was exploited in the paradigm by always presenting the agent of each scene on the left side of each picture (except in filler trials). This agent-left convention supported the participant in systematic and fast analysis of each picture as uncertainties about the agent's and the object's roles within each picture were reduced. The agent-left convention may have supported the listeners' left-to-right strategy. To correct for this, the test design was symmetrized: in random order, the target picture was presented equally often on the left and right sides. Subsequently, the fixation rate was averaged across all trials, averaging out any left-to-right picture reading strategy. One half was subtracted from the resulting averaged target fixation rate (which ranges between 0 and 1) in order to center it around 0. The result was then multiplied by 2. This resulted in the TDA, which assumed the

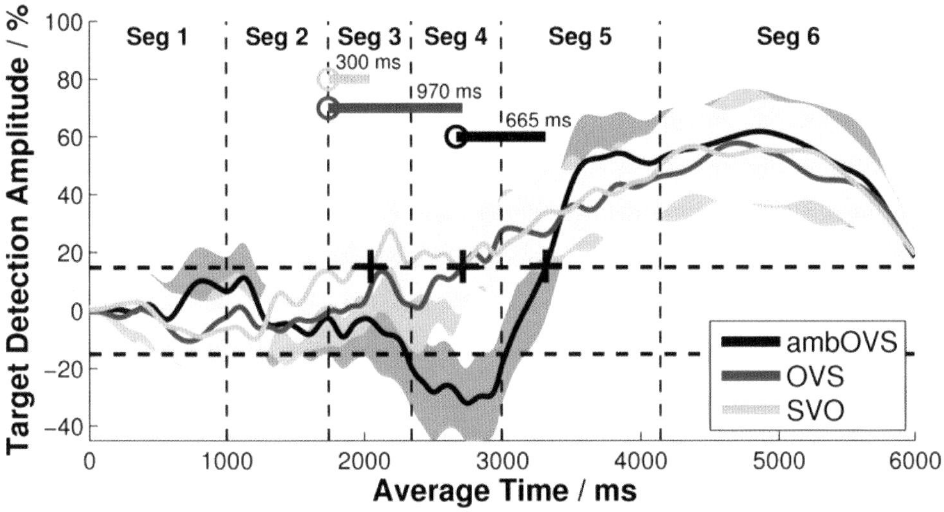

Figure 4. Mean target detection amplitude (TDA) for the verb-second structures. Mean target detection amplitude (TDA) averaged over all participants for the verb-second structures, i.e. the subject-verb-object (SVO), object-verb-subject (OVS), and the ambiguous object-verb-subject (ambOVS) structures. The shaded areas illustrate the 95% confidence intervals for each individual curve. The + signs at 2045 ms, 2715 ms, and 3315 ms denote the decision moments (DM) where the TDA first exceeded the threshold (15% of the TDA). The circles denote the point of target disambiguation (PTD): at 1745 ms for the SVO and OVS sentences and at 2650 ms for the ambOVS sentences. The horizontal lines denote the disambiguation to decision delay (DDD), which is the distance between the PTD and the DM.

value -1 for sole fixations of the competitor, 0 for random fixation, and 1 for sole fixations of the target. The calculation of the TDA was split into different processing steps, which allowed analysis of the fixation rates for left and right targets separately. Four different fixation rates FR(s | S, t) were considered, with s denoting the position of the fixated picture (with l for left side and r for right side), S denoting the position of the target picture (with L for left side and R for right side), and t denoting the time. Depending on the position of the target, the two fixation rates of the competitor pictures FR(r | L, t) and FR(l | R, t) were subtracted from the respective fixation rates of the target pictures FR(l | L, t) and FR(r | R, t). This gave the TDA for the left picture:

$$TDA(l,t) = FR(l|L,t) - FR(l|R,t)$$

and for the right picture:

$$TDA(r,t) = FR(r|R,t) - FR(r|L,t).$$

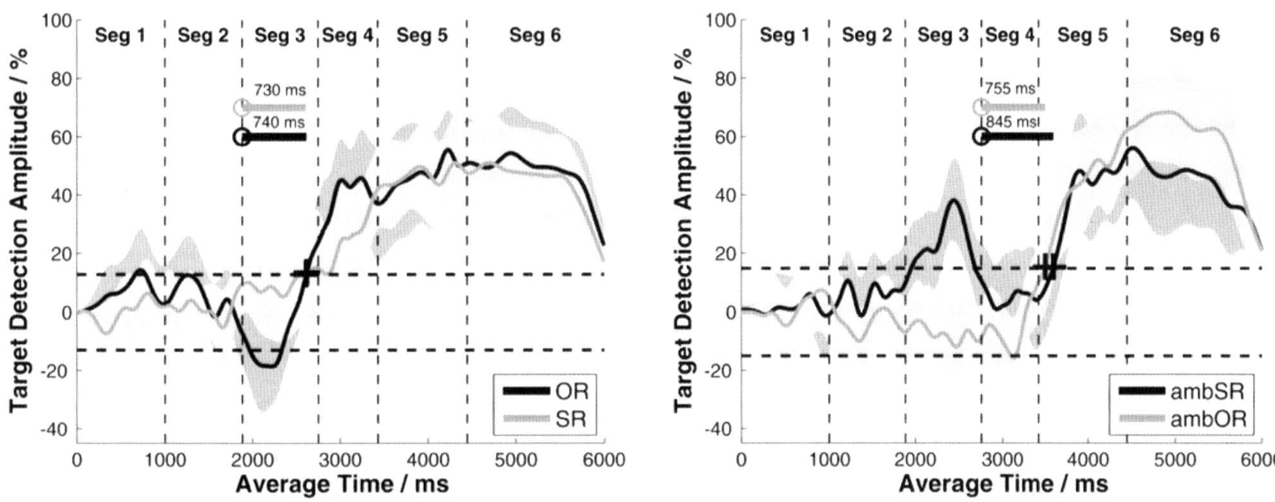

Figure 5. Mean target detection amplitude (TDA) for the relative-clause structures. Mean target detection amplitude (TDA) averaged over all participants for the relative-clause structures of the OLACS. The shaded areas illustrate the 95% confidence intervals for each curve. Left panel: unambiguous subject-relative clause (SR) vs. unambiguous object-relative clause (OR) sentences; DMs (+) at 2615 ms and 2625 ms, respectively. Right panel: ambiguous subject-relative clause (ambSR) vs. ambiguous object-relative clause (ambOR) sentences; DMs (+) at 3600 ms and 3510 ms, respectively. Circles denote the points of target disambiguation (PTD): at 1885 ms for the SR and OR sentences and at 2755 ms for the ambSR and ambOR sentences.

Table 3. Picture recognition rates and reaction times.

	Verb-second structures		
Sentence structure	**Recognition rate/rau**	**Reaction time/ms**	**Decision moment/ms**
SVO	97.6±5.1	2057±477	2045(Δt = 645)
OVS	105.8±8.1	1956±421	2715 (Δt = 1380)
ambOVS	81.0±4.3	1944±300	3315 (Δt = 275)
	Relative-clause structures		
Sentence structure	**Recognition rate/rau**	**Reaction time/ms**	**Decision moment/ms**
SR	101.4±8.8	2029±411	2615 (Δt = 1515)
OR	91.6±9.9	1965±447	2625 (Δt = 335)
ambSR	100.9±8.7	2084±643	3600 (Δt = 895)
ambOR	96.2±4.4	1898±367	3510 (Δt = 340)

Picture recognition rates and reaction times obtained from the keyboard responses, and the calculated decision moments (DM) for each sentence structure. The mean picture recognition rates in rationalized arcsine units (rau), reaction times (ms), and DMs (ms) were calculated over all participants for both verb-second and relative-clause structures of the OLACS corpus. The calculated DMs are listed for each sentence structure with the corresponding width Δt (in milliseconds) of the confidence interval at the 15% threshold along the timeline.

The position-independent total TDA was expressed using the sum of the two side-dependent TDA(s,t):

$$TDA(t) = TDA(l,t) + TDA(r,t).$$

The total TDA(t) was a function of time and quantified the tendency to fixate on the target picture within the arrangement of alternative pictures. Positive values indicated more fixations on the target picture and negative values indicated more fixations on the competitor picture. A value near zero reflected the inability to differentiate between the two pictures at a given point in time. The TDA(t) was computed for all 17 participants, resulting in a set M of 17 values for each sentence structure at a given point in time t:

$$M_{TDA} = TDA_1(t), \ldots, TDA_{17}(t).$$

C. Post-processing

To compute the time-smoothed mean value and estimate the 95% confidence interval of the TDA, this set was input to a post-processing stage, as depicted in Figure 3.

A bootstrapping resampling procedure was applied [35,36] to estimate the mean value and 95% confidence interval of the average TDA across participants for the different OLACS sentence structures without assuming any underlying distribution. This type of bootstrapping procedure has been successfully applied before to analyze eye-tracking data [48]. This bootstrapping was necessary because the underlying distribution of the mean value across the set MTDA at a given point in time was unknown and could vary across different sentence structures. For each time point, a sample from MTDA was randomly selected with replacement 17 times and averaged to provide a random estimate of the mean value <TDA(t)> across participants. This process was repeated 10,000 times, resulting in a resampled data set containing 10,000 values that approximated the estimated distribution of <TDA(t)>. From this distribution, the 95% confidence intervals and the mean value <TDA(t)> were obtained. Finally, a Gaussian smoothing filter with a kernel size of 25 samples was applied in order to reduce the random fluctuations of the <TDA(t)>. The resulting signal was called TDA (see e.g. Figure 4).

D. Calculation of the decision moment (DM) and the disambiguation to decision delay (DDD)

The decision moment (DM) was defined as the point in time from which the mean TDA exceeded the 15% threshold for at least 200 ms. The threshold was chosen as 15% TDA because small fluctuations in the TDA are not relevant for the investigation of speech processing. The time between the PTD and the DM was calculated for each sentence structure and defined as disambiguation to decision delay (DDD). This DDD is interpreted as a measure of processing time: The greater the DDD, the longer the processing time and the slower the speed of sentence processing.

Results and Discussion

A. Picture recognition rates and reaction times

The picture recognition rates–the percentage of correctly identified target pictures (by pushing the correct button)–for each sentence structure (see Table 3) were averaged across all participants. Before conducting further analyses, picture recognition rates were transformed to rationalized arcsine units (rau) according to [49].

To investigate the effect of sentence structure on picture recognition, a one-way repeated measures ANOVA was conducted for both groups of sentence structures. The factor sentence structure was significant for both groups of sentence structures (verb-second: $F(2;32) = 36.2$, $p<0.001$; relative-clause: $F(3;48) = 7.4$, $p<0.001$). Multiple pairwise comparisons with Bonferroni correction revealed differences in picture recognition rates between the SVO and ambOVS structures ($p<0.001$), reflecting lower picture recognition rates for the ambOVS structure. The picture recognition rate for ambOVS sentences was lower than that for OVS sentences ($p<0.001$). For the relative-clause structures, the pairwise comparisons revealed significant differences between SR and OR structures ($p = 0.001$) and between OR and ambSR structures ($p = 0.002$).

In general, significantly lower picture recognition rates, in particular for the object-first sentence structures (ambOVS and OR structures) suggest that linguistic complexity affects picture recognition performance. This is not self-evident: all of the sentences were presented in quiet at a constant sound pressure level of 65 dB and were acoustically controlled for equal intelligibility (for detailed information, see [14]), so they should all have been equally understandable. For that reason, the differences in picture recognition rates found here are evidence that linguistic factors influence the processing of syntactically complex structures in combination with the visual stimuli.

The reaction times were measured offline: participants were asked to press the response button after the end of the sentence. To investigate the effect of sentence structure on reaction time, a one-way repeated-measures ANOVA was conducted for both groups of sentence structures. The factor sentence structure was not significant for either group, indicating that sentence complexity did not affect reaction time within this paradigm. Note that the offline measures, recognition rate and reaction time, did not follow the same pattern across sentence structures, suggesting different response strategies and criteria. However, this effect was not considered further because the online measures used in this paper took place markedly before the (offline) button press. In addition, only correct trials were considered for the online analysis.

B. Eye-fixation data

The target detection amplitude (TDA) functions for the verb-second and relative-clause structures are depicted in Figures 4 and 5, respectively. The dashed vertical lines reflect the averaged segment borders. The time points corresponding to these segment borders are shown for both groups of sentence structures in Table 2. The dashed horizontal lines in Figures 4 and 5 indicate the thresholds of ±15% TDA. The decision moment (DM) is the point in time at which the TDA exceeded the threshold for at least 200 ms; it is indicated with a plus sign for each sentence structure. The DM was interpreted as the moment at which participants recognized the target, since they fixated the target picture significantly more freuquently than the competitor. The circles indicate the PTD corresponding with the words denoted in Table 1. The horizontal lines starting at the PTDs depict the disambiguation to decision delay (DDD).

Verb-second structures. Figure 4 shows the TDAs for the three sentence structures with verb-second structures. The TDAs fluctuated between the thresholds (±15% TDA) around zero during the first two segments for all three sentence structures: neither target nor competitor picture was fixated preferably. Since the PTDs for the two unambiguous sentence structures (SVO, OVS) did not occur until the beginning of segment 3, the DM was not expected before the beginning of segment 3. The fact that the TDA fluctuated around zero during the first segments indicated the success of the symmetrizing method in averaging out any systematic strategy of the participants. If the tendency of fixating the left picture first would not have been compensated for, the TDA would have differed significantly from zero.

The early case marking of the first noun phrase, *Der kleine Junge*$_{PTD}$ ('The$_{\text{nom}}$ little$_{\text{nom}}$ boy$_{\text{nom}}$;' see Table 1), in the SVO structure allowed an early thematic role assignment, so participants were able to identify the noun phrase referent, *Junge*$_{PTD}$ ('boy$_{\text{nom}}$') as the agent and to recognize the target even before the end of the spoken noun. This was indicated by an early DM during segment 3, with a DDD of 300 ms, for the SVO structure.

The first noun phrase, *Den lieben Vater*$_{PTD}$ ('The$_{\text{acc}}$ nice$_{\text{acc}}$ father' see Table 1), of the unambiguous OVS structure also provided role information at the very beginning of the spoken sentence. But despite the early PTD, the DM of the OVS structure was observed during segment 4, one segment after the first noun, *Vater*$_{PTD}$ ('father'), was spoken. Thus, the DDD for the OVS structure was about 970 ms. So although the 95% confidence intervals of the SVO and OVS structures overlapped slightly at the DMs, their DDDs differed by more than 600 ms.

Object-first sentences with a late PTD, as in the ambOVS structure, had a markedly different TDA time course. The DM of the ambOVS structure occurred during segment 5, after the onset of the second article, *der*$_{PTD}$ ('the$_{\text{nom}}$' Table 1), which disambiguated the sentence in segment 4. This resulted in a DDD of about 665 ms. Note that the DDD for the ambOVS structure was about 300 ms shorter than that of the unambiguous sentence structure, OVS. In addition, a strongly negative TDA was observed for the ambOVS structure at the end of segment 3, indicating that participants were preferentially fixating on the competitor picture. The negative TDAs were interpreted as a temporary misinterpretation arising out of listeners' preferences for subject-before-object word order. German shows a general preference of subject-before-object word order [41,42]. So listeners expected a subject-before-object sentence structure and tended to interpret the first noun phase, *Die liebe Königin* ('The$_{amb}$ nice$_{amb}$ queen$_{fem,\ amb}$' see Table 1), as the subject of the sentence. As a result, the competitor was fixated more frequently at the beginning of the sentence. This temporary misinterpretation only occurred before the sentence had been disambiguated by the article of the second noun phrase, *der*$_{PTD}$ ('the$_{nom}$').

Relative-clause structures. The left panel of Figure 5 shows the average TDAs of the unambiguous relative-clause structures (SR and OR structures). For both structures, the TDAs fluctuated around zero during the first two segments, indicating that the target was not recognized. For both sentence structures, the case-marking relative pronoun, der$_{\text{PTD}}$ ('who$_{\text{nom,\ sg}}$') or den$_{\text{PTD}}$ ('who$_{\text{acc,\ sg}}$' see Table 1), of the embedded phrase disambiguated the sentence; this is indicated by the PTD at the very beginning of segment 3. The DMs of both sentence structures occurred at the end of segment 3 and the DDDs varied between 730 ms and 740 ms.

The right panel of Figure 5 shows the TDAs of the two ambiguous relative-clause structures (ambSR and ambOR). It is clear that the embedded verbs (*fangen*$_{PTD}$ 'catch$_{\text{3pl}}$' and *fängt*$_{PTD}$ 'catches$_{\text{3sg}}$' Table 1) resolved the roles of agent and object: the PTD was located at the beginning of segment 4. The DMs were observed in segment 5, with a DDD of 755 ms for the ambOR structure and 845 ms for the ambSR structure. Note that for the unambiguous structures, the first article of the embedded sentence (*der*$_{PTD}$ 'who$_{nom,sg}$' or *den*$_{PTD}$ 'who$_{\text{acc,sg}}$' see Table 1), which had an average length of about 135 ms, disambiguated the spoken sentence. In contrast, the disambiguating word for the ambiguous sentence structure was the embedded verb (*fangen*$_{PTD}$ 'catch$_{\text{3pl}}$' and *fängt*$_{PTD}$ 'catches$_{\text{3sg}}$' see Table 1), with an average length of about 575 ms. For most of these embedded verbs the disambiguating information about the agent/object role assignment was not given until the suffix. Since the PTD was defined as the onset of the disambiguating word, the different word lengths (135 ms vs. 575 ms) had to be accounted for when comparing the DDDs of the different relative-clause structures. After subtracting the length of the disambiguating word, the remaining DDD was much smaller for the ambiguous structures than for the unambiguous structures.

Participants were not expected to discriminate between the two pictures before the PTD, so the TDAs of the two sentence structures should not differ markedly before the PTD. Surprisingly, a significant positive TDA was observed for the ambSR structure shortly after the relative pronoun *die* ('the$_{amb}$,' see Table 1) in segment 3. If this unexpected early increase in the TDA had been caused by the participants' subject-first preference, then it should have also been reflected in the time course of the ambOR structure. For instance, if the plural form of the noun used for the ambiguous subject-relative and object-relative clauses had helped the participants to recognize the target earlier, this should have been indicated in the TDA of both sentence structures. It would have appeared as an early increase in the TDA for the ambSR structure and a decrease in the TDA for the ambOR structure. However, this was not the case: no significant decrease in the TDA was observed in segment 3 or at any later point in time.

There is some evidence that this unexpected effect was caused by the presence of more acoustical cues in the ambSR sentences. Carroll and Ruigendijk [46] pointed out that there was a small but significant difference in the speech rate between the words in segment 2 in the ambSR and ambOR structures. The participants may have used the slower speech of the ambSR sentences to differentiate between the two sentence structures even before the PTD was reached. However, further investigations are needed to identify the reason for the early increase. With the rationale of this study and an audiological application in view, the ambSR structure is not recommended for further studies using the eye-tracking paradigm.

C. Precision of the estimated decision moment

In order to define the temporal precision of the DM, the temporal width Δt of the confidence interval of the TDA was determined at the DM (Table 3). That is, the width Δt of the confidence interval was calculated at the point in time at which the TDA began to exceed the 15% threshold for a period that lasted at least 200 ms. The width Δt varied from about 275 ms to 1515 ms across the seven different sentence structures. Sentence structures with a steep slope at the DM exhibited a small Δt. The steepest slopes were measured for the ambiguous sentence structures. While Δt was the smallest for the object-first sentences with ambiguous structures (ambOVS and ambOR; $\Delta t<500$ ms), for unambiguous subject-first sentence structures (SVO and SR) Δt showed high variability, due to the flat slope of the TDA at the DM. Possible differences in the process of recognizing the target between unambiguous and ambiguous sentence structures may have influenced the time course of the TDA and caused a smaller Δt for the ambiguous structures. Different decision-making processes are discussed in the following section.

General Discussion

An eye-tracking paradigm was introduced with a time-resolved statistical data analysis technique that enabled online analysis of the time course of the sentence comprehension process. The main objective of this study was to evaluate the paradigm for a group of listeners with normal hearing using a speech intelligibility test that was audiologically controlled with respect to speech intelligibility and linguistic complexity. The novel data analysis technique was designed to detect time-dependent effects in speech comprehension at various levels of linguistic complexity even at high speech intelligibility levels. The technique was designed with a potential application in audiological research in mind.

An increase in processing time could indicate that people have trouble in everyday communication situations, since the speech rate can be about 140–180 words per minute in ordinary conversations [50]. A person who is slow at sentence processing may miss speech information later in the conversation because he/she is still processing a "backlog" of past sentences or words. This slower sentence processing is interpreted as an indicator of increased cognitive processing demands even at high speech intelligibility levels. Speech intelligibility tests, in which speech recognition performance is recorded sentence by sentence, failed to detect these increased processing demands at high intelligibility. In the long run, however, this slowing down and an increased processing effort may prevent people from participating in a conversation. So far, there is no established method in audiological research that allows this kind of online analysis of speech comprehension. The results reported in this study highlighted another important advantage of the online measure: misinterpretations could be detected while the speech was presented; offline measures of processing time may be insensitive to these difficulties in sentence comprehension since participants can overcome them before the sentence is completed.

A. Effect of sentence structure on TDA and processing time

In general, processing time was expected to be increased for sentences with a higher level of linguistic complexity. Different levels of linguistic complexity were achieved using the OLACS material by altering word order, embedding relative clauses, and introducing ambiguity. In general, the results indicated that the DDD, which was interpreted as a measure of processing time, greatly depended on the sentence structure. Word order had a strong effect on sentence processing time for the verb-second structures. Longer processing times were found for the non-canonical compared to the canonical sentence structure, indicated by an increase in the DDD of almost 600 ms. An increase in processing time indicated additional cognitive processing costs, which were expected to arise from the non-canonical word order. Increased processing costs caused by non-canonical word order have been reported in many other psycholinguistics studies [39,41,44,46]. As expected, sentence processing was slower for embedded structures: the DDD was 300 ms for the SVO structure and 730 ms for the SR structure. Interestingly, no increase in processing time was observed for the object-relative (OR) structure compared to the subject-relative (SR) structure. It is possible that the additional processing cost of the embedded sentence structure covered any smaller differences in processing time caused by changes in word order.

Several earlier studies already reported that sentence structure complexity caused processing difficulties, increasing the cognitive processing load during speech comprehension. This was revealed using different measures, such as reaction times, recognition scores, and pupil size [9,10,50]. Tun and colleagues [10] presented different sentences structures and examined participants' reaction times when answering comprehension questions. They reported an increase in reaction time for complex sentence structures, indicating an imposed cognitive processing effort due to linguistic complexity even at a high intelligibility level. Piquardo et al. [51] reported that pupil size increased significantly during storing and processing of complex object-before-subject sentence structures compared to syntactically less complex subject-before-object sentence structures. They interpreted the pupillary enlargement as an indicator of the engagement of cognitive effort during the processing of the complex sentences. However, a significant effect of sentence structure on pupil size could only be measured *after* the verbal presentation of the sentence. The results of the current study supported most of these findings, underscoring the validity of this paradigm. The DDD greatly depended on sentence structure: syntax-related difficulties during sentence processing were observed by measuring processing time. In contrast to measures such as reaction times or pupil size, used in the previously mentioned studies, the proposed eye-tracking paradigm taps into sentence processing while the sentence is being spoken. Early literature about the visual world paradigm reported that participants had difficulties *during* speech comprehension either on the sentence or the word processing level [e.g., 19, 21, 26]. The fact that sentence structure had no significant effect on offline reaction times (measured by participants' button press) in this paradigm strengthens the assertion that the proposed online measure of processing speed is more sensitive for detecting processing difficulties.

Processing was expected to be slower for ambiguous sentence structures than for unambiguous structures. Interestingly, this was not the case; instead, sentence processing time was actually smaller for the ambiguous sentence structures than for their unambiguous counterparts. This was particularly evident for the ambOVS structure. Furthermore, negative TDAs indicated more fixations towards the competitor picture and were interpreted as a temporary misinterpretation of the agent and object roles. Temporal processing difficulties have been reported by Knoeferle and colleagues using the visual world paradigm [26]. They assessed online the participants' processing difficulties that arose from their expectations of thematic roles in German SVO and OVS sentence structures. The negative TDA values in the current study indicate that the eye movements and the time curve of the TDA was influenced not only the speech signal but also by the listeners' preferences and expectations. Only after the PTD did the participants realize that they had identified the wrong picture as the target picture; they then had to adjust their decision and choose the other picture; this decision is indicated by a steep increase in the TDA. This temporary misinterpretation of the sentence led to a sudden acceleration in the decision-making process: the participant just had to choose the other picture. This may make processing faster than for unambiguous sentence structures, and is reflected in the smaller DDDs.

B. Audiological application and further research

As discussed in the previous section, our results are largely consistent with other studies, especially in psycholinguistic research investigating linguistic aspects in sentence processing. Those studies did not address audiological aspects. Moreover, (psycho-) linguistic aspects of the speech material have been considered to a lesser extent in the audiological research field to date. The data presented demonstrate the value of the paradigm for assessing aspects of cognitive processing in a speech comprehension task. The paradigm presented here was developed as a combination of methods from both research fields: recording eye-fixation data during sentence processing, which is typically used in psycholinguistic studies, and using a sentence corpus that was developed for speech intelligibility measurements. This combination may provide a useful tool for diagnostic purposes in audiology.

Modern hearing aids offer several signal-processing technologies for adapting to different environments, depending on the type of hearing impairment. These include, for instance, dynamic range compression and noise reduction. Research concerning the benefit of hearing aid signal processing traditionally focused on the effects on speech recognition scores or intelligibility measures (such as the SRT). However, speech reception measures often lack the sensitivity to test the benefits of hearing aid algorithms or acclimatization effects of the user. One reason is that SRTs for standard speech intelligibly tests are typically at negative signal-to-noise ratios (SNRs). However some hearing aid algorithms, such as noise reduction algorithms, often require positive SNRs for optimum performance [52–54]. In this situation, speech intelligibility is high and speech intelligibility tests in audiology suffer from ceiling effects. In addition, several studies propose to focus less on improving speech intelligibility measures and more on the effort during speech processing [55,56]. The effects of these signal-processing technologies on the effort required for speech understanding is still an active field of research.

In any case, the opportunity to assess the processing speed of hearing-impaired listeners would be a valuable tool for the individualization of hearing aid fitting. Individual processing efforts in speech perception have been tested using subjectively rated efforts. Brons et al. [55] investigated subjectively rated effort of participants for different hearing aids and the effect of their noise-reduction outputs on the effort. They showed that hearing aid settings influenced the effort involved in listening to speech in noise. In addition, they reported that effort may change between conditions for which speech intelligibility remains constant. Minimizing listening effort is a desirable goal for fitting and adjusting hearing devices and should be supported by an effective and objective way of testing processing effort in audiology. The standard measures and methods used in audiology do not provide an effective and objective way of testing sentence processing and processing effort. The proposed objective measure of processing speed may be used for the design, selection and fitting of hearing devices to the individual listener so that they can be adapted to the individual processing speed and/or processing effort in perceiving speech in acoustically difficult situations. Furthermore, the eye-tracking method introduced here is able to detect differences in processing time that arise from sentence complexity. This could also be relevant for diagnostic purposes, enabling differentiation between peripheral, sensorineural deficits in speech comprehension and more cognitive, centrally located deficits.

However, this study is only the first step towards the application of this paradigm in audiology. Note that the scope of this manuscript includes presenting the proposed method and evaluating it with the OLACS sentence corpus. A systematic study of the influence of bottom-up vs. top-down processing in background noise or hearing impairment is beyond the scope of this study, and several issues need to be clarified before the method can be broadly applied:

1) Further studies are needed to examine the interaction of sensory factors, such as hearing loss and masking noise, with the linguistic factors investigated in this study. By applying different noise types, the effect of energetic, modulation, and informational masking on speech processing and the required effort at controlled speech intelligibly levels should be investigated systematically. In addition, it has been shown that speech intelligibility can also be influenced by the rate of speech [57], so the sensitivity of the proposed paradigm to changes in speech rates is a relevant aspect that should be addressed in future studies.
2) To gain better insight into how individual factors, such as hearing loss, might affect processing speed, it is important to assess speech processing in individual participants. The results of the current study indicate that the TDA varied widely across participants. The confidence intervals shown here include both inter-individual and intra-individual test-retest variance. A more precise TDA time course and DM could be estimated for a single participant by increasing the number of sentences per sentence structure.
3) For clinical studies, it is important to have a relatively small number of trial repetitions, so the number of sentence structures tested should be reduced for this purpose. In general, the set of verb-second structures showed strong effects on processing speed in response to changes in word order. In

contrast, the expected word order effects were not seen for the relative-clause sentence structures. Consequently, of the seven different sentence structures from the OLACS corpus, the verb-second structures are the most promising for analyzing processing time and are likely to be sufficient for audiological applications.

Conclusions

This study developed and evaluated an eye-tracking paradigm that provides a time-resolved, online measure of sentence processing, revealing the influence of linguistic complexity. Experimental data from 17 participants with normal hearing tested in quiet showed that the proposed method was able to detect syntax-related delays during sentence processing using speech material that was optimized for use in audiology. As the results were in line with findings of other psycholinguistic studies, it can be concluded that the method proposed here is valid. Moreover, the experimental data showed that the proposed methods can be relevant with regard to audiological research:

1. The target detection amplitude (TDA) provides a statistically supported, time-resolved measure that directly reflects the participants' comprehension of the sentence. This measure can even be negative, which indicates a temporary misinterpretation of the presented sentence. This underlines the advantage of an online measure that provides information about the time course of speech processing.
2. The eye-tracking paradigm reveals effects of linguistic complexity on processing time that were not found in offline measures of processing speed, such as reaction time, assessed by pressing a button. Processing time was influenced by sentence structures in a systematic way, even though all measurements were performed at the same high level of intelligibility. This indicates that the proposed measure provides information about cognitive processes in speech understanding that go beyond classical speech intelligibility measures.
3. The highest contrast in processing time was observed for the SVO, OVS, and ambOVS sentence structures. Thus the verb-second structures provide a reasonable subset for practical applications, for example in audiology.

In conclusion, the paradigm presented here has a strong potential for use in audiology, where measures revealing differences in speech processing at high levels of intelligibility are highly desired.

Acknowledgments

The authors wish to thank Verena Uslar, Rebecca Carroll, Mirko Hanke, Esther Ruigendijk, and Cornelia Hamann for cooperation in developing the sentence material and discussion of the study. The authors also wish to thank Albena Kaptebileva for drawing the graphical material and Ewen MacDonald, Tobias May, and Darrin K. Reed for proofreading. We would like to thank Torsten Dau for his support and Gerald Kidd for helpful advice concerning a former version of this manuscript.

Author Contributions

Conceived and designed the experiments: DW TB BK. Performed the experiments: DW. Analyzed the data: DW. Contributed reagents/materials/analysis tools: DW TB BK. Wrote the paper: DW TB BK.

References

1. Laroche C, Soli S, Giguere C, Lagace J, Vaillancourt V, et al. (2003) An approach to the development of hearing standards for hearing-critical jobs. Noise Health 6: 17–37.
2. Ozimek E, Warzybok A, Kutzner D (2010) Polish sentence matrix test for speech intelligibility measurement in noise. Int J Audiol 49: 444–454.
3. Haumann S, Hohmann V, Meis M, Herzke T, Lenarz T, et al. (2012) Indication criteria for cochlear implants and hearing aids: Impact of audiological and non-audiological findings. Audiol Research 2: 55–64.
4. Zokoll MA, Hochmuth S, Warzybok A, Wagener KC, Buschermöhle M, et al. (2013) Speech-in-noise tests for multilingual hearing screening and diagnostics. Am J Audiol 22: 175–178.
5. Plomp R, Mimpen AM (1979) Improving the reliability of testing the speech reception threshold for sentences. Audiol 18(1): 43–52.
6. Hagerman B (1982) Sentences for testing speech intelligibility in noise. Scand Audiol 11(2): 79–87.
7. Kollmeier B, Wesselkamp M (1997) Development and evaluation of a German sentence test for objective and subjective speech intelligibility assessment. J Acoust Soc Am 102(4): 2412–2421.
8. Nilsson M, Soil SD, Sullivan JA (1994) Development of the hearing in noise test for the measurement of speech reception thresholds in quiet and in noise. J Acoust Soc Am 95(2): 1085–1099.
9. Wingfield A, McCoy SL, Peelle JE, Tun PA, Cox LC (2006) Effects of adult aging and hearing loss on comprehension of rapid speech varying in syntactic complexity. J Am Ac Audiol 17: 487–497.
10. Tun PA, Benichov J, Wingfield A (2010) Response latencies in auditory sentence comprehension: Effects of linguistic versus perceptual challenge. Psychol Aging 25(3): 730–735.
11. Kalikow DN, Stevens KN (1977) Development of a test of speech intelligibility in noise using sentence materials with controlled word predictability. J Acoust Soc Am 61: 1337–1351.
12. Boothroyd A, Nittrouer S (1988) Mathematical treatment of context effects in phoneme and word recognition. J Acoust Soc Am 84(1): 101–114.
13. Uslar VN, Ruigendijk E, Hamann C, Brand T, Kollmeier B (2011) Sentence complexity effects in a German audiometric sentence intelligibility test: May we ignore psycholinguistics when testing speech in noise? Int J Audiol 50: 621–631.
14. Uslar VN, Carroll R, Hanke M, Hamann C, Ruigendijk E, et al. (2013) Development and evaluation of a linguistically and audiologically controlled sentence intelligibility test. J Acoust Soc Am 134(4): 3039–3056.
15. Pratt J, Dodd M, Welsh T (2006) Growing older does not always mean moving slower Examining aging and the saccadic motor system. J Motor Behav 38: 373–382.
16. Cerella J, Hale S (1994) The rise and fall in information-processing rates over the life span. Acta Psychol 86: 109–197.
17. Cooper RM (1974) The control of eye fixation by the meaning of spoken language: A newmethodology for the real-time investigation of speech perception, memory, and language processing. Cognitive Psychol 6: 84–107.
18. Huettig F, Rommers J, Meyer AS (2011) Using the visual world paradigm to study language processing: A review and critical evaluation. Acta Psychol 137: 151–171.
19. Tanenhaus MK, Spivey-Knowiton MJ, Eberharda KM, Sedivy JC (1995) Integration of visual and linguistic information in spoken language comprehension. Science 268: 1632–1634.
20. Eberhard KM, Spivey-Knowlton MJ, Sedivy JC, Tanenhaus MK (1995) Eye movements as a window into real-time spoken language comprehension in natural contexts. J Psycholinguist Res 24(6): 409–436.
21. Allopenna PD, Magnuson JS, Tanenhaus MK (1998) Tracking the time course of spoken word recognition using eye movements: Evidence for continuous mapping models. J Mem Lang 38: 419–439.
22. Altmann GTM, Kamide Y (1999) Incremental interpretation at verbs: Restricting the domain of subsequent reference. Cognition 73: 247–264.
23. Snedeker J, Trueswell JC (2004) The developing constraints on parsing decisions: The role of lexical-biases and referential scenes in child and adult sentence processing. Cognitive Psychol 49(3): 238–299.
24. Altmann GTM, Kamide Y (2007) The real-time mediation of visual attention by language and world knowledge: Linking anticipatory (and other) eye movements to linguistic processing. J Mem Lang 57: 502–518.
25. Kamide Y, Altmann GTM, Haywood SL (2003) The time course of prediction in incremental sentence processing: Evidence from anticipatory eye movements. J Mem Lang 49: 133–156.
26. Knoeferle P (2007) Comparing the time-course of processing initially ambiguous and unambiguous German SVO/OVS sentences in depicted events. In: van Gompel R, Fischer M, Murray W, Hill R, editors. Eye Movements: A Window on Mind and Brain. Oxford: Elsevier. pp. 517–533.
27. Knoeferle P, Crocker MW (2006) The coordinated interplay of scene, utterance, and world knowledge: Evidence from eye tracking. Cognitive Science 30(3): 481–529.
28. Knoeferle P, Crocker MW (2007) The influence of recent scene events on spoken comprehension: Evidence from eye movements. J Mem Lang 57: 519–543.
29. Knoeferle P, Crocker MW, Scheepers C, Pickering MJ (2005) The influence of the immediate visual context on incremental thematic role-assignment: Evidence from eye-movements in depicted events. Cognition 95: 95–127.

30. Chambers CG, Tanenhaus MK, Eberhard KM, Filip H, Carlson GN (2002) Circumscribing referential domains during real-time sentence comprehension. J Mem Lang 47: 30–49
31. Huettig F, McQueen JM (2007). The tug of war between phonological, semantic, and shape information in language-mediated visual search. J Mem Lang 57: 460–482.
32. Barr DJ, Gann TM, Russell SP (2011) Anticipatory baseline effects and information integration in visual world studies. Acta Psychol 137: 201–207.
33. Arnold JE, Fagnano M, Tanenhaus MK (2003) Disfluencies signal theee, um, new information. J Psycholinguist Res 32: 25–36.
34. Kaiser E, Trueswell JC (2008) Interpreting pronouns and demonstratives in Finnish: Evidence for a form-specific approach to reference resolution. Lang Cogn Process 23(5): 709–748.
35. Efron B, Tibshirani RJ (1993) An introduction to the bootstrap. New York: Chapman and Hall. 436 p.
36. van Zandt T (2002) Analysis of response time distributions. In: Wixted JT, editor. Stevens' handbook of experimental psychology: Vol.4. Methodology in experimental psychology, (third edition). New York: Wiley. pp. 461–516.
37. McMurray B, Clayards MA, Tanenhaus MK, Aslin RN (2008) Tracking the time course of phonetic cue integration during spoken word recognition. Psychometric Bulletin & Review 15(6): 1064–1071.
38. Toscano J, McMurray B (2012) Cue-integration and context effects in speech: Evidence against speaking-rate normalization. Atten Percept Psychophys 74(6): 1284–1301.
39. Bader M, Bayer J (2006) Case and linking in language comprehension: Evidence from German. Berlin: Springer 319 p.
40. Weskott T, Hörnig R, Fanselow G, Kliegl R (2011) Contextual licensing of marked OVS word order in German. Linguistische Berichte 225: 3–18.
41. Bader M, Meng M (1999) Subject-object ambiguities in German embedded clauses: An across-the-board comparison. J Psycholinguist Res 28(2): 121–143.
42. Gorrell P (2000) The subject-before-object preference in German clauses. In: Hemforth B, Konieczny L, editors. German sentence processing. Dordrecht: Kluwer Academic Publishers. pp. 25–63.
43. Fanselow G, Lenertová D,Weskott T (2008) Studies on the acceptability of object movement to spec, CP. In: Steube A, editor. Language, Context & Cognition: The discourse potential of underspecified structures. Berlin: De Gruyter. pp. 413–438.
44. Gibson E (2000) The dependency locality theory: A distance-based theory of linguistic complexity. In: Miyashita Y, Marantz A, O'Neil W, editors. Image, Language, Brain. Cambridge, MA: Massachusetts Institute of Technology Press, pp. 95–126.
45. Gordon PC, Hendrick R, Levine WH (2002) Memory load interference in syntactic processing. Psychol Science 13(5): 425–430.
46. Carroll R, Ruigendijk E (2013) The effect of syntactic complexity on processing sentences in noise. J Psycholinguist Res 42(2): 139–59.
47. Altmann GTM (1998) Ambiguity in sentence processing. Trends Cogn Sci 2: 146–152.
48. Ben-David BM, Chambers CG, Danemana M, Pichora-Fuller MK, Reingold EM, et al. (2011) Effects of aging and noise on real-time spoken word recognition: Evidence from eye movements. J Speech Lang Hear Res 54: 243–262.
49. Sherbecoe RL, Studebaker GA (2004) Supplementary formulas and tables for calculating and interconverting speech recognition scores in transformed arcsine units. Int J Audiol 43: 442–448.
50. Wingfield A, Tun PA (2007) Cognitive supports and cognitive constraints on comprehension of spoken language. J Am Ac Audiol 18(7): 548–558.
51. Piquado T, Isaacowitz D, Wingfield A (2010) Pupillometry as a measure of cognitive effort in younger and older adults. Psychophysiology 47: 560–569.
52. Marzinzik M (2000) Noise reduction schemes for digital hearing aids and their use for the hearing impaired. [dissertation], Oldenburg: Carl von Ossietzky Universität, 132 p.
53. Fredelake S, Holube I, Schlüter A, Hansen M (2012) Measurement and prediction of the acceptable noise level for single-microphone noise reduction algorithms. Int J Audiol 51(4): 299–308.
54. Bentler RA (2005) Effectiveness of directional microphones and noise reduction schemes in hearing aids: A systematic review of the evidence. J Am Ac Audiol 16(7):473–484.
55. Brons I, Houben R, Dreschler WA (2013) Perceptual effects of noise reduction with respect to personal preference, speech intelligibility, and listening effort. Ear Hear 34(1): 29–41.
56. Sarampalis A, Kalluri S, Edwards B, Hafter E (2009) Objective measures of listening effort: Effects of background noise and noise reduction. J Speech Lang Hear Res 52: 1230–1240.
57. Schlueter A, Lemke U, Kollmeier B, Holube I (2014) Intelligibility of time-compressed speech: The effect of uniform versus non-uniform time-compression algorithms. J Acoust Soc Am 135(3): 1541–1555.

12

Prevalence of p.V37I Variant of GJB2 in Mild or Moderate Hearing Loss in a Pediatric Population and the Interpretation of its Pathogenicity

So Young Kim[1], Gibeom Park[2], Kyu-Hee Han[1], Ahreum Kim[1], Ja-Won Koo[3,4], Sun O. Chang[1,4], Seung Ha Oh[1,4], Woong-Yang Park[5,6], Byung Yoon Choi[3,4]*

1 Department of Otorhinolaryngology-Head and Neck Surgery, Seoul National University Hospital, Seoul National University College of Medicine, Seoul, Korea, **2** Department of Biomedical Sciences, Seoul National University College of Medicine, Seoul, Korea, **3** Department of Otorhinolaryngology-Head and Neck Surgery, Seoul National University Bundang Hospital, Seoul National University College of Medicine, Seongnam, Korea, **4** Sensory Organ Research Institute, Seoul National University Medical Research Center, Seoul, Korea, **5** Department of Molecular Cell Biology, Sungkyunkwan University School of Medicine, Suwon, Korea, **6** Translational Genomics Laboratory, Samsung Genome Institute, Samsung Medical Center, Seoul, Korea

Abstract

A p.V37I variant of GJB2 has been reported from subjects with moderate or slight hearing loss especially in East Asian populations. This study aimed to estimate the prevalence of the p.V37I variant among such subjects and prove, epidemiologically, its pathogenic potential to cause mild hearing loss. A total of 380 subjects from 201 families with hearing loss were enrolled. From them, 103 families were selected who had autosomal recessive inheritance or sporadic occurrence of hearing loss and who were younger than 15 years old. *GJB2* sequencing was carried out for the probands of all 103 families. The prevalence of the p.V37I variant was compared between the subtle, mild or moderate hearing loss (group I) and the severe or profound hearing loss (group II) groups. Where possible, a targeted next generation sequencing of 82 deafness genes was performed from the p.V37I carrier to exclude the existence of other pathogenic genes. Five (4.8%) of 103 probands were found to carry p.V37I. The carrier frequency of p.V37I among group I (18.2%) was significantly higher than that of group II (1.2%) or the reported Korean normal hearing control group (1.0%). Detection of the p.V37I variant of GJB2 in 18.2% of Koreans with mild hearing loss strongly suggests its contribution to the pathogenesis of milder hearing loss, which might justify sequencing of *GJB2* from these subjects in the Korean population.

Editor: Yury E. Khudyakov, Centers for Disease Control and Prevention, United States of America

Funding: The authors declare no conflict of interest related to funding sources, or financial holdings that might raise questions about possible sources of bias. This study was supported by the Korea Healthcare Technology Research & Development Project, Ministry for Health, Welfare and Family Affairs, Republic of Korea (No. A080588 and No. A111377) and Seoul National University Bundang Hospital research fund 06-2011-024 (to BYC). The funders had no role in study design, data collection and analysis, decision to publish, or preparation of the manuscript.

Competing Interests: The authors have declared that no competing interests exist.

* E-mail: choiby@snubh.org

Introduction

Despite significant heterogeneity of genetic deafness, *GJB2* (encoding Gap junction beta-2 protein, also known as connexin 26) causes more than 50% of autosomal recessive nonsyndromic deafness in many populations [1,2]. More than 100 different pathogenic mutations and 24 polymorphisms have been identified within the *GJB2* gene (http://davinci.crg.es/deafness/) [3]. The mutational spectra often vary among different ethnic groups. For example, in Caucasians, the 35delG mutation accounts for up to 85% of the *GJB2* mutant alleles [2,4,5]. By contrast, the 235delC mutation is prevalent in Koreans [6], Japanese [7], Chinese [8] and Taiwanese [9].

The p.V37I is another *GJB2* variant that is frequently found in East Asian populations [10–13]. The variant resides in transmembrane M1 domain in beta connexins [14]. The p.V37I variant has been frequently observed to be associated with mild to moderate hearing loss [15,16].

The p.V37I variant was originally described as an innocent polymorphism because it was identified in unaffected heterozygous control subjects [14]. However, with the increasing number of identified hearing impaired subjects carrying the homozygous p.V37I or the heterozygous p.V37I in a *trans* configuration with other pathogenic mutation of *GJB2*, the possibility of a pathogenic role of the variant has been raised [17–19]. Recent functional studies have produced somewhat contradictory results regarding the pathogenicity of the p.V37I variant. Functional studies of electrical conductance between paired Xenopus oocytes demonstrated that the p.V37I mutant protein is non-functional, implying that the variant is a pathogenic mutation [20]. In contrast with the null function of the variant proposed by Bruzzone et al. (2003), other recent studies demonstrated only a partially reduced function of the p.V37I mutant protein [21,22]. These studies showed that the penetrance of the p.V37I variant was only about 1/10 relative to known pathogenic *GJB2* mutations [22].

Recently, an epidemiological study of a Chinese population by Li et al. (2012) demonstrated that the p.V37I variant, either in compound heterozygosity with other truncating mutations of *GJB2* or in homozygosity, may cause subclinical subtle hearing loss at birth, and this hearing loss may progress and become apparent at later age. In that paper, they showed that the genotype is present in a substantial portion (20%) of post natal permanent childhood hearing impairment (PCHI) [23]. Rarer detection of p.V37I variant allele in severe to profound hearing loss than what was predicted from the prevalence of this allele in normal hearing controls in the Korean population [6,12,13] strongly suggests that p.V37I variant contributes to milder hearing loss.

To the best of our knowledge, there has been no study estimating the prevalence of the p.V37I variant according to the degree of hearing loss. Therefore, we conducted a genetic test to estimate genetic loads of the p.V37I variants according to the degree of sensorineural hearing loss.

Methods

Ethical Considerations

The Institutional Review Boards (IRBs) at the Seoul National University Bundang Hospital (SNUBH) (IRB-B-1007-105-402) and the Seoul National University Hospital (SNUH) (IRBY-H-0905-041-281) approved the study. We obtained a written informed consent from all the participants in this study. In case of children participants, the written informed consent was obtained from the parents or guardians on behalf of them.

Study Participants

Clinical phenotype evaluations included medical and developmental history interviews, physical examinations, pure tone audiometry and imaging studies (Temporal bone CT and/or MR images), whenever possible. An initial cohort of 380 subjects from 201 families with varying degrees of hearing loss were collected at the otolaryngology clinics of SNUH and SNUBH from September 2010 through though March 2012. The 380 subjects were subjected to preselection based upon the presence of autosomal recessive inheritance or sporadic occurrence of hearing loss. Ten milliliters of whole blood was obtained from all probands in the 201 families and, if possible, their siblings and parents for the segregation study. Families segregating hearing loss in an autosomal dominant, a maternally transmitted or X-linked manner were excluded. To exclude any bias resulting from presbycusis, subjects were excluded if they were older than 15 years of age at their initial visit. Individuals with syndromic, unilateral hearing loss, or with inner ear anomalies, such as enlarged vestibular aqueduct or incomplete partition type III, were also excluded from this study. This preselection resulted in the number of study families being reduced to 103.

Clinical Evaluation

The following demographic data were collected for each patient: sex, birth date, date of initial otolaryngological consultation, and major comorbidities or syndromic features. The ethnicity of all subjects was Korean. Where available, the temporal bone CT or magnetic resonance imaging findings were also taken. For example, anomalies in the seventh nerve, cochlear anomaly or enlarged vestibular aqueduct syndromes were all recorded.

Audiometric Evaluation

All subjects underwent audiological evaluation. Hearing levels were determined by pure-tone audiometry. We performed serial audiograms regularly to detect any noticeable aggravation of hearing after their participation in this study and to provide timely auditory rehabilitation. In addition, if necessary, we traced back the previous hearing status by obtaining the clinical information from the private practitioner who referred patients to our center. Initial audiograms conducted in our center were reviewed, and the pure-tone average (PTA) was calculated for each ear. The pure-tone thresholds at 0.5, 1, 2, and 4 kHz were recorded, and the pure-tone average across these frequencies was calculated and reported as decibels of hearing loss. In six cases where pure-tone audiometry was not performed because of the subjects' young age, auditory brainstem response threshold (ABRT) evaluations and/or auditory Steady-State Response(ASSR) were recorded, and mean thresholds at frequencies in the 0.5-to 4-kHz range were averaged to approximate the PTA. The hearing level of the better ear calculated by four-tone average (0.5, 1, 2, and 4 kHz) was labeled as subtle (16–25 dB), mild (26–40 dB), moderate (41–70 dB), severe (71–95 dB), or profound (>95 dB). This cohort was then screened by visual examination of audiometric data and classified into two groups: Subtle, mild or moderate sensorineural hearing loss (SNHL) (group I) versus severe or profound SNHL (group II) (Figure 1).

PCR and Sanger Sequencing of *GJB2*

As a first step toward molecular genetic diagnosis of the 103 families, we performed bidirectional nucleotide sequence analysis of the two exons of *GJB2* (GenBank Accession NM_004004.5). The two exons and flanking sequences of *GJB2* were PCR-amplified and sequenced as previously described [12]. Mutation nomenclature and numbering were based upon NM_004004.5, a cDNA for *GJB2*. The names of all variants were checked using Mutalyzer (http://www.LOVD.nl/mutalyzer/). Novel splice site variants and synonymous changes were considered non-pathogenic when they were detected in the normal Korean population or BDGP (http://www.fruitfly.org/seq_tools/splice.html) and ESEfinder (http://rulai.cshl.edu/cgi-bin/tools/ESE3/esefinder.cgi?process = home) software did not predict a change that creates or eliminates a splicing acceptor or donor site. We have submitted our novel variants of *GJB2* to the LSDB database (https://research.cchmc.org/LOVD2/variants.php?select_db = GJB2&action = view&view = 0000808).

Targeted Capture of Exons and Flanking Sequences of 82 Deafness Genes and Massively Parallel Sequencing of DNA Libraries

For two subjects (SH42-94 and SB51-95) carrying the p.V37I variant of *GJB2* as one of two mutant alleles, they were further evaluated by targeted capture of exons and flanking sequences of 82 deafness genes, followed by massively parallel sequencing of DNA libraries, as previously described [24]. We have deposited our whole sequencing data in our private SNUH-SNUBH sequencing database and have submitted the novel variants of *TRIBOP*, *TMC1* and *DSPP* that we detected by next generation sequencing to the LSDB databases (http://grenada.lumc.nl/LOVD2/mendelian_genes/variants.php?select_db = TRIOBP&action = view&view = 0059473,https://research.cchmc.org/LOVD2/variants.php?select_db = TMC1&action = view&view = 0000809,http://grenada.lumc.nl/LOVD2/mendelian_genes/variants.php?select_db = DSPP&action = view&view = 0059474).

Breakpoint PCR for Detection of known Deletions Involving GJB6

To exclude the possibility of large genomic deletions that may be in a *trans* configuration with p.V37I, we conducted a multiplex breakpoint PCR assay for the single heterozygous carriers of the p.V37I allele designed to detect known reported large genomic deletions (del(GJB6-D13S1830) and del(GJB6-D13S1854)) [25,26]. The sequences of the primers and PCR conditions were as previously reported [25]. Water was used as a negative control,

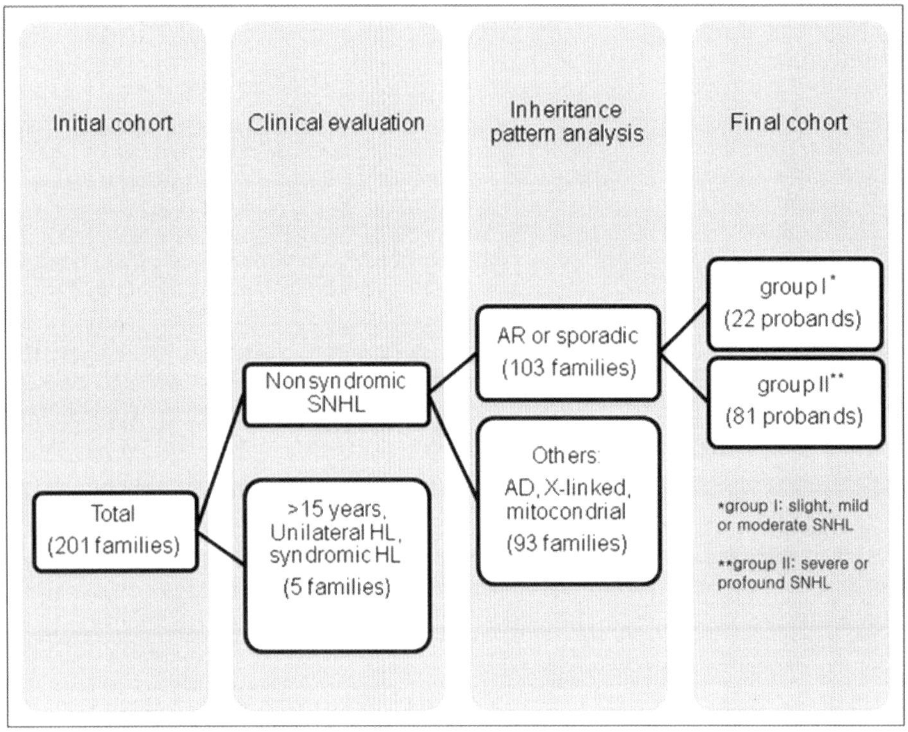

Figure 1. Schematic flow chart of this study. An initial cohort of 201 families underwent genetic studies. Among them, subjects with nonsyndromic SNHL (sensorineural hearing loss) and autosomal recessive (AR) or sporadic inheritance patterns were selected. Based on the degree of hearing loss, final cohorts were classified into two groups: slight, mild or moderate SNHL (group I); severe or profound SNHL (group II).

and two single heterozygous carriers of the p.V37I, SB80-141 in group I, and SHJ1 in group II were examined.

Statistical Analysis

The SPSS15 statistical package was used for the analysis (SPSS Inc., Chicago, IL, USA). Fisher's exact test and logistic regression analysis were used to compare the prevalence of the p.V37I variant among different subject groups. For control groups, we assembled a composite cohort of 3418 ethnically matched Korean normal hearing subjects from three independent studies (Han et al. 2008; Kim et al. 2011; Park et al. 2000).

Odds ratios and confidence intervals were calculated by logistic regression analysis; p-values ≤ 0.05 were considered statistically significant.

Results

One hundred and three families satisfied our inclusion criteria by showing either autosomal recessive inheritance pattern or sporadic occurrence of the hearing loss (Figure.1). Twenty-two of the 103 families showed moderate or slight hearing loss (group I), while the other 81 families manifested severe hearing loss (group II) (Figure.1). Five (4.8%) of 103 probands carried the p.V37I variant of *GJB2*. The variant was detected in a *trans* configuration with a known pathogenic variant in three subjects and as a mono-allelic variant in two subjects.

Among the 22 probands from group I segregating milder hearing loss, four subjects (18.2%) carried the p.V37I variant of *GJB2*, either as one of two mutant alleles (three subjects) or as a single heterozygote (one subject). In contrast, only one (1.2%) of the 81 probands from group II with a severe hearing loss carried the p.V37I variant (as a single heterozygote) (Table 1). The prevalence of p.V37I allele in group I was significantly higher than that in group II ($p = 0.008$, Fisher's exact test). It was also higher than that of the published Korean normal hearing control group ($p = 0.001$, Fisher's exact test) (Table 1). However, the prevalence of the p.V37I allele in group II was not significantly different to that of the published Korean normal hearing control ($p = 0.731$, Fisher's exact test).

Breaking down the four subjects from group I (SH42-94, SB51-95, SB80-141 and SHJ12) who carried the p.V37I variant, three subjects (SH42-94, SB51-95, SHJ12) carried the p.V37I allele in a *trans* configuration with another mutant allele of *GJB2* in the other homologous chromosome, as a compound heterozygote. SB80-141 carried the p.V37I allele as the only variant (Figure 2B). The p.R143W allele was in a *trans* configuration with the p.V37I in the other homologous chromosome for two compound heterozygotes (SB51-95 and SHJ12), while c.235delC was in a *trans* configuration with p.V37I in one subject (SH42-94) with subtle hearing loss. Rapid progression of hearing loss over a 5 month period was noted from SHJ12 carrying the p.V37I and p.R143W mutant alleles (Figure 3). Hearing loss of these four subjects was first detected at an average of 6.33 years old (Table 1).

We further verified that the hearing loss could be accounted for by the p.V37I allele of *GJB2*, and not by other known deafness genes by targeted next generation sequencing (panel sequencing) of 82 known deafness genes (including *GJB2*, *GJB3* and *GJB6*). For two subjects (SH42-94 and SB51-95), the other 81 known deafness genes were excluded as causes of the observed hearing loss (Figure 2B, Table 2, and Table S1). Two and three novel SNPs were detected from SH42-94 and SB51-95, respectively (Table 2). However, no potentially pathogenic candidate variants compatible with recessive inheritance of hearing loss were found from the two subjects (Table 2). Unfortunately, we were not able to perform

Table 1. Differences in prevalence of p.V37I variant and inheritance patterns.

		Group I*	Group II**	Control group[†]
AR or sporadic (family)		22	81	3418
p.V37I carrier (n)		4	1	39
Allele frequency		0.091	0.006	0.005
Onset of hearing loss (mean value)		6.33 yr	<1 yr	–
Fisher's exact test (p-value)	vs Group II	0.008	–	–
	vs Control	0.001	0.731	–

*Group I: slight, mild or moderate degree of hearing loss;
**Group II: Severe or profound degree of hearing loss;
[†]Control group: adapted from three independent studies with the same ethnic background (Han et al., 2008; Kim et al., 2011, Park et al, 2000).

targeted next generation sequencing of the 82 deafness genes for SB80-14 carrying the p.V37I as the only variant since the parents of SB80-14 were reluctant for the next generation sequencing at that moment. Instead, the possibility of the presence of at least two reported large deletions (del(GJB6-D13S1830) and del(GJB6-D13S1854)) in a *trans* configuration with the p.V37I from SB80-141 and SHJ1 was excluded; no band compatible with the presence of the two large deletions, despite a clear amplification from the exon 1 of GJB6, was observed (Figure 4).

One subject (SHJ1) carrying a single heterozygous p.V37I allele from group II was a monozygotic twin. The monozygotic twin brother of SHJ1 carried the same p.V37I allele but had completely normal hearing, indicating that detection of the p.V37I allele in this subject with profound deafness is probably incidental (Table 1).

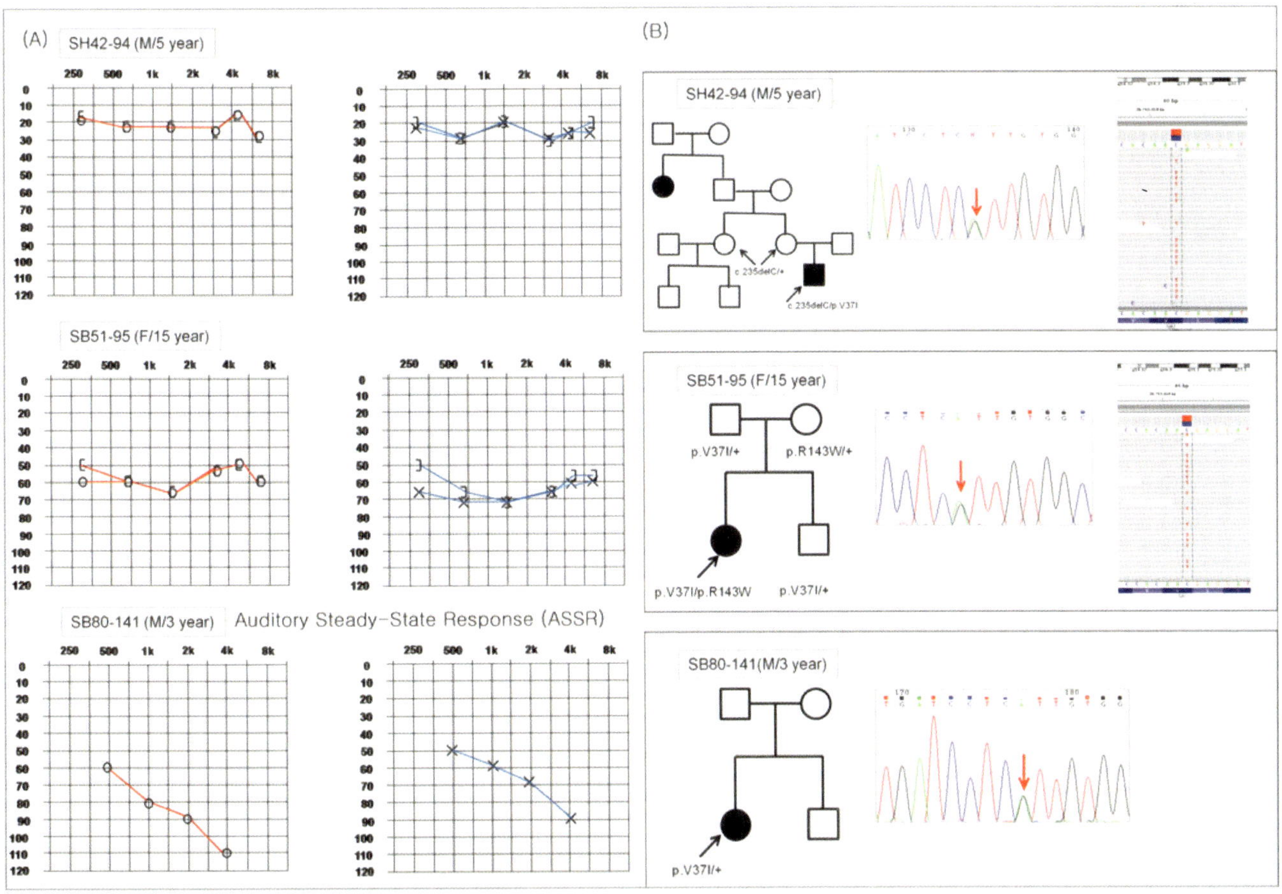

Figure 2. Three families with the p.V37I variant and moderate or slight hearing loss. Two subjects (SH42-94, SB51-95) carried the p.V37I allele *in a trans* configuration with another mutant allele of *GJB2*, as a compound heterozygote and the other subject (SB80-141) carried the p.V37I allele as the only variant. (A) Detailed data of each subject's pure tone audiometry at their initial visit. (B) Detailed data of each subject's pedigree and Sanger sequencing traces. Next generation sequencing trace of p.V37I variant of *GJB2* from two subjects (SH42-94, SB51-95) are shown. The Auditory Steady-State Response (ASSR) result of SB80-141 at the initial visit is shown due to poor cooperation in pure tone audiometry test.

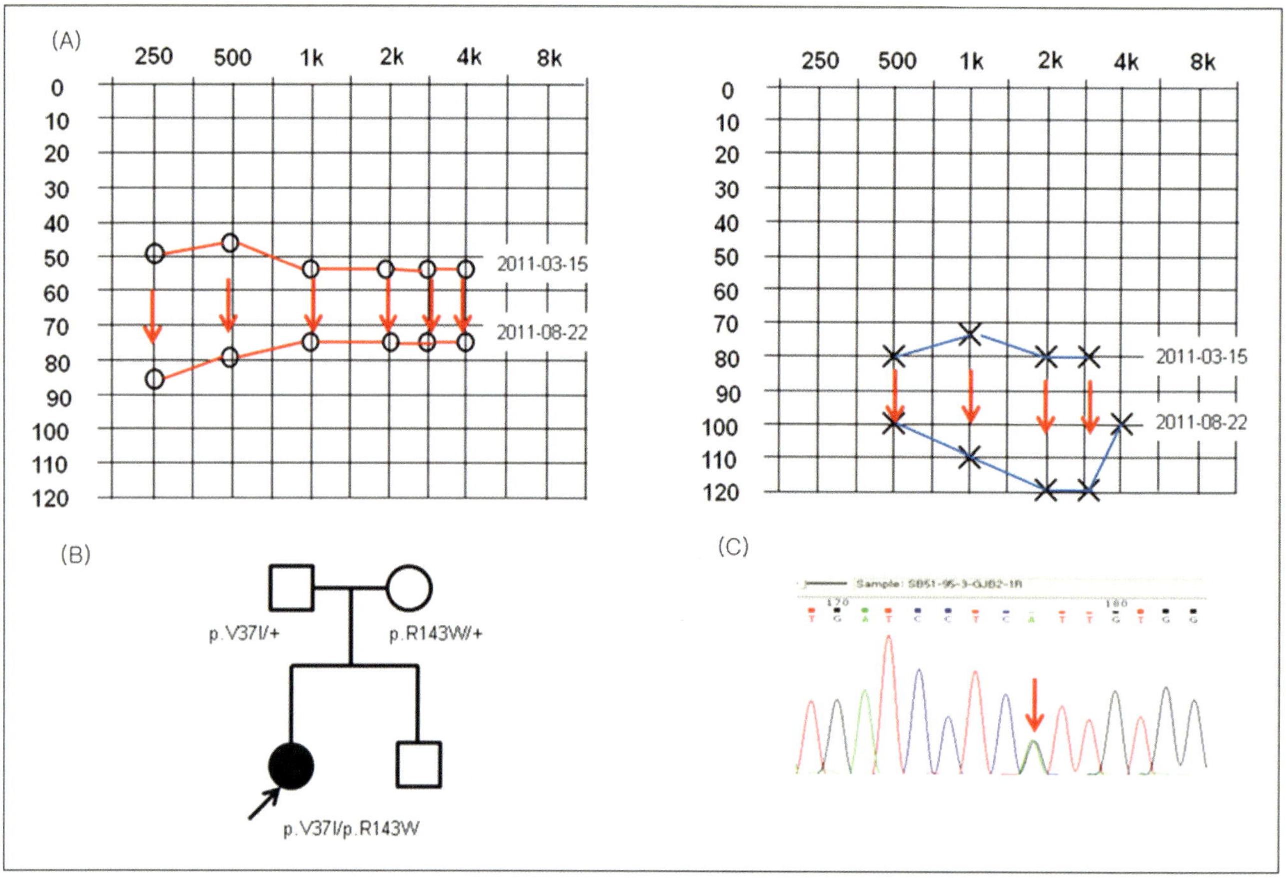

Figure 3. Progressive hearing loss shown in a family. (A) Pure tone audiometry (at initial visit, and at follow up visit 5 months later) (B) Subjects' pedigree and (C) Sanger sequencing traces are shown. Rapid progression of hearing loss over 5 months was noted in SHJ12 carrying the p.V37I and p.R143W mutant alleles.

Discussion

To the best of our knowledge, the frequency of the p.V37I allele has never been reported in an exclusive group with only mild hearing loss. The carrier frequency of the p.V37I allele was calculated as 18.2% among Korean subjects with moderate or slight hearing loss in this study. This figure is strikingly high, considering that the carrier frequency of the p.V37I variant from Korean normal hearing control populations ranged from 0.88 to 1.25% [12,13]. This figure is also comparable to what was reported in a recent study by Li et al. (2012) in a Chinese Han population. They showed that p.V37I exclusive genotype of *GJB2* was present in 20% of postnatal permanent childhood hearing impairment subjects [23]. However, they did not specify the degree of hearing loss for the postnatal permanent childhood hearing impairment subjects. Delayed onset hearing loss is likely to manifest as mild or moderate hearing loss rather than severe or profound hearing loss, because postnatal permanent childhood hearing impairment subjects were defined when they passed the newborn hearing screening or the pediatric hearing tests, but developed bilateral hearing loss before the age of 9 years. This implies that the frequency of p.V37I carrier would be around 20%, overall, in Southeast Asian populations with mild to moderate postlingual hearing loss. Our study cohort excluded families segregating autosomal dominant hearing loss and subjects older than 15 years of age, leaving only pediatric hearing impaired subjects, mostly without any family history of hearing loss, in our final cohort. The high carrier rate, up to 18.2%, of the p.V37I variant from this selected cohort may justify genetic testing focusing upon the p.V37I variant of GJB2, when the pediatric subjects show moderate or slight hearing impairment without any sign of syndromic hearing impairments or any inner ear anomaly, and if they show sporadic or autosomal recessive hereditary patterns.

The significantly higher prevalence of the p.V37I variant of *GJB2* in the mild hearing loss group compared with the severe hearing loss group and the reported Korean normal hearing control group, provides strong genetic evidence of its contribution to the pathogenesis of mild hearing loss, rather than more severe or profound hearing loss. This agrees with previous descriptive reports where p.V37I homozygotes and c.235delc/p.V37I compound heterozygotes had mild to moderate nonsyndromic hearing loss [19,26] [27].

The significantly variable degree of hearing loss among the p.V37I carriers in our cohort (Figure 2A) led us to hypothesize that the phenotype detected in some p.V37I carriers in the literature might be caused by other autosomal deafness genes, and that the detection of p.V37I in these patients was incidental. Our families were not large enough to perform linkage analysis to identify a candidate locus. In this study, we tried to minimize such a possibility by target exome sequencing of 82 deafness genes from two carriers of p.V37I (SH42-94 and SB51-95) with substantially different degrees of hearing loss between them (see Figure 2A). After completing our filtering strategy, two or three coding region

Table 2. Variants detected by targeted next generation sequencing of 82 deafness genes from two subjects (SH42-94, SB51-95) carrying p.V37I variant of GJB2.

Patient	freq(38)	Type	Gene	Annotation	Chr	Start	End	Ref	Var	Genotype	Quality score	1000 g	dbsnp135
SH42-94	2	Nonsyn	DSPP	NM_014208:exon5:c.C3429A:p.D1143E	4	88537243	88537243	C	A	Hetero	10.26	–	–
	2	fs. Del	GJB2	NM_004004:exon2:c.235delC:p.L79fs	13	20763486	20763486	G	–	Hetero	99	0.0023	rs80338943
	2	Nonsyn	GJB2	NM_004004:exon2:c.G109A:p.V37I	13	20763612	20763612	C	T	Hetero	99	0.01	rs72474224
	2	Nonsyn	TRIOBP	NM_001039141: exon7:c.C1494G:p.D498E	22	38120057	38120057	C	G	Hetero	71.06	–	–
SB51-95	2	Nonsyn	DSPP	NM_014208:exon5: c.C3429A:p.D1143E	4	88537243	88537243	C	A	Hetero	99	–	–
	1	Nonsyn	TMC1	NM_138691: exon10:c.C505G:p.P169A	9	75357411	75357411	C	G	Hetero	99	–	–
	2	Nonsyn	GJB2	NM_004004:exon2:c.C427T:p.R143W	13	20763294	20763294	G	A	Hetero	99	0.0005	rs80338948
	2	Nonsyn	GJB2	NM_004004:exon2:c.G109A:p.V37I	13	20763612	20763612	C	T	Hetero	99	0.01	rs72474224
	2	Nonsyn	TRIOBP	NM_001039141:exon7: c.C1494G:p.D498E	22	38120057	38120057	C	G	Hetero	77.16	–	–

variants remained, except *GJB2* variants, but none of the variants were compatible with a recessive inheritance pattern. More specifically, p.D1143E in DSPP and p.D498E in TRIOBP (Table 2) were identified as polymorphisms in the Korean population. However, it is still possible that a totally different gene not included in the 82 deafness genes or a non-coding region mutation in the 82 deafness genes may be responsible for the milder phenotype of some p.V37I carriers, especially when p.V37I is detected as the single variant.

Two single heterozygotes (SB80-141 from group I and SHJ1 from group II) of p.V37I were detected in our cohort. We suggest a different interpretation of the genotype depending upon the degree of hearing loss. Based upon our data, p.V37I detected as a single heterozygote is most likely to contribute to the phenotype if hearing loss is mild or moderate. It is not surprising that a substantial portion of DFNB1 patients carry only one detectable mutation of *GJB2* [25,28]. There could be other mutations within the DFNB1 locus, outside of the *GJB2* coding regions, such as a large deletion involving *GJB6* [25,29]. We used breakpoint PCR to detect the reported large genomic deletions in the DFNB1 locus, but none were detected (Figure 4). Unreported novel deletions within this locus might reside in a *trans* configuration with p.V37I in SB80-141 from group I. In contrast, the detection of this variant in congenital profound hearing loss, such as in SHJ1 in our study, is most likely to be fortuitous and a search for other etiologies is necessary. First, a monozygotic twin brother of SHJ1, who also carries the p.V37I allele, has perfectly normal hearing, strongly suggesting this allele has nothing to do with the observed hearing loss in SHJ1. Non-penetrance of the p.V37I allele could also be possible. However, our interpretation favors the fortuitous detection of this allele in congenital profound deafness, which agrees with our data that the carrier frequency of the variant (1.2%) in group II was not significantly different from that of the reported Korean normal hearing control group.

Occasionally, the p.V37I variant can be expressed as progressive hearing loss, especially in combination with other pathogenic mutations of *GJB2* in a *trans* configuration. Our subject SHJ12, carrying p.V37I and p.R143W, showed a rapid progression of hearing loss over 5 months (Figure.3), eventually requiring cochlear implantation. Such patients tend to show delayed onset

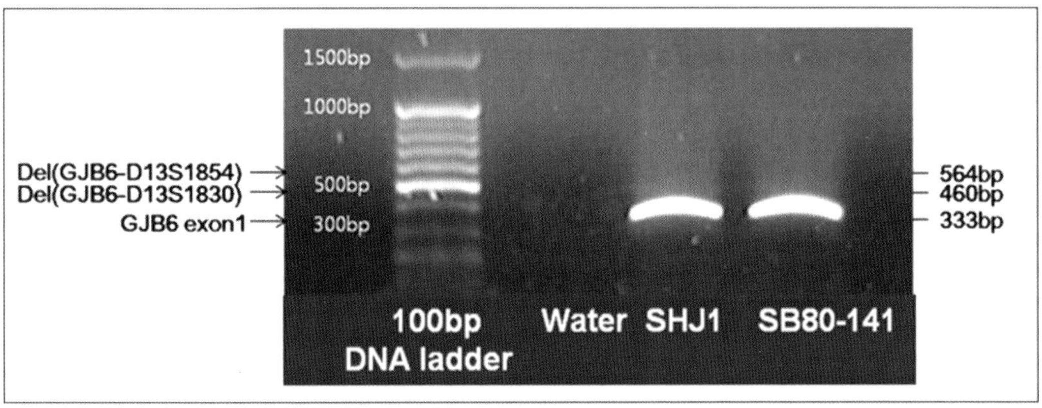

Figure 4. Multiplex breakpoint PCR to detect del(GJB6-D13S1830) and del(GJB6-D13S1854)) from two single heterozygous carriers of p.V37I (SHJ1 and SB80-141). A 564 bp band and a 460 bp band, indicative of the amplification of the del (GJB6-D13S1854) breakpoint junction and del (GJB6-D13S1830) breakpoint junction, respectively, were absent in SHJ1 and SB 80–141, despite a positive band being amplified from the control region, GJB6 exon 1.

of hearing loss, which cannot be detected by the newborn hearing screening test. Therefore, delayed diagnosis and delayed hearing rehabilitations can result. Thus, regular follow up is required in moderate or slight hearing loss with the p.V37I variant of *GJB2*. Some researchers advocate newborn genetic screening (NGS) [12,30] to avoid missing subjects with delayed on-set hearing loss related to this mutant allele. However, the carrier rate of this allele in normal controls is as high as 1.2% in the Korean population, making it difficult to interpret the result (especially when p.V37I is detected as only a single heterozygous allele) without information on the exact hearing status, not just an information of 'pass' or 'refer' obtained by the new born hearing screening. More practically, we suggest checking the p.V37I variant of *GJB2* in children with mild to moderate hearing impairment that segregates in a manner compatible with autosomal recessive inheritance. Further study is needed to elucidate the function of the p.V37I mutation, not only the p.V37I phenotype, but also any genetic interaction with other pathogenic or causative variants.

Conclusions

Our study strongly suggests that the p.V37I variant of *GJB2* contributes to the pathogenesis of milder hearing loss and may justify sequencing of *GJB2* from subjects with mild to moderate degree of hearing loss in the Korean population.

Author Contributions

Conceived and designed the experiments: GBP ARK WYP BYC. Performed the experiments: GBP ARK WYP BYC. Analyzed the data: SYK KHH BYC. Contributed reagents/materials/analysis tools: SYK KHH ARK JWK SOC SHO BYC. Wrote the paper: SYK ARK WYP BYC.

References

1. Van Camp G, Willems PJ, Smith RJ (1997) Nonsyndromic hearing impairment: unparalleled heterogeneity. Am J Hum Genet 60: 758–764.
2. Zelante L, Gasparini P, Estivill X, Melchionda S, D'Agruma L, et al. (1997) Connexin26 mutations associated with the most common form of non-syndromic neurosensory autosomal recessive deafness (DFNB1) in Mediterraneans. Hum Mol Genet 6: 1605–1609.
3. Lalaiants MR, Bliznets EA, Markova TG, Poliakov AV, Tavartkiladze GA (2011) [The results of audiological examination of children presenting with sensorineural loss of hearing due to GJB2 gene mutations during the first year of life]. Vestn Otorinolaringol: 31–35.
4. Gasparini P, Rabionet R, Barbujani G, Melchionda S, Petersen M, et al. (2000) High carrier frequency of the 35delG deafness mutation in European populations. Genetic Analysis Consortium of GJB2 35delG. Eur J Hum Genet 8: 19–23.
5. Denoyelle F, Weil D, Maw MA, Wilcox SA, Lench NJ, et al. (1997) Prelingual deafness: high prevalence of a 30delG mutation in the connexin 26 gene. Hum Mol Genet 6: 2173–2177.
6. Park HJ, Hahn SH, Chun YM, Park K, Kim HN (2000) Connexin26 mutations associated with nonsyndromic hearing loss. Laryngoscope 110: 1535–1538.
7. Kudo T, Ikeda K, Kure S, Matsubara Y, Oshima T, et al. (2000) Novel mutations in the connexin 26 gene (GJB2) responsible for childhood deafness in the Japanese population. Am J Med Genet 90: 141–145.
8. Liu Y, Ke X, Qi Y, Li W, Zhu P (2002) Connexin26 gene (GJB2): prevalence of mutations in the Chinese population. J Hum Genet 47: 688–690.
9. Wang T, Lerer I, Gueta Z, Sagi M, Kadouri L, et al. (2001) A deletion/insertion mutation in the BRCA2 gene in a breast cancer family: a possible role of the Alu-polyA tail in the evolution of the deletion. Genes Chromosomes Cancer 31: 91–95.
10. Chan DK, Schrijver I, Chang KW (2011) Diagnostic yield in the workup of congenital sensorineural hearing loss is dependent on patient ethnicity. Otol Neurotol 32: 81–87.
11. Tsukada K, Nishio S, Usami S (2010) A large cohort study of GJB2 mutations in Japanese hearing loss patients. Clin Genet 78: 464–470.
12. Han SH, Park HJ, Kang EJ, Ryu JS, Lee A, et al. (2008) Carrier frequency of GJB2 (connexin-26) mutations causing inherited deafness in the Korean population. J Hum Genet 53: 1022–1028.
13. Kim SY, Lee BY, Lim JH, Ryu HM, Yang JH, et al. (2011) Determination of the carrier frequencies of selected GJB2 mutations in the Korean population. Int J Audiol 50: 694–698.
14. Kelley PM, Harris DJ, Comer BC, Askew JW, Fowler T, et al. (1998) Novel mutations in the connexin 26 gene (GJB2) that cause autosomal recessive (DFNB1) hearing loss. Am J Hum Genet 62: 792–799.
15. Chan DK, Schrijver I, Chang KW (2010) Connexin-26-associated deafness: phenotypic variability and progression of hearing loss. Genet Med 12: 174–181.
16. Oguchi T, Ohtsuka A, Hashimoto S, Oshima A, Abe S, et al. (2005) Clinical features of patients with GJB2 (connexin 26) mutations: severity of hearing loss is correlated with genotypes and protein expression patterns. J Hum Genet 50: 76–83.
17. Palmada M, Schmalisch K, Bohmer C, Schug N, Pfister M, et al. (2006) Loss of function mutations of the GJB2 gene detected in patients with DFNB1-associated hearing impairment. Neurobiol Dis 22: 112–118.
18. Huculak C, Bruyere H, Nelson TN, Kozak FK, Langlois S (2006) V37I connexin 26 allele in patients with sensorineural hearing loss: evidence of its pathogenicity. Am J Med Genet A 140: 2394–2400.
19. Schrijver I, Chang KW (2006) Two patients with the V37I/235delC genotype: are radiographic cochlear anomalies part of the phenotype? Int J Pediatr Otorhinolaryngol 70: 2109–2113.
20. Bruzzone R, Veronesi V, Gomes D, Bicego M, Duval N, et al. (2003) Loss-of-function and residual channel activity of connexin26 mutations associated with non-syndromic deafness. FEBS Lett 533: 79–88.
21. Jara O, Acuna R, Garcia IE, Maripillan J, Figueroa V, et al. (2012) Critical role of the first transmembrane domain of Cx26 in regulating oligomerization and function. Mol Biol Cell.
22. Pollak A, Skorka A, Mueller-Malesinska M, Kostrzewa G, Kisiel B, et al. (2007) M34T and V37I mutations in GJB2 associated hearing impairment: evidence for pathogenicity and reduced penetrance. Am J Med Genet A 143A: 2534–2543.
23. Li L, Lu J, Tao Z, Huang Q, Chai Y, et al. (2012) The p.V37I exclusive genotype of GJB2: a genetic risk-indicator of postnatal permanent childhood hearing impairment. PLoS One 7: e36621.
24. Brownstein Z, Friedman LM, Shahin H, Oron-Karni V, Kol N, et al. (2011) Targeted genomic capture and massively parallel sequencing to identify genes for hereditary hearing loss in Middle Eastern families. Genome Biol 12: R89.
25. del Castillo FJ, Rodriguez-Ballesteros M, Alvarez A, Hutchin T, Leonardi E, et al. (2005) A novel deletion involving the connexin-30 gene, del(GJB6-d13s1854), found in trans with mutations in the GJB2 gene (connexin-26) in subjects with DFNB1 non-syndromic hearing impairment. J Med Genet 42: 588–594.
26. Cryns K, Orzan E, Murgia A, Huygen PL, Moreno F, et al. (2004) A genotype-phenotype correlation for GJB2 (connexin 26) deafness. J Med Genet 41: 147–154.
27. Snoeckx RL, Huygen PL, Feldmann D, Marlin S, Denoyelle F, et al. (2005) GJB2 mutations and degree of hearing loss: a multicenter study. Am J Hum Genet 77: 945–957.
28. Kenneson A, Van Naarden Braun K, Boyle C (2002) GJB2 (connexin 26) variants and nonsyndromic sensorineural hearing loss: a HuGE review. Genet Med 4: 258–274.
29. Lerer I, Sagi M, Ben-Neriah Z, Wang T, Levi H, et al. (2001) A deletion mutation in GJB6 cooperating with a GJB2 mutation in trans in non-syndromic deafness: A novel founder mutation in Ashkenazi Jews. Hum Mutat 18: 460.
30. Wu CC, Hung CC, Lin SY, Hsieh WS, Tsao PN, et al. (2011) Newborn genetic screening for hearing impairment: a preliminary study at a tertiary center. PLoS One 6: e22314.

Molecular and Clinical Characterization of the Variable Phenotype in Korean Families with Hearing Loss Associated with the Mitochondrial A1555G Mutation

Jae Woong Bae[1]¶, Dong-Bin Kim[1]¶, Jae Young Choi[2], Hong-Joon Park[3], Jong Dae Lee[4], Dong Gu Hur[5], Seung-Hyun Bae[1], Da Jung Jung[6], Sang Heun Lee[6], Un-Kyung Kim[1]*, Kyu Yup Lee[6]*

1 Department of Biology, College of Natural Sciences, Kyungpook National University, Daegu, South Korea, **2** Department of Otorhinolaryngology, Yonsei University College of Medicine, Seoul, South Korea, **3** Soree Ear Clinic, Seoul, South Korea, **4** Department of Otorhinolaryngology-Head and Neck Surgery, Soonchunhyang University College of Medicine, Bucheon, South Korea, **5** Department of Otorhinolaryngology-Head and Neck Surgery, Gyeongsang National University Hospital, Jinju, South Korea, **6** Department of Otolaryngology, College of Medicine, Kyungpook National University, Daegu, South Korea

Abstract

Hearing loss, which is genetically heterogeneous, can be caused by mutations in the mitochondrial DNA (mtDNA). The A1555G mutation of the 12S ribosomal RNA (rRNA) gene in the mtDNA has been associated with both aminoglycoside-induced and non-syndromic hearing loss in many ethnic populations. Here, we report for the first time the clinical and genetic characterization of nine Korean pedigrees with aminoglycoside-induced and non-syndromic hearing loss. These Korean families carry in the A1555G mutation of 12S rRNA gene and exhibit variable penetrance and expressivity of hearing loss. Specifically, the penetrance of hearing loss in these families ranged between 28.6% and 75%, with an average of 60.8%. These results were higher than the 29.8% penetrance that was previously reported in a Chinese population but similar to the 65.4% and 54.1% penetrance observed in a large Arab-Israeli population and nineteen Spanish pedigrees, respectively. The mutational analysis of the complete mtDNA genome in these families showed that the haplogroups of the Korean population, which belongs to the eastern Asian population, were similar to those of the Chinese population but different from the Spanish population, which belongs to the European-Caucasian population. The mtDNA variants that may act as modifier factors were also found to be similar to the Chinese population. Although the mtDNA haplogroups and variants were similar to the eastern Asian population, we did find some differing phenotypes, although some subjects had the same variants. This result suggests that both the ethnic background and environmental factors lead to a variable phenotype of the A1555G mutation.

Editor: Maria Moran, Instituto de Investigación Hospital 12 de Octubre, Spain

Funding: This work was supported by Biomedical Research Institute Grant, Kyungpook National University Hospital (2011) (K.Y. Lee). The funders had no role in study design, data collection and analysis, decision to publish, or preparation of the manuscript.

Competing Interests: The authors have declared that no competing interests exist.

* E-mail: kylee@knu.ac.kr (KYL); kimuk@knu.ac.kr (U-KK)

¶ These authors contributed equally to this work.

Introduction

Hearing loss is the most common sensorineural disorder in humans, affecting one in 1000 newborns and 10% and 50% of people aged 65 and 80 years or older, respectively [1]. It is genetically heterogeneous and can be caused by mitochondrial DNA (mtDNA) mutations [2]. MtDNA mutations have been reported in both non-syndromic and syndromic hearing loss such as Kearns-Sayre Syndrome (KSS) [3], myoclonic epilepsy and ragged red fibers (MERRF) [4], mitochondrial encephalopathy, lactic acidosis and stroke-like episodes (MELAS) [5], maternally inherited diabetes and deafness (MIDD) [6] and are associated with presbycusis [7,8].

The A1555G mutation of the 12S ribosomal RNA (rRNA) gene in the mtDNA is associated with both aminoglycoside-induced and non-syndromic hearing loss in many ethnic populations [9,10,11,12]. Transition of A to G results in an additional G–C pair in the 12S rRNA gene, which has been predicted to encode an aminoglycoside binding based on sequence similarity to the bacterium *Escherichia coli* [13,14]. In addition, sporadic aminoglycoside-induced hearing loss has been reported [15], and even without the use of antibiotics, non-syndromic hearing loss also occurs in ethnic families. Families with hearing loss caused by the A1555G mutation in the 12S rRNA gene have variable phenotypes, including varying severity, age of onset, and penetrance [2,9,16,17,18]. Penetrance appears to differ with the use of aminoglycosides, even within the same pedigree [19]. The variable phenotypes of hearing loss in persons carrying the A1555G mutation are difficult to explain because it is a single point mutation. Therefore, additional modifying factors, including the mtDNA haplogroup, nuclear DNA or mtDNA variations and aminoglycoside antibiotics, have been proposed to be associated with the variable phenotypic expression [18,20,21]. A nuclear modifier gene, tRNA 5-methylaminomethyl-2-thiouridylate methyltransferase (*TRMU*), has been identified, and this gene encodes a highly conserved mitochondrial protein related to transfer RNA

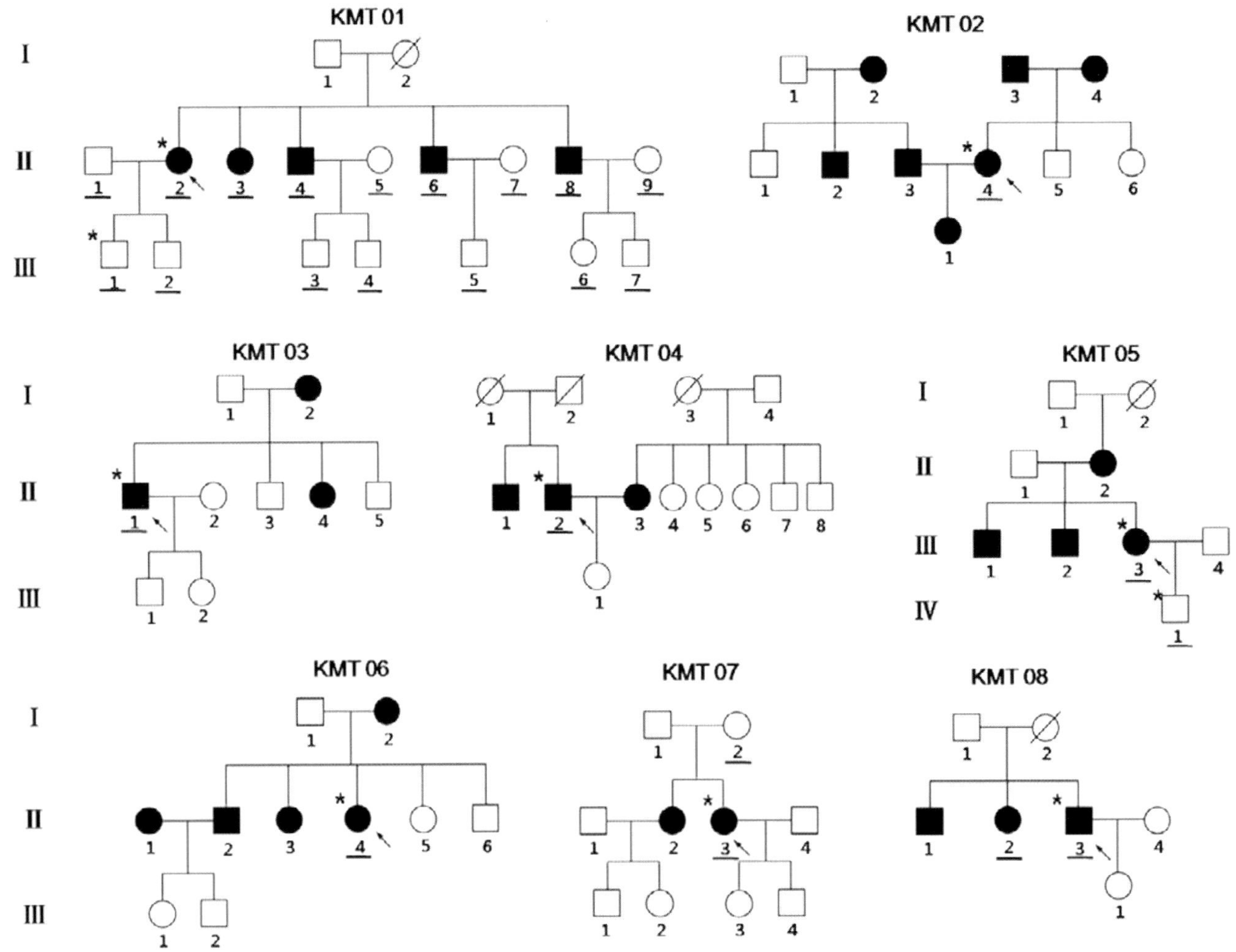

Figure 1. Eight Korean pedigrees presenting with nonsyndromic hearing loss were carrying the A1555G mtDNA mutation. Hearing-impaired individuals are indicated by filled symbols. Arrows denote probands. Subjects used for whole mtDNA sequence analysis are indicated by asterisks. Subjects used for the A1555G mutation screening are underlined.

(tRNA) modification [22]. The mtDNA variations that have been shown to influence the variable phenotype of hearing loss associated with the A1555G mutation are $tRNA^{Lys}$ T5802C [18] and G5821A [19], $tRNA^{Ser(UCN)}$ G7444A [23], $tRNA^{Arg}$ T10454C [24], $tRNA^{Glu}$ A14693G [24,25], $tRNA^{Thr}$ T15908C [24] and G15927A [18], and T12338C [18] in the ND5 gene. Ten eastern Asian haplogroups, including A, B, C, D, F, G, M, N, R and Y, have been detected in Chinese pedigrees carrying the A1555G mutation [26]. Seven European haplogroups have been detected in Spanish pedigrees, including H, I, J, K, T, U and K [27]. Notably, the frequency of the A1555G mutation is much higher in haplogroups D and H in the Chinese and Spanish populations, respectively, than the other haplogroups [26,27]. However, the A1555G mutation has been detected in all of the haplogroups, suggesting that the A1555G mutation in the mtDNA occurred sporadically and persisted over generations. Chinese pedigrees carrying the haplogroups C, Y and F2 have been shown to have higher penetrance than the pedigrees carrying the other haplogroups [26].

In the present study, we investigated the association of modifier factors and variable phenotypes of hearing loss in Korean pedigrees carrying the A1555G mutation. We performed clinical, molecular, and genetic characterizations of the pedigrees, including a sequence analysis of the complete mtDNA genome.

Subjects and Methods

Subjects and Audiological Evaluation

A total of 281 unrelated Korean subjects with non-syndromic hearing loss participated for the mtDNA A1555G mutation screening. All the subjects were subjected to appropriate audiological examinations, including pure-tone audiometry (PTA) and/or auditory brainstem response (ABR). The average of pure-tone audiometry (PTA) was calculated from the average of the audiometric thresholds at 500, 1000, 2000, and 3000 Hz. The severity of hearing loss was classified as follows: normal <26 decibels (dB), mild; 26–40 dB, moderate; 41–70 dB, severe; 71–90 dB, and profound; >90 dB. The subjects with the mtDNA A1555G mutation were subjected to a comprehensive history interview and physical examination to identify other symptoms and their history of aminoglycoside use. All subjects provided written informed consent according to the protocol approved by the Ethics Committee of Kyungpook National University Hospital prior to the study.

Table 1. Summary of clinical features and molecular data for nine patients carrying the A1555G mutation.

Patient no	Gender	Age at test	Age of onset (Pre- or Postlingual)	Audiometric configuration	Exposure to aminoglycosides	PTA (dB)*		Degree of Hearing loss	mtDNA haplogroup
						Right ear	Left ear		
KMT 01	F	51	-	Slope	No	90	93	Severe	D4b1b1a
KMT 02	F	26	Congenital (prelingual)	Slope	No	101	94	Severe	D4a
KMT 03	M	49	-	Slope	-	105	96	Profound	M7a1a
KMT 04	M	57	Childhood (postlingual)	-	-	111	112	Profound	D5a2a
KMT 05	F	41	R: Late childhood, L: 38 (postlingual)	Slope	No	104	101	Profound	D5b1b1
KMT 06	F	47	Late childhood (postlingual)	Slope	No	97	102	Profound	G1a1a
KMT 07	F	45	Childhood (postlingual)	Slope	Yes	73	67	Moderate	D4a
KMT 08	M	50	Congenital (prelingual)	Slope	No	103	117	Profound	M11b
KMT 09	F	67	Childhood (postlingual)	Slope	Yes	102	95	Profound	D4

*PTA, pure-tone audiometry; dB, decibels.

Mutation and Haplogroup Analysis of the mtDNA Genome

Genomic DNA was extracted from the peripheral blood of subjects using the Qiagen Flexigene DNA Extraction Kit (Qiagen, Hilden, Germany). PCR amplification of the mitochondrial 12S rRNA gene was performed using the following primers: forward, 5′- tggctttaacatatctgaacaca-3′, and reverse, 5′-ctcctaagtgtaagttgg-gtgct-3′. For the identification of the A1555G mutation, the PCR products were analyzed using PCR-RFLP with *Bsm*AI (New England Biolabs, Ipswich, MA, USA) [28]. To confirm the A1555G mutation, the PCR products were purified with the Exo-SAP enzyme (USB, Cleveland, OH, USA) and analyzed through direct sequencing on an ABI 3130 Genetic Analyzer (Applied Biosystems Corps., Foster City, CA, USA) using the Big-Dye Terminator Cycle Sequencing Kit (Applied Biosystems Corps., Foster City, CA, USA).

The complete mtDNA sequences of the subjects with the A1555G mutation were amplified (Table S1), purified with the Exo-SAP enzyme (USB, Cleveland, OH, USA), and analyzed through direct sequencing. All of the mtDNA sequences were compared with the updated consensus Cambridge Sequence (GenBank accession number: NC_012920).

Mutation Analysis of the *GJB2* and *TRMU* Genes

PCR amplification of the exon 2 of the *GJB2* gene was performed using the following primers: forward, 5′-gcattcgtcttttc-cagagc-3′, and reverse, 5′-cctcatccctctcatgctgt-3′. The PCR products were purified with the Exo-SAP enzyme (USB, Cleveland, OH, USA) and analyzed through direct sequencing. The results were compared with the sequence of the wild-type *GJB2* gene (GenBank accession number: NM_004004) to identify mutations. For the identification of the *TRMU* gene mutation G28T (A10S), the PCR amplification of exon 1 of the *TRMU* gene was performed using a previously reported primer, and the PCR products were analyzed using PCR-RFLP with *Bsp*1286I (New England Biolabs, Ipswich, MA, USA) [22]. The digested products were analyzed on a 2% agarose gel.

Results

Mutational Screening of the 12S rRNA Gene in Korean Subjects with Non-syndromic Hearing Loss

We performed a sequence analysis to identify the A1555G mutation in 281 Korean unrelated subjects with non-syndromic hearing loss, excluding those subjects with complete autosomal recessive inheritance patterns. First, the genomic DNA of each subject was amplified using the appropriate primers, and these products were digested using *Bsm*AI and analyzed on a 2% agarose gel. Nine of the subjects had the A1555G mutation, which was further confirmed using PCR and subsequent DNA sequence analysis. Next, we performed mutational screening for the A1555G mutation in the available matrilineal relatives of those subjects except for KMT09 family who was not available for pedigree data. The A1555G mutation was detected in all matrilineal relatives. The penetrance of hearing loss (affected matrilineal relatives/total matrilineal relatives) of the eight pedigrees ranged from 28.6% to 75%, with an average of 60.8% (Fig. 1) [17,19,23,24].

Clinical and Genetic Evaluation of the Nine Korean Pedigrees

We obtained a comprehensive history and performed physical and audiological examinations to identify any syndromic symptoms, the history of aminoglycoside use and genetic factors in all of

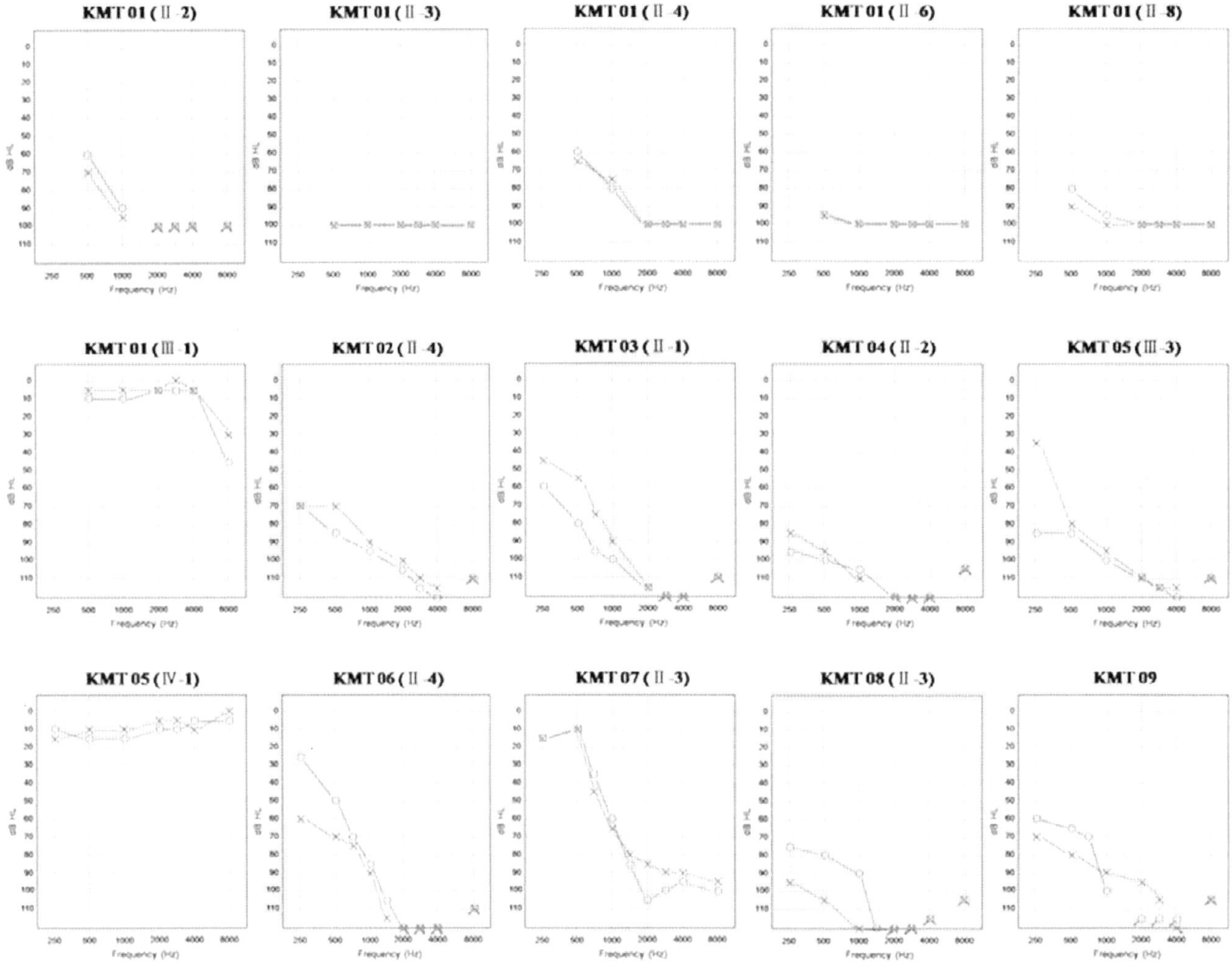

Figure 2. Air audiograms for pure tone audiometry (PTA) of the available subjects with the A1555G mutation. Arrows indicate no responses; Symbols, (X) left ear (O) right ear; dB HL, decibel hearing level.

the available subjects of the nine pedigrees carrying the A1555G mutation (Table 1). The results showed that the probands and members of the nine pedigrees showed no other clinical abnormalities, including diabetes, muscular diseases, visual dysfunction, and neurological disorders.

The probands of each pedigree exhibited hearing loss ranging from moderate to profound, with a slope-shaped pattern of audiological evaluation (Fig. 2). Only the probands of the KMT 07 and KMT 09 families had a history of exposure to aminoglycosides. For the age at onset, the probands of the KMT 02 and KMT 08 families showed prelingual hearing loss, and those of the KMT 04, KMT 07 and KMT 09 families had postlingual hearing loss (Table 1).

The examination of the clinical information of the KMT 01 pedigree (Fig. 1 and 2 and Table 1) revealed that subjects II-3 and II-6 of the proband's siblings (II-3, II-4, II-6, and II-8) had profound hearing loss with a flat-shaped pattern, and subjects II-4 and II-8 had severe hearing loss with a slope-shaped pattern. However, the proband's son, subject III-1, had normal hearing, with only high-frequency hearing loss (30 dB in the right ear and 40 dB in the left ear at 8000 Hz). Husband II-3 of proband II-4 in the KMT 02 family had acquired hearing loss, and the proband's daughter III-1 had congenital hearing loss. The reason for the hearing loss of subject III-1 was not known. Proband III-3 in the KMT 05 family had prelingual hearing loss in the right ear, but the hearing in the left ear became poor at 38 years of age. The onset of hearing loss in her siblings (III-1 and III-2) occurred during childhood and adulthood, respectively. In generations II and III, the penetrance of the A1555G mutation was 100%, but subject IV-1 had normal hearing. The proband's siblings II-1 and II-2 of the KMT 08 family all had hearing loss, and the hearing loss of proband II-3 and subject II-2 was congenital.

Haplogroup Analysis of the mtDNA Genome

To determine whether mtDNA variants or haplogroups modulated the variable phenotype of hearing loss in patients carrying the A1555G mutation, we performed a complete mtDNA sequence analysis of the probands and matrilineal members of the nine pedigrees. As shown in Table 2, the members of each pedigree had distinct mtDNA polymorphisms. Of the known nucleotide variations in the complete mtDNA sequence, we found thirty-five in the D-loop, six in the tRNA gene, nine in the 12S rRNA gene, and seven in the 16S rRNA gene. There were 83 variants in the protein-coding genes, including 56 silent variants and 27 missense variants. One novel variant of the 27 amino acid substitution variants was G3496A in the ND1 gene, which resulted

Table 2. mtDNA variants in nine Korean families with hearing loss.

			Conservation	KMT 01	KMT 01	KMT 02	KMT 03	KMT 04	KMT 05	KMT 05	KMT 06	KMT 07	KMT 07	KMT 08	KMT 09	
Gene	**Position**	**Replacement**	**(H/B/M/X)[a]**	**II-2**	**III-1**	**II-4**	**II-1**	**II-2**	**III-3**	**IV-1**	**II-4**	**II-3**	**I-2**	**II-3**		**Previously reported[b]**
D-loop	44	C>CC						CC								Yes
	73	A>G		G	G	G	G	G	G	G	G	G	G	G	G	Yes
	146	T>C												C		Yes
	150	C>T						T	T	T	T					Yes
	152	T>C				C						C	C		C	Yes
	183	A>G							G	G						Yes
	215	A>G												G		Yes
	228	G>A										A	A			Yes
	263	A>G		G	G	G	G	G	G	G	G	G	G	G	G	Yes
	310	T>CTC		CTC	CTC	CCTC	CTC	CTC	CCTC	CCTC	TC	CTC	CTC	CTC	CTC	Yes
	318	T>C												C		Yes
	326	A>G												G		Yes
	431	C>T		T	T											Yes
	456	C>T							T	T						Yes
	489	T>C		C	C	C	C	C	C	C	C	C	C	C	C	Yes
	515	Del AC		Del AC	Del AC		Del AC	Del AC								Yes
	681	T>C							C	C						Yes
	16092	T>C						C								Yes
	16129	G>A				A						A	A			Yes
	16164	A>G						G								Yes
	16182	A>C						C	C	C						Yes
	16183	A>C						C	C	C						Yes
	16189	T>C						C	C	C						Yes
	16209	T>C					C									Yes
	16223	C>T		T	T	T	T	T	T	T	T	T	T	T	T	Yes
	16266	C>T						T								Yes
	16287	C>T		T	T											Yes
	16319	G>A		A	A											Yes
	16324	T>C					C									Yes
	16325	T>C									C					Yes
	16357	T>C							C	C						Yes
	16362	T>C		C	C	C		C	C	C	C	C	C		C	Yes
	16399	A>G		G	G											Yes

Table 2. Cont.

			Conservation	KMT 01	KMT 01	KMT 02	KMT 03	KMT 04	KMT 05	KMT 05	KMT 06	KMT 07	KMT 07	KMT 08	KMT 09	
Gene	**Position**	**Replacement**	**(H/B/M/X)[a]**	**II-2**	**III-1**	**II-4**	**II-1**	**II-2**	**III-3**	**IV-1**	**II-4**	**II-3**	**I-2**	**II-3**		**Previously reported[b]**
	16497	A>G												G		Yes
	16519	T>C				C			C	C	C			C		Yes
12s rRNA	709	G>A	G/G/A/−								A					Yes
	750	A>G	A/G/G/−	G	G	G	G	G	G	G	G	G	G	G	G	Yes
	752	C>T						T								Yes
	1048	C>T							T	T						Yes
	1095	T>C												C		Yes
	1107	T>C	T/CT/T					C	C	C						Yes
	1310	C>T						T								Yes
	1438	A>G	A/A/A/G	G	G	G	G		G	G	G	G	G	G	G	Yes
	1462	G>A				A										Yes
	1555	A>G	A/A/A/A	G	G	G	G	G	G	G	G	G	G	G	G	Yes
16s rRNA	1811	A>G				G										Yes
	2626	T>C					C									Yes
	2706	A>G	A/G/A/A	G	G	G	G	G	G	G	G	G	G	G	G	Yes
	2772	C>T					T									Yes
	3010	G>A		A	A	A						A	A		A	Yes
	3107	Del C		Del C	Del C	Del C	Del C	Del C	Del C	Del C	Del C	Del C	Del C	Del C	Del C	Yes
	3206	C>T				T						T	T			Yes
ND1	3316	G>A (Ala to Thr)						A								Yes
	3496	G>A (Ala to Thr)	A/A/L/S						A	A						No
	3759	A>G							G	G						Yes
TQ	4386	T>C					C									Yes
ND2	4769	A>G		G	G	G	G	G	G	G	G	G	G	G	G	Yes
	4793	A>G									G					Yes
	4833	A>G (Thr to Ala)									G					Yes
	4859	T>C		C	C											Yes
	4883	C>T		T	T	T		T	T	T		T	T		T	Yes
	4958	A>G					G									Yes
	5108	T>C									C					Yes
	5147	G>A							A	A						Yes
	5153	A>G							G	G						Yes
	5178	C>A (Leu to Met)	L/T/T/T	A	A	A		A	A	A		A	A		A	Yes

Table 2. Cont.

			Conservation	KMT 01	KMT 01	KMT 02	KMT 03	KMT 04	KMT 05	KMT 05	KMT 06	KMT 07	KMT 07	KMT 08	KMT 09	
Gene	**Position**	**Replacement**	**(H/B/M/X)[a]**	**II-2**	**III-1**	**II-4**	**II-1**	**II-2**	**III-3**	**IV-1**	**II-4**	**II-3**	**I-2**	**II-3**		**Previously reported[b]**
	5276	A>G										G	G			Yes
	5301	A>G (Ile to Val)	I/I/M/L					G	G	G						Yes
TC	5802	T>C	T/T/T/C						C	C						Yes
NC5	5895	C>CC					CC								CC	Yes
CO1	6253	T>C (Met to Thr)							C	C						Yes
	6410	C>T		T	T											Yes
	6455	C>T					T									Yes
	6531	C>T												T		Yes
	6551	C>T	N/−/N/−									T	T			Yes
	6689	C>T		T	T											Yes
	7028	C>T		T	T	T	T	T	T	T	T	T	T	T	T	Yes
	7403	A>G							G	G						Yes
	7444	G>A (Ter to Lys)				A										Yes
CO2	7642	G>A												A		Yes
	7867	C>T									T					Yes
	8020	G>A		A	A											Yes
	8071	A>G						G								Yes
	8108	A>G (Ile to Val)	I/I/I/I											G		Yes
	8176	T>C						C								Yes
	8200	T>C									C					Yes
TK	8308	A>G					G									Yes
ATP8	8414	C>T (Leu to Phe)	L/F/M/W	T	T	T						T	T		T	Yes
	8473	T>C				C						C	C			Yes
ATP6	8701	A>G (Thr to Ala)	T/S/L/Q	G	G	G	G	G	G	G	G	G	G	G	G	Yes
	8860	A>G (Thr to Ala)	T/A/A/T	G	G	G	G	G	G	G	G	G	G	G	G	Yes
	9180	A>G						G	G	G						Yes
CO3	9254	A>G									G					Yes
	9531	A>G (Thr to Ala)													G	Yes
	9540	T>C		C	C	C	C	C	C	C	C	C	C	C	C	Yes
	9824	T>C					C									Yes
	9948	G>A (Val to Ile)							A	A						Yes
	9950	T>C												C		Yes
ND3	10084	T>C (Ile to Thr)		C	C											Yes

Table 2. Cont.

			Conservation	KMT 01	KMT 01	KMT 02	KMT 03	KMT 04	KMT 05	KMT 05	KMT 06	KMT 07	KMT 07	KMT 08	KMT 09	
Gene	**Position**	**Replacement**	**(H/B/M/X)[a]**	**II-2**	**III-1**	**II-4**	**II-1**	**II-2**	**III-3**	**IV-1**	**II-4**	**II-3**	**I-2**	**II-3**		**Previously reported[b]**
	10181	C>T		T	T											Yes
	10397	A>G						G	G	G						Yes
	10398	A>G (Thr to Ala)	T/T/T/A	G	G	G	G	G	G	G	G	G	G	G	G	Yes
	10400	C>T		T	T	T	T	T	T	T	T	T	T	T	T	Yes
TR	10438	A>G	A/A/A/G											G		Yes
ND4L	10685	G>A												A		Yes
ND4	10867	C>T	I/F/L/L	T	T											Yes
	10873	T>C		C	C	C	C	C	C	C	C	C	C	C	C	Yes
	11017	T>C					C									Yes
	11084	A>G (Thr to Ala)					G									Yes
	11719	G>A		A	A	A	A	A	A	A	A	A	A	A	A	Yes
	11914	G>A									A					Yes
	11944	T>C						C								Yes
	11969	G>A (Ala to Thr)												A		Yes
	12026	A>G (Ile to Val)						G								Yes
	12100	A>G	L/L/L/L												G	Yes
TH	12172	A>G		G	G											Yes
ND5	12705	C>T		T	T	T	T	T	T	T	T	T	T	T	T	Yes
	12771	G>A					A									Yes
	13074	A>G												G		Yes
	13278	A>G						G								Yes
	13528	A>G (Thr to Ala)		G	G											Yes
	13890	C>T												T		Yes
	13928	G>T (Ser to Ile)	S/T/S/T											T		Yes
ND6	14364	G>A					A									Yes
	14569	G>A									A					Yes
	14668	C>T		T	T	T						T	T		T	Yes
CYB	14766	C>T (Thr to Ile)	T/S/I/S	T	T	T	T	T	T	T	T	T	T	T	T	Yes
	14783	T>C		C	C	C	C	C	C	C	C	C	C	C	C	Yes
	14790	A>G (Asn to Ser)												G		Yes
	14979	T>C (Ile to Thr)	I/I/L/L			C						C	C			Yes
	15043	G>A		A	A	A	A	A	A	A	A	A	A	A	A	Yes
	15265	C>T												T		Yes

Table 2. Cont.

Gene	Position	Replacement	Conservation (H/B/M/X)[a]	KMT 01 II-2	KMT 01 III-1	KMT 02 II-4	KMT 03 II-1	KMT 04 II-2	KMT 05 III-3	KMT 05 IV-1	KMT 06 II-4	KMT 07 II-3	KMT 07 I-2	KMT 08 II-3	KMT 09	Previously reported[b]
	15301	G>A		A	A	A	A	A	A	A	A	A	A	A	A	Yes
	15323	G>A (Ala to Thr)									A					Yes
	15326	A>G (Thr to Ala)	T/M/I/I	G	G	G	G	G	G	G	G	G	G	G	G	Yes
	15440	T>C		C	C											Yes
	15497	G>A (Gly to Ser)									A					Yes
	15724	A>G							G	G						Yes
	15748	T>C							C	C						Yes
	15860	A>G (Ile to Val)									G					Yes
TT	15951	A>G		G	G											Yes

[a]Conservation of amino acids for polypeptides or nucleotides for RNAs in human (H), bovine (B), mouse (M), and *Xenopus laevis* (X).
[b]See the online mitochondrial genome database http://www.mitomap.org.

in the substitution of the amino acid alanine with threonine (Table 2).

Three major haplogroups, D, M and G, were detected in the mtDNA haplogroup analysis of the nine pedigrees. Haplogroups D4, D4b1b1a, D5a2a, D5b1b1, G1a1a, M7a1a and M11b were each found in seven pedigrees, and haplogroup D4a was found in two pedigrees. Haplogroup D was found in six pedigrees and was the most prevalent haplogroup in the nine pedigrees (Table 1).

Mutational Analysis of the *GJB2* and *TRMU* Genes

To assess the role of the *GJB2* gene in the variable phenotype or existence of the mutation in the patients carrying the A1555G mutation, we performed a sequence analysis of the *GJB2* gene in all of the subjects with the A1555G mutation. None of the subjects had mutations in the *GJB2* gene. Additionally, the A10S mutation of the *TRMU* gene has been reported to be a modifier gene in hearing loss with the A1555G mutation. We also analyzed the DNA of the subjects using PCR-RFLP, and the A10S mutation was not detected in any of the subjects (data not shown).

Discussion

The present study was performed in Korean subjects with non-syndromic clinically variable hearing loss carrying the A1555G mutation of the 12S rRNA gene in the mtDNA. To explain these variable phenotypes, we searched for mtDNA variants that acted as modifying factors of the variable phenotypes using complete mtDNA sequence analysis. First, the homoplasmic A1555G mutation of the 12S rRNA gene was detected in nine of the 281 unrelated subjects with non-syndromic hearing loss. Their pedigrees were characterized for clinical, genetic and molecular characteristics. The Korean pedigrees with hearing loss presented with wide penetrance and expressivity. The penetrance of the eight pedigrees (excluding the pedigree for KMT 09) ranged from 28.6% to 75%, with an average of 60.8%. These results were higher than the 29.5% penetrance observed in the previously reported Chinese population [26] but similar to the 65.4% and 54.1% penetrance of a large Arab-Israeli pedigree and nineteen Spanish pedigrees, respectively [9,29]. This result suggested that the penetrance of hearing loss with the A1555G mutation was variable even within the same eastern population and appeared to differ among ethnic groups.

Mitochondrial haplogroups have been reported to be associated with diseases, including blindness [30], ageing [31], male infertility[32], Alzheimer's [33], and diabetes [34]. In addition, mtDNA haplogroups have been shown to alter the phenotypic expression of syndromic and non-syndromic hearing loss. Lu et al. (2010) identified ten haplogroups in 69 pedigrees with hearing loss carrying the A1555G mutation: A, B, C, D, F, G, M, N, R and Y. Haplogroup D was found at a higher frequency in the hearing loss pedigrees than in 93 controls. In contrast, haplogroups A and M were found at lower frequencies in the hearing loss pedigrees than in the controls [26]. The mtDNA haplogroup analysis of the Spanish pedigrees revealed the following haplogroups: H, I, J, K, T, U, V and L [27,35]. These haplogroups did not overlap with the haplogroups of the eastern Asian population. In the study of the Spanish pedigrees, 45.1% of individuals in the control group and 76% of the individuals in the hearing loss group were of haplogroup H, revealing a significantly higher percentage of this haplogroup in the hearing loss group [27]. In the present study, three major haplogroups, D, M and G, were detected in the nine pedigrees. Haplogroups D4, D4b1b1a, D5a2a, D5b1b1, G1a1a, M7a1a and M11b were each present in seven pedigrees, and haplogroup D4a was present in two pedigrees. A study analyzing the mtDNA haplogroups of 593 Koreans showed the following haplogroups: 4.9% haplogroup D4 and D4a, 2% D4b1, 2.2% D5a2, 2.7% G1a1, 1.3% M7a1 and 0.8% M11 [36]. Mitochondrial DNA haplogroups are restricted among ethnic populations. Haplogroup D in the eastern Asian population and haplogroup H in the Europe-Caucasian population are associated with hearing loss with the A1555G mutation [26,27]. In the present study, haplogroup D was the most represented, similar to that found for the Chinese pedigrees. However, more pedigrees may be needed to estimate the association between an mtDNA haplogroup and hearing loss due to the mtDNA mutation.

Nuclear modifier genes have been reported to influence the variable phenotype of hearing loss with the A1555G mutation [22]. The mutant allele of the *MTO2* gene that encode mitochondrial proteins in yeast *S. cerevisiae* manifests a respiratory-deficient phenotype only when coupled with the paromomycin-resistance mitochondrial 15S rRNA 1409 C to T mutation [37]. This mutation corresponds to the human 12S rRNA 1494 C to T mutation. The *MTO2* gene is evolutionarily conserved and display sequence similarity to the human *TRMU* gene. Indeed, the missense mutation c.G28T (p.A10S) of the *TRMU* gene has been reported in hearing loss patients with the A1555G mutation in some ethnic populations [22]. However, the p.A10S mutation of the *TRMU* gene was not detected in the nine Korean pedigrees with hearing loss in this study.

Mitochondrial DNA variations have also been reported to influence the variable phenotype of mitochondrial disease, including the variable phenotype of hearing loss patients carrying the A1555G mutation. For example, the following mitochondrial tRNA variants may contribute to the phenotype: $tRNA^{Thr}$ G15927A [18], $tRNA^{Cys}$ T5802C [18], $tRNA^{Arg}$ T10454C [24], $tRNA^{Ser(AGY)}$ C12224T [26], $tRNA^{Cys}$ G5821A [19], $tRNA^{Glu}$ A14693G [24], $tRNA^{Thr}$ T15908C [24], T12338C [18] of ND5, G7444A [23] of $tRNA^{Ser(UCN)}$/CO1 and G11696A [26] of the ND4 gene. These mtDNA variants have been suggested to have significant effects on the penetrance and expressivity of hearing loss with the A1555G mutation. In this study, one novel mtDNA variant, G3496A of theND1 gene, was identified. Additionally, two variants of known modifier factors, $tRNA^{Cys}$ T5802C and G7444A of the $tRNA^{Ser(UCN)}$/CO1 gene, were identified. The G3496A variant, which causes a substitution of alanine to threonine at position 64 (p.A64T) of the ND1 gene, was analyzed for protein biochemical changes using the PolyPhen 2 (http://genetics.bwh.harvard.edu/pph2/), SNPs&GO (http://snps-and-go.biocomp.unibo.it/snps-and-go/) and Panther (http://www.pantherdb.org/tools/csnpScoreForm.jsp) programs. This substitution appears to have no association with the variable phenotype because all of the in silico tools predicted that this substitution is a benign polymorphism. The $tRNA^{Cys}$ T5802C variant, however, has been reported to alter the structure of tRNAs and lead to a defect in tRNA metabolism [18]. Another variant, G7444A of the $tRNA^{Ser(UCN)}$/CO1 gene, was not sufficient to produce a clinical phenotype [38]. Therefore, additional modifier factors, including nuclear backgrounds, environmental factors, and mitochondrial haplogroups, must alter the phenotypic manifestation. The variant G7444A of the $tRNA^{Ser(UCN)}$/CO1 gene has been detected in several haplogroups, including C4a, B4 and D4a [26,38], and was found in haplogroup D4a in this study. This result indicates that this variant was sporadic, similarly to the A1555G mutation. Additional studies are necessary to determine whether this variant affects the variable phenotype or is a simple polymorphism.

This study is the first to perform complete mtDNA sequencing to identify mtDNA haplogroups or variants in Korean pedigrees with non-syndromic hearing loss carrying the A1555G mutation. The haplogroups in the Korean population of the eastern Asian population are similar to those of the Chinese population but differ from the haplogroups of the Spanish populations of the Europe-Caucasian population. The mtDNA variants as modifier factors were also found to be similar to those of the Chinese population. The mtDNA haplogroups and variants are similar to the eastern Asian population but appear to have different phenotypes, although some subjects had the same variants [39,40]. These results suggest that both the ethnic population and environmental factors lead to the variable phenotype of the A1555G mutation. However, this observation requires further pedigree and clinical evaluations to fully elucidate the mechanisms of the phenotypic manifestation of the A1555G mutation.

Author Contributions

Conceived and designed the experiments: U-KK KYL. Performed the experiments: JWB D-BK S-HB. Analyzed the data: JWB D-BK U-KK KYL. Contributed reagents/materials/analysis tools: JYC H-JP JDL DGH DJJ SHL KYL. Wrote the paper: JWB D-BK U-KK KYL.

References

1. Morton NE, Shields DC, Collins A (1991) Genetic epidemiology of complex phenotypes. Ann Hum Genet 55: 301–314.
2. Prezant TR, Agapian JV, Bohlman MC, Bu X, Oztas S, et al. (1993) Mitochondrial ribosomal RNA mutation associated with both antibiotic-induced and non-syndromic deafness. Nat Genet 4: 289–294.
3. Moraes CT, DiMauro S, Zeviani M, Lombes A, Shanske S, et al. (1989) Mitochondrial DNA deletions in progressive external ophthalmoplegia and Kearns-Sayre syndrome. N Engl J Med 320: 1293–1299.
4. Shoffner JM, Lott MT, Lezza AM, Seibel P, Ballinger SW, et al. (1990) Myoclonic epilepsy and ragged-red fiber disease (MERRF) is associated with a mitochondrial DNA tRNA(Lys) mutation. Cell 61: 931–937.
5. Goto Y, Nonaka I, Horai S (1990) A mutation in the tRNA(Leu)(UUR) gene associated with the MELAS subgroup of mitochondrial encephalomyopathies. Nature 348: 651–653.
6. Ballinger SW, Shoffner JM, Hedaya EV, Trounce I, Polak MA, et al. (1992) Maternally transmitted diabetes and deafness associated with a 10.4 kb mitochondrial DNA deletion. Nat Genet 1: 11–15.
7. Guan MX (2004) Molecular pathogenetic mechanism of maternally inherited deafness. Ann N Y Acad Sci 1011: 259–271.
8. Van Camp G, Smith RJ (2000) Maternally inherited hearing impairment. Clin Genet 57: 409–414.
9. Estivill X, Govea N, Barcelo E, Badenas C, Romero E, et al. (1998) Familial progressive sensorineural deafness is mainly due to the mtDNA A1555G mutation and is enhanced by treatment of aminoglycosides. Am J Hum Genet 62: 27–35.
10. Li Z, Li R, Chen J, Liao Z, Zhu Y, et al. (2005) Mutational analysis of the mitochondrial 12S rRNA gene in Chinese pediatric subjects with aminoglycoside-induced and non-syndromic hearing loss. Hum Genet 117: 9–15.
11. Usami S, Abe S, Akita J, Namba A, Shinkawa H, et al. (2000) Prevalence of mitochondrial gene mutations among hearing impaired patients. J Med Genet 37: 38–40.
12. Fischel-Ghodsian N, Prezant TR, Chaltraw WE, Wendt KA, Nelson RA, et al. (1997) Mitochondrial gene mutation is a significant predisposing factor in aminoglycoside ototoxicity. Am J Otolaryngol 18: 173–178.
13. Guan MX, Fischel-Ghodsian N, Attardi G (2000) A biochemical basis for the inherited susceptibility to aminoglycoside ototoxicity. Hum Mol Genet 9: 1787–1793.
14. Hamasaki K, Rando RR (1997) Specific binding of aminoglycosides to a human rRNA construct based on a DNA polymorphism which causes aminoglycoside-induced deafness. Biochemistry 36: 12323–12328.
15. Casano RA, Johnson DF, Bykhovskaya Y, Torricelli F, Bigozzi M, et al. (1999) Inherited susceptibility to aminoglycoside ototoxicity: genetic heterogeneity and clinical implications. Am J Otolaryngol 20: 151–156.

16. Matthijs G, Claes S, Longo-Mbenza B, Cassiman JJ (1996) Non-syndromic deafness associated with a mutation and a polymorphism in the mitochondrial 12S ribosomal RNA gene in a large Zairean pedigree. Eur J Hum Genet 4: 46–51.
17. Tang X, Yang L, Zhu Y, Liao Z, Wang J, et al. (2007) Very low penetrance of hearing loss in seven Han Chinese pedigrees carrying the deafness-associated 12S rRNA A1555G mutation. Gene 393: 11–19.
18. Chen B, Sun D, Yang L, Zhang C, Yang A, et al. (2008) Mitochondrial ND5 T12338C, tRNA(Cys) T5802C, and tRNA(Thr) G15927A variants may have a modifying role in the phenotypic manifestation of deafness-associated 12S rRNA A1555G mutation in three Han Chinese pedigrees. Am J Med Genet A 146A: 1248–1258.
19. Zhao L, Wang Q, Qian Y, Li R, Cao J, et al. (2005) Clinical evaluation and mitochondrial DNA sequence analysis in two Chinese families with aminoglycoside-induced and non-syndromic hearing loss. Biochem Biophys Res Commun 336: 967–973.
20. Guan MX, Fischel-Ghodsian N, Attardi G (1996) Biochemical evidence for nuclear gene involvement in phenotype of non-syndromic deafness associated with mitochondrial 12S rRNA mutation. Hum Mol Genet 5: 963–971.
21. Wang X, Lu J, Zhu Y, Yang A, Yang L, et al. (2008) Mitochondrial tRNAThr G15927A mutation may modulate the phenotypic manifestation of ototoxic 12S rRNA A1555G mutation in four Chinese families. Pharmacogenet Genomics 18: 1059–1070.
22. Guan MX, Yan Q, Li X, Bykhovskaya Y, Gallo-Teran J, et al. (2006) Mutation in TRMU related to transfer RNA modification modulates the phenotypic expression of the deafness-associated mitochondrial 12S ribosomal RNA mutations. Am J Hum Genet 79: 291–302.
23. Yuan H, Qian Y, Xu Y, Cao J, Bai L, et al. (2005) Cosegregation of the G7444A mutation in the mitochondrial COI/tRNA(Ser(UCN)) genes with the 12S rRNA A1555G mutation in a Chinese family with aminoglycoside-induced and nonsyndromic hearing loss. Am J Med Genet A 138A: 133–140.
24. Young WY, Zhao L, Qian Y, Li R, Chen J, et al. (2006) Variants in mitochondrial tRNAGlu, tRNAArg, and tRNAThr may influence the phenotypic manifestation of deafness-associated 12S rRNA A1555G mutation in three Han Chinese families with hearing loss. Am J Med Genet A 140: 2188–2197.
25. Ding Y, Li Y, You J, Yang L, Chen B, et al. (2009) Mitochondrial tRNA(Glu) A14693G variant may modulate the phenotypic manifestation of deafness-associated 12S rRNA A1555G mutation in a Han Chinese family. J Genet Genomics 36: 241–250.
26. Lu J, Qian Y, Li Z, Yang A, Zhu Y, et al. (2010) Mitochondrial haplotypes may modulate the phenotypic manifestation of the deafness-associated 12S rRNA 1555A>G mutation. Mitochondrion 10: 69–81.
27. Torroni A, Cruciani F, Rengo C, Sellitto D, Lopez-Bigas N, et al. (1999) The A1555G mutation in the 12S rRNA gene of human mtDNA: recurrent origins and founder events in families affected by sensorineural deafness. Am J Hum Genet 65: 1349–1358.
28. Li R, Greinwald JH, Jr., Yang L, Choo DI, Wenstrup RJ, et al. (2004) Molecular analysis of the mitochondrial 12S rRNA and tRNASer(UCN) genes in paediatric subjects with non-syndromic hearing loss. J Med Genet 41: 615–620.
29. Bykhovskaya Y, Shohat M, Ehrenman K, Johnson D, Hamon M, et al. (1998) Evidence for complex nuclear inheritance in a pedigree with nonsyndromic deafness due to a homoplasmic mitochondrial mutation. Am J Med Genet 77: 421–426.
30. Torroni A, Petrozzi M, D'Urbano L, Sellitto D, Zeviani M, et al. (1997) Haplotype and phylogenetic analyses suggest that one European-specific mtDNA background plays a role in the expression of Leber hereditary optic neuropathy by increasing the penetrance of the primary mutations 11778 and 14484. Am J Hum Genet 60: 1107–1121.
31. Coskun PE, Ruiz-Pesini E, Wallace DC (2003) Control region mtDNA variants: longevity, climatic adaptation, and a forensic conundrum. Proc Natl Acad Sci U S A 100: 2174–2176.
32. Ruiz-Pesini E, Lapena AC, Diez-Sanchez C, Perez-Martos A, Montoya J, et al. (2000) Human mtDNA haplogroups associated with high or reduced spermatozoa motility. Am J Hum Genet 67: 682–696.
33. van der Walt JM, Dementieva YA, Martin ER, Scott WK, Nicodemus KK, et al. (2004) Analysis of European mitochondrial haplogroups with Alzheimer disease risk. Neurosci Lett 365: 28–32.
34. Fuku N, Park KS, Yamada Y, Nishigaki Y, Cho YM, et al. (2007) Mitochondrial haplogroup N9a confers resistance against type 2 diabetes in Asians. Am J Hum Genet 80: 407–415.
35. del Castillo FJ, Rodriguez-Ballesteros M, Martin Y, Arellano B, Gallo-Teran J, et al. (2003) Heteroplasmy for the 1555A>G mutation in the mitochondrial 12S rRNA gene in six Spanish families with non-syndromic hearing loss. J Med Genet 40: 632–636.
36. Lee HY, Yoo JE, Park MJ, Chung U, Shin KJ (2006) Mitochondrial DNA control region sequences in Koreans: identification of useful variable sites and phylogenetic analysis for mtDNA data quality control. Int J Legal Med 120: 5–14.
37. Yan Q, Li X, Faye G, Guan MX (2005) Mutations in MTO2 related to tRNA modification impair mitochondrial gene expression and protein synthesis in the presence of a paromomycin resistance mutation in mitochondrial 15 S rRNA. J Biol Chem 280: 29151–29157.
38. Zhu Y, Qian Y, Tang X, Wang J, Yang L, et al. (2006) Aminoglycoside-induced and non-syndromic hearing loss is associated with the G7444A mutation in the mitochondrial COI/tRNASer(UCN) genes in two Chinese families. Biochem Biophys Res Commun 342: 843–850.
39. Dai P, Liu X, Han D, Qian Y, Huang D, et al. (2006) Extremely low penetrance of deafness associated with the mitochondrial 12S rRNA mutation in 16 Chinese families: implication for early detection and prevention of deafness. Biochem Biophys Res Commun 340: 194–199.
40. Young WY, Zhao L, Qian Y, Wang Q, Li N, et al. (2005) Extremely low penetrance of hearing loss in four Chinese families with the mitochondrial 12S rRNA A1555G mutation. Biochem Biophys Res Commun 328: 1244–1251.

14

Preservation of Auditory P300-Like Potentials in Cortical Deafness

Marianna Cavinato[1]*, Jessica Rigon[1], Chiara Volpato[1], Carlo Semenza[1,2], Francesco Piccione[1]

1 San Camillo Foundation, Institute of Care and Research, Venice, Italy, **2** Department of Neuroscience, University of Padova, Padova, Italy

Abstract

The phenomenon of blindsight has been largely studied and refers to residual abilities of blind patients without an acknowledged visual awareness. Similarly, "deaf hearing" might represent a further example of dissociation between detection and perception of sounds. Here we report the rare case of a patient with a persistent and complete cortical deafness caused by damage to the bilateral temporo-parietal lobes who occasionally showed unexpected reactions to environmental sounds despite she denied hearing. We applied for the first time electrophysiological techniques to better understand auditory processing and perceptual awareness of the patient. While auditory brainstem responses were within normal limits, no middle- and long-latency waveforms could be identified. However, event-related potentials showed conflicting results. While the Mismatch Negativity could not be evoked, robust P3-like waveforms were surprisingly found in the latency range of 600–700 ms. The generation of P3-like potentials, despite extensive destruction of the auditory cortex, might imply the integrity of independent circuits necessary to process auditory stimuli even in the absence of consciousness of sound. Our results support the reverse hierarchy theory that asserts that the higher levels of the hierarchy are immediately available for perception, while low-level information requires more specific conditions. The accurate characterization in terms of anatomy and neurophysiology of the auditory lesions might facilitate understanding of the neural substrates involved in deaf-hearing.

Editor: Lawrence M. Ward, University of British Columbia, Canada

Funding: The authors have no support or funding to report.

Competing Interests: The authors have declared that no competing interests exist.

* E-mail: marianna.cavinato@ospedalesancamillo.net

Introduction

Extensive bilateral lesions of the primary auditory cortex can produce a complete loss of hearing, known as cortical deafness. Bitemporal damage required to produce this deficit is rare and is most frequently caused by ischemic cerebrovascular accident [1,2].

There is a relatively limited research on this condition, likely because cortical deafness is typically transient and rapidly resolves in more selective hearing disorders, such as auditory agnosia or word deafness [3]. In some isolated cases, however, cortical deafness may be permanent [4].

Generally, cortical deafness is characterized by the complete disruption of central auditory processing, despite intact peripheral auditory function [2]. However, from the limited literature available, several authors have described the presence of residual auditory behaviors in completely deaf patients [2,5,6]. Relatives reported occasional unexpected reactions of patients to environmental sounds despite they denied hearing. This phenomenon has been likened to blindsight, referring to residual visual abilities of individuals without acknowledged awareness [7]. Similarly, "deaf-hearing" seems to imply a dissociation between detection and perception of sounds.

In the present report, we had the opportunity to study a patient with severe persistent cortical deafness caused by two consecutive strokes. The lesions extended into both Heschl's gyri, insulae and superior temporal gyri. Surprisingly, the patient showed some reactions to unexpected sounds, despite the lack of any startle response to loud noises. We adopted an electrophysiological approach involving auditory evoked potentials (AEPs) and event related potentials (ERPs) to assess auditory processing and perceptual awareness. Generally, auditory potentials are characterized by a time-resolution on the order of milliseconds and can therefore provide temporal correlates of the stages of information processing between stimulus and response. AEPs reflect the activation of auditory nerve and central auditory pathways up to the primary auditory cortex [8]. Differently, ERP recordings represent a valuable method to provide quantitative information about the perception and higher order processing of acoustic stimuli [9,10].

On the basis of these assumptions, the present study should provide a procedure by which electrophysiological methods can be used to study auditory unawareness or deaf-hearing.

Methods

Ethics statement

The present study was approved by the Research Ethics Committee (REC) of the Scientific Foundation "San Camillo" and was compliant with the declaration of Helsinki guidelines. Written informed consent to publication for case details was obtained from the patient and the healthy volunteers that participated in the study.

Case report

CDB, a 55-year-old, right-handed female with previously normal hearing was admitted to our Neurorehabilitation Unit for two consecutive strokes. The first ischemic attack occurred in December 2007 and involved the territories of the middle cerebral artery of the right hemisphere. A week later, a second infarction affected the areas of the middle artery of the left side of the brain.

On admission, the patient was alert and oriented in space and time, but often appeared agitated and perplexed. Neurologic examination showed no sensorimotor deficits, but she complained a complete loss of hearing. Her speech was characterized by a severe dysarthria; she was unable to respond to verbal questions or environmental sounds and startle response to loud noises could not be detected. She could understand and execute complex written instructions and recognize and use gestures for communication. Writing was performed hesitantly with much persuasion and showed graphemic errors and agrammatism. The T_1-weighted MRI scan showed bilateral lesions of the superior temporal gyrus and its subregions (planum polare, Heschl gyrus, planum temporale), the inferior parietal lobe and angular gyri and the insular cortex. On the right, the lesion extended into the inferior frontal gyrus.

During the first year in our Neurorehabilitation Unit, CDB showed consistent evidence of cortical deafness. Language functions were measured with the Aachen aphasia test (AAT) [11] and revealed that the patient could not understand speech, repeat words and write to dictation. She could recognize and name pictures and match written words with objects. She showed a good visual-spatial memory and the Weigl's test revealed normal executive functions. She presented with buccofacial and constructional apraxia. There were, however, no signs of ideomotor apraxia.

The patient mood progressively improved. She appeared to become aware of her deafness and was distressed by this. The agitation that the patient showed a few days after the lesion, tended to resolve gradually. Occasionally, her relatives reported that she unconsciously manifested some startle reactions with blinking and head-turning in the direction of unexpected sounds.

In two-year follow up we did not find improvements in the clinical features of the patient. She complained complete loss of hearing and she could only communicate through reading and writing. Three years after stroke, CDB showed substantially unchanged clinical and neuropsychological features, confirming a persistent cortical deafness. However, sporadic startle responses were reported.

The MRI scan confirmed the extensive area of infarction in the territory of the bilateral middle cerebral artery. MRI sections of the lesion are shown in Fig. 1. In addition, we compared the voxel-based structural data of the patient with the T1-weighted MRI scans of ten age-matched healthy controls. We used an automated technique of statistical parametric mapping (SPM) to the analysis of gray matter (GM) to detect functional abnormalities that were not accounted for by either visible or unsuspected structural abnormalities. At the corrected threshold of $p<0.05$, the SPM-based morphometric comparison revealed that the patient had a decrease of GM distribution in the bilateral caudate nucleus and the pulvinar thalamus, in addition to the lesional areas delineated with traditional MRI [12]. We planned to perform a functional magnetic resonance (fMRI), but the patient refused the procedure.

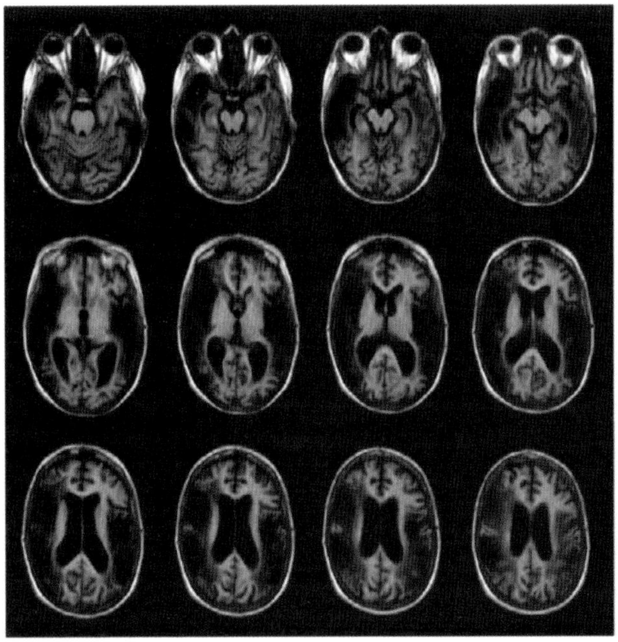

Figure 1. T1-weighted MRI scans of the patient. Consecutive sequences of axial T1-weighted MRI scan of the patient's brain three years after her strokes (right hemisphere is on the left side of the picture). Hypodense lesion massively extends from the bilateral superior temporal gyrus toward the transverse temporal gyrus, the pulvinar, thalamus and insula and the middle temporal gyrus. The right hemisphere was further damaged in the lentiform nucleus, the postcentral gyrus, the inferior frontal gyrus and the inferior parietal lobe.

Audiological testing

Audiological examination comprised pure tone audiometry and auditory evoked potentials.

Standard pure-tone air and bone conduction threshold audiometry tested for peripheral hearing impairment using tones of different frequencies with increasing sound pressure intensity, according to the guidelines recommended by the British Society of Audiology [13].

The audiological examination was completed with the auditory brainstem responses (ABRs) and further tests of the central auditory system: middle and long latency auditory evoked potentials (MLAEPs and LLAEPs, respectively). ABRs include short-latency potentials and are associated with the eighth nerve, cochlear nucleus, superior olive, and midbrain. They occur in the first 10 ms following stimulus onset. MLAEPs represent the earliest cortical response to acoustic stimulus and cover the 10–80 ms latency range, including Na, Pa, Nb and Pb components. Finally, N1, P2, and N2 components of LLAEPs occur between 80 and 200 ms after sound onset and are related to auditory system on primary and secondary cortical areas involved in the central auditory process.

Auditory responses were recorded with the patient rested on a bed in an acoustically shielded room. 1-kHz tone bursts were presented monaurally at a frequency of 10 Hz with alternating polarity (condensation and rarefaction clicks). The acoustic stimulus was applied monaurally via TDH-49 earphones. The estimation of auditory threshold was traced by the wave V detection which can be used as a robust indicator that the central nervous system detected an auditory stimulus [14]. The patient exhibited large and reproducible waves V at an intensity of 100 dB. Thus, we adopted the same stimulation intensity to evoke auditory responses. The contralateral ear was masked by 40 dB white noise in all trials. Recordings were derived from the vertex (Cz), referenced to the earlobes (A1 and A2). At least two runs, consisting of 2000 click presentations each, were obtained for all auditory evoked potentials. ABRs were set as follows: 10 ms epochs, bandpass filtering of 150–3000 Hz. Middle-latency response variables were: 80 ms epochs using band-pass of 5–

1000 Hz. Late auditory potentials were analysed in 500 ms epochs and band-pass of 0.5–30 Hz.

All auditory signals were inspected visually. All visual analyses were revised by one investigator aware of the patient but blinded to the patient's age and further clinical data. Auditory recordings classified as distorted or insufficient for interpretation were excluded. Individual waveforms were included in a grand average providing a better estimate of peak amplitudes and latencies.

Event-related potentials (ERPs)

In addition to audiological tests, the later, more cognitive stages of auditory processing were examined in an auditory oddball experiment.

Electroencephalogram (EEG) was recorded from a 32 channel electrode cap, according to the extended 10–20 method of electrode application, referred to linked earlobes with a forehead ground. Additional electrodes were placed below the right eye and at the outer canthus, for bipolar recordings or the electroocular activity (EOG). Stimuli were presented monaurally at 90 dB. Two sinusoid tones of 1000 and 2000 Hz served as frequent and rare tones, respectively. Probability of rare tones was 20% and probability of occurrence of frequent tones was 80%. The interstimulus interval was 1.0–1.3 sec. The experimental session was subdivided into four blocks consisting of 100 stimuli each, separated by 1-min breaks. Data were recorded with a band-pass of 0.15 to 70 Hz and digitized at 1000 Hz (NeuroScan Amplifier, Compumedics Neuroscan) for later off-line analysis. EEG data analysis was performed using EEGLAB 9.0.4, an open source Matlab toolbox. A notch filter was used to eliminate the frequencies centred on 50 Hz. The EEG data were segmented in epochs of 1200 ms including 200 ms pre-stimulus baseline, time-locked to the beginning of the stimulus presentation. Epochs including EEG excursions exceeding ±90 μV were rejected. After averaging, a further digital low-pass filter at 30 Hz was applied.

For assessment of the MMN, we computed the increase in the negativity of the evoked potential in response to the deviants as compared with the response to the standards occurring within a 100–300 ms time window.

P3 was measured relative to the pre-stimulus baseline and was defined as the largest positive component occurring after the N1-P2-N2 complex, within a latency window between 300 and 700 ms after a deviant stimulus was detected.

Auditory oddball ERP signals of the patient were compared with those of ten healthy controls matched for age and gender to gain insight into underlying mechanisms of P3 in cortical deafness. Healthy controls were submitted to the same data collection and analysis conditions as the patient. Topographic maps of P3 distribution were constructed using grand-average voltage information from all scalp electrodes.

Within and between group analysis was performed by the modified t-test described by Crawford and Howell (1998) [15]. Statistical analysis was restricted to P3 findings in terms of peak amplitude at central midline electrodes (Fz, Cz, and Pz), as well as overall brain electrical activity mapping when P3 component exhibited largest amplitude in both groups. Statistical significance was accepted when $p<0.05$.

Results

Audiological testing

Pure tone air and bone conduction audiometry indicated a complete sensorineural hearing loss bilaterally. The patient had no response at output limits of audiometry (110 decibels, dB) in the frequency range of 250–8000 Hz.

Figure 2 shows the grand-averaged waveforms of auditory evoked potentials for the two runs of stimulation. Brainstem auditory potentials of either ear evoked essentially normal responses suggesting the integrity of the auditory nerves and pathways up to the inferior colliculi of both sides.

Conversely, middle latency auditory responses (Na, Pa, Nb and Pb) and long latency potentials with N1, P2 and N2 could not be identified reliably.

Event-related potentials (ERPs)

The Mismatch Negativity could not be recorded in response to deviant stimuli. However, robust positive peaks in the latency

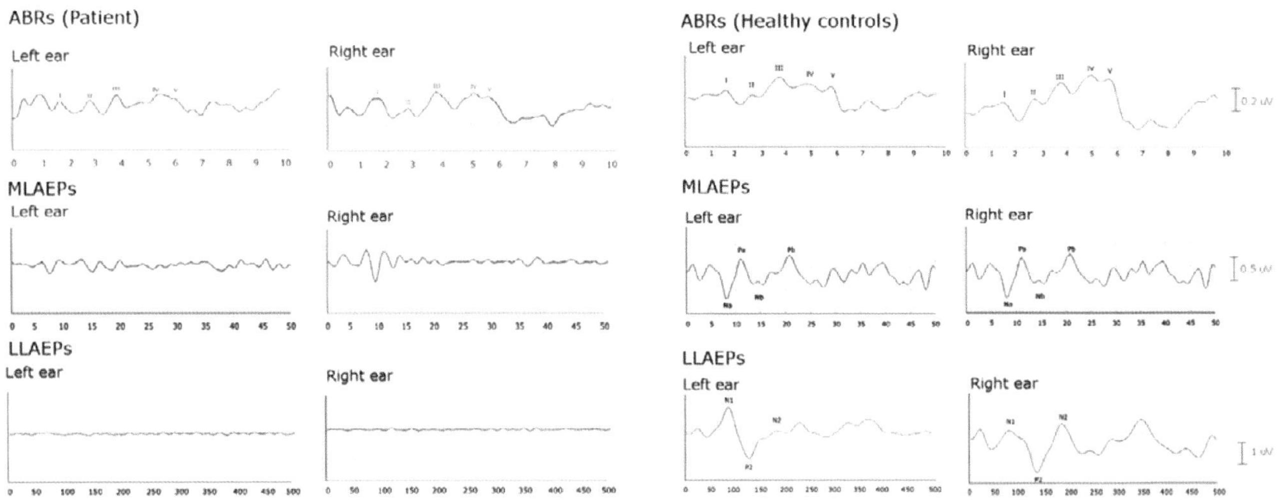

Figure 2. Grand-averaged auditory evoked potentials to sound onsets. Auditory brainstem responses (ABRs; top), middle-latency auditory evoked potentials (MLAEPs; middle), and long-latency auditory evoked potentials (LLAEPs; bottom) recorded by routine clinical protocols in the patient with cortical deafness (left) and in the control group (right). Note the integrity of brainstem auditory responses and the absence of bilateral middle- and long-latency evoked potentials, characterizing cortical deafness.

range of 650–700 ms were clearly seen following the right ear stimulation (Fig. 3B). Contralateral responses were abolished.

Statistical comparison between patient and controls revealed significant differences in P3 scalp distribution. In the within-group analysis, the control group showed a significantly larger right centro-parietal P3 in response to left ear stimulation (p = 0.0001), and a bilateral centro-temporal dominance in response to right ear stimulation (p = 0.01) (Fig. 3A). Differently, the patient exhibited the largest amplitude of P3 at the left posterior and central areas after right ear stimulation (p = 0.0001; p = 0.0001) (Fig. 3B). No P3 could be recorded in response to left ear stimuli. Finally, the between-group analysis showed a significantly lower P3 amplitude over the right fronto-temporal and central regions of the patient compared to controls ($p = 0.0001$; $p = 0.008$, respectively).

Discussion

In the present study, we reported the rare case of a patient with persistent cortical deafness. This disorder is characterized by bilateral temporo-parietal lesions involving the primary auditory areas and their radiations and implies the complete absence of auditory afferent input at the cortical level. In contrast, several authors have presented evidence of residual capacity of the damaged auditory system to process acoustic stimuli [2,5,6].

The goal of the present study was, therefore, a systematic examination of several levels of auditory function using auditory evoked potentials in the attempt to better evaluate the dissociation between perception and higher order processing of acoustic information.

Cortical deafness is generally associated with a damage of central auditory functions, in spite of normal peripheral hearing. Accordingly, our patient showed normal ABRs, expression of the integrity of the inner ear and cochlear nerve, as well as the auditory pathways within the brainstem. However, middle-latency responses were consistently absent to both right and left ear stimulation. The neural origin of MLAEPs is still a subject of controversy. Although some authors support the hypothesis of a subcortical involvement in the potential generation, it is generally assumed that MLAEPs arise from the medial geniculate and the supratemporal plane comprising the primary auditory area (A1), and the surrounding region of the superior temporal gyrus and the frontal and parietal operculum [16,17]. Thus, in our patient the extent of the brain damage and the absence of MLAEP waves provide evidence of a cortical origin of the mid-latency potentials.

Concerning the long-latency auditory potentials, recent neuro-imaging data have suggested that abnormalities in the P1, N1 and P2 components reflect lesions extended into the multi-modal areas of the inferior parietal lobule. This area appears to exert a critical modulatory influence over LLAEP generators outside of the superior temporal plane [18]. The absence of LLAEPs in our patient does not necessarily reflect a damage to primary auditory cortex, but also a damage to adjacent posterior areas.

Finally, we recorded two main components of ERPs: the Mismatch Negativity and the P3. Although we supposed to observe an absence of endogenous potentials, we found some unexpected results.

MMN could not be recorded in response to deviant sounds. Generally, the MMN appears in response to changes in sound stimulation and is known to reflect a relatively automatic comparison of incoming sounds to auditory cortex sensory-memory representations of the preceding repetitive stimuli [19]. Some authors have suggested that these representations might be explained by the transient adaptation of feature-specific neurons within the anterior and posterior parts of the primary auditory cortex that regulate the access to the conscious perception of sound [20,21]. In fact, numerous brain imaging studies on preattentive auditory deviance detection have demonstrated an initial contribution of the primary auditory cortex followed by the activation of the posterior superior temporal gyrus and the lateral planum temporale. These areas might be involved in the withdrawal of the details of the acoustic change [22,23]. Through the connections of the arcuate and superior longitudinal fascicle, the superior temporal gyrus is in communication with the inferior frontal gyrus. The activation of this region of the mid-ventrolateral prefrontal cortex might indicate a higher cognitive processing related to the judgement of sufficient novelty of auditory stimulus to require attentional resources [24]. The brain damage of CDB extended to the primary auditory cortex, the superior temporal gyrus, planum temporale and inferior frontal gyrus and could hamper sounds to access consciousness.

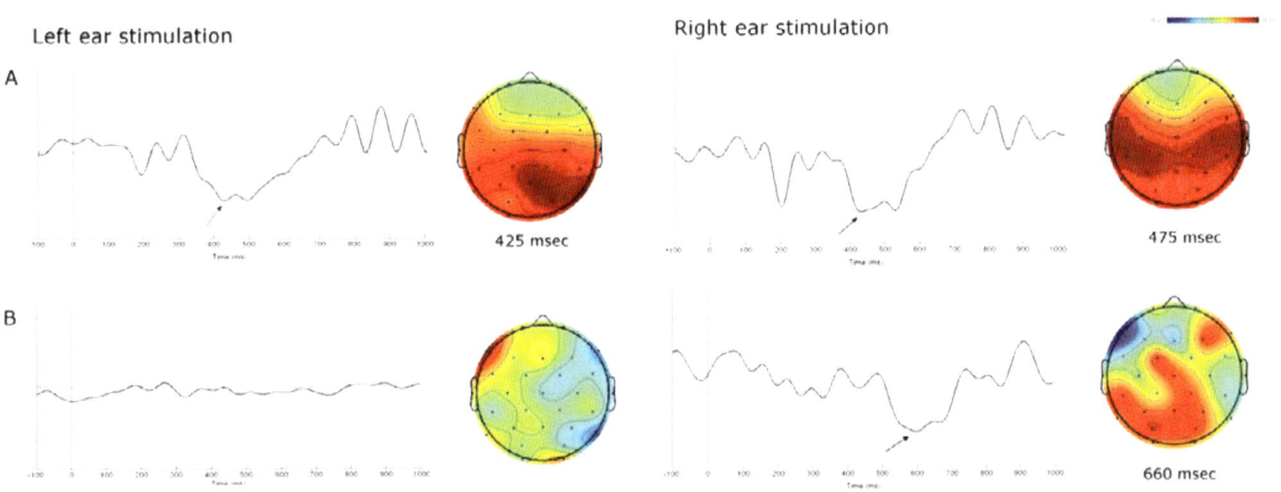

Figure 3. Grand-averaged event related potentials (ERPs) elicited by classic oddball at electrode Cz. Grand-averaged ERP waveforms at electrode Cz and thirty-one channel ERP topographical maps recorded in the patient (B) and controls (A). The latency is referred at the time point at which the positive peak between 300 and 700 ms latency is maximum at Cz electrode site. ERP waveform from the patient revealed a significantly higher P3 at the left posterior and central sites in response to right stimulation. No P3 could be recorded after left ear stimuli.

In contrast with the absence of the MMN, a reliable positive peak at 660 ms could be clearly detected in response to right ear stimulation. Because of its morphology and topographic distribution, we inferred that such late waveform could represent a P3-like potential.

P3 offers a covert and indirect measure of attentional resource allocation that represents an index of change detection [25]. P3 is related to the activity of associative cortical areas and is sensitive to complex processes around recalled information, stimulus significance, recognized auditory information and memory context updating [26,27]. The sources of P3 are believed to be located in heteromodal areas of the fronto-parietal cortex and their activation might reflect an attention switch to an environmental change encoded by the cerebral process generating the MMN [28,29]. The bilateral supramarginal gyrus, frontal operculum and insula seem to be mainly involved in the network for saliency detection in auditory modality [30]. However, some authors have demonstrated an asymmetrical cortical activation of P3 by using unilateral auditory stimulation. Among others, Gilmore and colleagues (2009) argued that in normal condition the right hemisphere is more prominently engaged during working memory and updating processes underlying P3 [31]. Accordingly, our healthy controls exhibited a right lateralized potential in response to left ear stimulation, and a bilateral distribution of ERPs to right ear stimulation. This denotes a more marked right side activation of P3 wave (Fig. 3A). In contrast, the patient showed robust P3-like components over the left posterior areas and a significantly lower distribution of the potentials over the right fronto-temporal and central areas in response to right ear stimulation. The left ear stimulation could not evoke any detectable responses. (Fig. 3B).

Depth recordings and lesion studies have implicated the frontal, temporal and inferior parietal lobes in the generation of the auditory P3 [32]. The interaction of these structures seems to play a key role in the auditory perceptual awareness, and the right hemisphere seems to be mainly engaged during working memory updating processes [31,33]. Thus, the marked right fronto-parietal dysfunction of our patient, in particular the damage of the right inferior frontal gyrus and the inferior parietal lobe, might partially explain the dissociation between detection and perception of sounds. Several authors have demonstrated that ERPs can be elicited even when stimuli are presented outside conscious awareness [34,35]. Bernat et al. (2001) offer evidence that subliminal stimuli can evoke consistent P3 waves. They speculated that P3 could represent a link between unconscious and conscious awareness in the context updating processes [35]. In our patient the generation of P3-like potentials implied that deviant stimuli were selectively processed bypassing networks involved in conscious perception. Schönwiesner et al. (2007) and Pandya (1995) hypothesized that association areas in and adjacent to the auditory parabelt might form an independent circuit from thalamo-cortical projections in the auditory system [26,36]. These alternate pathways could be preserved in our patient and responsible for the generation of P3-like potentials.

In addition, the lack of awareness of auditory stimuli might be further aggravated by the bilateral functional abnormalities of the pulvinar. In fact, the auditory association area seems to be preferentially related to the pulvinar complex [36]. The thalamic pulvinar nucleus plays an important role in the coupling of sensory and attentional functions. As demonstrated by Hugdahl et al. (1991), a lesion of this structure might imply an auditory neglect that further affected the conscious awareness of sounds of CDB [37].

As a final consideration, our findings seem to be in contrast with the hypothesis of a hierarchical information processing of auditory stimuli. A large body of physiological and functional data suggests that processing of auditory information is implemented in a hierarchical manner [38]. Lower levels are considered responsible for extracting basic spectro-temporal features of the auditory signal. Higher cortical areas are involved in a higher level of information processing, such as abstraction, perception, reasoning, and learning. They are characterized by at least four different, hierarchically organized processing levels, each containing several segregated sub-regions: the primary areas that receive their input from the thalamus; surrounding lateral and medial "belt" areas, that receive input from primary areas; a parabelt area on the dorsal plane of the superior temporal gyrus; and higher-level areas in the superior temporal sulcus and the frontal lobe. From that, the higher level integrative functions evolved from and are dependent on the integrity of lower-level structures. In other words, simple processing operations are necessary prerequisites for more complex operations [39,40].

Our results are rather compatible with a growing body of literature demonstrating another line of thought, based on the reverse hierarchy theory (RHT) [41]. The reverse hierarchy theory provides a representational hierarchy to describe the interaction between sensory input and top-down processes to guide plasticity in primary sensory areas [42–44]. RHT asserts that neural circuits mediating a certain percept can be modified starting at the highest representational level and progressing to lower-levels in search of more refined high resolution information to optimize perception. RHT may be a plausible explanation for top-down influences on cortical levels of sensory processing [45]. This might further clarify the presence of higher order auditory cortical responses, even when more automatic components are lacking.

In conclusion, the paradoxical partial preservation of P3-like potentials in a patient with persistent cortical deafness suggests the integrity of independent neural circuits necessary to process auditory stimuli even in the absence of conscious awareness. Furthermore, electrophysiological techniques combined with functional neuroimaging could be of primary importance in demonstrating the activation of neural substrates underlying deaf-hearing.

Acknowledgments

The authors gratefully acknowledge the very helpful discussions with Drs Luciano Foscolo, Annalena Venneri and Luca Ghezzo.

Author Contributions

Conceived and designed the experiments: MC. Performed the experiments: MC JR. Analyzed the data: MC CV. Contributed reagents/materials/analysis tools: MC. Wrote the paper: MC CV CS FP.

References

1. Szirmai I, Farsang M, Csüri M (2003) Cortical auditory disorder caused by bilateral strategic cerebral bleedings. Analysis of two cases. Brain Lang 85: 159–65.
2. Tanaka Y, Kamo T, Yoshida M, Yamadori A (1991) 'So-called' cortical deafness. Clinical, neurophysiological and radiological observations. Brain 114: 2385–401.
3. Polster MR, Rose SB (1998) Disorders of auditory processing: evidence for modularity in audition. Cortex 34: 47–65.
4. Bahls FH, Chatrian GE, Mesher RA, Sumi SM, Ruff RL (1988) A case of persistent cortical deafness: clinical, neurophysiologic, and neuropathologic observations. Neurology 38: 1490–3.

5. Michel F, Peronnet F, Schott B (1980) A case of cortical deafness: clinical and electrophysiological data. Brain Lang 10: 367–77.
6. Garde MM, Cowey A (2000) "Deaf hearing": unacknowledged detection of auditory stimuli in a patient with cerebral deafness. Cortex 36: 71–80.
7. Kentridge RW, Heywood CA, Weiskrantz L (1999) Attention without awareness in blindsight. Proc Biol Sci 266: 1805–11.
8. Celesia GG (1976) Organization of auditory cortical areas in man. Brain 99: 403–14.
9. Picton TW (1992) The P3 wave of the human event-related potential. J Clin Neurophysiol 9: 456–79.
10. Näätänen R, Alho K (1995) Mismatch negativity a unique measure of sensory processing in audition. Int J Neurosci 80: 317–37.
11. Huber W, Weniger D, Poeck K, Willmes K (1980) The Aachen Aphasia Test Rationale and construct validity. Nervenarzt 51: 475–82.
12. Ashburner J, Friston KJ (2000) Voxel-based morphometry. The methods. Neuroimage 11: 805–21.
13. Sparkes C, Clarke M, Gatehouse S, Lutman L, Marchbanks R, et al. (1995) Recommended procedure: computer coding of audiometric thresholds. Br J Audiol 29: 355–8.
14. Kochhar A, Hildebrand MS, Smith RJ (2007) Clinical aspects of hereditary hearing loss. Genet Med 9: 393–408.
15. Crawford JR, Howell DC (1998) Comparing an individual's test score against norms derived from small samples. Clin Neuropsychol 12: 482–6.
16. Woods DL, Clanvorth CC, Knight RT, Simpson GV, Naeser MA (1987) Generators of middle- and long-latency auditory evoked potentials: implications from studies of patients with bitemporal lesions. Electroencephal Clin Neurophysiol 68: 132–48.
17. Celesia GG (1976) Organization of auditory cortical areas in man. Brain 99: 403–14.
18. Godey B, Schwartz D, de Graaf JB, Chauvel P, Liégeois-Chauvel C (2001) Neuromagnetic source localization of auditory evoked fields and intracerebral evoked potentials: a comparison of data in the same patients. Clin Neurophysiol 112: 1850–9.
19. Näätänen R, Paavilainen P, Rinne T, Alho K (2007) The mismatch negativity (MMN) in basic research of central auditory processing: a review. Clin Neurophysiol 118: 2544–90.
20. Jääskeläinen IP, Ahveninen J, Bonmassar G, Dale AM, Ilmoniemi RJ, et al. (2004) Human posterior auditory cortex gates novel sounds to consciousness. Proc Natl Acad Sci U S A 101: 6809–14.
21. Braun A, McArdle J, Jones J, Nechaev V, Zalewski C, et al. (2008) Tune deafness: processing melodic errors outside of conscious awareness as reflected by components of the auditory ERP. PLoS One 3: e2349.
22. Schönwiesner M, Novitski N, Pakarinen S, Carlson S, Tervaniemi M, et al. (2007) Heschl's gyrus, posterior superior temporal gyrus, and mid-ventrolateral prefrontal cortex have different roles in the detection of acoustic changes. J Neurophysiol 97: 2075–82.
23. Molholm S, Martinez A, Ritter W, Javitt DC, Foxe JJ (2005) The neural circuitry of pre-attentive auditory change-detection: an fMRI study of pitch and duration mismatch negativity generators. Cereb Cortex 15: 545–51.
24. Giard MH, Perrin F, Pernier J, Bouchet P (1990) Brain generators implicated in the processing of auditory stimulus deviance: a topographic event-related potential study. Psychophysiology 27: 627–40.
25. Gray HM, Ambady N, Lowenthal WT, Deldin P (2004) P3 as an index of attention to self-relevant stimuli. J Exp Soc Psychol 40: 216–224.
26. Donchin E, McCarthy G (1980) Event-related brain potentials in the study of cognitive processes. Proceedings of Symposium on Neurological Bases of Language Disorders in Children: Methods and Direction for Research. C. Ludlow, ME. Doran-Quine, eds. Washington, D.C.: Government Printing Office, NINCDS Monograph #22, 109–128.
27. Van Hooff JC, Brunia CH, Allen JJ (1996) Event-related potentials as indirect measures of recognition memory. Int J Psychophysiol 21: 15–31.
28. Näätänen R (1990) The role of attention in auditory information processing as revealed by event-related potentials and other brain measures of cognitive function. Behav Brain Sci 13: 201–288.
29. Näätänen R, Tervaniemi M, Sussman E, Paavilainen P, Winkler I (2001) "Primitive intelligence" in the auditory cortex. Trends Neurosci 24: 283–8.
30. Linden DE, Prvulovic D, Formisano E, Völlinger M, Zanella FE, et al. (1999) The functional neuroanatomy of target detection: an fMRI study of visual and auditory oddball tasks. Cereb Cortex 9: 815–23.
31. Gilmore CS, Clementz BA, Berg P (2009) Hemispheric differences in auditory oddball responses during monaural versus binaural stimulation. Int J Psychophysiol 73: 326–33.
32. O'Donnell BF, McCarley RW, Potts GF, Salisbury DF, Nestor PG, et al. (1999) Identification of neural circuits underlying P3 abnormalities in schizophrenia. Psychophysiology 36: 388–98.
33. Eriksson J, Larsson A, Ahlström KR, Nyberg L (2006) Similar frontal and distinct posterior cortical regions mediate visual and auditory perceptual awareness. Cereb Cortex 17: 760–5.
34. Yingling CD (2001) Neural mechanisms of unconscious cognitive processing. Clin Neurophysiol 112: 157–8.
35. Bernat E, Shevrin H, Snodgrass M (2001) Subliminal visual oddball stimuli evoke a P3 component. Clin Neurophysiol 112: 159–71.
36. Pandya DN (1995) Anatomy of the auditory cortex. Rev Neurol (Paris) 51: 486–94.
37. Hugdahl K, Wester K, Asbjornsen A (1991) Auditory neglect after right frontal lobe and right pulvinar thalamic lesions. Brain Lang 41: 465–73.
38. Felleman DJ, Van Essen DC (1991) Distributed hierarchical processing in the primate cerebral cortex. Cereb Cortex 1: 1–47.
39. Howard RC (2001) Bringing brain events to mind: functional systems and brain event-related potentials. J Psychophysiol 15: 69–79.
40. Kotchoubey B, Lang S, Bostanov V, Birbaumer N (2002) Is there a mind? Psychophysiology of unconscious patients. News Physiol Sci 17: 38–42.
41. Ahissar M, Hochstein S (2004) The reverse hierarchy theory of visual perceptual learning. Trends Cogn Sci 8: 457–64.
42. Nahum M, Nelken I, Ahissar M (2008) Low-level information and high-level perception: the case of speech in noise. PLoS Biol 6: e126.
43. Shamma S (2008) Characterizing auditory receptive fields. Neuron 58: 829–31.
44. Hochstein S, Ahissar M (2002) View from the top: hierarchies and reverse hierarchies in the visual system. Neuron 36: 791–804.
45. Banai K, Abrams D, Kraus N (2007) Sensory-based learning disability: Insights from brainstem processing of speech sounds. Int J Audiol 46: 524–32.

15

Exome Sequencing Identifies a Founder Frameshift Mutation in an Alternative Exon of *USH1C* as the Cause of Autosomal Recessive Retinitis Pigmentosa with Late-Onset Hearing Loss

Samer Khateb[1], Lina Zelinger[1], Tamar Ben-Yosef[2], Saul Merin[1†], Ornit Crystal-Shalit[3], Menachem Gross[4], Eyal Banin[1*], Dror Sharon[1*]

1 Department of Ophthalmology, Hadassah - Hebrew University Medical Center, Jerusalem, Israel, **2** Genetics Department, Rappaport Faculty of Medicine, Technion - Israel Institute of Technology, Haifa, Israel, **3** Department of Ophthalmology, Meir Medical Center, Kfar-Saba, Israel, **4** Department of Otolaryngology - Head and Neck Surgery, Hadassah - Hebrew University Medical Center, Jerusalem, Israel

Abstract

We used a combined approach of homozygosity mapping and whole exome sequencing (WES) to search for the genetic cause of autosomal recessive retinitis pigmentosa (arRP) in families of Yemenite Jewish origin. Homozygosity mapping of two arRP Yemenite Jewish families revealed a few homozygous regions. A subsequent WES analysis of the two index cases revealed a shared homozygous novel nucleotide deletion (c.1220delG) leading to a frameshift (p.Gly407Glufs*56) in an alternative exon (#15) of *USH1C*. Screening of additional Yemenite Jewish patients revealed a total of 16 homozygous RP patients (with a carrier frequency of 0.008 in controls). Funduscopic and electroretinography findings were within the spectrum of typical RP. While other *USH1C* mutations usually cause Usher type I (including RP, vestibular dysfunction and congenital deafness), audiometric screening of 10 patients who are homozygous for c.1220delG revealed that patients under 40 years of age had normal hearing while older patients showed mild to severe high tone sensorineural hearing loss. This is the first report of a mutation in a known USH1 gene that causes late onset rather than congenital sensorineural hearing loss. The c.1220delG mutation of *USH1C* accounts for 23% of RP among Yemenite Jewish patients in our cohort.

Editor: Anneke I. den Hollander, Radboud University Nijmegen Medical Centre, The Netherlands

Funding: This study was financially supported by the Foundation Fighting Blindness USA (BR-GE-0510-0490-HUJ to DS), by the legacy heritage biomedical program of the Israeli Science Foundation (grant number 612/09 to DS and TBY), and the Yedidut 1 research grant (to EB). The funders had no role in study design, data collection and analysis, decision to publish, or preparation of the manuscript.

Competing Interests: The authors have declared that no competing interests exist.

* E-mail: banine@cc.huji.ac.il (EB); dror.sharon1@gmail.com (DS)

† Deceased.

Introduction

Retinitis pigmentosa (RP) [MIM #268000] is the most common inherited retinal degeneration with an estimated worldwide prevalence of about 1:4000 [1,2]. The disease is highly heterogeneous and can be inherited in autosomal dominant, autosomal recessive (AR), and X-linked modes. In most cases, RP is nonsyndromic (e.g. no other clinical features are evident), but in about 20–30% of cases the patients manifest a syndrome, such as Usher syndrome (USH) which also causes vestibular and hearing impairment to varying degrees, Bardet-Biedl syndrome (BBS), and others [3]. At present, 36 genes have been associated with arRP and 10 with USH (https://sph.uth.tmc.edu/RetNet/home.htm). An interesting group of retinal disease genes can cause both syndromic and nonsyndromic phenotypes, not always with a clear disease mechanism: for example, *USH2A* mutations can cause the USH phenotype but also RP alone [4,5,6,7,8]; *USH1C* and *MYO7A* mutations have been associated with the USH phenotype but also hearing impairment alone [9,10].

The Yemenite Jewish (YJ) population is ancient (over 2,000 years) and comprised of several small communities. Most members of this population immigrated back to Israel between 1950 and 1955. In 2010, Israeli residents of YJ descent comprised about 2.5% (140,000) of the Israeli Jewish population. Up to date, a single founder mutation in the *CERKL* gene (c.238+1G>A) has been reported by us as the cause of inherited widespread retinal degeneration with early macular involvement in about 30% of cases of YJ origin [11].

In order to identify additional causes of RP in this population, we recruited 36 families of YJ origin with isolate/AR retinal degenerations (33 with RP and three with cone-rod degeneration). The set of RP families of YJ origin comprises 16% of our cohort of Israeli Jewish patients (33/205) which is much higher than the fraction of YJ among all Israeli Jews. This difference can by explained by founder mutations that are relatively common among YJ, causing higher prevalence of disease. We identified the *CERKL* founder mutation (c.238+1G>A) in 13 of the YJ families. We performed homozygosity mapping using whole-genome single nucleotide polymorphism (SNP) arrays in six patients who belong to two YJ families followed by whole exome sequencing (WES) analysis. Using this method we identified a novel frameshift mutation in an alternative exon of *USH1C* as the cause of RP with late onset hearing loss rather than the classic USH1 phenotype which manifests with profound congenital hearing loss and vestibular dysfunction.

Materials and Methods

Subjects and Clinical Evaluation

The tenets of the Declaration of Helsinki were followed and prior to donation of a blood sample, a written informed consent was obtained from all individuals who participated in this study, after explanation of the nature and possible consequences of the study. The research was approved by the institutional review board (IRB) at the Hadassah medical center. DNA was extracted

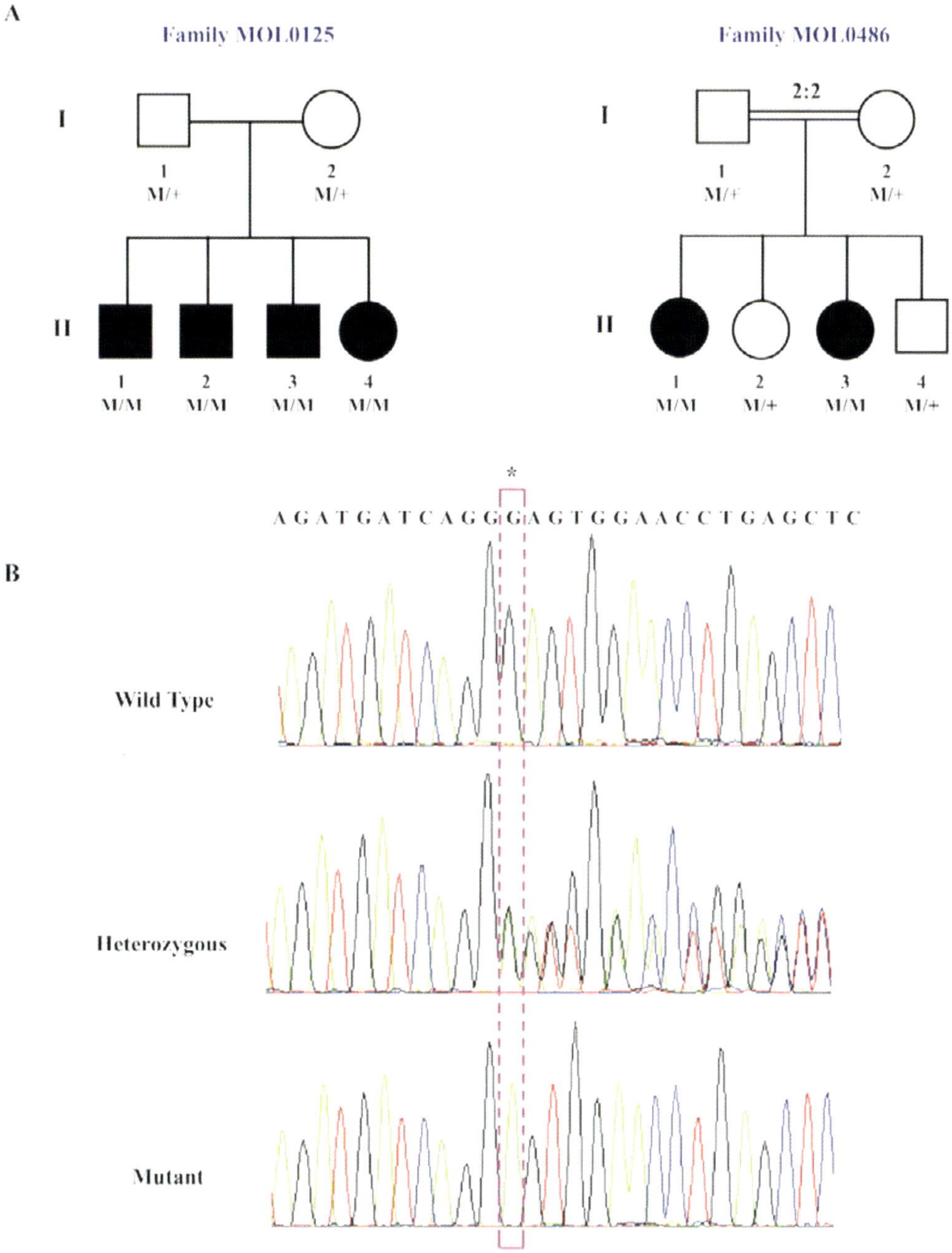

Figure 1. Family trees and segregation analysis of the *USH1C* c.1220delG mutation. A. Structure of the two families that were selected for whole exome sequencing. The family number is indicated above the corresponding family tree. Filled symbols represent affected individuals, whereas clear symbols represent unaffected individuals. Generation numbers are depicted on the left and individual numbers below each symbol. The *USH1C* genotype is presented as: M/M, homozygous for the c.1220delG mutation; M/+, heterozygous; +/+, homozygous for the wildtype allele. Index cases are marked with an arrow. B. Sequence chromatograms of part of *USH1C* exon 15 of a control individual (top), a heterozygote (middle), and a patient who is homozygous for the mutation (bottom). The c.1220delG mutation (boxed) results in a frameshift (p.Gly407Glufs*56).

Table 1. Data on sequence variants identified by the whole exome sequencing analysis.

Sample	Total no. of variants	No. of missense, nonsense and splicing variants	Variants in conserved regions and not in segmental duplications	Variants with MAF <0.5%	After exclusion of unlikely pathogenic missense changes	No. of variants fitting the disease model	No. of variants within linked regions
MOL0125 II:4	233,572	21,326	9,055	2,880	1,476	311	2*
MOL0486 II:1	232,065	20,469	8,245	2,536	1,252	277	2**

*- The two variants are: c.1220delG in *USH1C* and c.218_219insC in *VPS11*. The latter was found in about 73% of ethnicity-matched exomes and is therefore predicted to be a population-specific polymorphism.
**- The two variants are: c.1220delG in *USH1C* and c.705_706delTT in *PKD1L2*. The latter was found in about 20% of ethnicity-matched exomes and is therefore predicted to be a population-specific polymorphism.

from the index patient as well as from other affected and unaffected family members using the FlexiGene DNA kit (QIAGEN).

Ocular evaluation included a full ophthalmologic exam, Goldmann perimetry, electroretinography (ERG), color vision testing using the Ishihara 38-panel and Farnsworth-Munsell D-15 tests, color and infrared fundus photos, optical coherence tomography (OCT), and fundus autofluorescence (FAF) imaging performed as previously described [12].

Audiological screening included a comprehensive questionnaire (collecting information regarding any history of exposure to noise, ototoxic agents, and genetic factors related to hearing impairment), as well as physical and audiometric examinations. An age-appropriate audiological examination was performed including pure-tone audiometry (250 Hz to 12,000 Hz), tympanometry, and transient-evoked otoacoustic emission (TEOAE) for each ear. We used the following scale to grade the degree of sensorineural hearing loss (SNHL): slight- 16 to 25 dB hearing loss, mild- 26–40 dB, moderate- 41–55 dB, moderately severe- 56–70 dB, severe- 71–90 dB, and profound- >90 dB hearing loss [13]. Specific types of SNHL were determined by audiometric curve patterns: ascending (hearing loss greater at the lower frequencies), flat, descending (hearing loss greater at the higher frequencies), and "U-shaped" (hearing loss at mid-frequencies) curves. Otoacoustic emissions (OAEs) have been suggested as a sensitive measure of cochlear function with the potential for preclinical detection of damage [14]. TEOAE tests were conducted on the same day as the pure tone test. A response at three frequencies of 3 dB or greater above the background with a minimum of 70% reproducibility at each frequency and 90% or greater stability was required for passing the TEOAE test. TEOAE examination was categorized as either pass or fail for each ear.

Genetic Analyses

Whole genome SNP analysis was performed on six patients with nonsyndromic arRP who belong to two different YJ families, using either the Affymetrix 10K or 6.0 microarrays and data analysis was performed using HomozygosityMapper (http://www.homozygositymapper.org/). WES analysis was performed at Otogenetics corporation using Roche NimbleGen V2 (44.1 Mbp) paired-end sample preparation kit and Illumina HiSeq2000 at a 31x coverage. Sequence reads were aligned to the human genome reference sequence (build hg19) and variants were called and annotated using the DNAnexus software package. Dataset files including the annotated information were analyzed using ANNOVAR according to the dbSNP database (build 135) with the following filtering steps: autosomal recessive inheritance; variant type including missense, nonsense, and splice-site; not within segmental duplications; minor allele frequency (MAF) less than 0.5%; SIFT score <0.05 when available; PolyPhen2 score >0.85 when available. Primers for *USH1C* exon 15 (Table S1) were designed using the Primer3 software [15] and Sanger sequencing of PCR products was used to verify the mutation and to screen additional patients and controls. Retinal RNA was isolated from human retina using TRI-reagent (Sigma-Aldrich) and RNA derived from different human tissues was purchased (Clontech; cat. #636643, lot No. 8101369A). cDNA was synthesized using the Verso cDNA kit (Thermo) in accordance with the manufacturer's protocol. PCR specific primers (Table S1) were designed with Primer3 to amplify two parts of the *USH1C* mRNA: exons 14 through 16 and exons 14 through 23. RT-PCR of a *PGM1* fragment was used as a control (Forward: TGGTGCTCTGGACCGGGTGG; Reverse: GCACTCCCAGTGCCGCTCAG).

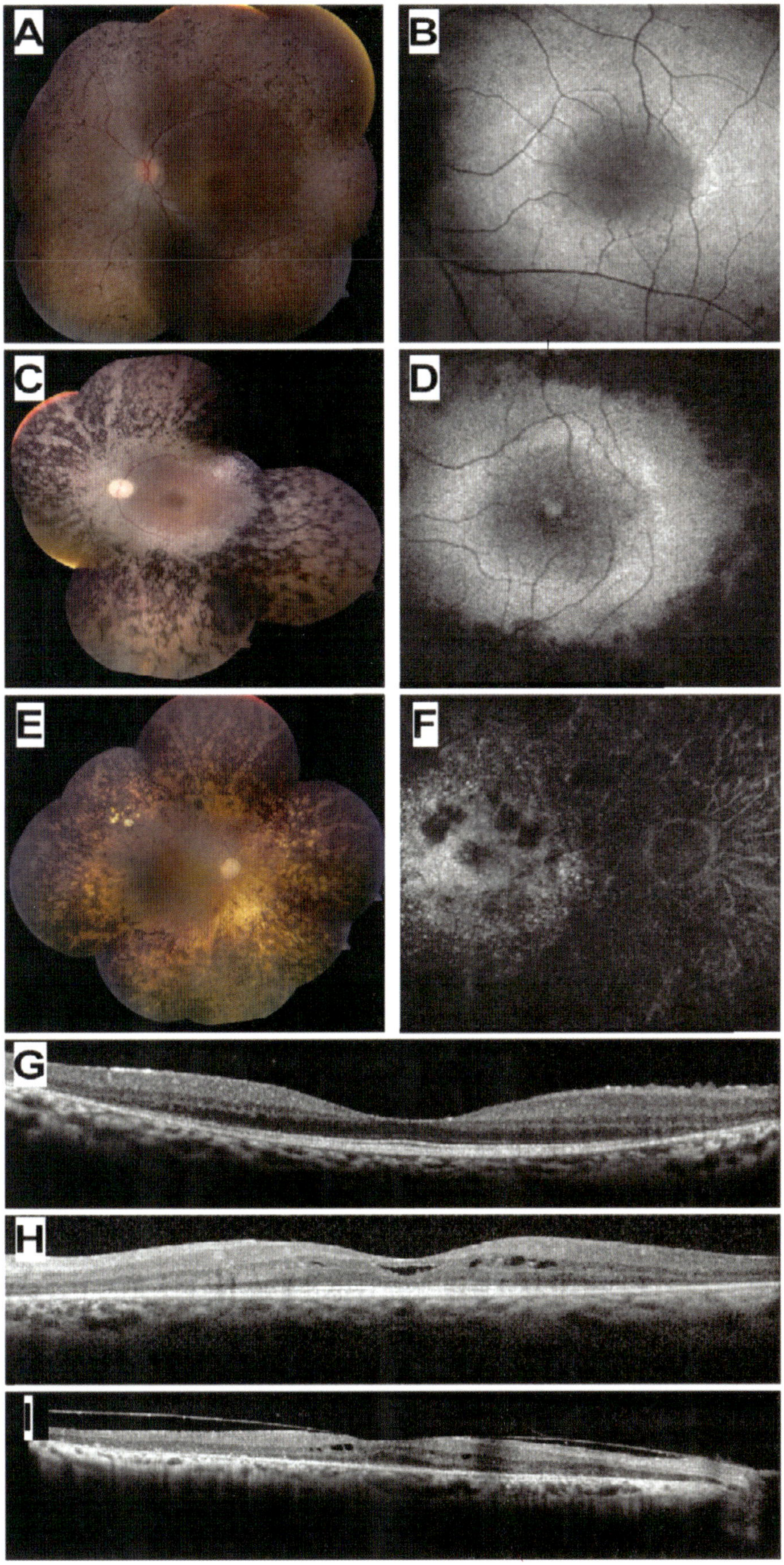
A
B
C
D
E
F
G
H
I

Figure 2. Ocular Phenotype of patients who are homozygous for the *USH1C* c.1220delG mutation. (A, C, E) Color fundus photographs of three patients aged 13 (MOL0486 II:3), 33 (TB16-R12), and 72 (MOL1023-1) years old, respectively. Note the increasing severity of fundus changes with age, and the presence of dense bone spicule-like pigmentation. (B, D, F) Corresponding fundus autofluorescence imaging of the macular area in the three patients shown in A,C,E. Note hyeprfluorescent rings around the foveas in the younger patients, and hypofluorescent areas of atrophy that encroach upon the macula in the 33 year-old patient and invade the macula in the 72 year-old. (G, H, I) Horizontal optical coherence tomography (OCT) cross-sections through the fovea in the 13 yo (panel G), 33 yo (H) and 72 yo (I) *USH1C* patients showing progressive loss of retinal and particularly photoreceptor layer thickness with age. Intra-retinal cysts of fluid (cystoid macular edema) are evident in two of the cases (H, I).

Results

Whole Genome SNP Analysis

We performed homozygosity mapping using whole genome SNP arrays in six patients who belong to two YJ families. Family MOL0125 is non-consanguineous with four affected siblings and family MOL0486 is consanguineous (the parents are first cousins) with two affected sisters (Fig. 1A). The index case of MOL0125 was screened for mutations using the APEX-based Asper arRP array (an arrayed primer extension-based genotyping process, including most of the arRP mutations thus far reported) and was homozygote for the wild-type allele in all tested nucleotides. Homozygosity mapping in MOL0486 revealed 6 and 5 homozygous regions (>10 Mb) in the two affected sisters, MOL0486 II:1 and MOL0486 II:3, respectively. Two of these regions were shared between the two affected sisters, the largest being a 38.98-Mb region on chromosome 11 between the markers rs1395558 and rs724759 (Table S2). A similar analysis of the four patients in MOL0125 did not reveal any large homozygous regions. The largest shared homozygous region was identified on chromosome 11 (Table S2) including 296 consecutive homozygous SNPs. This region was relatively small (about 1 Mb) including 9 genes, one of which is *USH1C*. We therefore could not exclude the possibility that the patients are compound heterozygous for two different mutations in the same gene.

Whole Exome Analysis

Aiming to identify the genetic cause of disease in the two studied families, we performed WES analysis on one patient from each family (Table S3). For MOL0486 II:1, we produced 4.77 gigabases (Gb) of paired-end 100-nucleotide sequence reads, 88% of which were mapped to gene regions. A total of 933.93 million bases were covered with an average coverage of 30.17 reads per nucleotide (Table S3). Alignment of these reads to hg 19 revealed a total of 232,065 variants that underwent a series of filters (Table 1) to exclude sequence changes that are unlikely to be pathogenic. A total of 277 variants passed the filters, only one of which was within a genomic region that was homozygously shared by the two affected individuals in the whole genome SNP array analysis: a deletion of guanine (c.1220delG) leading to a frameshift (p.Gly407Glufs*56) in an alternative exon (#15) of *USH1C*.

In parallel, we performed a similar analysis of MOL0125 II:4. WES produced sequence reads in a total length of 4.51 Gb, 92% of the reads were mapped to gene regions with an average coverage of 31.17 reads per nucleotide (Table S3). The analysis revealed a total of 233,572 variants, only 311 remained (Table 1) after applying the same filters used in family MOL0486. As mentioned above, this family was nonconsanguineous and homozygosity mapping did not reveal large homozygous regions, we therefore considered both homozygous changes and two heterozygous changes affecting the same gene. The filtering based on disease model revealed only one possible mutation in *USH1C* as described above.

The combined whole genome SNP array and WES analysis in the two families revealed the same mutation- c.1220delG in *USH1C*. The *USH1C* mutation is part of a shared homozygous haplotype of 27 SNPs that is shared by the two index cases of families MOL0125 and MOL0486, indicating a founder mutation. We confirmed this mutation by Sanger sequencing (Fig. 1B) and it fully cosegregated with the phenotype in the two families (Fig. 1A).

Mutation Analysis

Screening the c.1220delG mutation in a set of 119 ethnically-matched (YJ) normal controls revealed one heterozygous individual, thus indicating a carrier frequency of 0.008 (95% confidence interval 0.002–0.045) in this population. We subsequently screened a set of 35 unrelated YJ patients with retinal degenerations (21 of whom had nonsyndromic RP) for the c.1220delG mutation and identified six additional index RP cases who were homozygous for the mutation. Statistical analyses between patient and control groups showed a significant difference (Table S4).

Clinical Evaluation

Aiming to clinically characterize patients with the c.1220delG mutation, we performed full ophthalmologic examinations and audiometric testing in most of the patients. Ocular evaluation of 12 patients showed a spectrum of findings (Table S5). Visual acuity ranged from 0.2 to 1.0, usually being better at younger ages. Funduscopic findings also showed worsening with age, including waxy-appearance of the optic nerve head, attenuation of retinal blood vessels, and increasing, prominent bone spicule-like pigmentation which already extended from the mid-periphery to encroach upon the posterior poles in patients in their twenties and early thirties (Fig. 2A, C, E). There was relative preservation of the macular area, but FAF imaging showed increased involvement with age (Fig. 2B, D, F). OCT imaging in early disease showed a relatively preserved photoreceptor layer in the foveal area, with a decline in outer nuclear layer (ONL) thickness with increasing distance from the fovea (Fig. 2G). In older patients, the ONL showed thinning also in the foveal area and cystoid macular edema was evident in some cases (Fig. 2H, I). ERG responses ranged from severely reduced to non-detectable in patients in their teens and twenties, and non-detectable at older ages (Table S5). Visual fields were markedly constricted in patients in their twenties (Fig. S1).

Audiometric testing revealed variable degrees of SNHL in four out of 10 examined patients, ranging from mild to severe symmetric hearing impairment (Table S6). Normal hearing was found in most participants under the age of 40 at all examined frequencies (250–12,000 Hz; see an example in Fig. 3A). Older patients did show SNHL, mainly at high frequencies (4,000–12,000 Hz). For example, patient MOL0887-3, at 44 years of age, showed moderate to severe hearing loss with a descending audiogram (Fig. 3B). An analysis of high-frequency thresholds versus age (Fig. 3C, D) showed normal hearing function in most patients (five out of six) below 40 years of age, while patients above 40 years showed higher tendency for SNHL (three out of four patients). Normal TEOAE responses were found in all participants who showed normal hearing on audiometry. All patients reported normal vestibular function.

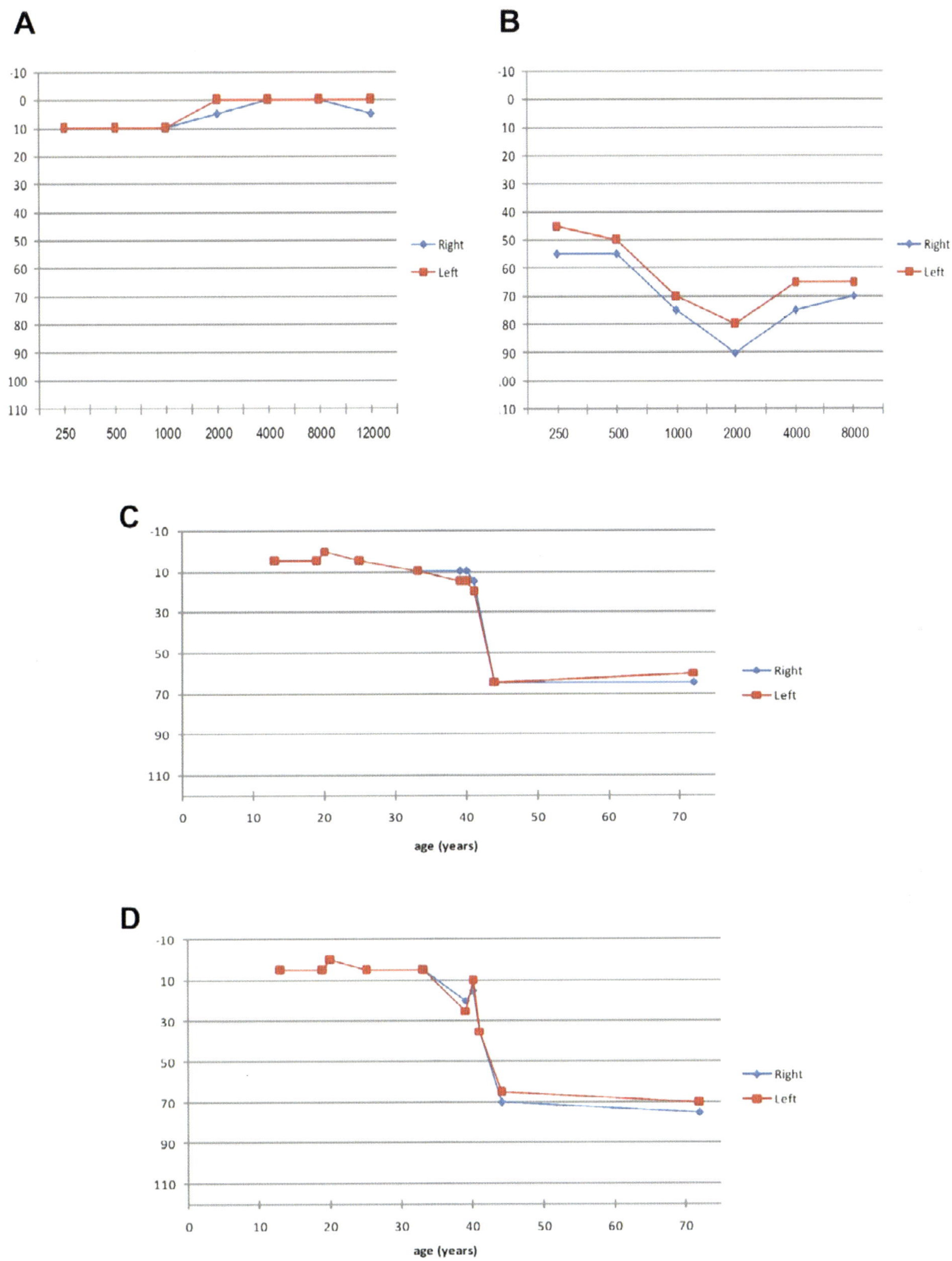

Figure 3. Audiometric results of patients who are homozygous for the *USH1C* c.1220delG mutation. A. Patient MOL0486 II:3 (13 yo) with normal hearing function. B. Patient MOL0887-3 (44 yo) with severe SNHL, particularly at higher frequencies (descending pattern). C,D. Hearing threshold versus age at a frequency of 4,000 Hz (C) and 8,000 Hz (D). At younger ages, normal hearing function is evident, but after the age of 40 years, sensitivity is markedly reduced. For each of the 10 patients, the data from both the right and left ears is presented, showing symmetry between both ears.

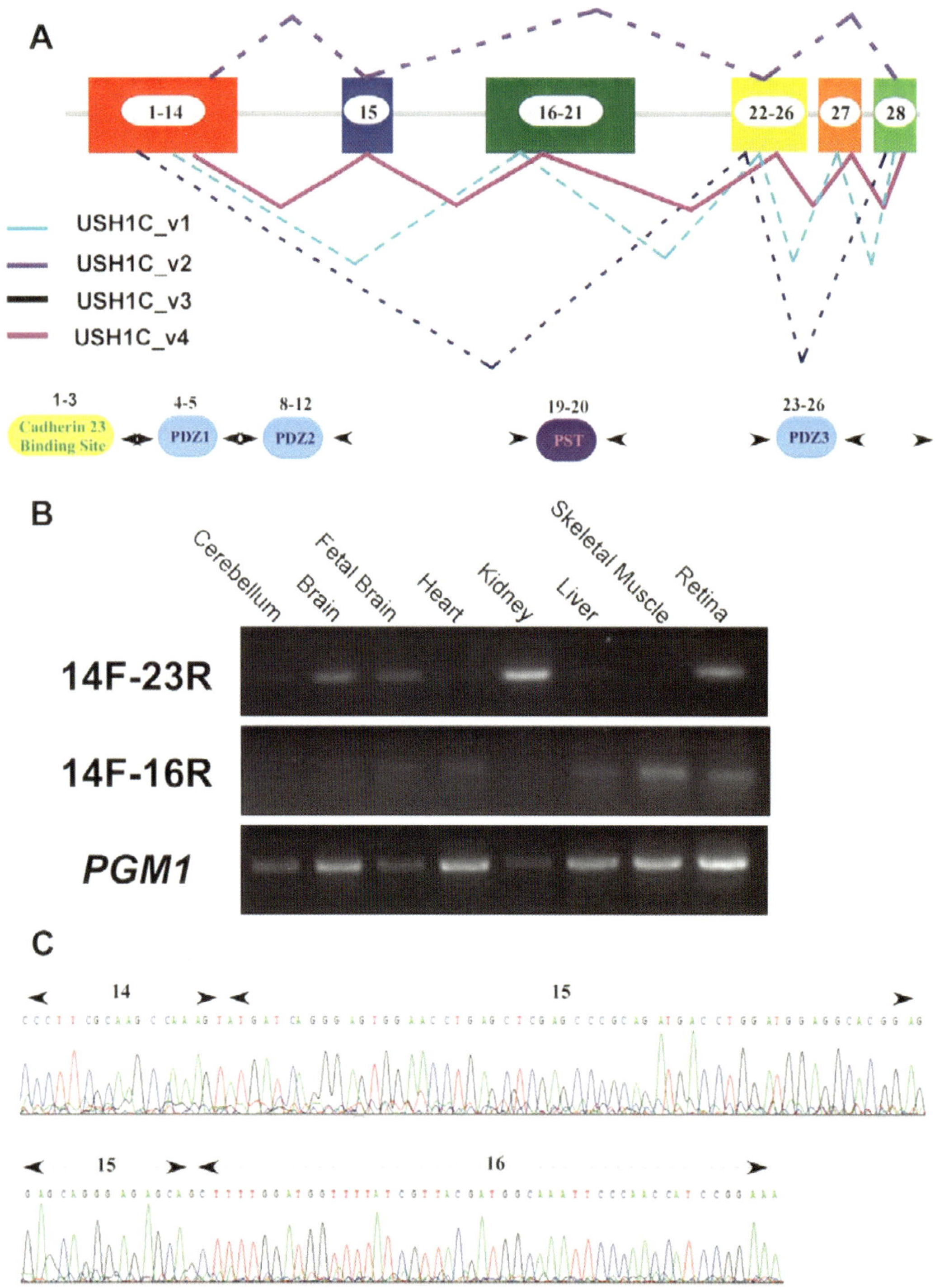

Figure 4. ***USH1C* alternatively-spliced transcripts.** A. *USH1C* can produce four different transcripts through alternative splicing. The scheme represents the full-length open reading frame (ORF) of *USH1C* and the alternatively-spliced transcripts that can be produced. Exon numbers are depicted within boxes. Previously reported transcripts are dashed and the novel transcript (USH1C_v4) is presented with a solid line. The bottom panel shows the USH1C functional domains and the corresponding coding exons. B. RT-PCR analysis of *USH1C* splicing variants. A PCR product of 249 bp (top panel) amplified by the 14F and 23R primers (Table S1), representing the most common *USH1C* splicing isoform, USH1C_v2, is depicted in different human tissues. The newly discovered transcript (USH1C_v4) is depicted in the middle panel (a PCR band of 189 bp amplified by primers 14F and 16R; Table S1) showing a relatively low expression level. Both PCR products were sequenced and verified in a few tissues, including the retina. *PGM1* RT-PCR was used as a control (bottom panel). C. Sequence chromatogram of the newly-identified *USH1C* splicing isoform. The splicing variant (USH1C_v4) contains all *USH1C* coding exons and the new splicing event (exon14-exon15-exon16) is depicted.

Expression Analysis

The human *USH1C* gene contains 28 coding exons along a genomic region of ~37 Kb and is known to produce three splice variants [16] (variants USH1C_v1, USH1C_v2, and USH1C_v3; Table S7 and Fig. 4A). To characterize the expression of *USH1C* in human tissues, we analyzed all available *USH1C* EST sequences deposited at NCBI and noted three regions that are affected by alternative splicing: exon15, exons 16–21, and exon 27. Out of the 15 sequences encompassing exon 15, the vast majority (13 sequences) included exon 15 but not exons 21–26. Therefore, the most common *USH1C* variant is USH1C_v2 (also known as variant a and PDZ-73; see Table S7 for more information). RT-PCR analysis using a set of primers that are specific for this variant (primers 14F and 23R, see Table S1) revealed a variable expression level in most studied human tissues (Fig. 4B, top panel). Extensive RT-PCR analysis of this region revealed a novel splice-variant, USH1C_v4 (Table S7 and Fig. 4C) that includes all *USH1C* coding exons and is ubiquitously expressed at relatively low levels (Fig. 4B; middle panel using primers 14F and 16R, see Table S1).

Discussion

We report here of the identification of a novel *USH1C* founder mutation in YJ patients with arRP. Some of the patients, mostly those above the age of 40 years, developed variable degrees of high tone SNHL. This *USH1C* mutation together with the previously reported *CERKL* founder mutation [11], account for about 50% of RP cases in this ethnic group.

USH1C encodes for harmonin, a scaffolding protein that is required for normal mechanosensory function in cochlear hair cells [17]. Its role in photoreceptors is not yet clear, although it may be involved in maintenance of the synaptic structure or in mediating the release of synaptic vesicles [18]. Mutations in *USH1C* were previously reported to cause the following phenotypes: Usher syndrome type 1 (characterized by congenital profound SNHL, vestibular dysfunction, and RP) [19,20], nonsyndromic profound SNHL at the DFNB18 locus [9,21], and sector RP with early-onset SNHL [22]. A complete list of mutations can be obtained from https://grenada.lumc.nl/LOVD2/Usher_montpellier/home.php?select_db=USH1C. Most patients with *USH1C* mutations suffer from typical USH1, usually due to null (including nonsense, frameshift, and splicing) mutations on both gene copies. The only exception is a patient who is a compound heterozygous for a null and a missense mutation but no clinical data were presented by the authors [23]. A few patients with less severe phenotypes (sector RP with early onset deafness and nonsyndromic profound deafness) carry mutation(s) that are expected to have a milder effect on protein amount or function. Two siblings who suffer from sector RP and hearing loss from the age of 4 years (but were able to develop language) were reported to be compound heterozygotes for a missense (p.Arg103His) and a canonical splice-site mutation (c.2227-1G>A) [22]. Nonsyndromic deafness was reported in only two families so far: patients from the original DFNB18 family were homozygous for a "leaky" splice-site mutation (IVS12+5G>C) that might affect the splicing of exons 11 and 12 [9], and patients from a Chinese family were homozygous for a missense change (p.Pro608Arg) but no functional assay was performed to prove the pathogenicity of this change [21]. Most of the mutations identified in *USH1C* so far (except for p.Pro608Arg and c.2227-1G>A) are located within the first 13 exons, which are present in all *USH1C* transcripts reported to date. The most common *USH1C* transcript, USH1C_v2, lacks exons 16–21 and exon 27, while two relatively rare variants (USH1C_v1 and USH1C_v3) lack exon 15. The founder mutation we report here causes a typical form of RP with prominent bone spicule-like pigmentation at relatively early ages, which is later complicated by late-onset SNHL. In the literature, the vast majority of *USH1C* patients were reported to manifest early and profound hearing loss, while the patients we report here maintain normal hearing until the age of about 40 years. This might be explained by partial compensation of harmonin function by the rare splicing variants that lack exon 15 (USH1C_v1 and USH1C_v3) and are therefore unlikely to be affected by the mutation. A relatively high expression or a more prominent role of these isoforms in the human cochlea versus the retina might explain the relatively mild and delayed hearing loss.

The data we report here together with previously reported studies suggest that mutations in *USH1C* may cause nonsyndromic hearing loss or RP (usually the typical form and rarely the sectorial form) with a variable effect on hearing (usually congenital profound deafness with vestibular dysfunction and rarely late-onset hearing loss). *USH1C* therefore should be considered a candidate gene in patients with USH1, nonsyndromic hearing loss, young (<40 years) RP patients with normal hearing function, and RP patients with mild or late-onset hearing loss. To the best of our knowledge, this is the first report showing that a mutation in a gene known to cause the USH1 phenotype can cause RP with late onset hearing loss.

Supporting Information

Figure S1 Goldmann perimetry of two patients who are homozygous for the *USH1C* c.1220delG mutation. A. A 20 year-old patient (MOL0125 II:4) presented in 2007 with severely restricted visual fields which became worse 4 years later. B. The visual field of a 25 year-old patient (MOL0125 II:2) was markedly reduced in 2006 with additional progression 3 years later. The visual fields represent an average of both eyes.
(DOCX)

Table S1 Primer sequences used to amplify the *USH1C* exon 15 from gDNA samples and the various transcripts of *USH1C*.

Table S2 Homozygosity mapping analysis of arRP families.

Table S3 Summary of original exome sequencing data.

Table S4 Statistical analysis of the c.1220delG mutation frequency.

Table S5 Ocular data of patients with the c.1220delG *USH1C* gene mutation.

Table S6 Hearing function tests: Audiometry and Transient Evoked Otoacoustic Emissions (TEOAEs).

Table S7 Splice-variants produced by the human *USH1C* gene.

Acknowledgments

The authors would like to dedicate this paper to the memory of Prof. Saul Merin who passed away during the preparation of this manuscript. We thank the patients and their families for their participation in the study. The authors thank Israel Barzel for excellent and generous assistance. We thank the audiology unit at Hadassah Medical Center for the assistance with the audiometric evaluation.

Author Contributions

Conceived and designed the experiments: SK EB DS. Performed the experiments: SK LZ. Analyzed the data: SK OCS LZ TBY SM EB MG. Contributed reagents/materials/analysis tools: TBY SM EB. Wrote the paper: SK EB MG DS.

References

1. Haim M (2002) Epidemiology of retinitis pigmentosa in Denmark. Acta Ophthalmol Scand Suppl: 1–34.
2. Bunker CH, Berson EL, Bromley WC, Hayes RP, Roderick TH (1984) Prevalence of retinitis pigmentosa in Maine. Am J Ophthalmol 97: 357–365.
3. Hartong DT, Berson EL, Dryja TP (2006) Retinitis pigmentosa. Lancet 368: 1795–1809.
4. Rivolta C, Sweklo EA, Berson EL, Dryja TP (2000) Missense Mutation in the USH2A Gene: Association with Recessive Retinitis Pigmentosa without Hearing Loss. Am J Hum Genet 66: 1975–1978.
5. Kaiserman N, Obolensky A, Banin E, Sharon D (2007) Novel USH2A mutations in Israeli patients with retinitis pigmentosa and Usher syndrome type 2. Arch Ophthalmol 125: 219–224.
6. Aller E, Najera C, Millan JM, Oltra JS, Perez-Garrigues H, et al. (2004) Genetic analysis of 2299delG and C759F mutations (USH2A) in patients with visual and/or auditory impairments. Eur J Hum Genet 12: 407–410.
7. Xu W, Dai H, Lu T, Zhang X, Dong B, et al. (2011) Seven novel mutations in the long isoform of the USH2A gene in Chinese families with nonsyndromic retinitis pigmentosa and Usher syndrome Type II. Mol Vis 17: 1537–1552.
8. Sandberg MA, Rosner B, Weigel-DiFranco C, McGee TL, Dryja TP, et al. (2008) Disease course in patients with autosomal recessive retinitis pigmentosa due to the USH2A gene. Invest Ophthalmol Vis Sci 49: 5532–5539.
9. Ahmed ZM, Smith TN, Riazuddin S, Makishima T, Ghosh M, et al. (2002) Nonsyndromic recessive deafness DFNB18 and Usher syndrome type IC are allelic mutations of USHIC. Hum Genet 110: 527–531.
10. Weil D, Kussel P, Blanchard S, Levy G, Levi-Acobas F, et al. (1997) The autosomal recessive isolated deafness, DFNB2, and the Usher 1B syndrome are allelic defects of the myosin-VIIA gene. Nat Genet 16: 191–193.
11. Auslender N, Sharon D, Abbasi AH, Garzozi HJ, Banin E, et al. (2007) A common founder mutation of CERKL underlies autosomal recessive retinal degeneration with early macular involvement among Yemenite Jews. Invest Ophthalmol Vis Sci 48: 5431–5438.
12. Beit-Ya'acov A, Mizrahi-Meissonnier L, Obolensky A, Landau C, Blumenfeld A, et al. (2007) Homozygosity for a novel ABCA4 founder splicing mutation is associated with progressive and severe Stargardt-like disease. Invest Ophthalmol Vis Sci 48: 4308–4314.
13. Clark JG (1981) Uses and abuses of hearing loss classification. ASHA 23: 493–500.
14. Engdahl B, Tambs K (2002) Otoacoustic emissions in the general adult population of Nord-Trondelag, Norway: II. Effects of noise, head injuries, and ear infections. Int J Audiol 41: 78–87.
15. Rozen S, Skaletsky HJ (2000) Primer3 on the WWW for general users and for biologist programmers. In: Krawetz S, Misener S, editors. Bioinformatics Methods and Protocols: Methods in Molecular Biology. Totowa, NJ: Humana Press. pp. 365–386.
16. Scanlan MJ, Williamson B, Jungbluth A, Stockert E, Arden KC, et al. (1999) Isoforms of the human PDZ-73 protein exhibit differential tissue expression. Biochim Biophys Acta 1445: 39–52.
17. Grillet N, Xiong W, Reynolds A, Kazmierczak P, Sato T, et al. (2009) Harmonin mutations cause mechanotransduction defects in cochlear hair cells. Neuron 62: 375–387.
18. Lillo C, Kitamoto J, Williams DS (2006) Roles and interactions of usher 1 proteins in the outer retina. Adv Exp Med Biol 572: 341–348.
19. Bitner-Glindzicz M, Lindley KJ, Rutland P, Blaydon D, Smith VV, et al. (2000) A recessive contiguous gene deletion causing infantile hyperinsulinism, enteropathy and deafness identifies the Usher type 1C gene. NatGenet 26: 56–60.
20. Verpy E, Leibovici M, Zwaenepoel I, Liu XZ, Gal A, et al. (2000) A defect in harmonin, a PDZ domain-containing protein expressed in the inner ear sensory hair cells, underlies Usher syndrome type 1C. NatGenet 26: 51–55.
21. Ouyang XM, Xia XJ, Verpy E, Du LL, Pandya A, et al. (2002) Mutations in the alternatively spliced exons of USH1C cause non-syndromic recessive deafness. Hum Genet 111: 26–30.
22. Saihan Z, Stabej Ple Q, Robson AG, Rangesh N, Holder GE, et al. (2011) Mutations in the USH1C gene associated with sector retinitis pigmentosa and hearing loss. Retina 31: 1708–1716.
23. Roux AF, Faugere V, Le Guedard S, Pallares-Ruiz N, Vielle A, et al. (2006) Survey of the frequency of USH1 gene mutations in a cohort of Usher patients shows the importance of cadherin 23 and protocadherin 15 genes and establishes a detection rate of above 90%. J Med Genet 43: 763–768.

A Systematic Review of Studies Measuring and Reporting Hearing Aid Usage in Older Adults since 1999: A Descriptive Summary of Measurement Tools

Elvira Perez[1,2]*, Barrie A. Edmonds[1,2]

1 National Biomedical Research Unit in Hearing, National Institute for Health Research (NIHR), Nottingham, United Kingdom, 2 School of Clinical Sciences, University of Nottingham, Nottingham, United Kingdom

Abstract

Objective: A systematic review was conducted to identify and quality assess how studies published since 1999 have measured and reported the usage of hearing aids in older adults. The relationship between usage and other dimensions of hearing aid outcome, age and hearing loss are summarised.

Articles were identified through systematic searches in PubMed/MEDLINE, The University of Nottingham Online Catalogue, Web of Science and through reference checking. Study eligibility criteria: (1) participants aged fifty years or over with sensori-neural hearing loss, (2) provision of an air conduction hearing aid, (3) inclusion of hearing aid usage measure(s) and (4) published between 1999 and 2011.

Results: Of the initial 1933 papers obtained from the searches, a total of 64 were found eligible for review and were quality assessed on six dimensions: study design, choice of outcome instruments, level of reporting (usage, age, and audiometry) and cross validation of usage measures. Five papers were rated as being of high quality (scoring 10–12), 35 papers were rated as being of moderate quality (scoring 7–9), 22 as low quality (scoring 4–6) and two as very low quality (scoring 0–2). Fifteen different methods were identified for assessing the usage of hearing aids.

Conclusions: Generally, the usage data reviewed was not well specified. There was a lack of consistency and robustness in the way that usage of hearing aids was assessed and categorised. There is a need for more standardised level of reporting of hearing aid usage data to further understand the relationship between usage and hearing aid outcomes.

Editor: Iris Schrijver, Stanford University School of Medicine, United States of America

Funding: The National Biomedical Research Unit in Hearing is funded by the National Institute for Health Research. The funders had no role in study design, data collection and analysis, decision to publish, or preparation of the manuscript.

Competing Interests: The authors have declared that no competing interests exist.

* E-mail: elvira.perez@nottingham.ac.uk

Introduction

In the UK, it is estimated that 41.7% of adults aged 50 years or over has some form of hearing loss [1]. Presbycusis (age-related sensorineural hearing loss) is the most common type of hearing loss and it affects 25–43% of people aged between 65 and 74 years and 40–63% of those aged over 75 years [2], [3]. The most common form of treatment for hearing loss in adults is the provision of a hearing aid. It is estimated that about six million people in the UK could benefit from using a hearing aid, but only 1.4 million people in the UK who currently own hearing aids wear them regularly [4]. Hearing loss increases the need for more formal support (e.g., meals on wheels) in the elderly and it impacts negatively on independence by increasing reliance on community/family support [5]. Hearing loss also has an impact on communication, social interaction and self-sufficiency [6]. If left untreated (either through non-detection of the problem or non-adherence with the treatment) hearing loss can further precipitate social, physical and psychological decline [7] and will likely result in wasted resources (i.e., clinical time and un-used hearing aids). Consequently, when hearing aids are prescribed for the treatment of hearing loss it is important to ensure that patients are provided with regular follow up appointments to monitor their success [8].

The success of hearing aid provision as a treatment for hearing loss, like any health-care intervention, largely depends on two factors. First, the intervention should be capable of providing the patient with a favourable change in their condition. Second, the patient must comply with the intervention programme in order to have a chance of receiving that benefit. Indeed, there are a number of tools available for monitoring patient outcomes following provision of a hearing aid which seek to determine how often a hearing aid is used, whether the patient has experienced any changes in speech understanding, or other changes to quality of life. The amount of time spent wearing a hearing aid has been reported to be positively associated with the benefit that the hearing aid provides (i.e., an improvement in speech understanding) and levels of patient satisfaction [9], [10]. However, Humes et al [11] performed a principal component analysis of seven dimensions of hearing aid outcome (i.e., subjective benefit, aided performance, usage, objective benefit, speech in noise, handicap benefit and judgements of sound quality) which indicated that hearing aid usage is a distinct and relatively independent dimension of hearing aid outcome.

Bentler and Kramer [12] in an overview of audiological-focused self-report outcome measures identified three self-report inventories, out of 33, that assessed hearing aid usage: the Hearing Problem Inventory [13], the Hearing Aid User Questionnaire (HAUQ) [14], and the Glasgow Hearing Aid Benefit Profile (GHABP) [15]. In the last decade, however, the number of outcome instruments has increased considerably. Moreover, there has been a step change in hearing aid technology available in this period which has enabled more sophisticated devices (e.g., the advent of hearing aids capable of digital signal processing) to enter the market. Furthermore, audiology departments in the UK adopted a modernised hearing service which has allowed for greater levels of patient-clinician interaction, provision of digital hearing aids and the option of bilateral fittings. However, there are currently no recognised guidelines in the UK for managing the rehabilitation of patients with hearing loss using hearing aids nor is there a gold standard outcome measure for evaluating the success of auditory rehabilitation. Consequently, one of the dilemmas faced by clinicians and researchers is how to assess hearing aid usage and which methods to use. Self-reports measures are criticised because they are subject to socially desirable responses and may provide inaccurate responses. However, it has also been argued that objective alternatives (i.e., hearing aid data logs and battery consumption) are not free from error either, as users can forget to turn off the devices [16].

In this manuscript, we provide a descriptive overview of studies that were published since 1999 pertaining to usage of hearing aids in older listeners with sensori-neural hearing loss. We examined how usage has been measured and reported and how usage of hearing aids related to other dimensions of hearing aid outcomes. Information about study design, outcome instruments, measures of usage, and cross validation of data was extracted from research manuscripts identified using a systematic search. The purpose of this systematic review was consolidate this information into one source, to grade the quality of the evidence reported, and to identify trends in the data reported that might inform clinical guidelines or the direction of future research. We hope that clinicians and researches will find the review interesting and of help when deciding on how they should measure and report hearing aid usage in future reports.

Methods

The Preferred Reporting Items for Systematic reviews and Meta-Analyses (PRISMA) statement checklist [17] was used to improve the reporting of this systematic review as suggested by the NHS Centre for Reviews and Disseminations [18].

Search strategy

A systematic search strategy, following the principles published by the NHS Centre for Reviews and Dissemination [18] was used to identify potential articles. The University of Nottingham Online Catalogue, PubMed/MEDLINE, and Web of Science (including Science Citation Index Expanded, Social Sciences Citation Index, Arts & Humanities Citation Index, and Conference Proceedings Citation Index- Science) electronic databases were searched for peer-reviewed articles published between 1999–2011 using the search term "hearing aid" in conjunction with each of the following terms: "outcome", "use", "usage", "non-use", "compliance", "satisfaction" and "benefit". Database searches were conducted in April 2010 and updated in September 2011. Further 'hand searches' of the key subject journals (to identify articles published since August 2011 that may not yet have been registered on a database) were conducted in October 2011.

Inclusion criteria and study selection

The objective of this review was to examine the reporting of hearing aid usage as an outcome measure and the factors that contribute to hearing aid usage. The author's current research interests lie with the auditory rehabilitation of presbycusic patients. In order to align the scope of this review with these research interests, we restricted eligibility of studies for review using a set of pre-specified inclusion criteria. Studies had to include participants aged fifty years or over with sensori-neural hearing loss, that had been provided with an air conduction hearing aid for the treatment of their hearing loss. Although no limitations were placed on the nature of the primary outcome measure reported, studies were only included if a measure of hearing aid usage was recorded. In addition, no constraints were placed on acceptable study design. While randomised control trials would be preferred as they give the highest level of evidence, it was anticipated that not many studies would meet this criteria.

Titles and abstracts of articles identified by the search strategy were screened to determine whether the study matched the inclusion criteria. Where evidence for inclusion of a manuscript was in doubt from the title and abstract, the full text was screened. The reference lists of all manuscripts matching the inclusion criteria were searched to find additional manuscripts for inclusion in the review.

Data extraction

Data extraction was performed independently by both authors using an electronic reporting form developed specifically for this purpose; any differences in reporting were reconciled by jointly revisiting each publication. The reporting form was used to capture the following information: aims, study design, sample size, sampling issues, audiometric data and participant's age at time of outcome, timing of post-fitting follow-ups, outcome instruments, usage assessments, usage data and associations with other variables.

Quality assessment criteria

All studies that met the inclusion criteria were subjected to a quality assessment exercise. Our approach to quality assessment was informed by NHS guidelines for systematic reviews [18]. The quality of each study was determined against six pre-specified criteria: i) study design, ii) use of appropriate outcome measures (i.e. standardised questionnaires and tests), iii) reporting of usage data, iv) cross validation of usage estimates (i.e. were estimates of usage obtained using multiple alternative methods or repeated measures over a number of visits), v) reporting of participant age and vi) reporting of audiometric data. While the first criterion assesses the overall methodological quality of the studies reviewed, the other criteria influence the reader's confidence in the reported usage effects in older adults with hearing loss.

Each study was given an overall grading of high, moderate, low or very low which reflected our confidence in the reported effect [19]. The grade awarded to each study was based on a number of points accrued on the six quality criteria: *High* (10–12 points), *Moderate* (7–9 points), and Low (4–6 points) and Very low (0–3 points). For each criterion, studies were awarded *0* points if the information regarding the criterion was absent or flawed on a number of levels, *1* point was awarded if the study partially met the criterion or the implementation was partially flawed, and *2* points were awarded if the study fulfilled the criterion to a high standard. Studies were independently scored by both authors and a final score was agreed after discussion. Specific examples of how points were awarded to studies for each of the six criteria are given in the relevant portions of the Results section.

It should be noted that each criterion is given equal weighting in the overall grade. That is, we consider each of the criteria as important as the next for the purpose of addressing the aims of this review. As such, studies that were graded as 'Low' or 'Very Low' quality use a combination of methods or reporting techniques which on-the-whole reduced our confidence in the results reported or limited the degree to which the results could be interpreted in the context of this review. Studies that were graded as being of 'High Quality' on-the-other-hand incorporated methods or levels of reporting which on-the-whole strengthened our confidence in the usage data reported and its relevance to the topic of hearing aid usage in older adults while. If a reader is interested in only a subset of the quality criteria used here, then the overall grading could be ignored entirely or replaced with a grading system that gives greater weight to one or more of the quality criteria.

Results

Search results

The systematic search of electronic databases produced 1933 items of which 46 met the inclusion criteria for this review (see Figure 1). A further 18 eligible papers were obtained by searching

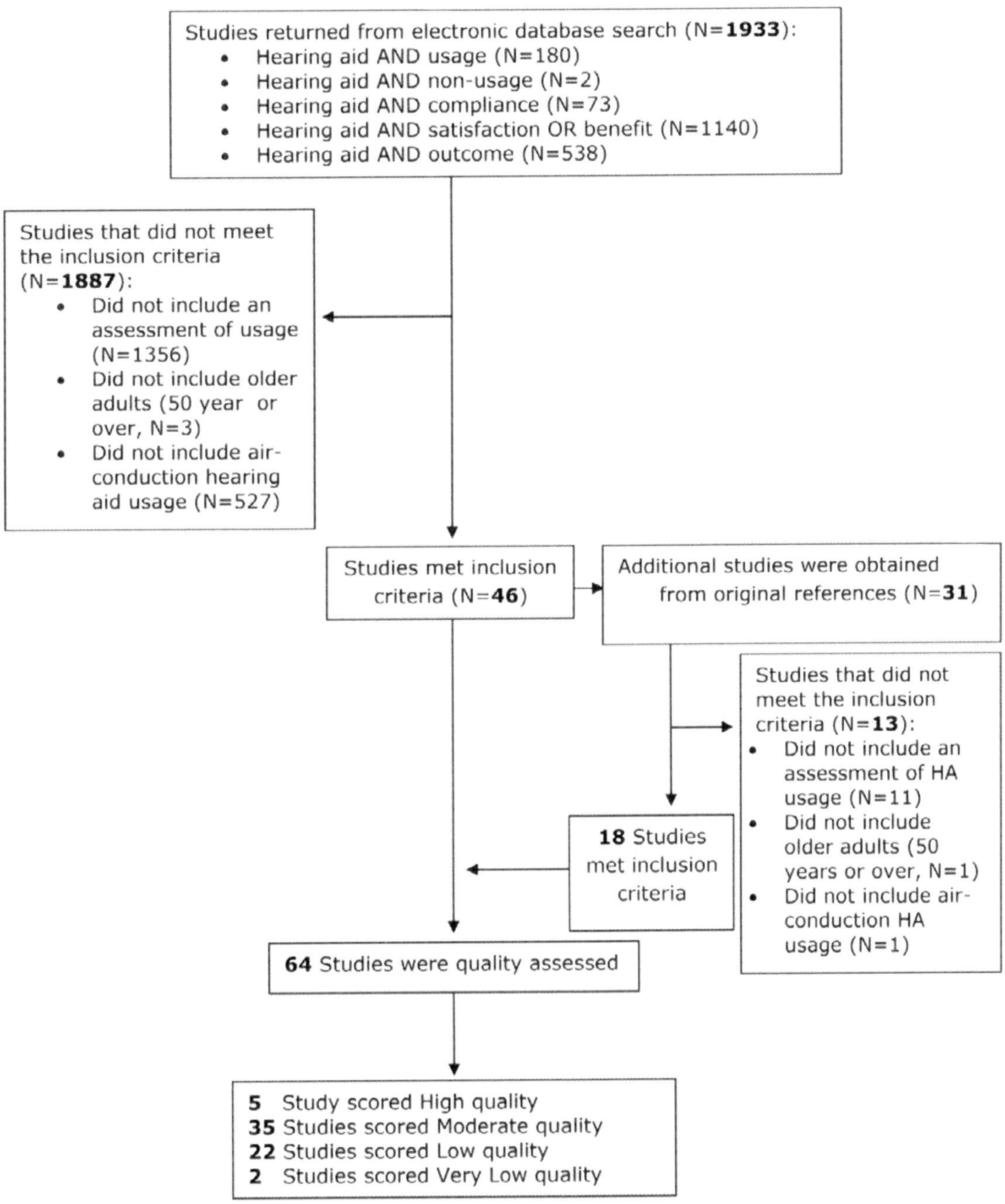

Figure 1. Flow diagram to illustrate the systematic review process undertaken.

the references of the original 46 giving a total of 64 research papers. The selected studies originated from 16 countries: Australia (n = 10), Canada (n = 1), China (n = 1), Denmark (n = 3), Finland (n = 4), Germany (n = 2), Hong Kong (n = 1), New Zealand (n = 2), Nigeria (n = 1), Norway (n = 1), Taiwan (n = 1), The Netherlands (n = 1), UK (n = 6), USA (n = 27), Sweden (n = 2), and Switzerland (n = 1). The information obtained at the data extraction stage is summarised in Table S1.

Quality assessment

Study design. In clinical or therapeutic settings, randomisation is the 'gold standard' design [20] and systematic reviews often only include randomized trials [21]. When participants are not randomly allocated to groups, the detection of sampling bias is crucial for assessment of the quality of study design. Our review identified 54 observational studies of which eight were cross-sectional studies, eight randomised control trials and one crossover clinical trial. Thirty-eight studies did not specify whether any steps were taken to adjust for sampling bias. Twenty studies used only a single clinic and six studies only recruited male veterans. Other studies, however, included as many as twelve private clinics and seven public hospitals to recruit participants [22] or randomly selected participants from the public of a specific geographical area [23]. Other methods employed in order to minimise sampling bias included: contacting non-respondents, analysing potential differences between the results of different hearing clinics and surveys, randomly selected the hearing clinics involved and recruiting participants via a range of media (i.e., newspapers, advertisements, flyers, printed announcements in church bulletins, or word of mouth).

When grading the quality of evidence for study design, a score of 2 was awarded to randomised control trials (see Table S2). A score of 1 was awarded to all other study designs. A score of 0 was reserved for studies with serious methodological and design issues. In consideration of the evidence outlined above, eleven studies employed a high quality study design (scored *2* points) which utilised randomisation, control groups were a population-based study or other measures to minimise bias. A total of 30 studies were rated as medium quality as they implemented a non-optimal design but took steps to identify and address possible sources of bias. A score of 0 was awarded to 24 studies because they used a severely flawed design that failed to provide any adjustments for sample bias or randomisation of conditions.

Outcome instruments. A large number of validated and non-validated tests and techniques were used to evaluate dimensions of hearing aid outcome (see Figure 2a for the top ten most used outcome instruments). The majority of the studies reviewed focused on dimensions of satisfaction, benefit or residual handicap as the primary outcome measure for their research question rather than hearing aid usage. Hearing aid usage was the primary outcome measure in 10 studies [16], [23], [24], [25], [26], [27], [28], [29], [30], [31]. Of the top six outcome instruments, the Glasgow Hearing Aid Benefit Profile (GHABP, [15]) and International Outcome Instrument - Hearing Aids (IOI-HA, [32]) are multi-dimensional instruments, the Abbreviate Profile for Hearing Aid Benefit (APHAB, [33]) focuses on subjective benefit, the Satisfaction and Amplification in Daily Life (SADL, [34]) focuses on satisfaction, the Hearing Handicap Inventory for the Elderly (HHIE, [35]) focuses on handicap, and the speech reception tests like the Connected Speech Test (CST, [36]) or City University of New York Nonsense Syllable Test (CUNY NST, [37]) assesses benefit objectively in the form of percentage correct, other test like the QuickSIN [38] provide a threshold for speech intelligibility (typically signal-to-noise ratio in decibels for identifying 50% of items correctly).

In grading the quality of studies based on the choice of outcome measures, we looked for evidence of multiple standardised or validated tests of outcome in our quality assessment. A total of 32 studies included multiple standardised outcome measures and were rated as being of high quality. A score of *1* was awarded to 25 studies that employed a range of non-standardised tests or only a single standardised test to determine hearing aid outcomes. Seven studies scored *0* points as hearing aid outcome was determined purely on the basis of a single non-standardised outcome measure.

Assessment of hearing aid usage. Hearing aid usage was assessed with standardised questionnaires in 32 of the studies reviewed, 21 studies included custom questionnaires; interview was the third most popular method for assessing usage, diaries and hearing aid data logs the fourth, while battery consumption was used in only one of the studies reviewed (see figure 2b). Data logs likely reflect the relatively recent addition of such functionality in hearing instruments. We would expect to see greater use of this digital logging feature in future studies.

The most popular standardised questionnaires for measuring usage (see Figure 2b) were the IOI-HA [32], the APHAB [33] and the GHABP [15].

Reporting hearing aid usage

Both IOI-HA and GHABP categorise usage on a 5-point scale, but differ in their approach. The GHABP asks the patient to reflect on what *proportion of time for a given activity* that they use their hearing aid (acceptable response are: all of the time, about ¾ of the time, about ½ of the time, about *a* ¼ *of the* time, never/not at all). The IOI-HA assesses the *average amount of time* spent wearing a hearing aid (i.e. 'on an average day, how many hours did you use the device? Acceptable responses are: >8 hr/day, 4–8 hr/day, 1–4 hr/day, <1 hr/day, none). The distinction is subtle but potentially very important. The GHABP focuses very much on the situations important to the patient, but gives data that is difficult to compare against other studies and measures of usage (e.g., what does wearing a hearing for ¾ of the time spent watching television really mean?). The IOI-HA is perhaps less patient-needs focused, but gives data that is clearly comparable with other studies (8 hours is always 8 hours). The APHAB is a 24-item self-assessment questionnaire that reports patient's communication difficulties. It produced scores for 4 subscales; easy of communication, reverberation, background noise and aversiveness. APHAB includes a daily hearing aid section in which participants have to circle the most appropriate answer (less than 1 hour per day, 1 to 4 hours per day, 4 to 8 hours per day or 8 to 16 hours per day).

If one compares the data presented in Figure 2a with that of 2b a number of discrepancies can be observed in the number instances an outcome instrument is reported. For instance, the SADL which consists of 15 items on hearing aid performance and user satisfaction, and four additional questions concerning hearing aid experience and use, featured in a total of 11 of the studies reviewed. However, only two of these studies reported the amount of time spent wearing a hearing aid in the format dictated by the SADL: the other nine studies either reported usage in the format of another outcome instrument or failed to report usage in any form.

Custom questionnaires and structured interviews included open questions (e.g., 'How many hours a day do you use your hearing aid?) or were built around specific duration-based categories. The format of patient diaries was not well described nor was the method used to interpret entries, but they were usually

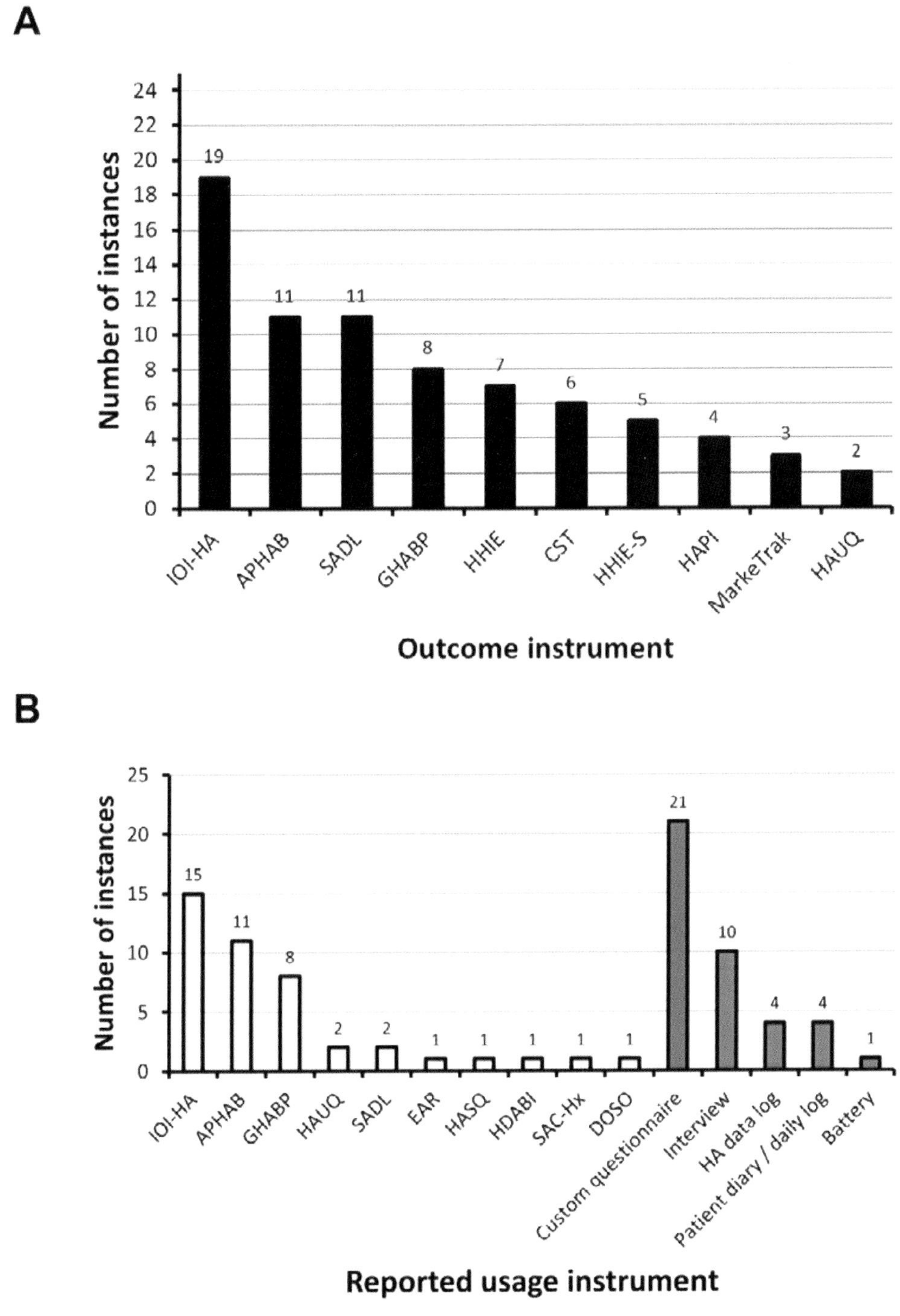

Figure 2. Reported instances of outcome and usage instruments. Panel A shows the top ten most used outcomes measures. Panel B shows the range of methods employed for assessing hearing aid usage. White bars indicate standardised questionnaires; grey bars indicate non-standardised methods. Abbreviations: **IOI-HA** International Outcome Inventory - Hearing Aids [32], **APHAB** Abbreviated Profile of Haring Aid Benefit [57], **SADL** Satisfaction with Amplification in Daily Life [34], **GHABP** Glasgow Hearing Aid Benefit Profile [15], **HHIE** Hearing Handicap Inventory for the Elderly [59], **CST** Connected Speech Test [36], [56], **HHIE-S** screening version [62], **HAPI** Hearing Aid Performance Inventory [54], **MarkeTrak** [63,64] and **HAUQ** Hearing Aid Users Questionnaire [55], **EAR** Effectiveness of Auditory Rehabilitation [60], **HASQ** Hearing Aid Status Questionnaire [58], **HDABI** Hearing Disability and Aided Benefit Interview [15], **SAC-Hx** Self-Assessment of Communication [40] and **DOSO** Device Oriented Subjective Outcome Scale [61].

complemented by estimates of usage obtained from questionnaires like the GHABP [15], digital data logs or interviews [24].

Data regarding the usage of hearing aids was graded by employing an approach which awarded points for clear and unambiguous presentation of data. A total of 38studies recorded usage as duration in hours per day or categorized usage with a numerical value and scored *2* points for this criterion. A score of *1* was awarded to 16 studies because they categorized usage using only descriptive labels (e.g., occasionally or all of the time). Ten studies scored *0* points because they categorized usage with binary labels or did not report the amount of time participants used their hearing aids despite having collected the data (i.e., the data and format of that data was not reported in the manuscript).

Cross-validation of usage data. In order to further strengthen our confidence in the usage data reported, we asked whether or not efforts had been made to check the reliability/validity of the data collected. Seven studies scored *2* points for the cross-validation of usage data by combining subjective estimates (e.g., self-report diary) and objective measures (i.e., device memory or battery usage) or by assessing patients on multiple visits. Thirteen studies scored *1* point for cross validation as they compared data from two different self-report questionnaires. The remaining 44 studies did not provide any cross-validation of hearing aid usage data and scored *0* points for this criterion.

Reporting of participant age. In order to appreciate the relevance of each study for understanding auditory habilitation in older adults, we examined the way in which the age of participants was reported. Our strategy was to award points to studies for clear and unambiguous reporting of the data. A total of 48 studies scored *2* points for reporting data pertaining to the age of participants to a high standard (i.e., they reported the mean and standard deviation or analysed participants' data by age group). A total of 14 studies provided some details about the age of participants (e.g., minimum, maximum or range of ages) but no measures of the variance (scored *1* point). Age was not reported in two studies [39], [40]] that included war veterans (scoring *0* points).

Reporting of audiometric data. Audiometric data derived from pure tone hearing thresholds are necessary to establish the degree of hearing loss, and further explore how this variable might relate to usage. In order to fully understand the relevance of each study to older adults with hearing loss we examined the way in which audiometric thresholds were reported. Again, we rated the quality of studies on this criterion based on the level of reporting. Twenty-six studies scored *2* points for reporting audiometric data to a high standard including means and standard deviations per frequency band. Twenty-four provided some audiometric aspects like pure-tone average (scoring *1* point). Audiometric data was not reported in fourteen studies (scoring *0* points).

Factors associated with the usage of hearing aids

Previous research ([41], not reviewed) showed a significant positive correlation between hearing aid use and increasing hearing loss in the elderly. However, our review indicates that this result is not reflected in the majority of studies. Thirteen studies assessed the impact of hearing loss at fitting on usage of hearing aids, but hearing loss was found to be significantly related to usage in only three of these studies [28], [42], [31].

The relationship between age and hearing aid usage was assessed in only eight studies. Two studies [28] and [43] showed a decrease in hearing aid usage with increasing age (>75 years) due to low benefit expectations, a reduction in dexterity to handle the hearing aid, or acquirement of alternative coping mechanisms (e.g., turning the volume up on the television). Five studies did not find any association between age and hearing aid usage and only one [31] found age as a significant predictor of hearing aid usage where older adults (80+) had the highest incidence of hearing aid use (25%). Complementarily, Vuorialho et al. [44] reported that the proportion of individuals with hearing aids was greater in the retired population than in the general population.

A number of the studies reviewed ([45], [46], [47]) suggested that usage was not strongly correlated with improvements in technical aspects of hearing aids made over the last decade or so. Rather, Bertoli et al. [28] suggested that difficulty in handling aids is one of the most important factors contributing to non-regular use of hearing aids. Indeed, a number of studies reviewed here ([48], [22], [45], [49]) showed that the efforts of manufacturers towards making hearing aids smaller, easier to handle and aesthetically more attractive can reduce the risk of non-regular use.

Lupsako et al. [23] noted that in countries where hearing aid provision is not state funded, hearing aid possession was positively correlated with income. However, Stephens et al. [25] found no significant differences in usage between private- and NHS-funded hearing aids. This suggests that whilst affordability might prove to be an initial barrier to the uptake of a hearing aid it has little bearing on continued use of the device. Other studies ([22], [29], [31], [50]), however, have reported that attitude towards rehabilitation, high cost, comfort, pre-fitting expectations and greater acceptance of hearing loss were found to be significantly related to hours of use.

Discussion

Being able to determine whether a hearing aid is used regularly and effectively is an important measure of outcome. After all, what benefit is a hearing aid that provides improved speech intelligibility if it is never used? Equally, why wear a hearing aid if it does not provide any benefit? It has been recommended ([8], [51]) that regular follow up appointments in which the patient's progress with the device are required in order to improve patient outcomes. It is particularly important in older adults, where there is an increased risk of social isolation, that hearing loss does not go untreated; once a patient has been identified as having a hearing loss this invariably leads to the provision of hearing aids. The aim of this systematic review was to summarise the evidence available in the literature on how hearing aid usage in older adults has been measured in the last decade.

Our review identified fifteen different metrics for evaluating the usage of hearing aids; there was little consistency in the way that usage was recorded in the studies reviewed. Thus, it is fair to say that there is no standard tool for evaluating hearing aid usage. There was a dichotomy in the literature between those studies interested in the amount of time spent (i.e., hours per day) wearing a hearing aid, and those that focused on how regularly/frequently a hearing aid was used. Others used a mixed model asking what proportion of time a hearing aid was used in a specific situation. Tools like the IOI-HA [32] report a fixed number of hours which can be compared across listeners and studies fairly simply. The GHABP [15], on the other hand, takes a much more individualised approach which might better reflect the needs of the patient, but makes it very difficult to compare one patient with another. Both approaches have their merits and flaws so it is important to consider exactly which aspects of the patient's behaviour you are trying to capture.

One might have thought that distinguishing between 'users' and 'non-users' would be fairly straightforward, but this has not been the case. For instance, Gussekloo et al. [44] reported that 241 of 367 participants with severe hearing loss "did not make use of a hearing aid". However, it was unclear from the text whether this response indicated "I do not own a hearing aid" or "I own a hearing aid, but do not wear it". Similarly, the criteria for defining what constitutes 'regular' usage appeared somewhat arbitrary, as studies that employed such terminology tended not to specify the equivalent numerical cut-off point for these nominal categories. For this reason, we believe that having usage linked to a numerical value (e.g., hours per day or days per week) would prove to be extremely useful. The differences in data types (binary, ordinal, and interval) mean that it was impossible to calculate a definitive estimate of the proportion of patients that use their hearing aids or the amount of time that they spend wearing their hearing aids.

Typically, the success of hearing aid provision in the studies reviewed was determined by assessing how much benefit (e.g., objective and subjective ratings of speech intelligibility) a patient experienced. Our review suggests that the relationship between usage and other outcome domains is highly complex. Although a number of studies found that hearing aid usage was correlated with other outcome measures like benefit and satisfaction [9], [14], [28], [47] no single dimension was consistently shown to depend on the amount of time spent using a hearing aid. It is also noteworthy that while some patients may only require the use of hearing aids for specific situations and feel very satisfied, others may rely heavily on their hearing aids, using them throughout the day, but report low levels of satisfaction ([22], [29]).

We would like to reiterate arguments made in an earlier report [51] that recommended estimates of the time spent using a hearing aid should be cross validated. Ideally, this would involve a combination of objective (e.g., battery consumption or hearing aid data log) and subjective (e.g., diary or questionnaire) measures. If a numerical value of how many hours per day a patient wears a hearing aid (as suggested above) is not covered by a clinic's preferred self-report assessment tool then cross-validation would be one way of capturing that information. For instance, where the preferred clinical tool is the GHABP one might also consider including data from the hearing aid's data log. If an objective measure of usage is unavailable for cross validation, then a consensus approach using a second self-report questionnaire that does provide a numerical estimate of usage might be a reasonable solution. However, it should be remembered that self-reported usage measures are vulnerable to both over and under estimation (see [16], [24]).

While the usage of hearing aids does not guarantee successful patient outcomes, it is important to ensure that patients are using their hearing aids regularly and that the device makes a difference to the patient's ability to listen and communicate effectively. A number of studies reviewed asked patients how much they thought their life had changed as a result of a hearing aid, and many asked how much time was spent wearing hearing aids in particular situations. However, none of the outcome instruments identified in this review determined how much time was spent in that situation before receipt of a hearing aid. One might argue that a more useful measure of hearing aid outcome would be to determine how much *more* time people can spend doing the things they like as a result of wearing a hearing aid. It has been suggested that counselling [52] and motivational interviewing techniques [53] might improve not only the uptake of hearing aids, but also promote the continued use of the hearing instruments. Such a patient-centred, individualised approach paired with an objective measure of hearing aid usage in targeted situations might prove useful in planning and monitoring the auditory rehabilitation of patients receiving hearing aids.

Overall, we found that the level of reporting in the studies reviewed was inconsistent and of variable quality. There is a need for higher levels of evidence in the form of RCTs to study the impact of hearing aids as a treatment for hearing loss, and in particular for monitoring advances in service and technology on the uptake and compliance with hearing aid provision. Only with greater standardisation and precision in the level of reporting will future reviews of the literature be able to perform greater levels of analysis (e.g., meta-analysis) and provide firm guidelines on auditory habilitation with hearing aids.

In order to monitor auditory rehabilitation of patients provided with hearing aids it is important to determine that the patient is using the device regularly and effectively. Our review demonstrates that there is currently no standard method or format for reporting the amount of time spent using hearing aids. However, if one wants to be able to compare how much time is spent wearing hearing aids then outcome metrics do need to be standardised; a common metric would allow for meta-analysis and cross-comparisons to be undertaken.

While it is not likely, nor necessarily appropriate, that a single tool or method be adopted by clinical practices to evaluate compliance and success of hearing aid provision, it might be possible to reduce heterogeneity in reporting of usage data in research studies or health service evaluations by ensuring that when descriptive labels like regular and non-regular are to be used to characterize usage that they are clearly defined in terms of hours or days. Additionally, the assessment of hearing aid usage should be cross-validated by obtaining estimates with a number of different, preferably objective, assessment tools, and over multiple time courses in order to improve confidence in self-report estimates.

Supporting Information

Table S1 Summary of the data extraction from the 64 studies selected. *Data estimated from figures HL: Hearing loss, PTA: Pure tone audiometry; sd: standard deviation; RCT = randomised control trial; OCS = observational case series; ROC = retrospective observational cohort.

Table S2 Quality assessment and grading results. Scoring codes are: 2 (study meets criterion to a high standard); 1 (study partially meets criterion); 0 (study does not meet criterion or relevant information is absent). The grading of the quality of evidence is: High (13–16), Moderate (8–12), and Low (4–7) and Very low (0–3) [19]. Abbreviations: Hearing loss (HL).

Acknowledgments

We are thankful to Heather Fortnum and Derek Hoare for constructive comments and Phil Gander, Robert Risley, Daniel Rowan and 'H' for their support.

Author Contributions

Conceived and designed the experiments: EP BE. Performed the experiments: EP BE. Analyzed the data: EP BE. Contributed reagents/materials/analysis tools: EP BE. Wrote the paper: EP BE. Revised the manuscript: EP BE.

References

1. Davis AC, Smith P, Ferguson M, Stephens D, Gianopoulus I (2007) Acceptability, benefit and costs of early screening for hearing disability: a study of potential screening tests and models. Health Technol Assess 11: 3–5.
2. Cacciatore F, Napoli C, Abete P, Marciano E, Triassi M, et al. (1999) Quality of life determinants and hearing function in an elderly population: Osservatorio Geriatrico Campano Study Group. Gerontology 45: 323–328.
3. Lopez-Torres J, Boix C, Tellez J, Lopez MA, del Campo JM, et al. (2009) Functional status of elderly people with hearing loss. Archives of Gerontology and Geriatrics 49: 88–92.
4. Action for Hearing Loss (2011) Facts and figures on deafness and tinnitus. Taking Action on Hearing Loss in the 21st century, June 2011.
5. Schneider J, Gopinath B, Karpa M, McMahon C, Rochtchina E, et al. (2010) Hearing loss impacts on the use of community and informal supports. Age Ageing 39: 458–464.

6. Dalton D, Cruickshanks K, Klein B, Klein R, Wiley T, et al. (2003) The impact of hearing loss on quality of life in older adults. Gerontologist 43: 661–668.
7. Kramer S, Goverts S, Dreschler W, Boymans M, Festen J (2002) International Outcome Inventory for Hearing Aids (IOI-HA): results from The Netherlands. Int J Audiol 41: 36–41.
8. Goggins S, Day J (2009) Pilot study: Efficacy of recalling adult hearing-aid users for reassessment after three years within a publicly-funded audiology service. Int J Audiol 48: 204–210.
9. Uriarte M, Denzin L, Dunstan A, Sellars J, Hickson L (2005) Measuring hearing aid outcomes using the Satisfaction with Amplification in Daily Life (SADL) questionnaire: Australian data. J Am Acad Audiol 16: 383–402.
10. Roup C, Noe C (2009) Hearing aid outcomes for listeners with high-frequency hearing loss. Am J Audiol 18: 45–52.
11. Humes L, Garner C, Wilson D, Barlow N (2001) Hearing aid outcome measures following one month of hearing aid use by the elderly. J Speech Hear Res 443: 469–486.
12. Bentler R, Kramer S (2000) Guidelines for choosing a self-report outcome measure. Ear and Hearing 21: 37S–49S.
13. Hutton CL (1980) Responses to a Hearing Problem Inventory. Journal of the Academy of Rehabilitative Audiology 13: 133–154.
14. Dillon H, Birtles G, Lovegrove R (1999) Measuring the outcomes of a national rehabilitation program: Normative data for the client oriented scale of improvement (COSI) and the hearing aid user's questionnaire (HAUQ). J Am Acad Audiol 10: 67–79.
15. Gatehouse S (1999) Glasgow hearing aid benefit profile: derivation and validation of a client-centered outcome measure for hearing aid services. J Am Acad Audiol 10: 80–103.
16. Taubman L, Palmer C, Durrant J, Pratt S (1999) Accuracy of hearing aid use time as reported by experienced hearing aid wearers. Ear Hear 20: 299–305.
17. Moher D, Liberati A, Tetzlaff J, Altman DG, The PRISMA Group (2009) Preferred Reporting Items for Systematic Reviews and Meta-Analyses: The PRISMA Statement. PLoS Med 6(6): e1000097. doi:10.1371/journal.pmed1000097.
18. NHS Centre for Research and Dissemination, Systematic Reviews (2009) CRD's guidance for undertaking reviews in health care. York. University of York.
19. Atkins D, Best D, Briss PA, Eccles M, Falck-Ytter Y, et al. (2004) Grading quality of evidence and strength of recommendations. BMJ 328(7454): 1490.
20. Oxman A (2004) Grading quality of evidence and strength of recommendations. Br Med J 328: 1490–1494.
21. Liberati A, Altman DG, Tetzlaff J, Mulrow C, Gotzsche PC, et al. (2009) The PRISMA statement for reporting systematic reviews and meta-analyses of studies that evaluate health care interventions: explanation and elaboration. J Clin Epidemiol 62(10): e1–34.
22. Jerram JC, Purdy SC (2001) Technology, expectations, and adjustment to hearing loss: predictors of hearing aid outcome. J Am Acad Audiol 12: 64–79.
23. Lupsakko T, Kautiainen H, Sulkava R (2005) The non-use of hearing aids in people aged 75 years and over in the city of Kuopio in Finland. Eur Arch Otorhinolaryngol 262: 165–169.
24. Maki-Torkko E, Sorri M, Laukli E (2001) Objective assessment of hearing aid use. Scand Audiol 30: 81–82.
25. Stephens D, Lewis P, Davis A, Gianopoulos I, Vetter N (2001) Hearing aid possession in the population: Lessons from a small country. Audiology 40: 104–111.
26. Smeeth L, Fletcher A, Ng ESW, Stirling S, Nunes M, et al. (2002) Reduced hearing, ownership, and use of hearing aids in elderly people in the UK - the MRC Trial of the Assessment and Management of Older People in the Community: a cross-sectional survey. Lancet 359: 1466–1470.
27. Bratt G, Rosenfield M, Williams D (2007) NIDCD/VA hearing aid clinical trial and follow-up: Background. J Am Acad Audiol 18(4): 274–281.
28. Bertoli S, Staehelin K, Zemp E, Schindler C, Bodmer D, et al. (2009) Survey on hearing aid use and satisfaction in Switzerland and their determinants. Int J Audiology 48: 183–195.
29. Hartley D, Rochtchina E, Newall P, Golding M, Mitchell P (2010) Use of Hearing Aids and Assistive Listening Devices in an Older Australian Population. J Am Acad Audiol 21(10): 642–653.
30. Williams V, Johnson C, Danhauer J (2009) Hearing Aid Outcomes: Effects of Gender and Experience on Patients' Use and Satisfaction. J Am Acad Audiol 20(7): 422–432.
31. Gopinath B, Mitchell P, Schneider J, Hartley D, Teber E, et al. (2011) Incidence and Predictors of Hearing Aid Use and Ownership among Older Adults with Hearing Loss. Annals of Epidemiology 21(7): 497–506.
32. Cox R, Hyde M, Gatehouse S, Noble W, Harvey D, et al. (2000) Optimal outcome measures, research priorities, and international cooperation. Ear Hear 21(4 Suppl): 106S–115S.
33. Cox R, Alexander G (1995) The abbreviated profile of hearing aid benefit. Ear Hear 16: 176–186.
34. Cox R, Alexander G (1999) Measuring satisfaction with amplification in daily life: the SADL scale. Ear Hear 20: 306–320.
35. Ventry I, Weinstein B (1982) The Hearing Handicap Inventory for the Elderly: a new tool. Ear and Hearing 3(3): 128–34.
36. Cox R, Alexander G, Gilmore C, Pusakulich K (1988) Use of Connected Speech Test (CST) with hearing-impaired listeners. Ear Hear 9: 198–207.
37. Levitt H, Resnick S (1978) Speech reception by the hearing impaired: Methods of testing and development of meterials. Scand Audiol Suppl 6: 107–129.
38. Killion MC, Niquette PA, Gudmundsen GI, Revit LJ, Banerjee S (2004) Development of a quick speech-in-noise test for measuring signal-to-noise ratio loss in normal-hearing and hearing-impaired listeners. J Acoust Soc Am 116(4 Pt 1): 2395–2405.
39. Gnewikow D, Ricketts T, Bratt G, Mutchler L (2009) Real-world benefit from directional microphone hearing aids. J Rehabil Res Dev 46(5): 603–618.
40. Ivory P, Hendricks B, Van Vliet D, Beyer C, Abrams H (2009) Short-term hearing aid benefit in a large group. Trends Amplif 13(4): 260–280.
41. Brooks DN (1985) Factors relating to the under-use of postaural hearing aids. Br J Audiol 19(3): 211–217.
42. Brannstrom KJ, Wennerstrom I (2010) Hearing aid fitting outcome: clinical application and psychometric properties of a Swedish translation of the international outcome inventory for hearing aids (IOI-HA). J Am Acad Audiol 21(8): 512–521.
43. Gussekloo J, de Bont LE, von Faber M, Eekhof J, Laat J, et al. (2003) Auditory rehabilitation of older people from the general population–the Leiden 85-plus study. Br J Gen Pract 53: 536–540.
44. Vuorialho A, Sorri M, Nuojua I, Mulhi A (2006) Changes in hearing aid use over the past 20 years. Eu Arch Oto-Rhino-Laryng 263: 355–360.
45. Parving A, Sibelle P (2001) Clinical study of hearing instruments: A cross-sectional longitudinal audit based on consumer experiences. Audiology 40: 43–53.
46. Humes L, Alhstrom J, Bratt G, Peek B (2009) Studies of hearing-aid outcome measures in older adults: A comparison of technologies and an examination of individual differences. Sem Hear 30: 112–128.
47. Humes L, Humes L, Wilson D (2004) A comparison of single-channel linear amplification and tow-channel wide-dynamic-range-compression amplification by means of an independent-group design. Am J Audiol 13: 39–53.
48. Arlinger S, Billermark E (1999) One year follow-up of users of a digital hearing aid. Br J Audiol 33: 223–232.
49. Keidser G, Hartley D, Carter L (2008) Long-term usage of modern signal processing by listeners with severe or profound hearing loss: a retrospective survey. Am J Audiol 17: 136–146.
50. Hickson L, Timm M, Worrall L, Bishop K (1999) Hearing aid fitting: outcomes for older adults. Aust J Audiology 21(1): 11.
51. Brooks DN (1996) The time course of adaptation to hearing aid use. Br J Audiol 30: 55–62.
52. Vuorialho A, Karinen P, SorriM (2006) Effect of hearing aids on hearing disability and quality of life in the elderly. Int J Audiol 45(7): 400–405.
53. Beck D, Harvey A (2009) Creating successful professional-patient relationships. Audiology Today 12.
54. Walden B, Demorest M, Hepler E (1984) Self-report approach to assessing benefit derived from amplification. J Speech Hear Res 27: 49–56.
55. Forster S, Tomlin A (1988) Hearing Aid Usage in Queensland. Paper presented at the Audiological Society of Australia Conference.
56. Cox R, Alexander G, Gilmore C (1987) Development of the connected speech test (CST). Ear Hear 8: 119S–126S.
57. Cox R, Rivera I (1992) Predictability and reliability of hearing aid benefit measured using the PHAB. J Am Acad Audiol 3(4): 242–254.
58. Boothroyd A, Noffsinger D Hearings status questionnaire (HASQ).
59. Weinstein B (1986) Validity of a screening protocol to identifying elderly people with hearing problems. ASHA 28: 41–45.
60. Yueh B, McDowell JA, Collins M, Souza P, Loovis C, et al. (2005) Development and validation of the effectiveness of corrected auditory rehabilitation scale. Arch Otolaryngol Head Neck Surg 131(10): 851–856.
61. Cox R, Alexander G, Xu J (2009) Development of the Device Oriented Subjective Outcome Scale (DOSO). Annual Meeting of the American Auditory Society. http://www.memphis.edu/ausp/harl/publications.htm#posters.
62. Wechsler D (1981) The Wechsler Adult Intelligence Scale-Revised. New York: The Psychological Corporation.
63. Kochkin S (2000) MarkeTrak V: Consumer satisfaction revisited. Hear J 53(1): 38–55.
64. Kochkin S (2005) MarkeTrak VII: Customer satisfaction with hearing instruments in the digital age. Hear J 58(9.

State-and Trait-Related Alterations of Motor Cortex Excitability in Tinnitus Patients

Martin Schecklmann[1]*, Michael Landgrebe[2], Tobias Kleinjung[3], Elmar Frank[1], Rainer Rupprecht[1], Philipp G. Sand[1], Peter Eichhammer[1], Göran Hajak[2], Berthold Langguth[1]

1 Department of Psychiatry and Psychotherapy, University Regensburg, Regensburg, Germany, **2** Department of Psychiatry, Psychosomatic Medicine and Psychotherapy, Social Foundation Bamberg, Bamberg, Germany, **3** Department of Otorhinolaryngology, University of Zurich, Zurich, Switzerland

Abstract

Chronic tinnitus is a brain network disorder with involvement of auditory and non-auditory areas. Repetitive transcranial magnetic stimulation (rTMS) over the temporal cortex has been investigated for the treatment of tinnitus. Several small studies suggest that motor cortex excitability is altered in people with tinnitus. We retrospectively analysed data from 231 patients with chronic tinnitus and 120 healthy controls by pooling data from different studies. Variables of interest were resting motor threshold (RMT), short-interval intra-cortical inhibition (SICI), intra-cortical facilitation (ICF), and cortical silent period (CSP). 118 patients were tested twice - before and after ten rTMS treatment sessions over the left temporal cortex. In tinnitus patients SICI and ICF were increased and CSP was shortened as compared to healthy controls. There was no group difference in RMT. Treatment related amelioration of tinnitus symptoms were correlated with normalisations in SICI. These findings confirm earlier studies of abnormal motor cortex excitability in tinnitus patients. Moreover our longitudinal data suggest that altered SICI may reflect a state parameter, whereas CSP and ICF may rather mirror a trait-like predisposing factor of tinnitus. These findings are new and innovative as they enlarge the knowledge about basic physiologic and neuroplastic processes in tinnitus.

Editor: Andreas Reif, University of Wuerzburg, Germany

Funding: The authors have no support or funding to report.

* E-mail: martin.schecklmann@medbo.de

Introduction

Tinnitus is associated with neural changes in both the auditory pathway (increase of spontaneous stochastic firing rate, hyperactivity, alterations of the tonotopic map), and in non-auditory brain areas [1]. Tinnitus related changes of brain activity and connectivity (e.g. [2,3]) seem to reflect pathologically altered brain networks, which develops as a response to abnormal sensory input [4]. Based on these findings repetitive transcranial magnetic stimulation (rTMS) was introduced as a treatment approach in tinnitus [5].

In addition TMS can also be used as a diagnostic tool for the assessment of motor cortex excitability by quantifying contractions of peripheral muscles induced by stimulation of the corresponding motor cortex representation. Assessment of motor cortex excitability in a longitudinal study design before and after a specific therapeutic intervention (e.g. multiple sessions of rTMS) enables to describe treatment-related neuroplastic changes.

Several pilot studies suggest that tinnitus is related to alterations in motor cortex excitability. ICF was found to be enhanced in 19 patients with tinnitus in contrast to 19 controls [6] and CSP was found to be shortened (37 patients vs. 12 controls) [7]. However, it is not known whether these findings are state or trait parameters. They could either represent cross-modal plasticity like changes accompanying tinnitus, or unspecific general neural mechanisms reflecting individual predisposition factors for developing tinnitus.

Moreover it has been shown, that rTMS over the temporal cortex can induce changes in motor cortex excitability. Five days of active low-frequency rTMS over auditory cortex lead to prolongation of the CSP in 18 healthy subjects [8], whereas sham rTMS had not such effects. Clinical benefit of the same protocol in ten patients with tinnitus was positively correlated with changes in SICI, ICF, and CSP [9].

Here, we aimed to investigate in a retrospective analysis whether the observed alterations of cortical excitability can be replicated in a large sample of patients with tinnitus and controls. In order to address the open question whether such changes represent state or trait markers, we analysed longitudinal data before and after a therapeutic intervention.

Materials and Methods

Ethics Statement

All participants gave written informed consent after a comprehensive explanation of the procedures. All studies whose data contributed to this analysis were approved by the Ethics Committee at the University of Regensburg. All experiments were conducted in accordance with the last revision of the Declaration of Helsinki.

Subjects

Patients presenting with a phantom sound of at least two month duration were recruited and investigated at the Tinnitus center Regensburg (Germany) which is a collaboration of the Department of Otolaryngology and the Department of Psychiatry and Psychotherapy of the University Hospital of Regensburg (Germany). Measurements of cortical excitability were performed in 231 patients (172 (74.5%) males; 49.5±12.2 (20–83) years) with chronic tinnitus (duration 93±95 (2–476) months). 44 (19%) out of 208 patients reported a purely left-sided, 37 (16%) a purely right-sided tinnitus, and 127 (55%) patients described their tinnitus as bilateral or originating within the head. Tinnitus distress was assessed by the German version [10] of the Tinnitus questionnaire (TQ) [11]. TQ overall scores ranged from 3 to 79 (41±18). Patients suffering from Menière's disease, presenting conductive hearing loss or displaying hints of objective tinnitus were not included. 132 patients underwent a complete otologic and audiologic examination including pure tone audiometry, tympanometry, stapedius reflex tests, and otomicroscopy. For the other subjects no standardized audiometry data were available. Mean hearing level in the frequency range from 125 to 8000 Hz was 17±12 dB HL (0–61). As patients were measured in the context of clinical trials of rTMS only patients were included that were eligible for rTMS treatment. Thus, patients with cardiac pacemakers, history of seizures, suspected diagnosis of organic brain damage or any other severe somatic, neurologic, or psychiatric diagnosis were not included.

Healthy volunteers (n = 120; 57 (47.5%) males; age: 28.2±7.5 (19–55) years) were recruited through advertisements and by requesting the hospital staff. All healthy participants were free of medication and free of any mental disorder as verified during an interview by board-certified psychiatrists (B.L., E.F. and P.E.). Controls did significantly differ from patients with respect to age ($t = 17.5$; $df = 349$; $p<0.001$) and gender ($\eta^2 = 25.3$; $df = 1$; $p<0.001$).

Procedures

For measurement of cortical excitability, the participants were seated in a reclining chair. TMS was delivered by two Magstim 200 stimulators (Magstim Co., UK) connected via a Bistim module to a figure-of-eight coil (double-circular-70-mm coil). The coil was held tangential to the skull and with the handle pointing backwards and about 45° away from the midline. The optimal coil position for stimulation was defined as the position above the left motor cortex for eliciting MEPs of maximal amplitude in abductor digiti minimi muscle with a slightly supra-threshold stimulus. Once this position was found, it was marked on a scientific head cap and the coil was held in this position by the investigator.

MEPs of the abductor digiti minimi of the right hand were recorded with surface electrodes. The analogue signal was registered, band-pass filtered between 20 Hz and 10 kHz, then digitised at a frequency of 5 kHz and analysed off-line. The employed hardware setup required the analogue signal to be acquired with a band-pass filter between 20 Hz and 10 kHz and a digitization frequency of 5 kHz. Whereas these suboptimal filter settings yield the possibility of aliasing effects (according to the Nyquist theorem, a 2.5 kHz low pass filter should have been applied to the analogue signal), the small signal amplitudes for high frequencies render it unlikely that the recording setup may have biased or altered the present findings [12].

Resting and active motor threshold were determined according to Rossini and colleagues [13]. Resting motor threshold (RMT) was determined as the lowest stimulation intensity that evoked in at least four out of eight consecutive trials a MEP of at least 50 μV in the resting abductor digiti minimi. Active motor threshold was determined only for conduction of the double-pulse rTMS paradigms (ICI and ICF) and was not included in analysis due to high variability. Active motor threshold was defined as the lowest stimulation intensity that evoked in at least four out of eight consecutive trials a MEP of at least 250 μV during isometric contraction of the abductor digiti minimi at about 20% of maximum voluntary contraction. A constant level of voluntary contraction was maintained by audiovisual feedback of the electromyographic (EMG) activity. MEP amplitudes were measured peak-to-peak.

Short-interval intra-cortical inhibition and intracortical facilitation were measured with a paired-pulse TMS protocol [14]. The intensity of the first (conditioning) stimulus was set at 90% of the active motor threshold. The second (test) stimulus was delivered at an intensity that produced MEPs of about 1 mV in the resting abductor digiti minimi. Interstimulus intervals (ISIs) were 2 ms and 15 ms to measure short-interval intra-cortical inhibition (reduction of amplitude) and intracortical facilitation (increase of amplitude), respectively [14]. The conditioned stimuli and the control condition (test pulse alone) were each tested 10 times in a random order (inter-sweep-interval: 4 s). The effect of conditioning stimuli on MEP amplitude at each ISI was determined as the ratio of the average amplitude of conditioned MEP to the average amplitude of unconditioned test MEP.

Cortical silent period was measured in 10 trials (stimulus intensity: 150% resting motor threshold; inter-sweep-interval: 5 s) in the moderately active abductor digiti minimi muscle on the non-rectified recording of every individual sweep and then averaged [15]. Participants were instructed to contract this muscle at 30% maximum strength. A constant level of voluntary contraction was maintained by audiovisual feedback of the electromyographic (EMG) activity. The onset of the cortical silent period was defined as the end of the MEP when activity dropped consistently below pre-stimulus EMG level. The end of the cortical silent period was defined as first reappearance of voluntary EMG activity. In conclusion, TMS variables of interest were resting motor threshold (RMT), cMEP/uMEP ratio of 2 ms and 15 ms interstimulus intervals (SICI and ICF, respectively), and cortical silent period (CSP).

Study Procedures

The therapeutic intervention consisted of 10 rTMS sessions on consecutive weekdays. Treatment effects were evaluated by change in TQ between the first and the last day of treatment. Motor cortex excitability was examined on these days, too. We analyzed longitudinal data of 118 patients participating in three different treatments [16,17] and receiving three different active stimulation protocols (1000 stimuli over auditory cortex with 1 Hz: n = 76; 4000 stimuli over auditory cortex with 1 Hz: n = 26; 2000 stimuli over left frontal cortex with 20 Hz and 2000 stimuli over auditory cortex with 1 Hz: n = 23). 1 Hz stimulation was performed over the left auditory cortex. In single cases of positron emission guided stimulation the right auditory cortex was stimulated instead. Stimulation intensity was set to 110% RMT.

Statistics

Firstly, we were interested in differences in motor cortex excitability between patients with tinnitus and healthy controls. We contrasted both groups with two-sided Student t-tests. As groups were not comparable for age and gender, we also contrasted both groups with an analysis of variance (ANOVA) with group as between-subjects factor and age and gender as covariate (ANCOVA). As we included data from former studies [6,8,9] we controlled for this fact by including a dummy coded variable as third covariate. Data of 28 (11.1%) patients and 17 (14.2%) controls overlapped with former studies. To evaluate the role of hearing loss, we correlated mean hearing level for the left and right ear with measures of motor cortex excitability in a sub-group of 132 patients.

Secondly, we were interested if rTMS induced clinical amelioration was associated with changes in motor cortex excitability. Thus, we correlated changes/differences in the TQ with changes/differences in excitability parameters. This analysis would shed light on the question if tinnitus-related changes in motor cortex excitability represent state or trait markers of tinnitus. As three different treatments were included we were interested in the interrelationship of kind of treatment with correlations. Thus, we repeated the correlation analysis with partial correlations using kind of treatment as control variable.

As we had four variables of interest (RMT, SICI, ICF, and CSP), only p-values below a Bonferroni corrected significance level of 0.0125 (0.05/4 = 0.0125) were presented as significant. Statistical analyses were performed with SPSS 18.0.0 (SPSS, USA).

Results

Firstly, group contrasts of two big samples of patients with tinnitus (n = 231) and healthy controls (n = 120) revealed significant differences in short-interval intra-cortical inhibition (SICI), intra-cortical facilitation (ICF; with a statistical trend), and cortical silent period (CSP). Patients with tinnitus showed increased SICI (by definition, lower values of SICI correspond to enhanced inhibitory function), increased intra-cortical facilitation, and shortened cortical silent period (table 1). As groups differed with respect to age and gender and we included data from previous publications, we controlled for these potential confounders by ANCOVAs. Effects were still significant. We did not find significant effects for resting motor threshold (RMT). Correlations between hearing level and RMT (right: r = 0.015; p = 0.866; left: r = 0.076; p = 0.389), SICI (right: r = 0.136; p = 0.120; left: r = 0.103; p = 0.239), ICF (right: r = −0.139; p = 0.112; left: r = −0.116; p = 0.186), and CSP (right: r = −0.001; p = 0.993; left: r = 0.034; p = 0.701) were not significant.

Secondly, for a sub-group of patients (n = 118) data of motor cortex excitability were available at two different time points before and after a therapeutic intervention. Here we found that a change in tinnitus severity correlated significantly with changes in SICI, i.e., the higher the improvement the higher the decrease in SICI (r = 0.234; n = 116; p = 0.011). A scatter plot (figure 1) indicated three outliers with high SICIs (negative values of the abscissa). Excluding these patients from the analysis did also reveal a significant correlation (r = 0.188; n = 113; p = 0.046). There were no significant correlations of RMT (r = 0.062; n = 116; p = 0.509), ICF (r = 0.124; n = 116; p = 0.183), or CSP (r = 0.043; n = 115; p = 0.648). Partial correlations with kind of treatment as covariate indicates no systematic differences in results (RMT: r = 0.056; n = 112; p = 0.551; SICI: r = 0.237; n = 111; p = 0.011; ICF: r = 0.121; n = 111; p = 0.200; CSP: r = 0.04; n = 112; p = 0.640) which means that correlations were comparable for all three kind of treatments.

Discussion

Motor cortex excitability as measured by short-interval intra-cortical inhibition (SICI), intra-cortical facilitation (ICF), and cortical silent period (CSP) appeared to be altered in tinnitus patients (table 1). SICI and ICF were increased, and CSP was shortened. These findings confirm findings from previous studies that demonstrated increased ICF [6] and shortened CSP [7] in smaller samples of tinnitus patients.

SICI and CSP are measures for inhibitory and ICF of facilitatory processes in the motor system. Tinnitus is known to be related to neural changes along the auditory pathway emerging from a dysbalance of inhibitory and excitatory neurons [18]. Activity in the central auditory pathways is further modulated by inter-connected extra-auditory areas such as frontal regions as parts of "noise-cancellation" or top-down inhibition processes [3,19,20]. However in current pathophysiological models of tinnitus the motor system is not considered to be directly involved [4]. Notably the findings of abnormal motor cortex excitability [6,7] do not prove specific involvement of the motor cortex in tinnitus pathophysiology, since these findings may reflect global changes. On the other hand there are several hints for a possible involvement of the motor cortex in tinnitus. In primates the relevance of the motor system for auditory perception has been demonstrated repeatedly [21,22]. Moreover, electroencephalographic studies revealed alterations in oscillatory activity in the supplementary motor area related to different aspects of tinnitus [23].

Several confounding factors may potentially influence motor cortex excitability in tinnitus patients. First, the influence of hearing loss has to be considered as a confounding factor. Hearing loss results in sensory deprivation and is considered to be the most relevant risk factor for tinnitus. At the same time sensory

Table 1. Descriptive and statistical data of motor cortex excitability for the group contrasts.

	tinnitus	controls	t-test	ANCOVA#
resting motor threshold	43.21±7.84	43.50±7.53	t = 0.328; df = 346; p = 0.743; d = 0.037	t-test not significant
short-interval intra-cortical inhibition	0.47±0.37	0.58±0.30	t = 2.801; df = 349; p = 0.005; d = 0.316*	F = 3.202; df = 1,346; p = 0.009*
intra-cortical facilitation	1.47±0.78	1.29±0.37	t = 2.385; df = 349; p = 0.018; d = 0.269+	F = 3.400; df = 1,346; p = 0.010*
cortical silent period (s)	0.11±0.05	0.13±0.04	t = 4.612; df = 335; p < 0.001; d = 0.541*	F = 2.843; df = 1,332; p = 0.008*

*significant at a Bonferroni corrected threshold with p-values displayed uncorrected;
+near significant at a Bonferroni corrected threshold with p-values displayed uncorrected;
#indicates group effects of an ANCOVA (analysis of variance) with age, gender, and former analysis as covariate.

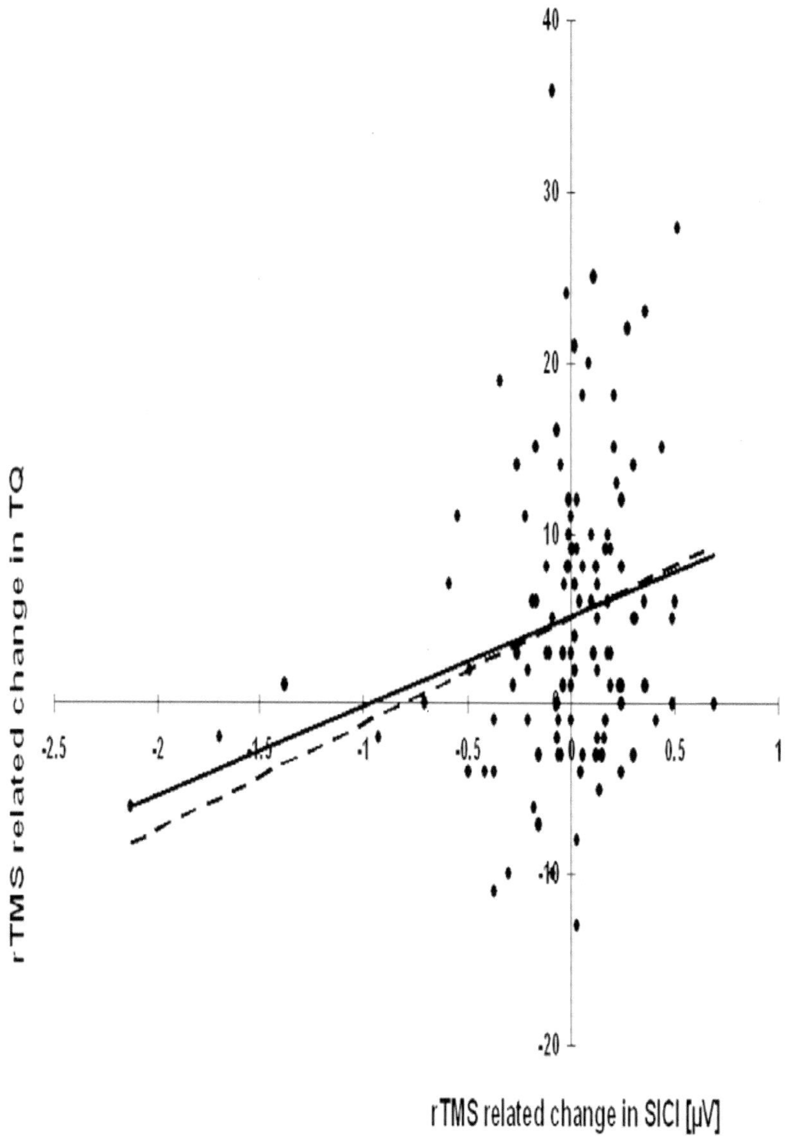

Figure 1. Scatter plot for the significant Pearson correlation between the repetitive transcranial magnetic stimulation (rTMS) induced change in short-interval intra-cortical inhibition (SICI) and rTMS induced change in tinnitus questionnaire (TQ) including the regression line for the whole sample (continuous line) and for the sample without the three outliers (dashed line).

deprivation may have a direct influence on motor cortex excitability. Increased ICF has been reported after experimental somatosensory deafferentiation [24] and in limb amputees [25,26]. Sensory deprivation in the auditory system could induce changes in the motor system via mechanisms of cross-modal plasticity (see below). In order to control for hearing loss we analysed the subsample for which audiometric data were available (132 patients; 57% of the whole sample). However, we did not find significant correlations between hearing level and motor cortex excitability. Other influencing factors might be co-morbid pain syndromes and the ability to influence the tinnitus percept by somatic manoeuvres [27]. This is more frequently the case in tinnitus patients with temporomandibular joint complaints [28,29]. Whether the ability to modulate tinnitus by somatic manoeuvres has an impact on motor cortex excitability could not be analysed in the present study, since these data were not available. Further limitations of this analysis are that we did not control for conditions which are known to interfere with motor cortex excitability and plasticity or with tinnitus or both. For example, mental diseases such as anxiety or affective disorders are known in tinnitus as co-morbid condition [30] but also in modulating motor cortex excitability [12]. The same is the case for medication (e.g., GABAergic drugs) which can interfere with TMS related measures [31] and tinnitus [32]. Insomnia [33] and also hyperacousis [34] also are closely related to tinnitus. With respect to insomnia it could be demonstrated that selective REM and complete night sleep deprivation is accompanied by changes in SICI [35,36]. Thus, further studies might control for this limitation by asking for hours of sleep per night. More generally, level of education/intelligence, sex [37], age [38], and TMS procedures such as differences in maximum voluntary contraction for AMT, stimulation intensity and ISI for SICI, no use of neuronavigation might also have influence on the presented findings. We statistically controlled the factors age and sex by redoing the group contrasts with ANCOVAs. Methodologically, future studies might try to control for these demographic factors by matching the groups with respect to these variables. TMS parameters generally should be reported in detail [39]. Thus, future studies should carefully control for these conditions.

Alterations of motor cortex excitability in a cross-sectional group comparison between tinnitus patients and controls could be either a consequence or a pre-condition of tinnitus or both. This could be evaluated by large-sampled prospective studies in non-tinnitus sufferers. Another approach for disentangling state and trait markers is to evaluate the influence of treatment effects. Here the cross-sectional comparison between tinnitus patients and controls was complemented by a longitudinal data analysis in order to identify to which extent the observed alterations of motor cortex excitability in tinnitus patients reflect an alteration of inhibitory-excitatory cortical processes predisposing for tinnitus, or a consequence of tinnitus.

By analysing longitudinal data before and after rTMS treatment we found a significant association of treatment-related change in TQ with change in SICI, i.e., the higher amelioration of symptoms the higher the decrease in inhibition (figure 1). Pending confirmation by further studies our findings suggest that the increase of SICI might display a state-like factor for tinnitus severity, whereas increased ICF and shortened CSP might display rather trait-like factors. Speculatively, increased ICF and shortened CSP may reflect neural hyper-excitability as a general risk factor for developing a hyper-excitability disorder such as tinnitus. The increased SICI in contrast might reflect a compensatory effort related to the severity of tinnitus.

Alternatively, the increased SICI may reflect a direct consequence of tinnitus. Neural changes in the auditory system could induce changes in the motor system via mechanisms of cross-modal plasticity. Functional imaging and transcranial magnetic stimulation studies suggest multisensory association areas as neural basis for cross-modal or multisensory integration. However, recent findings in synaesthesia - an example for the incorporation of one modality in two modalities - changed the focus of research from a single core region to network properties and connectivity [40]. Also primary visual and auditory areas were identified as synaesthesia relevant [41]. Another example for the cross-modal functioning of the brain is transfer of processes from a sensory system to a deprived sensory system, e.g., deaf people show active auditory cortex during visual stimulation [42,43]. Considered mechanisms may take place via multi-sensory association areas, via direct cortico-cortical connections, or via subcortical interplay of the corresponding sensory systems at the thalamic level [42]. In tinnitus and other neuropsychiatric disorders, the model of thalamo-cortical dysrhythmia considers altered thalamic activity due to faulty signals in afferent neurons as the core symptom. This altered thalamic activity in turn is generating altered cortical activity which again induces symptoms such as phantom perceptions [44]. The exact mechanism might be best evaluated by connectivity methodology in future studies; dynamic causal modelling would enable the modelling of the direction of information flow of assumed network hubs.

Our findings fit well to concepts and findings in tinnitus with respect to trans-synaptic chemical signalling. Inhibitory-excitatory dysbalance in tinnitus is considered to be related to altered activity of inhibitory-acting γ-aminobutyric acid (GABA) and excitatory-acting glutamate or *N*-methyl-d-aspartate (NMDA) [32]. Evidence comes from pharmacological treatments [32], animal models [45], and genetic analyses [46]. GABA and NMDA are also involved in motor cortex excitability and plasticity [31,47]. Based on our findings it is tempting to speculate that the identified "trait-markers" *increased ICF* and *shortened CSP* reflect globally increased glutamatergic and reduced GABA-B transmission, respectively. Support for this theory comes from a recent genetic study providing preliminary evidence for a role of genetic variations of the GABA-B receptor in the pathophysiology of tinnitus [46].

In conclusion, present data show that tinnitus is accompanied by excitability and plasticity changes in the motor cortex. This finding sheds light on neglected areas in tinnitus research and highlights the inter-connectedness of the brain.

Acknowledgments

The authors wish to thank Sandra Pfluegl and Helene Niebling for technical assistance.

Author Contributions

Conceived and designed the experiments: ML TK EF PGS PE GH BL. Performed the experiments: ML EF PGS PE BL. Analyzed the data: MS BL. Contributed reagents/materials/analysis tools: TK RR PGS PE GH BL. Wrote the paper: MS ML TK PE GH BL.

References

1. Adjamian P, Sereda M, Hall DA (2009) The mechanisms of tinnitus: perspectives from human functional neuroimaging. Hear Res 253: 15–31.
2. Maudoux A, Lefebvre P, Cabay JE, Demertzi A, Vanhaudenhuyse A, et al. (2012) Auditory resting-state network connectivity in tinnitus: a functional MRI study. PLoS One 7: e36222.
3. Schlee W, Hartmann T, Langguth B, Weisz N (2009) Abnormal resting-state cortical coupling in chronic tinnitus. BMC Neurosci 10: 11.
4. De Ridder D, Elgoyhen AB, Romo R, Langguth B (2011) Phantom percepts: tinnitus and pain as persisting aversive memory networks. Proc Natl Acad Sci U S A 108: 8075–8080.
5. Langguth B, Schecklmann M, Lehner A, Landgrebe M, Poeppl TB, et al. (2012) Neuroimaging and neuromodulation: complementary approaches for identifying the neuronal correlates of tinnitus. Front Syst Neurosci 6: 15.
6. Langguth B, Eichhammer P, Zowe M, Kleinjung T, Jacob P, et al. (2005) Altered motor cortex excitability in tinnitus patients: a hint at crossmodal plasticity. Neurosci Lett 380: 326–329.
7. Khedr EM, Rothwell JC, Ahmed MA, Awad EM, Galal O (2008) Cortical excitability and transcallosal inhibition in chronic tinnitus: transcranial magnetic study. Neurophysiol Clin 38: 243–248.
8. Eichhammer P, Kleinjung T, Landgrebe M, Hajak G, Langguth B (2007) TMS for treatment of chronic tinnitus: neurobiological effects. Prog Brain Res 166: 369–375.
9. Langguth B, Kleinjung T, Marienhagen J, Binder H, Sand PG, et al. (2007) Transcranial magnetic stimulation for the treatment of tinnitus: effects on cortical excitability. BMC Neurosci 8: 45.
10. Göbel G, Hiller W (1994) [The tinnitus questionnaire. A standard instrument for grading the degree of tinnitus. Results of a multicenter study with the tinnitus questionnaire]. HNO 42: 166–172.
11. Hallam RS, Jakes SC, Hinchcliffe R (1988) Cognitive variables in tinnitus annoyance. Br J Clin Psychol 27 (Pt 3): 213–222.
12. Schecklmann M, Landgrebe M, Frank E, Sand PG, Eichhammer P, et al. (2012) Is motor cortex excitability associated with personality factors? A replication study. Int J Psychophysiol 83: 323–327.
13. Rossini PM, Barker AT, Berardelli A, Caramia MD, Caruso G, et al. (1994) Non-invasive electrical and magnetic stimulation of the brain, spinal cord and roots: basic principles and procedures for routine clinical application. Report of an IFCN committee. Electroencephalogr Clin Neurophysiol 91: 79–92.
14. Kujirai T, Caramia MD, Rothwell JC, Day BL, Thompson PD, et al. (1993) Corticocortical inhibition in human motor cortex. J Physiol 471: 501–519.
15. Wolters A, Ziemann U, Benecke R (2008) The cortical silent period. In: Wasserman EM, Epstein CM, Ziemann U, Walsh V, Paus T et al., editors. The Oxford Handbook of Transcranial Stimulation. Oxford: University Press.
16. Lehner A, Schecklmann M, Landgrebe M, Kreuzer PM, Poeppl TB, et al. (2012) Predictors for rTMS response in chronic tinnitus. Front Syst Neurosci 6: 11.
17. Langguth B, Landgrebe M, Frank E, Schecklmann M, Sand PG, et al. (2012) Efficacy of different protocols of transcranial magnetic stimulation for the treatment of tinnitus: Pooled analysis of two randomized controlled studies. World J Biol Psychiatry.

18. Eggermont JJ, Roberts LE (2004) The neuroscience of tinnitus. Trends Neurosci 27: 676–682.
19. Rauschecker JP, Leaver AM, Muhlau M (2010) Tuning out the noise: limbic-auditory interactions in tinnitus. Neuron 66: 819–826.
20. Schecklmann M, Landgrebe M, Poeppl TB, Kreuzer P, Manner P, et al. (2013) Neural correlates of tinnitus duration and Distress: A positron emission tomography study. Hum Brain Mapp 34: 233–240.
21. Graziano MS, Reiss LA, Gross CG (1999) A neuronal representation of the location of nearby sounds. Nature 397: 428–430.
22. Lemus L, Hernandez A, Romo R (2009) Neural encoding of auditory discrimination in ventral premotor cortex. Proc Natl Acad Sci U S A 106: 14640–14645.
23. Vanneste S, De Ridder D (2012) The auditory and non-auditory brain areas involved in tinnitus. An emergent property of multiple parallel overlapping subnetworks. Front Syst Neurosci 6: 31.
24. Ziemann U, Hallett M, Cohen LG (1998) Mechanisms of deafferentation-induced plasticity in human motor cortex. J Neurosci 18: 7000–7007.
25. Chen R, Corwell B, Yaseen Z, Hallett M, Cohen LG (1998) Mechanisms of cortical reorganization in lower-limb amputees. J Neurosci 18: 3443–3450.
26. Schwenkreis P, Witscher K, Janssen F, Dertwinkel R, Zenz M, et al. (2000) Changes of cortical excitability in patients with upper limb amputation. Neurosci Lett 293: 143–146.
27. Sanchez TG, Rocha CB (2011) Diagnosis and management of somatosensory tinnitus: review article. Clinics (Sao Paulo) 66: 1089–1094.
28. Vielsmeier V, Strutz J, Kleinjung T, Schecklmann M, Kreuzer PM, et al. (2012) Temporomandibular joint disorder complaints in tinnitus: further hints for a putative tinnitus subtype. PLoS One 7: e38887.
29. Vielsmeier V, Kleinjung T, Strutz J, Burgers R, Kreuzer PM, et al. (2011) Tinnitus with temporomandibular joint disorders: a specific entity of tinnitus patients? Otolaryngol Head Neck Surg 145: 748–752.
30. Zoger S, Svedlund J, Holgers KM (2006) Relationship between tinnitus severity and psychiatric disorders. Psychosomatics 47: 282–288.
31. Ziemann U (2004) TMS and drugs. Clin Neurophysiol 115: 1717–1729.
32. Salvi R, Lobarinas E, Sun W (2009) Pharmacological Treatments for Tinnitus: New and Old. Drugs Future 34: 381–400.
33. Cronlein T, Langguth B, Geisler P, Hajak G (2007) Tinnitus and insomnia. Prog Brain Res 166: 227–233.
34. Baguley DM (2003) Hyperacusis. J R Soc Med 96: 582–585.
35. Kreuzer P, Langguth B, Popp R, Raster R, Busch V, et al. (2011) Reduced intra-cortical inhibition after sleep deprivation: a transcranial magnetic stimulation study. Neurosci Lett 493: 63–66.
36. Placidi F, Zannino S, Albanese M, Romigi A, Izzi F, et al. (2013) Increased cortical excitability after selective REM sleep deprivation in healthy humans: a transcranial magnetic stimulation study. Sleep Med 14: 288–292.
37. De Gennaro L, Bertini M, Pauri F, Cristiani R, Curcio G, et al. (2004) Callosal effects of transcranial magnetic stimulation (TMS): the influence of gender and stimulus parameters. Neurosci Res 48: 129–137.
38. Petitjean M, Ko JY (2013) An age-related change in the ipsilateral silent period of a small hand muscle. Clin Neurophysiol 124: 346–353.
39. Chipchase L, Schabrun S, Cohen L, Hodges P, Ridding M, et al. (2012) A checklist for assessing the methodological quality of studies using transcranial magnetic stimulation to study the motor system: an international consensus study. Clin Neurophysiol 123: 1698–1704.
40. Rothen N, Terhune DB (2012) Increased resting state network connectivity in synesthesia: evidence for a neural basis of synesthetic consistency. J Neurosci 32: 13641–13643.
41. Dovern A, Fink GR, Fromme AC, Wohlschlager AM, Weiss PH, et al. (2012) Intrinsic network connectivity reflects consistency of synesthetic experiences. J Neurosci 32: 7614–7621.
42. Bavelier D, Neville HJ (2002) Cross-modal plasticity: where and how? Nat Rev Neurosci 3: 443–452.
43. Merabet LB, Pascual-Leone A (2010) Neural reorganization following sensory loss: the opportunity of change. Nat Rev Neurosci 11: 44–52.
44. Llinas RR, Ribary U, Jeanmonod D, Kronberg E, Mitra PP (1999) Thalamocortical dysrhythmia: A neurological and neuropsychiatric syndrome characterized by magnetoencephalography. Proc Natl Acad Sci U S A 96: 15222–15227.
45. Guitton MJ, Dudai Y (2007) Blockade of cochlear NMDA receptors prevents long-term tinnitus during a brief consolidation window after acoustic trauma. Neural Plast 2007: 80904.
46. Sand PG, Langguth B, Itzhacki J, Bauer A, Geis S, et al. (2012) Resequencing of the auxiliary GABA(B) receptor subunit gene KCTD12 in chronic tinnitus. Front Syst Neurosci 6: 41.
47. Ziemann U, Meintzschel F, Korchounov A, Ilic TV (2006) Pharmacological modulation of plasticity in the human motor cortex. Neurorehabil Neural Repair 20: 243–251.

Effects of Temperature on Auditory Sensitivity in Eurythermal Fishes: Common Carp *Cyprinus carpio* (Family Cyprinidae) versus Wels Catfish *Silurus glanis* (Family Siluridae)

Isabelle Pia Maiditsch, Friedrich Ladich*

Department of Behavioural Biology, University of Vienna, Vienna, Austria

Abstract

Background: In ectothermal animals such as fish, -temperature affects physiological and metabolic processes. This includes sensory organs such as the auditory system. The reported effects of temperature on hearing in eurythermal otophysines are contradictory. We therefore investigated the effect on the auditory system in species representing two different orders.

Methodology/Principal Findings: Hearing sensitivity was determined using the auditory evoked potentials (AEP) recording technique. Auditory sensitivity and latency in response to clicks were measured in the common carp *Cyprinus carpio* (order Cypriniformes) and the Wels catfish *Silurus glanis* (order Siluriformes) after acclimating fish for at least three weeks to two different water temperatures (15°C, 25°C and again 15°C). Hearing sensitivity increased with temperature in both species. Best hearing was detected between 0.3 and 1 kHz at both temperatures. The maximum increase occurred at 0.8 kHz (7.8 dB) in *C. carpio* and at 0.5 kHz (10.3 dB) in *S. glanis*. The improvement differed between species and was in particular more pronounced in the catfish at 4 kHz. The latency in response to single clicks was measured from the onset of the sound stimulus to the most constant positive peak of the AEP. The latency decreased at the higher temperature in both species by 0.37 ms on average.

Conclusions/Significance: The current study shows that higher temperature improves hearing (lower thresholds, shorter latencies) in eurythermal species from different orders of otophysines. Differences in threshold shifts between eurythermal species seem to reflect differences in absolute sensitivity at higher frequencies and they furthermore indicate differences to stenothermal (tropical) species.

Editor: Jacob Engelmann, Universitat Bielefeld, Germany

Competing Interests: The authors have declared that no competing interests exist.

* Email: friedrich.ladich@univie.ac.at

Introduction

Physiological and metabolic processes of ectothermal animals are affected in any environment that is characterized by major and rapid temperature changes. Many fish species occur in habitats in which the water temperature changes either quickly such as in shallow waters or slowly or not at all such as in oceans or deep lakes. Fishes can also experience rapid temperature changes when moving to different water depths, or slower changes with season, during which the acclimation time is longer [1,2]. Ambient temperature affects the speed of metabolic and physiological processes such as respiration, the immune system or growth [3,4,5]. Furthermore, temperature affects the behaviour including the locomotory activity [1,6,7].

Ambient temperature is also known to affect the sensitivity of sensory systems such as the lateral line [8] and the auditory system. Influences of temperature on the auditory system have been studied in many ectothermal taxa such as insects [9,10] amphibians [11,12,13] and reptiles [14,15]. In general, a decrease in body temperature results in a decline in auditory sensitivity.

Fish rely on sound production and hearing for orientation, intraspecific communication or prey and predator detection [16,17,18,19,20]. A few studies described influences of ambient temperature on sound characteristics and hearing sensitivity in fish. The sound duration and the fundamental frequency tend to increase with temperature, whereas the pulse period decreased [21,22,23,24,25,26].

Dudok van Heel [27] observed that the detectable frequency range broadened with increasing temperature in the European minnow *Phoxinus phoxinus*. Fay and Ream [28] showed that higher temperature boosts the spontaneous activity and sensitivity in the auditory neuron of the goldfish *Carassius auratus*. Auditory sensitivity decreased at lower temperature within hours in the walleye pollock *Theragra chalcogramma* [29]. Among catfishes, Wysocki et al. [2] investigated the effects of temperature on hearing in the eurythermal channel catfish *Ictalurus punctatus* and the stenothermal pictus catfish *Pimelodus pictus*, and Papes and Ladich [26] conducted similar experiments on the Striped Raphael Catfish *Platydoras armatulus*Interestingly, thresholds shifts seem to be more pronounced in the eury- than in the stenothermal catfish species from the Amazonian river system.

Temperatures affect hearing thresholds as well as the resolution of temporal patterns of acoustic information in ectothermal animals. Interpeak latencies increased in anurans when the temperature dropped below 20°C [30]. The influence of ambient water temperature on temporal processing and latencies in fish has been demonstrated by Papes and Ladich [26] in the thorny catfish *P. armatulus*. Wysocki and Ladich [31] showed that representatives of several fish families were able to detect pulse periods of less than 2 ms. This ability enables fish to detect the temporal resolution of conspecific sounds [32,33].

The goal of this study was to investigate the effect of ambient temperature on the auditory system of two eurythermal species representing different otophysan orders. It was designed to answer the questions how eurythermal species are affected by temperature and how this differs compared to stenothermal (tropical) species. The Common carp *Cyprinus carpio* (order Cyrpiniformes)and the Wels catfish *Silurus glanis* (order Siluriformes) were chosen because they represent two different orders and because they possess improved hearing abilities (due to peripheral hearing structures), which are more likely affected by temperature changes [2]. Both species inhabit freshwaters in Eurasia and can survive under a wide range of temperatures from 0°C to 30°C [34,35,36,37]. We also investigated the change in latencies in response to single-click stimuli and thus temporal processing of acoustic signals in both species at different temperatures.

Materials and Methods

Ethics statement

Experiments were performed with permission of the Austrian Federal Ministry of Science and Research (GZ 66.006/0023-II/10b/2008).

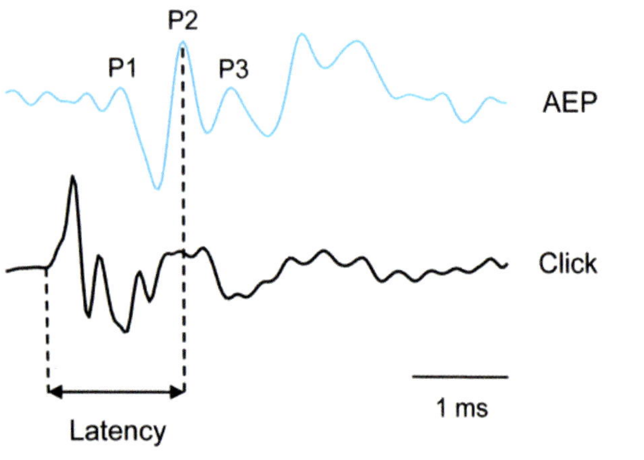

Figure 1. Oscillograms of an AEP and a click stimulus. AEP of a *S. glanis* in response to the click stimulus presented 28 dB above hearing threshold. The first, second and third positive peak (P1, P2, P3) are labelled. The double-headed arrow indicates the latency measured from the onset of the click stimulus to the second positive peak (P2).

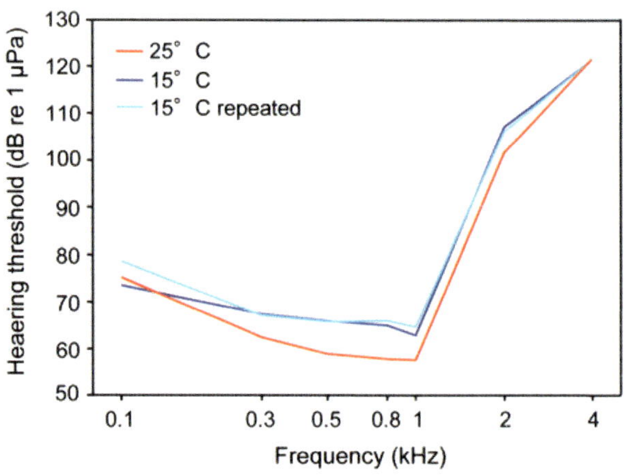

Figure 2. Auditory evoked potential audiogram at 15°C and 25°C. Mean hearing thresholds of *C. carpio* kept 15°C, 25°C and 15°C repeated. N = 9.

Animals

Nine Common carps, *Cyprinus carpio* Linnaeus 1758 [11.3–12.8 cm standard length (SL) 40–64 g body mass (BM)] and eight Wels catfish, *Silurus glanis* Linnaeus 1758 [23.0–30.6 cm SL, 103–211 g BM] were used for his study. *S. glanis* were obtained from a fish hatchery (Fischzucht Pottenbrunn, Pottenbrunn, Austria), *C. carpio* from a private fish pond near Vienna.

Fish were kept in glass tanks (110×55×30 cm or 100×50×50 cm) with a sand bottom equipped with plastic tubes, roots and artificial plants. External filters were used and a 12 h: 12 h L:D cycle was maintained. *S. glanis* were fed frozen food (chironomid larvae) and *C. carpio* were fed commercially prepared food (Tetra Pond; www.tetra-fish.com) as well as frozen food (chironomid larvae). The baseline temperature was 20±1°C.

The fishes were acclimated to the baseline temperature (20°C) for more than one month before experiments started. The temperature in the holding tanks was controlled using a cooling system (Hailea HC-300A and HC-130A; Guangdong Heilea Group CO., Ltd.) and submersible heaters. Temperature was controlled daily. The temperature of the holding water was changed at a rate of 1°C per day until the test temperature of 15°C or 25°C was reached. Fish had an acclimation time of at least three weeks to each experimental temperature before hearing measurements started. First, fish were acclimated and measured at 15°C, followed by 25°C and finally again at 15°C for control purposes. Fish had more than three weeks rest after each hearing test.

At each water temperature the audiograms of eight *S. glanis* and nine *C. carpio* were measured. In *S. glanis*, individuals were recognized based on different colour patterns. Individuals of *C. carpio* were marked on their fins.

Auditory sensitivity measurements

Auditory sensitivity was measured using the auditory evoked potential (AEP) recording technique [38,39,40].

The test subjects were immobilized during the hearing test using Flaxedil (gallamine triethiodide; Sigma-Aldrich, Vienna, Austria). The dosage used was 9–24 µg g^{-1} for *S. glanis* and 4–7 µg g^{-1} for *C. carpio* and allowed the fish to breath during the experiment. A respiration pipette was inserted into the animals' mouth. Respiration was achieved by a temperature-controlled gravity-fed circulation system.

Table 1. Mean (± S.E.) hearing thresholds of *C. carpio* measured at 15°C, 25°C and 15°C repeated. N = 9.

Frequency kHz	15°C dB re 1 μPa	25°C dB re 1 μPa	15°C repeated dB re 1 μPa
0.1	73.4±1.3	75.1±1.1	78.7±1.3
0.3	67.3±1.0	62.3±1.2	67.1±1.1
0.5	65.9±0.9	58.8±1.1	65.8±0.6
0.8	64.9±1.1	57.7±1.6	66±1.2
1	62.8±1.3	57.4±0.6	64.7±0.7
2	107±2.0	101.4±1.7	106±1.1
4	121.2±1.3	121.3±0.7	121.2±0.5

The fish were secured in a plastic tub (45×35 cm; 18 cm height). The bottom was covered with fine sand. The temperature was maintained at either 15±1°C or 25±1°C using cooling packs or a submersible heater. The fish's head was positioned just below the water surface. The plastic tub was positioned on an air table (TCM Micro-g 63-540), which rested on a vibration-isolated concrete plate. The entire setup was enclosed in a soundproof room constructed as a Faraday cage (interior dimensions: 3.2×3.2×2.4 m).

For AEP recordings, silver electrodes (0.32 mm diameter) were placed in the midline of the skull. The recording electrode was positioned over the region of the medulla and the reference electrode cranially between the nares; both were pressed firmly against the skin, which was covered with a small piece of Kimwipes tissue paper to keep it moist, in order to ensure proper contact during experiments. Shielded electrodes leads were attached to the differential input of a preamplifier (Grass P-55, Grass Instruments, West Warwick, RI, USA; gain 10,000x, high-pass at 30 Hz, low-pass at 1 kHz). A ground electrode was placed in the water. Stimuli presentation and AEP-waveform recording were specified using a modular rackmount system (TDT System 3, Tucker-Davis Technologies, Gainesville, FL, USA) running TDT BioSig RP Software.

Sound stimuli

Sound stimuli were generated using TDT SigGen RP software and fed through a power amplifier (Alesis RA 300, Alesis Corporation, Los Angeles, CA, USA) to a dual-cone speaker (Tannoy System 600, frequency response 50 Hz to 15 kHz±3 dB), which was placed 1 m above the tub. Sound stimuli were presented as tone bursts at a repetition rate of 21 per second.

Hearing thresholds were determined at frequencies of 0.1, 0.3, 0.5, 0.8, 1, 2 and 4 kHz, presented in random order. Rise and fall times were one cycle at 0.1 and 0.2 kHz, and two cycles at all other frequencies. All bursts were gated using a Blackman window. The stimuli were presented at opposite polarities (180° phase shifted) for each test condition and the corresponding AEPs were averaged by the BioSig RP software in order to eliminate stimulus artefacts. The sound pressure level (SPL) of tone-burst stimuli was reduced in 4 dB steps until the AEP waveform was no longer apparent. The lowest SPL for which a repeatable AEP trace could be obtained, which was determined by overlaying replicate traces, was considered the threshold. A hydrophone (Brüel & Kjaer 8101) was positioned near the right side of each fish (2 cm apart) to determine absolute SPLs values underwater close to the subjects. The absolute SPL was determined by analyzing the hydrophone recording at the threshold. Using Bio-Sig RP, the RMS voltage of the largest (i.e., center) sinusoid of a particular tone-burst recording was determined. This RMS voltage was then used to calculate the absolute SPL re 1 μPa based on the sensitivity of the hydrophone and the amplification factor of the hydrophone amplifier and of the TDT system.

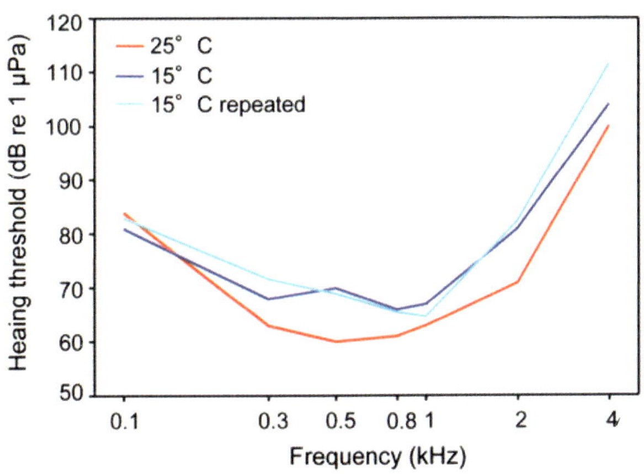

Figure 3. Auditory evoked potential audiogram at 15°C and 25°C. Mean hearing thresholds of *S. glanis* kept at 15°C, 25°C and 15°C repeated. N = 8.

Latency measurements

Latency measurements followed the method described by Wysocki and Ladich [31] and Papes and Ladich [26]. AEPs in response to a single click consisted of a series of negative and positive deflections. The positive AEP peaks were denominated with P for positive peaks (directed upwards) by ascending numbers. The latency was defined as time between the onset of the click stimulus and the most constant prominent peak of the AEP (P2) found in responses to this click stimulus in all individuals (Fig. 1).

The single click was presented 28 dB above hearing threshold in both species. Clicks were generated and presented using the TDT SigGen RP software. They were fed through a RP 2.1 realtime processor, a PA5 programmable attenuator, and a power amplifier (Alesis RA 300) to the air speaker (Tannoy System 600). Single clicks were presented to the animals at a repetition rate of 35 per second.

Statistical Analyses

All data were tested for normal distribution using the Kolmogorov-Smirnov-test, and when data were normally distributed, parametric statistical tests were applied. Audiograms obtained at three temperatures (15°C, 25°C and 15°C repeated)

Table 2. Mean (± S.E.) hearing thresholds of *S. glanis* measured at 15°C, 25°C and 15°C repeated. N = 8.

Frequency kHz	15°C dB re 1 μPa	25°C dB re 1 μPa	15°C repeated dB re 1 μPa
0.1	81.4±1.8	83.9±1.3	83±1.6
0.3	67.9±1.9	62.9±0.8	71.8±0.9
0.5	70.4±2.3	60±0.7	69±0.6
0.8	65.9±1.6	60.9±1.3	65.5±0.7
1	66.9±1.7	62.5±1.3	64.8±0.5
2	80.9±1.6	71.4±2.3	82.5±1.2
4	104±1.1	100.4±1.7	111.5±1.4

were compared by a two-factorial analysis of variance (ANOVA) using a general linear model where one factor was temperature and the other was frequency. The temperature factor alone should indicate overall differences in sensitivity between temperatures (and in combination with the frequency factor if different tendencies exist at different frequencies of the audiogram)s. A repeated measures ANOVA followed by a Bonferroni post hoc tests was calculated to determine differences between thresholds at each frequency. Differences between latencies were calculated using a Friedman-test followed by a Wilcoxon test. All statistical tests were run using SPSS 17.0. The significance level was set at $p \leq 0.05$.

Results

Auditory sensitivities

Cyprinus carpio. Hearing curves showed best hearing between 0.3 and 1 kHz at both temperatures and a rapid decline towards higher frequencies. A two-factorial ANOVA revealed that the auditory sensitivity was significantly lower at 15°C ($F_{2,168} = 36.9$, $p \leq 0.001$) and that there was a significant interaction between temperature and frequency ($F_{12,168} = 3.05$, $p \leq 0.001$). Thus, changes in auditory sensitivity showed different trends at different frequencies (Table 1, Fig. 2). A Bonferroni post-hoc test showed no significant difference between both 15°C audiograms, but significance between both 15°C and 25°C (15°C vs. 25°C: $p \leq 0.001$; 25°C vs. 15°C repeated: $p \leq 0.001$; 15°C vs. 15°C repeated: n.s.).

Silurus glanis. Hearing sensitivity curves showed best hearing between 0.3 and 1 kHz and a decline towards 4 kHz. Auditory sensitivities were significantly lower at the lower temperatures, as revealed by a two-factorial ANOVA ($F_{2,176} = 346.6$, $p < 0.001$), and there was a significant interaction between temperature and frequency ($F_{7,176} = 4.313$, $p \leq 0.001$). Therefore, changes in auditory sensitivity showed different trends at different frequencies (Table 2, Fig. 3).

Catfish had better hearing sensitivity at the higher temperature, especially above 300 Hz (Fig. 3). A Bonferroni post-hoc test showed a significant difference between 25°C and both 15°C audiograms but no difference between both 15°C audiograms (15°C vs. 25°C: $p \leq 0.001$; 25°C vs. 15°C repeated: $p \leq 0.001$; 15°C vs. 15°C repeated: n.s.).

Comparison between *C. carpio* and *S. glanis*. Both *C. carpio* and *S. glanis* showed no change in sensitivity at the lowest frequency measured (100 Hz) when the temperature increased from 15°C to 25°C (Repeated measures ANOVA). A significant increase was found at higher frequencies except for 4 kHz in the carp. In *C. carpio* the main change in sensitivity was observed between 0.3 and 2 kHz, whereas in the *S. glanis* changes of more than 5 dB were found up to 4 kHz (Table 3). The maximum increase occurred at 0.8 kHz (7.8 dB) in *C. carpio* and at 0.5 kHz (10.3 dB) in *S. glanis*.

A two-factorial ANOVA revealed that the improvement in hearing differed between the two species ($F_{1,105} = 6.35$, $p < 0.05$) and that there was an interaction between the difference and the frequency ($F_{6,105} = 6.72$, $p < 0.001$). Hearing sensitivity improved to a higher degree in *C. carpio* at 1 and in *S. glanis* at 2 and 4 kHz (Table 3).

Latencies in response to single clicks

Cyprinus carpio. AEP waveforms of *C. carpio* in response to a single-clicks consisted of a series of positive and negative

Table 3. Mean differences in hearing sensitivity of *C. carpio* and *S. glanis*, between the two tested temperatures (mean of 15°C and 15°C repeated) and 25°C.

Frequency kHz	*S. glanis* dB	*C. carpio* dB	Difference dB
0.1	1.7	0.9	0.8
0.3	6.9	4.9	2
0.5	9.7	7.1	2.6
0.8	4.8	7.8	−3
1	3.4	6.3	−2.9 *
2	10.3	5.1	5.2 *
4	7.4	0.1	7.3 *

The last column gives the difference in threshold changes between *S. glanis* and *C. carpio*. Asterisks indicate significant differences between species.

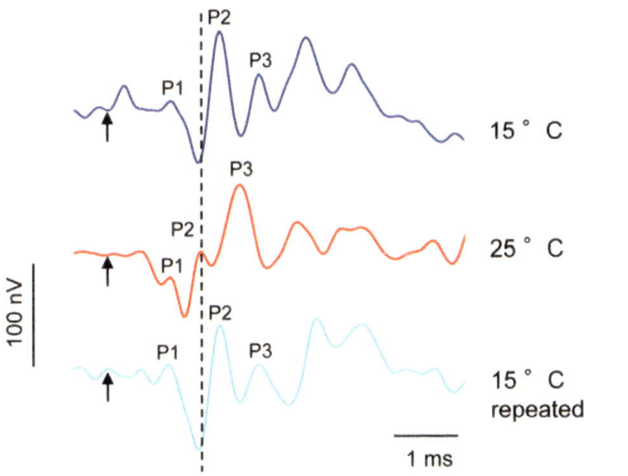

Figure 4. AEPs of one specimen of *C. carpio* in response to a single-click stimulus. Click stimulus presented 28 dB above hearing thresholds at both temperatures. Arrows indicate onset. The vertical dashed line indicates the position of the P2 peak at 25°C relative to the P2 peak at 15°C and 15°C repeated.

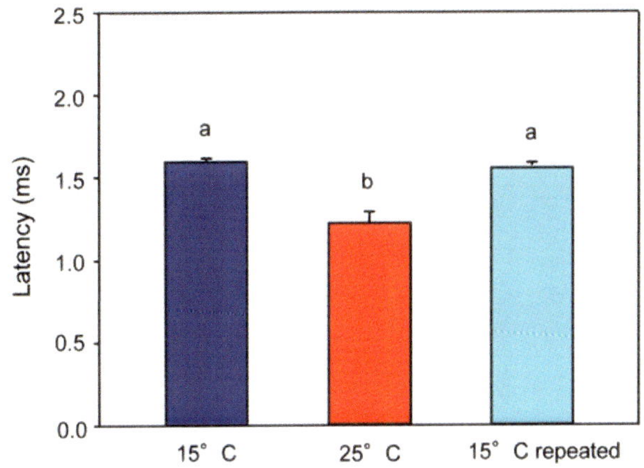

Figure 5. Latency between the onset of the click and the second positive peak. Mean (+ S.E.) latency of *C. carpio* kept at 15°C, 25°C and 15°C repeated. N = 9. Different letters (a, b) indicate significant differences between temperatures ($p \leq 0.05$).

deflections. AEPs started with a positive peak, followed by a negative peak at all three tested temperatures (Fig. 4). In this study, the main constant positive peak (P2) of the AEPs was analyzed.

The latency between the onset of the single-click stimulus and P2 differed between temperatures in *C. carpio* (Friedman test: $\chi^2 = 10.34$, df = 2, $p \leq 0.01$). Wilcoxon tests showed that the delay in the onset of P2 was significantly longer at lower temperature and that there was no significant difference between latencies in both 15°C tests (15°C vs. 25°C: $p \leq 0.05$; 25°C vs. 15°C repeated: $p \leq 0.05$; 15°C vs. 15°C repeated: n.s.) (Table 4, Fig. 5).

Silurus glanis. In *S. glanis*, similar to *C. carpio*, the AEP in response to a single-click stimulus consisted of a series of positive and negative peaks (Fig. 6). The delay between the onset of the single-click stimulus and the first constant prominent peak (P2) was similar in both 15°C tests and shorter at 25°C (Friedman test: $\chi^2 = 7.45$, df = 2, $p \leq 0.05$). A Wilcoxon test showed that the delay in the onset of P2 was significantly longer at lower temperature and that there was no significant difference between both 15°C measurements (15°C vs. 25°C: $p \leq 0.05$; 25°C vs. 15°C repeated: $p \leq 0.05$; 15°C vs. 15°C repeated: n.s.) (Table 4, Fig. 7).

Discussion

Hearing sensitivity in *C. carpio* as well as *S. glanis* is significantly higher at higher water temperatures, but the change in sensitivity differs between species. Temperature dependence of hearing sensitivity has been described in ectothermal animals besides fish such as in insects, amphibians and reptiles. In insects, the most sensitive hearing frequency, the spike rate and sensitivity increases [9,41,42]. Similar increases in hearing capability with temperature were shown in amphibians [11,43] and reptiles [44].

Effects of ambient temperature on the auditory system have been shown in several fish species [2,26,27,29], but the results of these studies vary. Dudok van Heel [27] showed that the detectable frequency range became wider in the European minnow, but he did not mention any change in absolute sensitivity. At higher temperature, the upper limit of frequency discrimination shifted in the minnow from 1200 Hz up to 1600 Hz. In a single specimen of the walleye pollock (*Theragra chalcogramma*), the hearing thresholds decreased by 8 dB at 350 Hz when temperature rose by 8° [29]. No acclimation periods were reported in the prior studies. Detailed studies involving at least three-week acclimation periods to different temperatures have only been conducted in otophysines so far.

Temperature effects on hearing sensitivity in eurythermal fish

Prior to this study, temperature effects on auditory sensitivity have been studied in detail in only one eurythermal fish. Eurythermal species can tolerate major changes in ambient water temperature. Wysocki et al. [2] observed major shifts in hearing thresholds in the North American channel catfish *I. punctatus* after acclimation to different temperatures. Changes in hearing sensitivity occurred especially at higher frequencies. Auditory sensitivity increased by 36 dB at 4 kHz when the temperature was raised from 10°C to 26°C. Here we compare the changes in sensitivity observed between 18°C and 26°C in *I. punctatus*, with those found in the present study in *C. carpio* und *S. glanis* between 15°C and 25°C. The two eurythermal catfish species studied, namely the channel catfish [2] and the European wels, showed a frequency-dependent increase in hearing sensitivity with increasing temperature. This trend was more pronounced in *I. punctatus*, whose sensitivity increased by 23 dB at 4 kHz (versus only 7 dB in *S. glanis*) (Fig. 8).

Interestingly, the temperature-dependent increase in sensitivity differed between both catfish species and the cypriniform, especially at 4 kHz. This points to major differences between otophysine families and orders. In fact *C. carpio* is less sensitive at 4 kHz than both catfish species with large unpaired swim bladders (25°C: 121 dB in *C. carpio* versus 100 dB in *S. glanis* and 81 dB in *I. punctatus*) [2]. The low sensitivity of *C. carpio* at 4 kHz is apparently unaffected by temperature. Moreover, the high sensitivity of *I. punctatus* at 4 kHz is affected much more than the lower sensitivity in *S. glanis* (23 dB change versus 7 dB). Thus, the differences in threshold shifts between eurythermal otophysines probably reflects the difference in the absolute sensitivity at higher frequencies.

Changes in ambient water temperature affect the auditory system of all eurythermal species investigated so far, although the degree of the sensitivity change differs considerably between species. Wysocki et al. [2] expected small changes in hearing in eurythermal fish species because they are adapted to a wide range

Table 4. Mean (± S.E.) latency of the second positive peaks (P2) of *C. carpio* and *S. glanis* measured at 15°C, 25°C and 15°C repeated calculated as the time period between the onset of a single click stimulus and the second positive peak.

Temperature	Latency (ms) *C. carpio*	Latency (ms) *S. glanis*
15°C	1.59±0.02	2.02±0.2
25°C	1.22±0.1	1.63±0.03
15°C repeated	1.55±0.02	2.02±0.2

of temperature in their habitats, which should lead to more resistance to temperature changes. Even so, differences were found in hearing ability between temperatures among all three species, especially at higher frequencies. Reasons could be that lower temperatures affect the auditory system more than higher ones and that fish are able to gain heat tolerance more rapidly than cold tolerance [2,45].

Comparison between stenothermal and eurythermal fish

Stenothermal species live in habitats characterized by small fluctuations in ambient temperatures (tropical regions) and should tolerate only small temperature changes. Wysocki et al. [2] and Papes and Ladich [26] observed that a temperature increase of 8°C (from 22°C to 30°C) resulted in only a small sensitivity improvement in two Amazonian catfish species from two different families. Both the pimelodid *Pimelodus pictus* and the doradid *Platydoras armatulus* showed a similar increase in hearing sensitivity of up to 5 dB (Fig. 8) even though the hearing curve is U-shaped in *P. armatulus* and ramp-like in *P. pictus*.

Cyprinus carpio showed smaller changes in sensitivity, especially at higher frequencies, similar to the stenothermal species. This similarity is, as discussed above, probably due to the low absolute thresholds of the carp at higher frequencies (threshold at 4 kHz at 22°C: *P. pictus*: 73 dB re 1 μPa, *P. armatulus:* 84 dB).

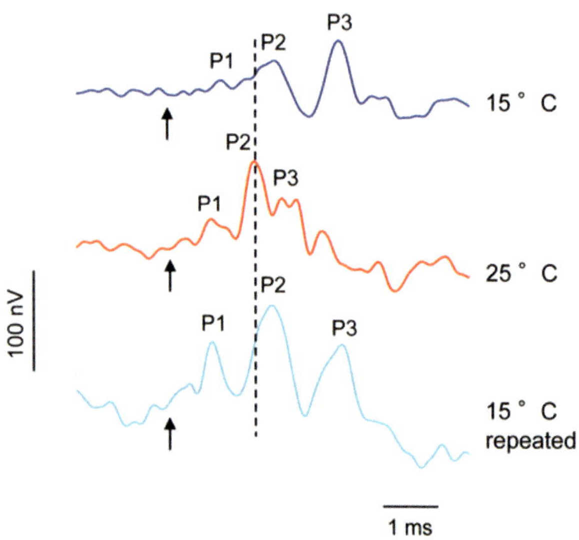

Figure 6. AEPs of one specimen of *S. glanis* in response to a single-click stimulus. Click stimulus was presented 28 dB above hearing thresholds at both temperatures. Arrows indicate onset of the single-click stimulus. The vertical dashed line indicates the position of the P2 peak at 25°C relative to the P2 peak at 15°C and 15°C repeated.

The comparison between the eurythermal and stenothermal catfishes indicates that the influence of temperature on the auditory system may differ depending upon whether a species is physiologically adjusted to tolerate a wide or narrow temperature range [2]. Eurythermal catfish species seem to respond more to temperature changes than stenothermal species. Nonetheless, note that the temperature increase from 15 (18)°C to 25 (26)°C in eurythermal species cannot directly be compared to an increase from 22°C to 30°C in stenothermal species.

In summary, all otophysines investigated so far showed higher hearing sensitivity when temperature increased [2,26,46]. This finding agrees with results of other studies on fish and amphibians, showing that temperature changes affects the inner ear and the central auditory pathways. Fay and Ream [28] and Smotherman and Narins [47] already suggested that warming water temperatures increase the cell's spontaneous activity, best frequency, as well as the cell's sensitivity and responsiveness in the goldfish as well as electrical resonance for hair cell tuning in the leopard frog. None of the studies conducted in fish within the last decade reported an increase of the frequency range detectable with increasing temperature. Thus, Dudok von Heel's [27] observation in the European minnow is not supported by recent studies.

Latencies in response to clicks and temporal processing

The auditory system of fish species, particularly of otophysan fishes, is well adapted for temporal processing of acoustic stimuli [31,32,33,48]. In the current study, the latency between the onset of a single-click stimulus and the second positive peak of the AEP decreased similarly in *C. carpio* and *S. glanis* when the temperature increased. Latencies became shorter by approximate-

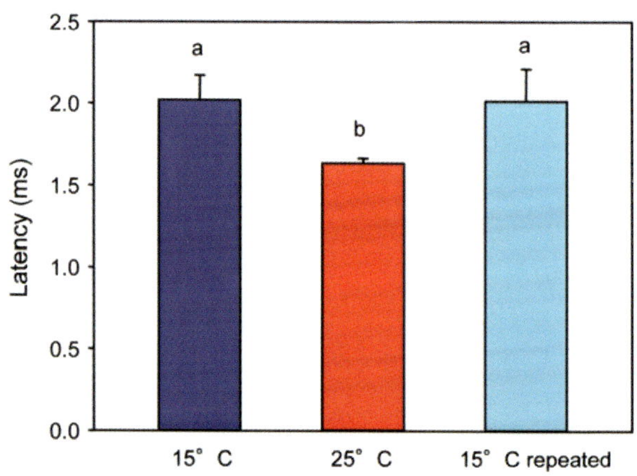

Figure 7. Latency between the onset of the click and the second positive peak. Mean (+ S.E.) latency of *S. glanis* kept at 15°C, 25°C and 15°C repeated. N = 8. Different letters (a, b) indicate significant differences between temperatures ($p \leq 0.05$).

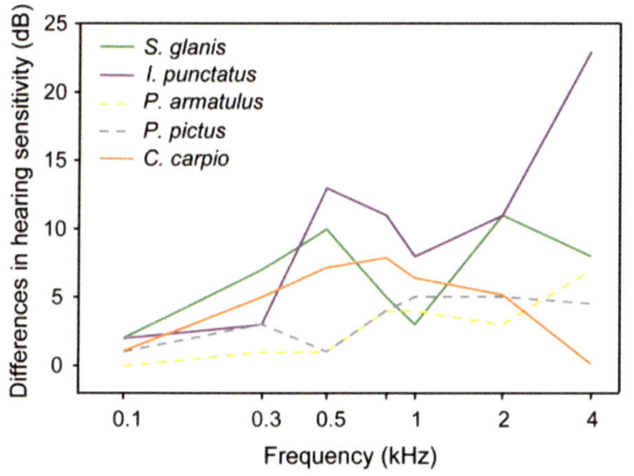

Figure 8. Comparison of the changes in hearing sensitivity in eurythermal (solid lines) and stenothermal (dashed lines) otophysines. *C. carpio* and *S. glanis* (recent study, 15°C vs. 25°C), *I. punctatus* (Wysocki et al., 2009: 18°C vs. 26°C), Amazonian catfishes *P. pictus* (Wysocki et al., 2009: 22°C vs. 30°C) and *P. armatulus* (Papes and Ladich, 2011; 22°C vs. 30°C).

ly 0.35 ms in *C. carpio* and 0.39 ms in *S. glanis*. A comparison of the P2 latencies between *C. carpio* and *S. glanis* revealed that the carp's P2 showed up faster by approximately 0.45 ms at 15°C and 0.41 ms at 25°C. This faster response to click stimuli in carps could point to differences in the temporal processing of short acoustic stimuli between otophysan families. The different latencies could furthermore reflect different auditory pathways between both species, indicating that P2s are generated in different brainstem nuclei [49]. Finally, the longer latencies in catfish could be because the tested catfish were twice as long as carps, resulting in longer distances between the swim bladder and the inner ear and in longer auditory pathways in the catfish (standard length: 11–13 cm in carps versus 23–31 cm in catfish).

A similar trend toward shorter latencies at higher temperatures has been found in the stenothermal doradid *P. armatulus*. Papes and Ladich [26] showed that the latency decreased in three out of four AEP peaks (P1, N2 and P2) at the higher temperature. However, a direct comparison of latencies between the silurid and the doradid catfish is not possible because AEP waveforms differ considerably between species and it is unclear if P2s are generated by the same brainstem nuclei. Furthermore, the *P. armatulus* specimens were half as long as the *S. glanis* (SL: 11–12 cm versus 23–31 cm), yielding the effects already mentioned above.

Note here also that different temperatures were used during tests (recent study, 15°C vs. 25°C; Papes and Ladich, [26]: 22°C vs. 30°C); this resulted in a 10°C difference between highest and lowest temperature in the current study versus an 8°C difference in the study of Papes and Ladich [26]. Nevertheless, latencies decreased when temperature rose. Papes and Ladich [26] already mentioned that this phenomenon could be an effect involving temperature dependence of spike conduction velocity, of spike shape or synaptic delay.

Wysocki and Ladich [31] showed that the minimum pulse period resolvable by the auditory system was below 1.5 ms. This enables otophysines and osphronemids (labyrinth fishes or gouramis) to process each pulse within a series of intraspecific sounds. Current data, however, do not indicate that the temporal resolution in fishes depends on temperature. Papes and Ladich [26] revealed that the minimum resolvable click period is unaffected by changes in temperature in *P. armatulus*.

Acknowledgments

We want to thank Lidia Eva Wysocki for her support with the latency measurements and analysis, Walter Lechner for help with threshold measurements, Heinz Tunner for providing carps and Michael Stachowitsch for scientific English proofreading.

Author Contributions

Conceived and designed the experiments: IPM FL. Performed the experiments: IPM. Analyzed the data: IPM FL. Contributed reagents/materials/analysis tools: FL. Contributed to the writing of the manuscript: IPM FL.

References

1. Zitek A, Schmutz S, Ploner A (2004) Fish drift in a Danube sidearm-system: II. Seasonal and diurnal patterns. J Fish Biol 65: 1339–1357.
2. Wysocki LE, Montey K, Popper AN (2009) The influence of ambient temperature and thermal acclimation on hearing in a eurythermal and a stenothermal otophysan fish. J Exp Biol 212: 3091–3099.
3. Huber M, Guderley H (1993) The effect of thermal acclimation and exercise upon the binding of glycolytic enzymes in muscle of the goldfish *Carassius auratus*. J Exp Biol 175: 195–209.
4. Sollid J, Weber RE, Nilsson GE (2005) Temperature alters the respiratory surface area of crucian carp *Carassius carassius* and goldfish *Carassius auratus*. J Exp Biol 208: 1109–1116.
5. David JA (2006) Water quality and accelerated winter growth of European catfish using an enclosed recirculating system. Water Envir J 20: 233–239.
6. Cossins AR, Friedlander MJ, Prosser CL (1977) Correlations between behavioural temperature adaptations of goldfish and the viscosity and fatty acid composition of their synaptic membranes. J Comp Physiol 120: 109–121.
7. Jones EA, Jong AS, Ellerby DJ (2008) The effects of acute temperature change on swimming performance in bluegill sunfish *Lepomis macrochirus*. J Exp Biol 211: 1386–1396.
8. Wiersinga-Post JEC, van Netten SM (2000) Temperature dependency of cupular mechanics and hair cell frequency selectivity in the fish central lateral line organ. J Comp Physiol A 186: 949–956.
9. Oldfield BP (1988). The effect of temperature on the tuning and physiology of insect auditory receptors. Hear Res 35: 151–158.
10. Franz A, Ronacher B (2002) Temperature dependence of temporal resolution in aninsect nervous system. J Comp Physiol A 188: 261–271.
11. Hubl L, Mohneke R, Schneider H (1977) Temperature dependence of auditory thresholds in two central European anurans, *Bombina variegata variegata* (L.) and *Rana ridibunda ridibunda* pall. (Amphibia), and its relation to calling. Behav Proc 2: 305–314.
12. Long GR, Van Dijk P, Wit HP (1996) Temperature dependence of spontaneous otoacoustic emissions in the edible frog (*Rana esculenta*). Hear Res 98: 22–28.
13. Egert D, Lewis ER (1995) Temperature-dependence of saccular nerve fiber response in the North American bullfrog. Hear Res 84: 72–80.
14. Eatock RA, Manley GA (1981) Auditory nerve fibre activity in the Tokay Gecko: II. Temperature effect on tuning. J Comp Physiol 142: 219–226.
15. Smolders JWT, Klinke R (1984) Effects of temperature on the properties of primary auditory fibres of the spectacled caiman, *Caiman crocodilus* (L.). J Comp Physiol 155: 19–30.
16. Fay RR, Popper AN (2000) Evolution of hearing in vertebrates: the inner ears and processing. Hear Res 146: 1–10.
17. Ladich F, Popper AN (2004) Parallel evolution in fish hearing organs. In: Evolution of the Vertebrate Auditory System. G. Manley, A.N. Popper and R.R. Fay (eds). Springer- Verlag, New York. pp. 95–227.
18. Ladich F, d Myrberg AA (2006) Agonistic behaviour and acoustic communication. In: Ladich F, Collin SP, Moller P, Kapoor BG, editors. Communication in Fishes. Enfield, NH: Science Publishers. pp. 122–148.
19. Wysocki LE (2006) Detection of communication sounds. In: Ladich, F, Collin, S.P, Moller, P, Kapoor, B.G., editors. Communication in Fishes. Enfield, N.H.: Science Publishers Inc. pp. 177–205.
20. Fay RR (2009) Sound scapes and the sense of hearing in fishes. Integr Zool 4: 26–32.
21. Torricelli P, Lugli M, Pavan G (1990) Analysis of sounds produced by male *Padogobius martensi* (Pisces, Gobiidae) and factors affecting their structural properties. Bioacoustics 2: 261–275.

22. Lugli M, Torricelli P, Pavan G, Millers PJ (1996) Breeding sounds of male *Padogobius nigricans* with suggestions for further evolutionary study of vocal behavior in gobioid fishes. J Fish Biol 49: 648–657.
23. Connaughton MA, Taylor MH, Fine ML (2000) Effects of fish size and temperature on weakfish disturbance calls: implications for the mechanism of sound generation. J Exp Biol 203: 1503–1512.
24. Amorim MCP (2005) Diel and seasonal variations of sound production in captive grey gurnards *Eutrigla gurnardus*. Acta Zool Sin 51: 1013–1022.
25. Amorim MCP, Vasconcellos RO, Marques JF, Almada F (2006) Seasonal variation of sound production in the Lusitanian toadfish *Halobatrachus didactylus*. J Fish Biol 69: 1892–1899.
26. Papes S, F Ladich (2011) Effects of temperature on sound production and auditory abilities in the Striped Raphael catfish *Platydoras armatulus* (Family Doradidae). PLOS ONE 6: e26479.
27. Dudok Van Heel WH (1956) Pitch discrimination in the minnow (*Phoxinus phoxinus*) at different temperature levels. Experientia 12: 75–77.
28. Fay RR, Ream TJ (1992) The effects of temperature change and transient hypoxia on auditory nerve fiber response in the goldfish (*Carassius auratus*). Hear Res 58: 9–18.
29. Mann DA, Wilson CD, Song J, Popper AN (2009) Hearing sensitivity of the Walleye pollock. Trans Amer Fish Soci 138: 1000–1008.
30. Carey MB, Zelick R (1993) The effect of sound level, temperature and dehydration on the brainstem auditory evoked potential in anuran amphibian. Hear Res 70: 216–228.
31. Wysocki LE, Ladich F (2002) Can fishes resolve temporal characteristics of sounds? New insights using auditory brainstem response. Hear Res 169: 36–46.
32. Wysocki LE, Ladich F (2003) The representation of conspecific sounds in the auditory brainstem of teleost fishes. J Exp Biol 206: 2229–2240.
33. Vasconcelos RO, Fonseca PJ, Amorim MCP, Ladich F (2011) Representation of complex vocalizations in the Lusitanian toadfish auditory system: evidence of fine temporal, frequency and amplitude discrimination. Proc Roy Soc London B. Biol Sci 278: 826–834.
34. Hilge V (1985) The influence of temperature on the growth of the European catfish (*Silurus glanis* L.). J Appl Ichthyol 1: 27–31.
35. Banarescu PM, Paepke HJ (2001) The Freshwater Fishes of Europe. Cyprinidae 2, Gasterosteidae. Vol. 5. Aula-Verlag, Wiebelsheim.
36. Itoi S, Kawahara S, Kondo H, Sakai T, Watabe S (2003) Changes in mitochondrial fatty acid composition following temperature acclimation of carp and their possible effects on F0F1-ATPase activity. Fish Physiol Biochem 29: 237–244.
37. Copp GH, Robert Britton J, Cucherousset J, Garcia-Berthou E, Kirk R, et al. (2009) Voracious invader or benign feline? A review of the environmental biology of European catfish *Silurus glanis* in its native and introduced ranges. Fish Fisher 10: 252–282.
38. Kenyon TN, Ladich F, Yan HY (1998) A comparative study of hearing ability in fishes: the auditory brainstem response approach. J Comp Physiol A 182: 307–318.
39. Wysocki LE, Ladich F (2005) Effects of noise exposure on click detection and the temporal resolution ability of the goldfish auditory system. Hear Res 201: 27–36.
40. Ladich F, Fay RR (2013) Auditory evoked potential audiometry in fish. Rev Fish Biol Fisher 23: 317–364.
41. Van Dijk P, Wit HP, Segenhout JM (1997) Dissecting the frog inner ear with Gaussian noise. II. Temperature dependence of inner ear function. Hear Res 114: 243–251.
42. Fonseca PJ, Correia T (2007) Effects of temperature on tuning of the auditory pathway in the cicada *Tettigetta josei* (Hemiptera, Tibicinidae). J Exp Biol 210: 1834–1845.
43. Walkowiak W (1980) Sensitivity, range and temperature dependence of hearing in the grass frog and fire-bellied toad. Behav Proc 5: 363–372.
44. Campbell HW (1969) The effects of temperature on the auditory sensitivity of lizards. Physiol Zool 42: 183–210.
45. Davies WD (1973) Rates of temperature acclimation for hatchery reared striped bass fry and fingerlings. Progr Fish-Culturist 35: 214–217.
46. Amoser S (2007) Acoustic communication in fishes: Influence of the habitat on sound detection. University of Vienna, Vienna.
47. Smotherman MS, Narins PM (1998) Effect of temperature on electrical resonance in leopard from saccular hair cells. J Neurophysiol 79: 312–321.
48. Myrberg AA, Spanier E, Ha SJ (1978) Temporal patterning in acoustical communication. In: Reese ES, Lighter FJ, editors. Contrasts in Behaviour. New York: Wiley & Sons. pp. 137–179.
49. Ladich F, Bass AH (2003) Audition. In: Arratia G, Kapoor BG, Chardon M, Diogo R, editors. Catfishes. Enfield, NH: Science Publishers Inc. pp. 701–730.

19

Auditory and Visual Health after Ten Years of Exposure to Metal-on-Metal Hip Prostheses

Jennifer R. Prentice[1], Christopher S. Blackwell[1], Naz Raoof[2], Paul Bacon[3], Jaydip Ray[3], Simon J. Hickman[4], J. Mark Wilkinson[1]*

1 Department of Human Metabolism, University of Sheffield, Sheffield, South Yorkshire, United Kingdom, **2** Department of Ophthalmology, Sheffield Teaching Hospitals NHS Foundation Trust, Sheffield, South Yorkshire, United Kingdom, **3** Department of Otolaryngology, Sheffield Teaching Hospitals NHS Foundation Trust, Sheffield, South Yorkshire, United Kingdom, **4** Department of Neurology, Sheffield Teaching Hospitals NHS Foundation Trust, Sheffield, South Yorkshire, United Kingdom

Abstract

Case reports of patients with mal-functioning metal-on-metal hip replacement (MoMHR) prostheses suggest an association of elevated circulating metal levels with visual and auditory dysfunction. However, it is unknown if this is a cumulative exposure effect and the impact of prolonged low level exposure, relevant to the majority of patients with a well-functioning prosthesis, has not been studied. Twenty four male patients with a well-functioning MoMHR and an age and time since surgery matched group of 24 male patients with conventional total hip arthroplasty (THA) underwent clinical and electrophysiological assessment of their visual and auditory health at a mean of ten years after surgery. Median circulating cobalt and chromium concentrations were higher in patients after MoMHR versus those with THA ($P<0.0001$), but were within the Medicines and Healthcare Products Regulatory Agency (UK) investigation threshold. Subjective auditory tests including pure tone audiometric and speech discrimination findings were similar between groups ($P>0.05$). Objective assessments, including amplitude and signal-to-noise ratio of transient evoked and distortion product oto-acoustic emissions (TEOAE and DPOAE, respectively), were similar for all the frequencies tested ($P>0.05$). Auditory brainstem responses (ABR) and cortical evoked response audiometry (ACR) were also similar between groups ($P>0.05$). Ophthalmological evaluations, including self-reported visual function by visual functioning questionnaire, as well as binocular low contrast visual acuity and colour vision were similar between groups ($P>0.05$). Retinal nerve fibre layer thickness and macular volume measured by optical coherence tomography were also similar between groups ($P>0.05$). In the presence of moderately elevated metal levels associated with well-functioning implants, MoMHR exposure does not associate with clinically demonstrable visual or auditory dysfunction.

Editor: William H. MeriganJr, Univ Rochester Medical Ctr, United States of America

Funding: This study was funded by Sheffield Musculoskeletal Biomedical Research Unit through its core grant from the National Institute of Health Research in the United Kingdom (NIHR). The funders had no role in study design, data collection and analysis, decision to publish, or preparation of the manuscript.

Competing Interests: The authors have declared that no competing interests exist.

* E-mail: j.m.wilkinson@sheffield.ac.uk

Introduction

More than 500,000 patients in the United States have received metal-on-metal hip prostheses, including metal-on-metal hip resurfacing (MoMHR), the majority of whom have well-functioning devices [1]. Cobalt and chromium are the principal metals released by MoMHR [2,3]. Ten-year steady state median blood cobalt and chromium concentrations in patients with well-functioning devices are between 1.5 and 2.3 µg/L, but remain 10-fold higher than physiological levels [4,5].

Case reports relating to prosthesis failure commonly include visual and auditory problems associated with grossly elevated blood metal concentrations [6,7,8,9,10,11]. Tower et al. described two cases in which prosthesis failure associated with hearing loss [10]. Ikeda et al. quantitated hearing loss by pure tone audiometry and demonstrated hearing thresholds of 52 and 45 dB in the right and left ears respectively (average over 0.5, 1, 2 and 4 kHz, normal <25) [11]. The patient described by Rizzetti et al. had bilateral absence of brainstem acoustic responses [8]. Assessment of visual loss within the case studies showed in one case undefined visual changes and hyper-intensity of the optic nerves and tracts on magnetic resonance imaging (MRI), and 'irregular' cortical visual responses when measuring visual evoked potentials in another subject. Whilst these cases highlight association between overt failure of prosthetic devices and auditory or visual dysfunction, the effect on these sensory systems of prolonged exposure to moderately elevated blood metal concentrations, relevant to the great majority of patients with these devices, has not been defined.

Between 2009 and 2010 we undertook a single-centre cross-sectional study to investigate the systemic effects of chronic metal exposure following MoMHR [12]. Thirty-five patients after MoMHR were individually matched by age, sex and time since surgery to patients who had received a conventional total hip arthroplasty (THA) using a non-metal-on-metal bearing at a mean of 8 years following surgery. Patients within both groups were in good self-reported health and had well-functioning prostheses. We identified differences in grey matter density in the occipital cortex and in the cross-sectional area of the optic chiasm in subjects receiving MoMHR versus those who had received a conventional THA, indicating an association between MoMHR exposure and subtle structural changes in the visual system of the brain [13]. Following these findings we recalled all 62 male participants in the study order to conduct a detailed auditory and visual assessment to determine whether chronic low elevated metal exposure in well-functioning MoMHR associates with demonstrable functional effects on these systems.

Patients and Methods

Ethics, design, setting, and participants

This extension study was approved by South Yorkshire Research Ethics Committee, and all patients provided written informed consent prior to participation. This single centre study was undertaken as an extension of a cross sectional study Investigation examining the systemic effects of metal exposure in MoMHR. In this extension study all men (n = 31 MoMHR and 31 age-matched THA patients) were invited to return for further visual and auditory assessment. Patients were recruited from the community between November 24th, 2009 and May 20th, 2010. The study design was reviewed by a statistician at Sheffield Clinical Trials Research Unit, and its conduct and dissemination of results were reviewed by Sheffield Lay Advisory Panel for Bone Research. The study inclusion and exclusion criteria are documented elsewhere [12]. Blood and plasma cobalt and chromium were measured by inductively-coupled plasma-mass spectroscopy (ICP-MS), as described previously [12]. Briefly, blood samples were collected via plastic cannulae using the last draw method directly into trace element collection tubes, and metal assays were performed by a laboratory that participates in national trace element measurement quality assurance schemes (TEQAS).

Auditory Outcomes

Clinical evaluation. All subjects were questioned about their auditory health including occupational noise exposure, tympanic membrane perforation, tinnitus and current respiratory infections. Otoscopic examination was performed by an otolaryngologist to determine the presence of any co-existent pathology. All Audiometric assessments were made in sound attenuated test rooms.

Subjective audiometric tests. Pure tone audiometry (PTA) was performed in accordance with the British Society of Audiology recommended procedures (The British Society of Audiology, 2011) using an Aurical Audiometer type 1081 and its associated OTO suite application software module v. 4.50.01 (GN Otometrics A/S). Air conduction (AC) thresholds were obtained using TDH39 headphones across the frequency range 0.25 to 8 kHz. If AC thresholds were raised above 20 dB hearing level (dBHL) then bone conduction thresholds were measured using a B-71 bone oscillator across frequencies 0.5 to 4 kHz. The integrated speech test module was used with the AB word lists and the 50 per cent speech recognition level measured for each ear [14].

Objective audiometric tests. Evoked oto-acoustic emissions were recorded to assess cochlear function whilst the electrophysiology tests of auditory brainstem response (ABR) and the auditory cortical response (ACR) were used to assess for retro-cochlear pathology in the auditory brainstem and auditory cortex respectively. Both Transient evoked otoacoustic emissions (TEOAEs) and distortion-product oto-acoustic emissions (DPOAEs) were recorded using a dual probe DP Echoport (ILO292-II USB interface) coupled with a laptop using the ILOv6 software (v 6.34.22.0). For the TEOAEs, non-linear type stimuli with a target level of 84 dB SPL were presented. Noise rejection threshold was set to 40 dB SPL and 360 sweeps were averaged. The resulting TEOAEs were analysed over a 2.5 to 20 millisecond time window and in half octave bands OAE power (1, 1.4, 2, 2.8 and 4 kHz). A response was judged to be present in a given half octave band if the signal was >-5 dBSPL with a signal to noise ratio >6 dB. For the DPOAEs, two primary tones at frequencies f_1 and f_2 were presented at levels L_1 and $L_2 = 70$ dB SPL with a fixed frequency ratio of f_2/f_1 at 1.22.

Oto-neurologic auditory brainstem evoked responses (ABRs) were recorded using a Biologic Navigator Pro AEP system. Subjects were asked to relax and if possible go to sleep in a reclined chair in order to minimise myogenic and movement artifacts. Alternating polarity 100 μs duration clicks at a repetition rate of 11.1 per second were presented at a stimulus level of 80dBnHL using TDH-39P headphones. Two channel evoked potential activity was recorded. Electrodes were placed on the forehead (common), vertex (jumpered to both channels) and on the left and right mastoids. EEG activity was sampled over 512 points for a 10.66 ms time epoch (0.5 ms blocking) and amplified with a gain setting of 150000. Filtering was from 100 to 3000 Hz with an artefact rejection level of ± 10 μV peak to peak. A minimum of two replicated averages each with a minimum of 1800 sweeps were recorded. The absolute ipsilateral Wave V latency for each ear was measured along with inter-aural latency differences [15]. A subjective threshold to the ABR test stimuli was also measured for each ear.

Auditory cortical evoked responses (ACR) were recorded using the same Biologic Navigator Pro AEP system and the same electrode configuration as used for ABR recordings. Subjects were sat up in a chair and asked to maintain an alert state by reading a magazine or newspaper. Rarefaction tone burst stimuli calibrated at 80 dB HL and at a frequency of 1000 Hz (10 cycle linear ramp and 50 cycle plateau) were presented at a repetition rate of 0.5 per second using TDH-39P headphones. EEG activity was sampled over 512 points for a 533 ms time epoch and amplified with a gain setting of 75000. Filtering was from 1 Hz (12 dB/octave) to 15 Hz with an artefact rejection level of ± 45 μV peak to peak. A minimum of two replicated averages each with a minimum of 40 sweeps were recorded. These replications were further averaged together to form a grand average and to optimise peak identification. The P1-N1-P2 sequence was identified and the amplitudes measured for both ipsilateral and contralateral recordings. A subjective threshold to the ACR test stimuli was also measured for each ear.

Visual Outcomes

Clinical evaluation. The ophthalmic evaluation comprised an ocular and targeted medical history, as well as an ocular examination made by an Ophthalmologist to exclude primary ocular pathology. All patients were examined for pupillary defects and underwent visual field testing to confrontation. Ocular motility examination, Goldmann applanation tonometry and slit lamp biomicroscopy were also undertaken. The dilated fundus was then examined by slit lamp biomicroscopy using 78D and 90D lenses.

Visual symptoms. The National Eye Institute Visual Functioning Questionnaire (NEI-VFQ) was used to measure self-reported visual function and general health implications [16]. The 10 question neuro-ophthalmic supplement was administered to identify visual defects due to neurological disorders [17]. These were administered before the rest of the evaluation and vision testing to avoid bias.

Subjective visual tests. Uniocular and binocular best corrected logMAR visual acuities were measured using Early

Table 1. Patient characteristics.

Characteristic	MoMHR (n = 24)	THA (n = 24)	P-value
Age at assessment (years)	62.5±7.1	62·6±7.5	0.95
Age at time of surgery (years)	52.3±7.2	52.9±8.6	0.79
Time since surgery (years)	10.2±1·8	9.7±2·5	0.49
*Serum cobalt (μg/L)	0.47 (0.36 to 1.05)	0.06 (0.04 to 0.08)	<0.0001
*Serum chromium (μg/L)	0.61 (0.47 to 2.31)	<0.1 (<0.1 to <0.1)	<0.0001
*Whole blood cobalt (μg/L)	0.43 (0.29 to 1.26)	0.05 (0.03 to 0.07)	<0.0001
*Whole blood chromium (μg/L)	0.48 (0.33 to 1.82)	0.10 (<0.1 to 0.13)	<0.0001

Data are mean ±SD or median (interquartile range). Analyses are MoMHR versus THA by Student's t-test or Mann Whitney test.

Treatment Diabetic Retinopathy Study (ETDRS) charts at 4 m. Binocular low contrast acuity was measured using 4 m ETDRS charts of 1.25% and 2.5% contrast and recorded as logMAR acuity. Colour vision was assessed binocularly using the Farnsworth-Munsell 100-hue test (Munsell Color Company, Grand Rapids, MI, USA) administered under simulated daylight (20 W Compact fluorescent light of 1152lm and 65,000K colour temperature) with no time limit imposed. Total error scores were calculated for each participant using the traditional scoring method [18]. Partial error scores for the blue-yellow colour axis and the red-green axis were also calculated for each participant. A square root transformation was used to normalize the distribution of error scores for the statistical analyses.

Objective visual tests. Retinal nerve fibre layer thickness and macular volume were then measured using Spectralis optical coherence tomography (OCT) (Heidelberg Engineering Ltd, Heidelberg, Germany). In both eyes, retinal nerve fibre (RNFL) thickness was measured using the Fast RNFL scanning protocol in which three circular 3.4 mm diameter scans, centred on the optic disc were taken, the mean of which was then used to express RNFL thickness. Macular volume was measured using the Fast Macular Thickness map protocol, and 6 mm by 6 mm (20° by 20°) of the macular was scanned by means of 25 vertical B scans centred on the fovea.

Statistical analysis

Between group analyses of PTA were made in each ear independently, and speech discrimination in the best ear and as the mean value for both ears. Auditory electrophysiology data was analysed as the mean value for both ears. OCT measurements were used for one randomly selected eye from each subject in both groups unless there was pre-existing ocular disease in one eye, when the measurement from the fellow unaffected eye was used, as described by Henderson et al. [19]. Between group analyses of continuous datasets were made using Students t-test or the Mann-Whitney test, as appropriate. Categorical data were analysed using the Chi-squared test. All tests were made 2-tailed with a critical p-value of 0.05, and made using IBM SPSS statistical software (version 20, IBM, Portsmouth, UK).

Results

Participants and metal levels

24 participants with MOMHR and 24 with THA agreed to participate in this extension study. The groups were well matched for age and time since surgery (Table 1). Median blood, plasma, and urinary cobalt and chromium were 5 to 10 fold higher in MoMHR versus THA patients ($P<0.0001$). However, blood median and interquartile range metal levels were below guidance threshold concentration of 7 μg/L suggestive of prosthesis malfunction, and set by the Medicines and Healthcare Products Regulatory Agency (MHRA) in the United Kingdom (MDA/2012/008, 28 February).

Auditory outcomes

Clinical audiological evaluation. The two groups were well matched based on audiological history findings except self-reported loud noise exposure, which was greater in the THA group with 19 cases compared to 11 in the MOMHR group (Table 2). No patients were excluded from auditory testing following clinical assessment.

Subjective audiometric tests. The PTA findings were similar between groups (Figure 1, $P>0.05$ for all comparisons). The median half peak levels for speech discrimination in the subjects best ear were 19 dB (interquartile range 13 to 24) in the MoMHR subjects versus 17 dB (14 to 20) in the THA subjects ($P=0.56$). The median half peak levels for speech discrimination expressed as the average of both ears were 21 dB (17 to 26) in the MoMHR subjects versus 20 dB (16 to 24) in the THA subjects ($P=1.00$).

Objective audiometric tests. The amplitude and signal-to-noise ratio of the otoacoustic emissions (TEOAE and DPOAE) for all the frequencies tested were similar between groups (Figure 2, $P>0.05$ all comparisons). When considering an emission to be present when the signal-to-noise-ratio is greater than 6 dB and the signal greater than −5 dB, the percentage of subjects gaining a positive test result were also similar. At higher frequencies fewer emissions were recorded for both groups. Auditory brainstem responses, expressed as latency time of wave V and the inter-aural latency differences were similar between the two groups (Table 3, $P>0.05$ for both comparisons). No difference was observed between the ACR parameters measured. The latency times of N1 and P2 peaks as well as the N1-P2 latency and amplitude were all similar (Table 3, $P>0.05$ for all comparisons).

Visual outcomes

Clinical visual evaluation. Unilateral primary ocular disease was identified in 8 participants. In the MOMHR group there were 2 subjects with amblyopia and 1 subject with a previous penetrating eye injury. In the THA group there were two 2 subjects with previous eye trauma, 1 subject with a previous retinal detachment, 1 subject with amblyopia and 1 subject with severe macular degeneration. These participants were excluded from the binocular tests of visual and contrast acuity, Farnsworth-Munsell

Table 2. Audiology medical history.

Characteristic	MoMHR (n = 24)	THA (n = 24)	P-value
Self-reported hearing loss	8 (33%)	10 (42%)	0.77
Previous otalgia	1 (4%)	1 (4%)	1.00
Loud noise exposure	11 (46%)	19 (79%)	0.04
Use of hearing aids	1 (4%)	0	1.00
Current tinnitus	5 (21%)	8 (33%)	0.52
Current balance problems	0	2 (8%)	0.49
Previous tinnitus	8 (33%)	14 (58%)	0.15
Previous balance problems	3 (13%)	3 (13%)	1.00
Ear surgery	0	0	1.00
Previous perforated tympanic membrane	2 (8%)	1 (4%)	1.00
Current ear infection	0	0	1.00

Data are number of patients (percentage). Analyses are MoMHR versus THA by Fisher's exact test.

100-Hue Test and the NEI-VFQ. For the OCT, which was performed on individual eyes, only the affected eye was excluded.

Visual symptoms. Patients in both groups had similar perceived visual functioning quality assessed by the NEI-VFQ and no evidence of neuro-ophthalmologic dysfunction using the neuro-ophthalmic supplement (Table 4, P>0.05 for all comparisons).

Subjective visual assessments. Both groups had similar logMAR binocular visual acuity and similar low contrast visual acuity (at 2.5% and 1.25%) (Table 4, P>0.05 all comparisons).

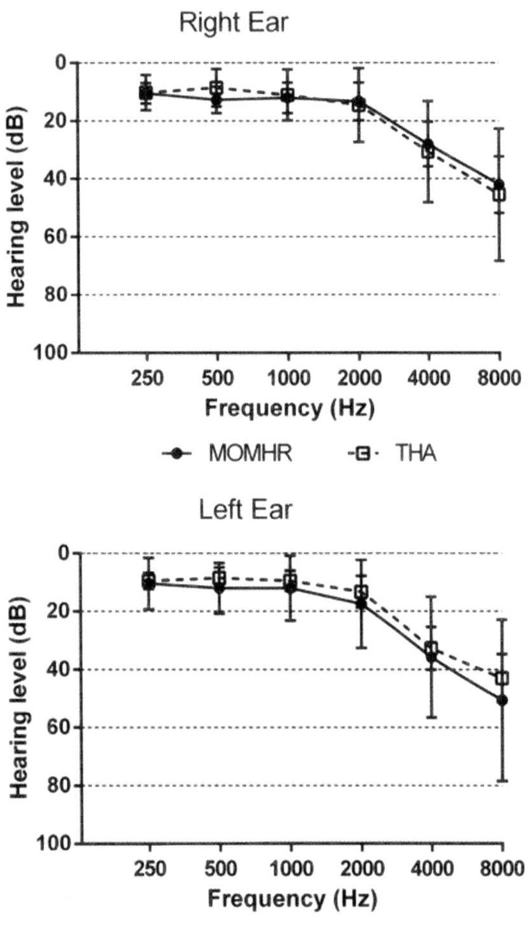

Figure 1. Pure Tone Audiogram hearing thresholds in MoMHR versus THA patients for (top panel) left and (bottom panel) right ears. Data are mean (95% confidence interval) hearing level threshold (dB). Analyses are MoMHR versus THA groups by Mann-Whitney test at each frequency, P>0.05 all comparisons.

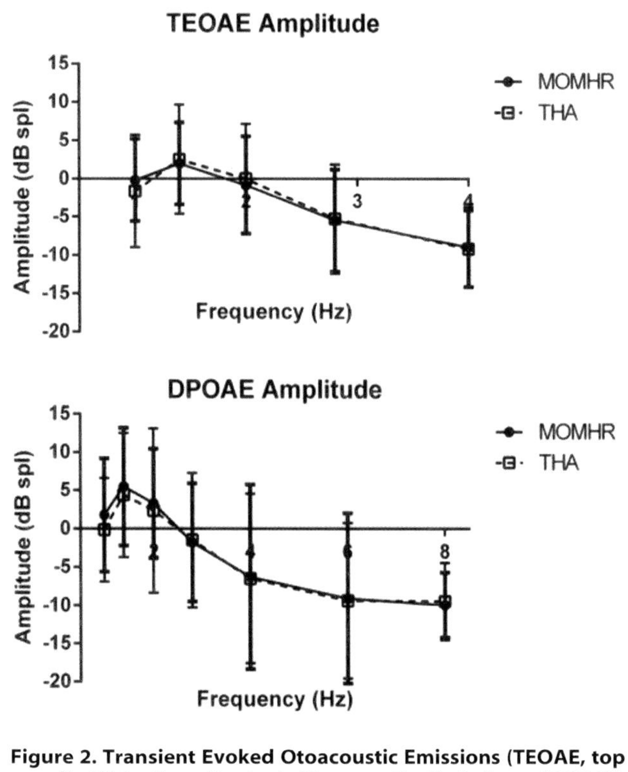

Figure 2. Transient Evoked Otoacoustic Emissions (TEOAE, top panel), Distortion Product Otoacoustic Emissions (DPOAE, bottom panel). Graphs show mean and standard deviation of the amplitude recorded for each of the frequencies tested. Analysis Students T-test, P>0.05 for all.

Table 3. Auditory responses.

Variable	MOMHR (n = 24)	THA (n = 24)
ABR Wave V latency (L-R) (ms)	0 (−0.06 to 0.12)	0.08 (−0.05 to 0.17)
ABR Wave V latency Mean (ms)	5.77 (5.62 to 5.93)	5.97 (5.74 to 6.09)
CERA N1 Latency (ms)	106.0±6.0	106.4±5.4
CERA P2 Latency (ms)	189.5±21.6	184.4±20.1
CERA N1-P2 latency (ms)	83.5±19.0	78.0±19.3
CERA N1-P2 amplitude (μV)	11.6±3.2	10.2±3.3

Values are mean ± standard deviation or median (interquartile range). Analyses are MoMHR versus THA by students t-test or Mann Whitney test; P>0.05, all comparisons. ABR = Auditory Brainstem Response, CERA = Cortical Evoked Response Audiometry.

Colour discrimination using the Farnsworth-Munsell 100-Hue test was similar between the two groups (Table 4, P>0.05). Both groups also showed poorer blue-yellow colour discrimination ability compared with red-green, consistent with the age-related decline in colour discrimination (Table 4, P>0.05).

Objective visual assessments. Both RNFL thickness and macular volume measured by OCT was similar between groups (Figure 3, P>0.05 for both comparisons).

Discussion

We studied visual and auditory health in patients chronically exposed to low levels of metal following MoMHR compared with age matched patients with the same duration of exposure to a conventional THA. This investigation followed the identification of structural differences in the brain between these patient groups [13], and aimed to determine whether these structural differences associated with quantifiable functional differences between the groups. Following exclusion of individuals with primary ocular or aural pathology, patients in both groups had similar auditory and visual function, as assessed by a range of clinical, subjective, and objective standardised tests.

This study was conducted in a clinically healthy population of patients. The MoMHR group is representative of the general MoMHR population, in that they are typically younger patients and male, and the majority received the most frequently used prosthesis brand, the Birmingham Hip Resurfacing (BHR). The patients also had well-functioning prostheses, representative of the majority of patients after MoMHR, reflected by good Oxford hip score and metal levels below the MHRA 7 μg/L threshold.

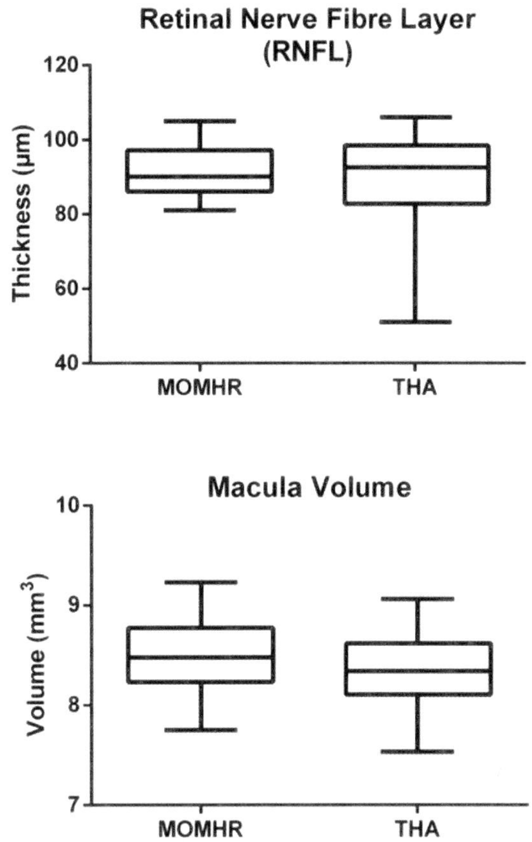

Figure 3. Box and whisker plots showing (top panel) difference in retinal nerve fibre layer thickness, and (bottom panel) differences in macular volume between the patient groups. All participants (n = 24) included as either non-pathological eye only or mean of right and left. All analyses are MOMHR versus THA by independent t-test (P>0.05 for both comparisons).

Case report and occupational exposure evidence suggests that exposure to high systemic levels of cobalt and chromium may result in damage to both the visual and auditory systems

Table 4. Visual function.

Test	MOMHR (n = 21)	THA (n = 19)
VFQ: 25 standard questions	98.2 (95.8 to 98.2)	97.4 (94.4 to 98.2)
VFQ: Neuro-ophthalmic supplement	97.5 (87.5 to 100)	97.5 (87.5 to 100)
Binocular visual acuity (LogMar)	−0.06 (−0.17 to −0.05)	−0.08 (−0.14 to 0.00)
Contrast visual acuity (LogMar): 2.5%	0.22 (0.20 to 0.33)	0.26 (0.22 to 0.42)
Contrast Visual Acuity (LogMar): 1.25%	0.44 (0.40 to 0.60)	0.42 (0.38 to 0.52)
Color discrimination: Total error score (TES)	52 (40 to 82)	80 (52 to 108)
Color discrimination: $\sqrt{TES}$	7.58±2.29	9.10±2.50
Color discrimination: Blue-yellow error score	32 (19 to 56)	39 (27 to 58)
Color discrimination: Red-green error score	27 (19 to 38)	30 (13 to 55)

Values are median (interquartile range). Analysis is MoMHR versus THA by Mann Whitney test; P>0.05, all comparisons. VFQ = Visual Functioning Questionnaire.

[6,7,8,10,11,20]. Two of the case reports describe high frequency hearing loss in association with patient reported hearing loss [10,11]. High frequency hearing loss is a normal feature of ageing in males (presbycusis), and this characteristic was present to a similar extent in both our patient groups. The further investigation of hearing loss by Rizzetti et al showed loss of auditory brainstem responses bilaterally [8]. Here we performed a much larger scale study and more detailed assessment and found no evidence of an association of MoMHR exposure with altered brainstem responses at metal levels experienced by the majority of patients. The investigation of individual cases of visual loss with high systemic metal levels has suggested optic nerve atrophy on funduscopy and optic nerve and tract hyper-intensity on MRI [8,10]. Using the principle that damage to the optic nerve and tracts should be reflected in degeneration of the retinal ganglion cells we investigated retinal structure using OCT but found no differences between the groups in our population with well-functioning prosthesis.

It is important to note the differences between our study population and those patients described in the case studies. In contrast to those patients described in the case studies who had failing prostheses with very high metal levels (up to several hundred µg/L), our study was designed specifically to determine whether prolonged exposure to low elevated metal levels is associated with subtle defects.

Hip resurfacing remains a treatment option in the young male patient with arthritis. The current FDA advice refers to visual and auditory problems associated with systemic metal levels and advises close monitoring of high risk patients (FDA, 2013). Our data suggest that patients with chronic exposure to lower concentrations of circulating metal typical of well-functioning prostheses does not associate with clinically detectable defects in visual or auditory function. However, it remains unclear whether such effects may become clinically present with longer-term exposure.

Author Contributions

Conceived and designed the experiments: JMW JRP NR PB JR SJH. Performed the experiments: CSB NR PB. Analyzed the data: JRP CSB NR SJH JMW. Wrote the paper: JRP NR PB JR SJH JMW.

References

1. Rising JP, Reynolds IS, Sedrakyan A (2012) Delays and difficulties in assessing metal-on-metal hip implants. N Engl J Med 367: e1.
2. Heisel C, Streich N, Krachler M, Jakubowitz E, Kretzer JP (2008) Characterization of the running-in period in total hip resurfacing arthroplasty: an in vivo and in vitro metal ion analysis. J Bone Joint Surg Am 90 Suppl 3: 125–133.
3. Daniel J, Ziaee H, Pradhan C, Pynsent PB, McMinn DJ (2007) Blood and urine metal ion levels in young and active patients after Birmingham hip resurfacing arthroplasty: four-year results of a prospective longitudinal study. J Bone Joint Surg Br 89: 169–173.
4. Hartmann A, Lutzner J, Kirschner S, Witzleb WC, Gunther KP (2012) Do Survival Rate and Serum Ion Concentrations 10 Years After Metal-on-Metal Hip Resurfacing Provide Evidence for Continued Use? Clin Orthop Relat Res.
5. Holland JP, Langton DJ, Hashmi M (2012) Ten-year clinical, radiological and metal ion analysis of the Birmingham Hip Resurfacing: from a single, non-designer surgeon. J Bone Joint Surg Br 94: 471–476.
6. Steens W, von FG, Katzer A (2006) Severe cobalt poisoning with loss of sight after ceramic-metal pairing in a hip–a case report. Acta Orthop 77: 830–832.
7. Oldenburg M, Wegner R, Baur X (2009) Severe cobalt intoxication due to prosthesis wear in repeated total hip arthroplasty. J Arthroplasty 24: 825 e815–820.
8. Rizzetti MC, Liberini P, Zarattini G, Catalani S, Pazzaglia U, et al. (2009) Loss of sight and sound. Could it be the hip? Lancet 373: 1052.
9. Apostoli P, Catalani S, Zaghini A, Mariotti A, Poliani PL, et al. (2013) High doses of cobalt induce optic and auditory neuropathy. Exp Toxicol Pathol 65: 719–727.
10. Tower SS (2010) Arthroprosthetic cobaltism: neurological and cardiac manifestations in two patients with metal-on-metal arthroplasty: a case report. J Bone Joint Surg Am 92: 2847–2851.
11. Ikeda T, Takahashi K, Kabata T, Sakagoshi D, Tomita K, et al. (2010) Polyneuropathy caused by cobalt-chromium metallosis after total hip replacement. Muscle Nerve 42: 140–143.
12. Prentice JR, Clark MJ, Hoggard N, Morton AC, Tooth C, et al. (2013) Metal-on-Metal Hip Prostheses and Systemic Health: A Cross-Sectional Association Study 8 Years after Implantation. PLoS One 8: e66186.
13. Clark MJ, Prentice JR, Hoggard N, Paley MN, Hadjivassiliou M, et al. (2014) Brain structure and function in patients after metal-on-metal hip resurfacing. Am J Neuroradiol (in press).
14. Boothroyd A (1968) Statistical theory of the speech discrimination score. J Acoust Soc Am 43: 362–367.
15. Jewett DL, Williston JS (1971) Auditory-evoked far fields averaged from the scalp of humans. Brain 94: 681–696.
16. Mangione CM, Lee PP, Gutierrez PR, Spritzer K, Berry S, et al. (2001) Development of the 25-item National Eye Institute Visual Function Questionnaire. Arch Ophthalmol 119: 1050–1058.
17. Raphael BA, Galetta KM, Jacobs DA, Markowitz CE, Liu GT, et al. (2006) Validation and test characteristics of a 10-item neuro-ophthalmic supplement to the NEI-VFQ-25. Am J Ophthalmol 142: 1026–1035.
18. Katz B (1995) The dyschromatopsia of optic neuritis: a descriptive analysis of data from the optic neuritis treatment trial. Trans Am Ophthalmol Soc 93: 685–708.
19. Henderson AP, Trip SA, Schlottmann PG, Altmann DR, Garway-Heath DF, et al. (2008) An investigation of the retinal nerve fibre layer in progressive multiple sclerosis using optical coherence tomography. Brain 131: 277–287.
20. Meecham HM, Humphrey P (1991) Industrial exposure to cobalt causing optic atrophy and nerve deafness: a case report. J Neurol Neurosurg Psychiatry 54: 374–375.

A Novel DFNA36 Mutation in *TMC1* Orthologous to the Beethoven (*Bth*) Mouse Associated with Autosomal Dominant Hearing Loss in a Chinese Family

Yali Zhao[1,2], Dayong Wang[1], Liang Zong[1], Feifan Zhao[1], Liping Guan[3], Peng Zhang[3], Wei Shi[1], Lan Lan[1], Hongyang Wang[1], Qian Li[1], Bing Han[1], Ling Yang[4], Xin Jin[3,5], Jian Wang[3], Jun Wang[3], Qiuju Wang[1]*

1 Chinese PLA Institute of Otolaryngology, Chinese PLA General Hospital, Beijing, China, **2** Beijing Institute of Otorhinolaryngology, Beijing Tongren Hospital, Capital Medical University, Beijing, China, **3** BGI-Shenzhen, Shenzhen, China, **4** BGI-Tianjin, Tianjin, China, **5** School of Bioscience and Biotechnology, South China University of Technology, Guangzhou, China

Abstract

Mutations in the transmembrane channel-like gene 1 (*TMC1*) can cause both DFNA36 and DFNB7/11 hearing loss. More than thirty DFNB7/11 mutations have been reported, but only three DFNA36 mutations were reported previously. In this study, we found a large Chinese family with 222 family members showing post-lingual, progressive sensorineural hearing loss which were consistent with DFNA36 hearing loss. Auditory brainstem response (ABR) test of the youngest patient showed a special result with nearly normal threshold but prolonged latency, decreased amplitude, and the abnormal waveform morphology. Exome sequencing of the proband found four candidate variants in known hearing loss genes. Sanger sequencing in all family members found a novel variant c.1253T>A (p.M418K) in *TMC1* at DFNA36 that co-segregated with the phenotype. This mutation in *TMC1* is orthologous to the mutation found in the hearing loss mouse model named *Bth* ten years ago. In another 51 Chinese autosomal dominant hearing loss families, we screened the segments containing the dominant mutations of *TMC1* and no functional variants were found. *TMC1* is expressed in the hair cells in inner ear. Given the already known roles of *TMC1* in the mechanotransduction in the cochlea and its expression in inner ear, our results may provide an interesting perspective into its function in inner ear.

Editor: Berta Alsina, Universitat Pompeu Fabra, Spain

Funding: This work was supported by the grants of the National Key Basic Research Program of China, No. 2014CB943001, the National Natural Science Foundation of China, Major Project, No. 81120108009. The funders had no role in study design, data collection and analysis, decision to publish, or preparation of the manuscript.

Competing Interests: The authors have declared that no competing interests exist.

* E-mail: wqcr@263.net

Introduction

Hearing loss is the most common sensory disorder affecting one in 1000 births [1] and the prevalence rises to 2.7 per 1000 by the age of four [2]. More than 60% of cases can be attributed to genetic causes and inherited across generations. Hereditary hearing loss is a highly heterogeneous disorder. So far, a total of 76 non-syndromic hearing loss genes have been identified, including 31 autosomal dominant, 47 autosomal recessive and four X-linked genes (http://hereditaryhearingloss.org). Among these genes, eight of them are inherited in both autosomal dominant and recessive patterns, such as *TMC1* (http://hereditaryhearingloss.org/).

TMC1 was identified as a causative gene for both autosomal dominant (DFNA36) and autosomal recessive (DFNB7/11) non-syndromic hearing loss by Kurima and colleagues in 2002[3]. Based on their results, Vreugde and colleagues screened the *Tmc1* gene and found the p.M412K mutation in a hearing loss mouse model named *Bth* which was arisen in a large-scale ENU mutagenesis program [4,5]. Since then, more than 30 autosomal recessive mutations in *TMC1* have been reported in DFNB7/11 families. *TMC1* is identified as a common gene associated with non-syndromic hearing loss with a frequency up to 6.6% in Turkey [3,6–17]. In contrast, only two amino acid residues with three mutations have been reported to be associated with autosomal dominant hearing loss [3,14,18,19]. One is the amino acid-572 with two mutations at this site, p.D572N and p.D572H. These two mutations have been observed in three unrelated North American families with non-syndromic, post-lingual, progressive sensorineural hearing loss [3,18,19]. The other residue is the amino acid-417 with mutation p.G417R [14]. This mutation is adjacent to the *Bth* mouse mutation in the *Tmc1* gene, which may have similar function consequences. However, the mutation orthologous to p.M412K in murine *Tmc1* has yet to been found in human hearing loss family since it has been reported in 2002 [5]. Here, in a large Chinese family (1304) of six-generation with autosomal dominant hereditary hearing loss, we identified a novel mutation of p.M418K in *TMC1* through sequencing the whole exome of the proband, which is important and beneficial to discover the pathologic mechanism of DFNA36 hearing loss caused by *TMC1* mutation.

Methods

Ethics Statement

The study was approved by the Committee of Medical Ethics of Chinese People's Liberation Army (PLA) General Hospital. All the

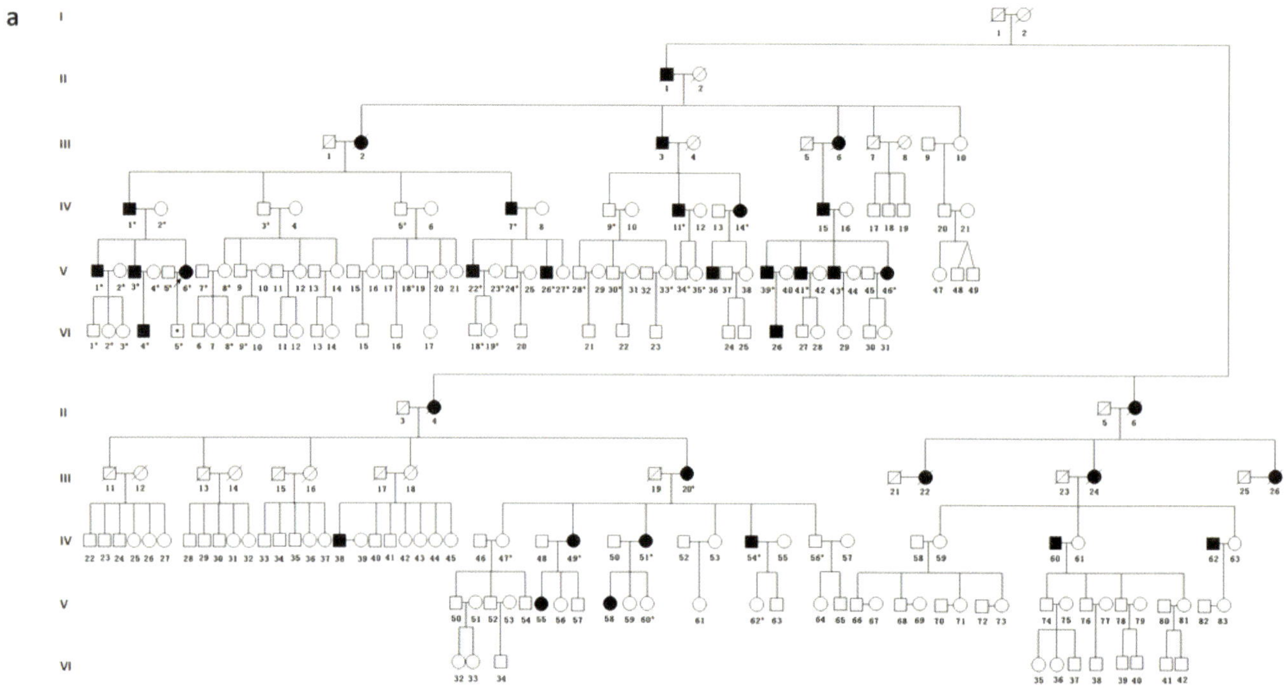

Figure 1. Pedigree of family 1304. Filled symbols for males (squares) and females (circles) represent affected individuals, and empty, unaffected ones. An arrow denotes the proband. A symbol with dot indicates the individual younger than the average age of onset, who is mutation carrier but does not present hearing loss (a mutation carrier). Symbols with asterisk are individuals who have had clinical and genetic tests.

samples were analyzed under the appropriate ethical approvals, and written informed consents were obtained from all subjects or caregivers. Next of kin, care takers or guardians consented on the behalf of minors/children participants whose capacity to consent was compromised.

Family Recruitment and Clinical Evaluations

Family 1304 were ascertained from the Department of Otolaryngology, Head and Neck Surgery, at the Institute of Otolaryngology of PLA, Chinese PLA General Hospital. Members of this family were interviewed by a team of experienced ear, nose and throat doctors, and physicians to identify either personal or

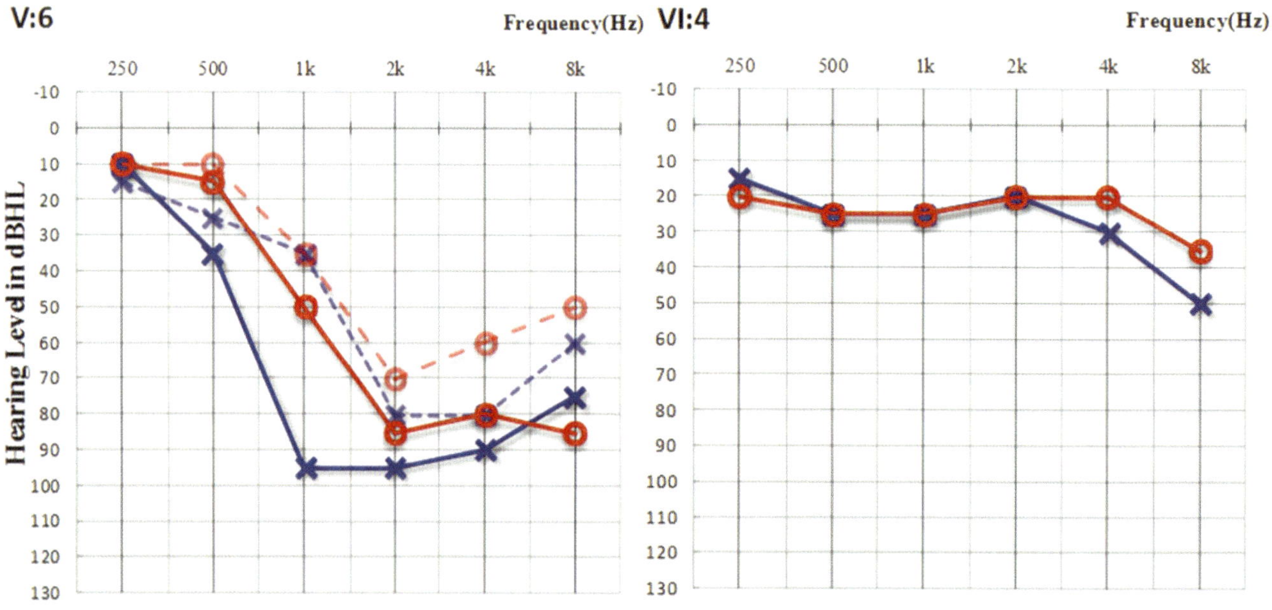

Figure 2. Audiograms of the proband (V:6) and the a five-year-old patient (VI:4). Symbols "o" and "x" denote air conduction pure-tone thresholds at different frequencies in the right and left ear. dB, decibels; Hz, Hertz. The dashed line represent the audiograms detected in 2005 when the proband (V:6) was 23 years old. Audiological examination with solid line was performed in 2012.

Table 1. Summary of the clinical data for all individuals with p.M418K in family 1304.

ID	Gender	Age of test (years)	Age of onset (years)	PTA	Severity of hearing loss	Tinnitus	Genotype
III:20	Female	70	NA	L:80.00 R:83.75	severe severe	L:durative R:durative	T/A
IV:1	Male	62	20	L:105.00 R:107.50	profound profound	L:durative R:durative	T/A
IV:7	Male	53	17	L:68.75 R:75.00	moderate severe	L:durative R:durative	T/A
IV:11	Male	44	24	L:83.75 R:71.25	severe severe	L:durative R:no	T/A
IV:14	Female	52	20	L:92.50 R:93.75	severe severe	L:no R:no	T/A
IV:49	Female	46	5	L:98.75 R:101.25	profound profound	L:durative R:durative	T/A
IV:51	Female	42	13	L:77.50 R:81.25	severe severe	L:durative R:durative	T/A
IV:54	Male	38	20	L:55.00 R:60.00	moderate moderate	L:durative R:durative	T/A
IV:60	Male	64	20	L:76.25 R:77.50	severe severe	L:durative R:durative	T/A
V:1	Male	37	18	L:80.60 R:93.75	severe severe	L:intermittence R:intermittence	T/A
V:3	Male	26	15	L:73.75 R:71.25	severe severe	L:durative R:durative	T/A
V:6	Female	23	13	L:55.00 R:43.75	moderate moderate	L:durative R:durative	T/A
V:22	Male	27	15	L:62.50 R:66.25	moderate moderate	L:intermittence R:intermittence	T/A
V:26	Male	20	15	L:62.50 R:66.25	moderate moderate	L:intermittence R:intermittence	T/A
V:39	Male	53	10	L:105.00 R:105.00	profound profound	L:durative R:durative	T/A
V:41	Male	45	28	L:73.75 R:82.50	severe severe	L:durative R:durative	T/A
V:43	Male	35	20	L:75.00 R:71.25	severe severe	L:durative R:durative	T/A
VI:4	Male	5	5	L:25.00	mild	L:no	T/A

Table 1. Cont.

ID	Gender	Age of test (years)	Age of onset (years)	PTA	Severity of hearing loss	Tinnitus	Genotype
				R:22.50	mild	R:no	
VI:5	Male	2	NA	L:NA	NA	NA	T/A
				R:NA	NA	NA	

PTA, Pure Tone Average. NA, Not Available. L, left ear; R, right ear; T/A in "Genotype" column indicates the genotype of the patient in the mutation of c.1253T>A (p.M418K).

family medical evidence of hearing loss, tinnitus, vestibular symptoms, use of aminoglycosides, and other clinical abnormalities. Audiometric evaluations included pure tone audiometry using Madsen Orbiter 922 audiometer (Denmark), auditory brainstem responses (ABR) and distortion product otoacoustic emissions (DPOAE) using SmartEP of Intelligent Hearing system (USA). The audiological data were evaluated based on the criteria established by European Working Group on Genetics of Hearing loss [20]. High resolution computed tomography (HRCT) was also performed on some subjects to verify whether the family members had other complications in addition to hearing disorders.

A total of 51 unrelated autosomal dominant hearing loss families were chosen as the other affected set for further analysis. In these families, mutations in common genes associated with hearing loss, such as *GJB2*, *SLC26A4* and mitochondrial DNA A1555G, were all excluded. As a comparison group, 100 unaffected individuals of matched geographical ancestry were recruited in this study.

DNA Sample and Exome capture

Peripheral blood samples were obtained and genomic DNA was extracted according to standard procedures. Qualified genomic DNA samples (6 ug) of the proband were sheared by sonication. Then the fragment of each shared genomic DNA sample was hybridized to the SureSelect Biotiny lated RNA Library (BAITS) for enrichment.

NGS, reads mapping and SNPs detection

The enriched libraries were loaded on the HiSeq 2000 platform to be sequenced. Raw image files were processed by Illumina Pipeline v1.6 for base-calling with default parameters and the sequences of each individual were generated as 90 bp paired-end reads. Then the sequenced raw data was aligned to the NCBI human reference genome (NCBI 36.3) using SOAPaligner [21]. After that, the duplicated reads were filtered out and the clean reads located in the target region were collected. The consensus of genotype and quality were estimated by SOAPsnp (version1.03) using the clean reads. The variations of low quality were filtered out according to the following criteria: (i) quality score $<$ 20 (Q20); (ii) average copy number at the allele site $>=2$; (iii) distance of two adjacent SNPs $<$5 bp; and (iv) sequencing depth $<$4 or $>$500.

Detection of insertions and deletions

Insertions and deletions (indels) in the exome regions were identified through the sequencing reads. We aligned the reads to the reference genome by Burrows-Wheeler Aligner (BWA0.5.8) [22], and passed the alignment results to the Genome Analysis Toolkit (GATK1.0.4705) to identify the breakpoints. Finally, we annotated the genotypes of insertions and deletions [23].

Sequencing analysis of candidate gene

Candidate variants located in previously reported hearing loss genes found in exome sequencing were screened in all available members from family 1304. Genotype of the variant c.1253T>A (p.M418K) in *TMC1* was found to be co-segregated with the hearing loss in family 1304. As the candidate gene, the variant in *TMC1* was screened in 100 unaffected individuals geographically matched. In addition, 51 unrelated autosomal dominant hearing loss families without *GJB2*, *SLC26A4* and mitochondrial DNA A1555G mutations were chosen as another affected set for further analysis. For this cohort, exon16, exon19 and their flank sequences containing all the four mutations associated with dominant

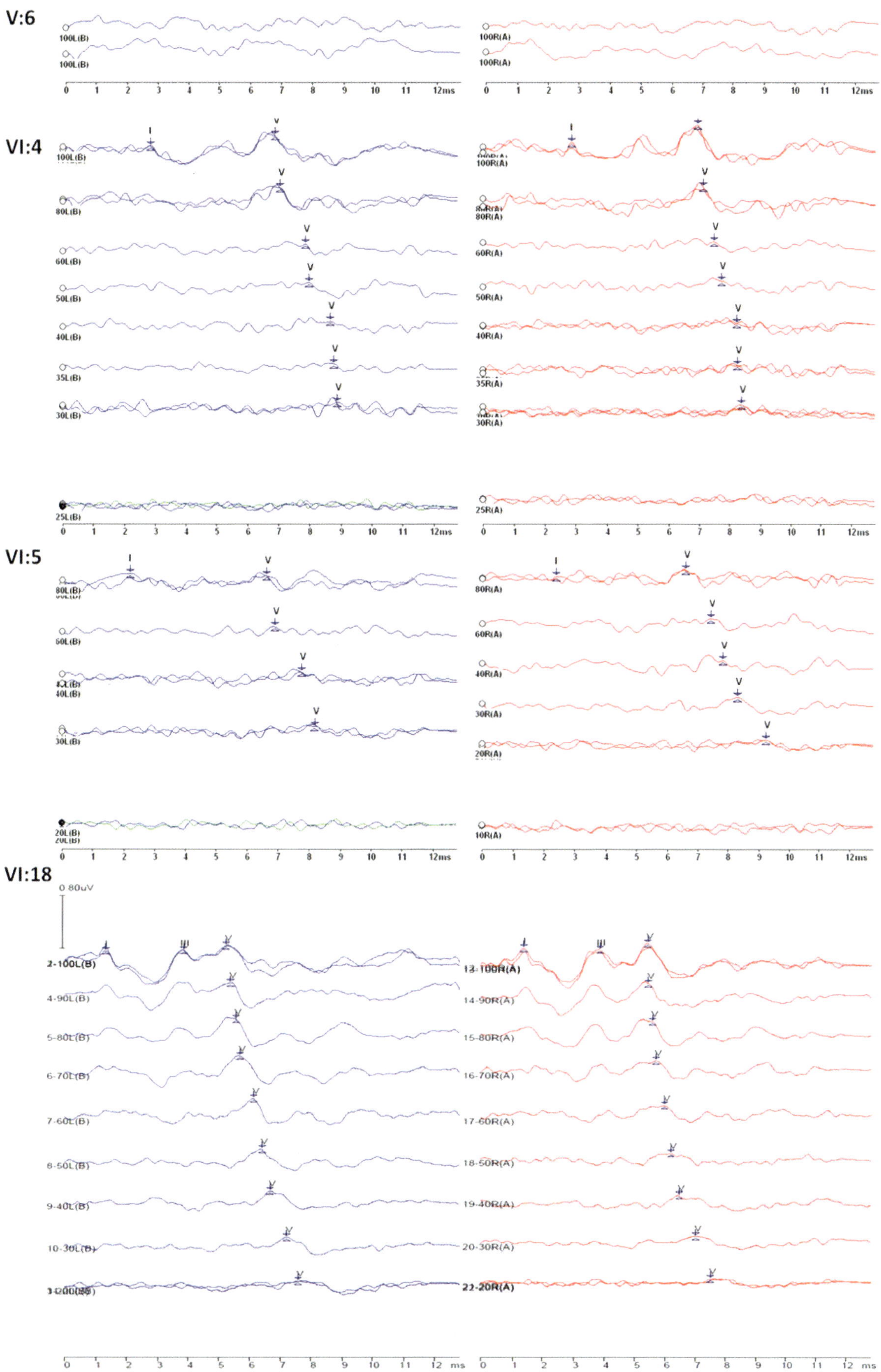
V:6
VI:4
VI:5
VI:18
0.80uV
100L(B)
100R(A)
12ms

Figure 3. ABR results performed to the proband (V:6), a five-year-old patient (VI:4), a two-year-old carrier (VI:5) of p.M418K and a five-year-boy (VI:18) with normal hearing and wildtype genotype. ABR was performed using click stimulus.

hearing loss were sequenced applying Sanger sequencing. Primer pairs were designed using the online Primer 3.0 software and synthesized by Invitrogen (Table S1, Beijing, China) to amplify each exon and boundaries.

Results

Clinical description

Family 1304 was a six-generation pedigree with 222 members, 35 of whom suffered hearing loss (Figure 1). This family was originated from Hebei province in North China. In this study, 48

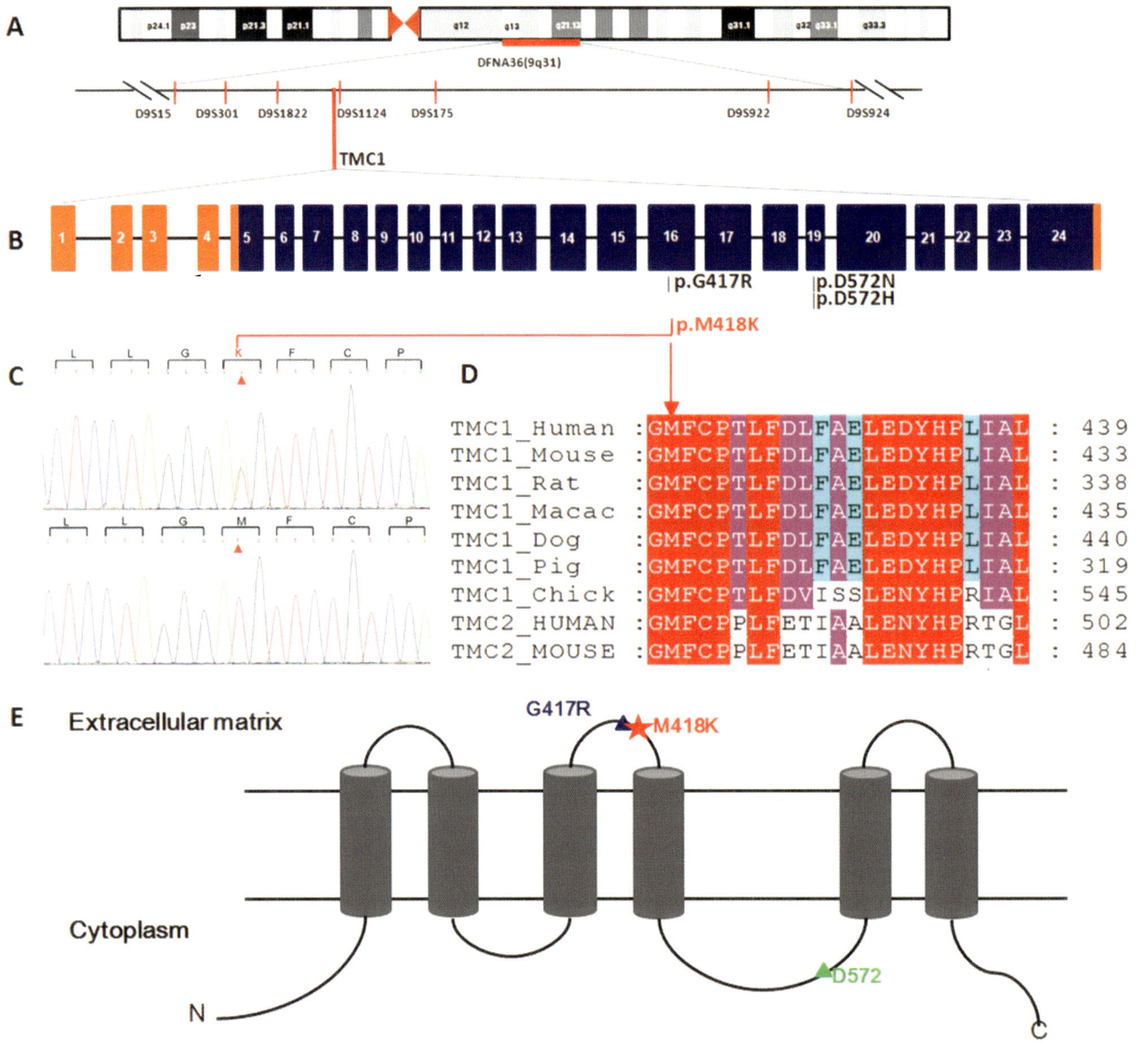

Figure 4. Gene identified in family 1304 with autosomal dominant progressive hearing loss. A: Schematic physical and genetic maps of DFNA36 locus on the 9q31chromosomal region. The *TMC1* gene is indicated. B: Schematic structure of *TMC1* gene. *TMC1* gene has 24 exons. Mutation of p.M418K and p.G417R locate in exon16, and mutation of p.D572N and p.D572H are in exon19. C: Sequencing chromatograms of *TMC1* showing the heterozygous substitution, c.1253A>T in affected individuals (upper panel) compared with that of normal control (lower panel). The mutated nucleotides are marked by triangles. The predicted amino acid changes and surrounding ones are indicated above the sequences. D: Multiple amino acid sequences alignment of *TMC1* and its paralog of *TMC2* using ClustalW software. The conservation analysis shows that p.M418K(arrow) mutation in *TMC1* located in a highly conserved position comparing with the corresponding sequences of human, mouse, rat, macaque, dog, pig, chick, human *TMC2* and mouse *Tmc2*. E: A schematic diagram of *TMC1* protein predicted by TMHMM2.0 containing six transmembrane domains, a cytoplasmic N and C termini. All reported DFNA36 mutations or residual are indicated. Mutation of p.M418K found in this study is located in the second extracellular loop between the third and the fourth transmembrane domain.

Table 2. Filter process for the variants found by whole exome sequencing.

Filter process	V:6
Functional_variations	7477
Against_dbSNP_132	1051
Against_dbSNP_1000 Genomes	723
Against_dbSNP_1000 Genomes _Hapmap 8	639
Against_dbSNP_1000 Genomes _Hapmap 8_YH	635
Variants in genes associated with hearing loss	4

The number of functional variants (non-synonymous/splice acceptor and donor site/insertions or deletions) is listed under various filters. Variants were filtered by presence in dbSNP, 1000 Genomes, HapMap 8 or YH.

members were under detailed physical examinations and audiometric evaluations (Figure 1), and 18 of them showed post-lingual, progressive, and symmetric sensorineural hearing loss with high frequency tinnitus (Figure 2, and Table 1). The onset age ranged from 5 to 28 years old. Hearing loss appeared to initially affect high frequencies with mild or moderate levels at the onset age and progressed to profound levels by the fifth or sixth decade. The low-frequency hearing deteriorated to profound levels and the audiometric graph changed to flat pattern eventually.

The proband (V:6) was a 23-year-old female suffering from hearing loss accompanied by tinnitus when she first visit the outpatient clinic in the year of 2005. She showed a severe hearing loss at 2 kHz and 4 kHz and a moderate hearing loss at 1 kHz and 8 kHz. Seven years later, the threshold increased about 15–30 dB HL at 1 kHz–8 kHz in the right ear, 10–15 dB HL at 2 kHz–8 kHz in the left ear (Figure 2). The threshold of the left ear at 1 kHz increased 60 dB HL within seven years. ABR could not be evoked in both ears (Figure 3). DPOAEs were absent at all frequencies. The youngest patient of this family (VI:4) was 5 years old. And behavior audiometry to him showed bilaterally mild hearing loss (Figure 2). The threshold of ABR was 30 dB nHL. The latencies of wave I, III and V were prolonged and the I-to-V interwave latencies were normal in both ears. The waveform morphology was abnormal and the amplitudes were lower compared to normal waveform morphology (Figure 3). DPOAEs were present from 2.5 kHz to 8 kHz and other frequencies were absent in the left ear, while in the right ear, it was evoked from 2 kHz to 8 kHz and other frequencies were not elicited. High resolution CT scan showed normal middle and inner ear structure, including normal vestibular aqueduct and internal auditory canal.

Exome sequencing

Whole exome of the proband was sequenced and an average of 4.7 billion bases of sequence were generated as paired-end, 90 bp reads, about 63.4% of the total bases were mapped to the targeted bases with a mean coverage of 53.7-fold. At this depth of coverage, 98.3% of the targeted regions were sufficiently covered to pass our thresholds for variant calling (Table S2, Figure S1 and Figure S2). A total of 38130 single nucleotide variants and 2220 indels were identified by exome sequencing (Table S3 and Table S4). Among these variants, we focused on non-synonymous (NS) variants, splice acceptor and donor site variants (SS), and short, frame-shift coding indels that were more likely to be pathogenic mutations than other variants. A total of 7477 variants following the above inclusion criteria were detected in the proband of family 1304 (Table 2). Hereditary hearing loss is a monogenic and always caused by rare variants, frequency of which may be rare or absent in the general population. Therefore, we compared all identified NS/SS/Indel variants in the proband against dbSNP132, the 1000 Human Genome Project (201003 released), eight previously exome-sequenced HapMap samples (HapMap 8), and YH SNPs (Table 2), and removed the shared SNPs. After this filter process, the candidate list reduced to 635 NS/SS/Indel variants. Four of the 635 NS/SS/Indel variants, p.M418K (*TMC1*), p. R382C (*ESRRB*), p.S385P (*ESPN*) and p.D2E (*WFS1*) located in the known hearing loss genes, which may attribute to the phenotypes of the family. Then these four variants were sequenced in all available members of family 1304 by Sanger sequencing. It was found that the mutation of c.1253T>A (p.M418K, NM_138691) in *TMC1* gene completely co-segregated with the phenotype and all 18 patients were heterozygous on this site (Figure 4A, 4B, 4C). In addition to the clinically diagnosed patients, there was a two-year-old boy (VI:5) who carried this mutation without hearing loss (Figure 1). This mutation was not detected in any of the 100 geographical matched controls. The other three candidate variants did not co-segregate with the members of family. To access the likelihood that whether the variant p.M418K in *TMC1* gene is functional or not, we used SIFT software (vision 4.0.3) to predict the biophysical consequences of this substitution and found that this variant is likely to be deleterious. Alignments of the amino acid sequences of *TMC1* in human species, mouse, rat, macaque, dog, pig and chick as well as with human *TMC2* and mouse *Tmc2* showed that the mutation is located in a highly conserved position, which is homologous to the p.M412K mutation in the *Bth* mouse inherited in autosomal dominant pattern (Figure 4D).

To further analyze the contribution of *TMC1* for autosomal dominant hearing loss, we successfully screened the exon16 and exon19 in another 51 autosomal dominant hearing loss families. No functional variants were found to be associated with hearing loss in these families.

Discussion

In this study, we identified a novel mutation p.M418K in *TMC1* in a Chinese family of six generation using the strategy of exome sequencing to the proband. Screening of this mutation in family members showed that all patients were heterozygous and individuals with normal hearing were homozygous in the wild type, which indicated that p.M418K in *TMC1* was responsible for the hearing loss in this autosomal dominant family. *TMC1*, the transmembrane cochlear-expressed gene 1, was reported as the causative gene for both dominant and recessive hearing loss at the DFNA36 and DFNB7/11 [3]. Patients in this family (1304) showed post-lingual, bilateral, symmetric sensorineural hearing loss initially affected the mid and high frequency with mild level, followed by progression to severe or profound levels along with increasing ages, which was consistent with the phenotype of DFNA36 families reported previously [3,14,18,19]. Alignments of the amino acid sequences of transmembrane channel-like gene 1 in different species showed that mutation in family 1304 was an orthologous to the p.M412K mutation reported in the hearing loss mouse model named Beethoven [5]. All these results strongly supported that the mutation of p.M418K in *TMC1* was associated with the hearing loss of patients in family 1304.

Notably, for the first time, our study reported a dominant mutation of *TMC1* in a large family from Chinese. During the past ten years, three dominant mutations in *TMC1* (p.D572N, p.D572H and p.G417R) from four DFNA36 hearing loss families have been reported [5,14,18,19], i.e., the mutation of p.D572N and p.D572H were found in North American families [5,18,19]. The p.G417R mutation was found in an Iranian family [14].

TMC1 is predicted to encode a transmembrane protein containing at least six membrane spanning domains, a cytoplasmic N- and C-termini, and a large cytoplasmic loop named TMC domain [24,25]. The mutation found in this study, p.M418K, and the adjacent DFNA36 mutation of p.G417R, lie within a predicted second extracellular loop between the third and the fourth transmembrane domain (Figure 4E) [14,24], while the amino acid, D572, is located in the region of TMC domain (Figure 4E) [24]. These dominant mutations must act via a gain-of-function or dominant-negative mechanism. The cluster of these dominant mutations of *TMC1* indicates that this region should be important for the proper function of the protein.

It's noteworthy that, for the first time, we have found a family in human with the mutation orthologous to p.M412K in *Tmc1* of *Bth* mouse model since it was found in 2002 [5]. The *Bth* mouse showed progressive loss of the Preyer reflex from around P30 with appeared normal structure of middle ear and inner ear[5], which was similar with the phenotype of late-onset and progressive hearing loss in family 1304. In-situ hybridization on mouse cochlear showed that *Tmc1* is expressed in both outer and inner hair cells from early stage of development [3,5]. It may be required for cochlear hair-cell mechanotransduction as the integral components of the mechanotransduction complex [26]. Studies on the mutant mice that expressing the $Tmc1^{Bth}$ allele implicated that *Tmc1* was the component of the mechanotransduction channel in auditory hair cells of the inner ear [27]. And cells with the p.M412K point mutation in *Tmc1* reduced calcium permeability and single-channel currents [27]. Therefore, *TMC1* should act as a pore-forming subunit of the transduction channel and be involved in determining permeation properties [27].

To summarize, we found ABRs of the patients carrying the p.M418K mutation in *TMC1* showed a prolonged latency and abnormal waveform morphology for wave I to V, which was most likely a direct and causative link, although the mechanism was still obscure. The identification of the p.M418K in *TMC1* in family 1304 makes the *Bth* mouse an excellent animal model to study the mechanism for autosomal dominant hearing loss caused by *TMC1* mutation.

Supporting Information

Figure S1 The distribution of per-base sequencing depth in target regions for each sample. Y-axis indicated the percentage of total target region under a given sequencing depth.

Figure S2 Cumulative depth distribution in target regions for each sample. X-axis denotes sequencing depth, and y-axis indicated the fraction of bases that achieves at or above a given sequencing depth. From the figure above, we can see about 75.50% of target region bases obtains at least 20x fold coverage, that is to say, about 75.50% of target region was covered by more than 20 reads. And about 89.10% of target region achieved at least 10x.

Table S1 Primer sequences for p.M418 in exon16 and p.D572 in exon19.

Table S2 Summary of effective data for exome sequencing. * The region near target refers to flanking region within 200 bp of target regions. ** Total effective reads is the same meaning as the unique mapped reads which was stated in the pipeline above. Here the effective reads consist of two parts: i) the reads have only one best hit in the alignment. These reads comes from the unique region of genome ii) the reads have multiple best hits on the genome (the number of hits between 1 and 20), and they were randomly aligned onto the target regions. These reads mainly come from low complex genomic region, such as repetitive sequences, and account for about 4% of total effective reads. *** Target regions used here refer to genomic regions that the Exome array actually covered. The aggregate length of target is about 37.8 Mb.

Table S3 Summary of SNPs in Exome Sequencing for each Sample. * Consensus genotype with quality score of at least 20. ** Intronic SNPs within 4 bp of exon/intron boundary. *** 5' UTR refers to 200 bp upstream of initiation codon, 3'UTR is defined as 200 bp downstream of termination codon.

Table S4 Summary of Indels in Exome Sequencing for each Sample.

Author Contributions

Conceived and designed the experiments: QW YZ. Performed the experiments: YZ. Analyzed the data: LG PZ LY XJ. Contributed reagents/materials/analysis tools: DW LZ FZ WS LL HW QL BH. Wrote the paper: YZ. Critical reading and discussion of manuscript: Jian Wang Jun Wang QW.

References

1. Morton NE (1991) Genetic epidemiology of hearing impairment. Ann N Y Acad Sci 630: 16–31.
2. Morton CC, Nance WE (2006) Newborn hearing screening—a silent revolution. N Engl J Med 354: 2151–2164.
3. Kurima K, Peters LM, Yang Y, Riazuddin S, Ahmed ZM, et al. (2002) Dominant and recessive deafness caused by mutations of a novel gene, TMC1, required for cochlear hair-cell function. Nat Genet 30: 277–284.
4. Hrabe de Angelis MH, Flaswinkel H, Fuchs H, Rathkolb B, Soewarto D, et al. (2000) Genome-wide, large-scale production of mutant mice by ENU mutagenesis. Nat Genet 25: 444–447.
5. Vreugde S, Erven A, Kros CJ, Marcotti W, Fuchs H, et al. (2002) Beethoven, a mouse model for dominant, progressive hearing loss DFNA36. Nat Genet 30: 257–258.
6. Kalay E, Karaguzel A, Caylan R, Heister A, Cremers FP, et al. (2005) Four novel TMC1 (DFNB7/DFNB11) mutations in Turkish patients with congenital autosomal recessive nonsyndromic hearing loss. Hum Mutat 26: 591.
7. Meyer CG, Gasmelseed NM, Mergani A, Magzoub MM, Muntau B, et al. (2005) Novel TMC1 structural and splice variants associated with congenital nonsyndromic deafness in a Sudanese pedigree. Hum Mutat 25: 100.

8. Santos RL, Wajid M, Khan MN, McArthur N, Pham TL, et al. (2005) Novel sequence variants in the TMC1 gene in Pakistani families with autosomal recessive hearing impairment. Hum Mutat 26: 396.
9. Kitajiri SI, McNamara R, Makishima T, Husnain T, Zafar AU, et al. (2007) Identities, frequencies and origins of TMC1 mutations causing DFNB7/B11 deafness in Pakistan. Clin Genet 72: 546–550.
10. Hilgert N, Alasti F, Dieltjens N, Pawlik B, Wollnik B, et al. (2008) Mutation analysis of TMC1 identifies four new mutations and suggests an additional deafness gene at loci DFNA36 and DFNB7/11. Clin Genet 74: 223–232.
11. Sirmaci A, Duman D, Ozturkmen-Akay H, Erbek S, Incesulu A, et al. (2009) Mutations in TMC1 contribute significantly to nonsyndromic autosomal recessive sensorineural hearing loss: a report of five novel mutations. Int J Pediatr Otorhinolaryngol 73: 699–705.
12. Ben Said M, Hmani-Aifa M, Amar I, Baig SM, Mustapha M, et al. (2010) High frequency of the p.R34X mutation in the TMC1 gene associated with nonsyndromic hearing loss is due to founder effects. Genet Test Mol Biomarkers 14: 307–311.
13. Hildebrand MS, Kahrizi K, Bromhead CJ, Shearer AE, Webster JA, et al. (2010) Mutations in TMC1 are a common cause of DFNB7/11 hearing loss in the Iranian population. Ann Otol Rhinol Laryngol 119: 830–835.
14. Yang T, Kahrizi K, Bazazzadeghan N, Meyer N, Najmabadi H, et al. (2010) A novel mutation adjacent to the Bth mouse mutation in the TMC1 gene makes this mouse an excellent model of human deafness at the DFNA36 locus. Clin Genet 77: 395–398.
15. Brownstein Z, Friedman LM, Shahin H, Oron-Karni V, Kol N, et al. (2011) Targeted genomic capture and massively parallel sequencing to identify genes for hereditary hearing loss in middle eastern families. Genome Biol 12: R89.
16. de Heer AM, Collin RW, Huygen PL, Schraders M, Oostrik J, et al. (2011) Progressive sensorineural hearing loss and normal vestibular function in a Dutch DFNB7/11 family with a novel mutation in TMC1. Audiol Neurootol 16: 93–105.
17. Duman D, Sirmaci A, Cengiz FB, Ozdag H, Tekin M (2011) Screening of 38 genes identifies mutations in 62% of families with nonsyndromic deafness in Turkey. Genet Test Mol Biomarkers 15: 29–33.
18. Kitajiri S, Makishima T, Friedman TB, Griffith AJ (2007) A novel mutation at the DFNA36 hearing loss locus reveals a critical function and potential genotype-phenotype correlation for amino acid-572 of TMC1. Clin Genet 71: 148–152.
19. Hilgert N, Monahan K, Kurima K, Li C, Friedman RA, et al. (2009) Amino acid 572 in TMC1: hot spot or critical functional residue for dominant mutations causing hearing impairment. J Hum Genet 54: 188–190.
20. Mazzoli M, Van Camp G, Newton V, Giarbini N, Declau F, et al. (2003) Recommendations for the description of genetic and audiological data for families with nonsyndromic hereditary hearing impairment. Audiol Med 1: 148–150.
21. Li R, Li Y, Kristiansen K, Wang J (2008) SOAP: short oligonucleotide alignment program. Bioinformatics 24: 713–714.
22. Li H, Durbin R (2010) Fast and accurate long-read alignment with Burrows-Wheeler transform. Bioinformatics 26: 589–595.
23. McKenna A, Hanna M, Banks E, Sivachenko A, Cibulskis K, et al. (2010) The Genome Analysis Toolkit: a MapReduce framework for analyzing next-generation DNA sequencing data. Genome Res 20: 1297–1303.
24. Keresztes G, Mutai H, Heller S (2003) TMC and EVER genes belong to a larger novel family, the TMC gene family encoding transmembrane proteins. BMC Genomics 4: 24.
25. Kurima K, Yang Y, Sorber K, Griffith AJ (2003) Characterization of the transmembrane channel-like (TMC) gene family: functional clues from hearing loss and epidermodysplasia verruciformis. Genomics 82: 300–308.
26. Kawashima Y, Geleoc GS, Kurima K, Labay V, Lelli A, et al. (2011) Mechanotransduction in mouse inner ear hair cells requires transmembrane channel-like genes. J Clin Invest 121: 4796–4809.
27. Pan B, Geleoc GS, Asai Y, Horwitz GC, Kurima K, et al. (2013) TMC1 and TMC2 are components of the mechanotransduction channel in hair cells of the mammalian inner ear. Neuron 79: 504–515.

21

Targeted High-Throughput Sequencing Identifies Pathogenic Mutations in KCNQ4 in Two Large Chinese Families with Autosomal Dominant Hearing Loss

Hongyang Wang[1]⁹, Yali Zhao[1]⁹¤, Yuting Yi[2]⁹, Yun Gao[1], Qiong Liu[1], Dayong Wang[1], Qian Li[1], Lan Lan[1], Na Li[1], Jing Guan[1], Zifang Yin[1], Bing Han[1], Feifan Zhao[1], Liang Zong[1], Wenping Xiong[1], Lan Yu[1], Lijie Song[2], Xin Yi[2], Ling Yang[2], Christine Petit[3,4,5,6], Qiuju Wang[1]*

1 Institute of Otolaryngology, Chinese PLA General Hospital, Medical School of Chinese PLA, Beijing, China, **2** BGI-Tianjin, Tianjin, China, **3** Unité de Génétique et Physiologie de l'Audition, Institut Pasteur, Paris, France, **4** UMRS 1120, Institut National de la Santé et de la Recherche Médicale (INSERM), Paris, France, **5** Université Pierre et Marie Curie (Paris VI), Paris, France, **6** Collège de France, Paris, France

Abstract

Autosomal dominant non-syndromic hearing loss (ADNSHL) is highly heterogeneous, among them, *KCNQ4* is one of the most frequent disease-causing genes. More than twenty *KCNQ4* mutations have been reported, but none of them were detected in Chinese mainland families. In this study, we identified a novel *KCNQ4* mutation in a five generation Chinese family with 84 members and a known *KCNQ4* mutation in a six generation Chinese family with 66 members. Mutation screening of 30 genes for ADNSHL was performed in the probands from thirty large Chinese families with ADNSHL by targeted region capture and high-throughput sequencing. The candidate variants and the co-segregation of the phenotype were verified by polymerase chain reaction (PCR) amplification and Sanger sequencing in all ascertained family members. Then we identified a novel *KCNQ4* mutation p.W275R in exon 5 and a known *KCNQ4* mutation p.G285S in exon 6 in two large Chinese ADNSHL families segregating with post-lingual high frequency-involved and progressive sensorineural hearing loss. This is the first report of *KCNQ4* mutation in Chinese mainland families. *KCNQ4*, a member of voltage-gated potassium channel family, is likely to be a common gene in Chinese patients with ADNSHL. The results also support that the combination of targeted enrichment and high-throughput sequencing is a valuable molecular diagnostic tool for autosomal dominant hereditary deafness.

Editor: You-Qiang Song, The University of Hong Kong, Hong Kong

Funding: This work was supported by the grants of the National Key Basic Research Program of China, No. 2014CB943001, the National Natural Science Foundation of China, Major Project, No. 81120108009. The funders had no role in study design, data collection and analysis, decision to publish, or preparation of the manuscript.

Competing Interests: The authors have declared that no competing interests exist.

* Email: wqcr@263.net

⁹ These authors contributed equally to this work.

¤ Current address: Department of Otolaryngology, Beijing Tongren Hospital, Beijing, China

Introduction

Hereditary hearing loss can be inherited in many patterns, such as autosomal dominant audosomal recessive, X-linked dominant, X-linked recessive, Y-linked pattern, among which ADNSHL has strikingly genetic heterogeneity. To date, more than 60 loci for ADNSHL have been mapped and only 30 corresponding genes have been identified (http://hereditaryhearingloss.org). During the past twenty years, linkage analysis and candidate gene sequencing has been proved to be a powerful tool to identify responsible genes for ADNSHL. However, limited number of samples in the clinical part, the large number of genes in the mapped region, and the large size of many genes restrained the application of this method. Recently, high-throughput sequencing, also known as next-generation sequencing (NGS) has been proved to be an ideal tool to decipher the genetic heterogeneity of deafness. More than ten deafness genes have been identified using NGS including *TPRN*, *GPSM2*, *HSD17B4*, *MASP1*, *CACAM1*, *HARS2*, *SMPX*, *DNMT1*, *ABHD12*, *TSPEAR*, *TNC* and *P2RX2* [1,2,3].

Among ADNSHL genes, *KCNQ4* (MIM*600101), one of the most frequent genes [4], was firstly identified as the causal gene for ADNSHL at DFNA2 by Kubisch and colleagues [5]. As a member of voltage-gated potassium channel family, *KCNQ4* plays a crucial role in potassium recycling in the inner ear. *KCNQ4* has six predicted transmembrane domains encoded by six exons (exon 2 to 7) and a P-loop between transmembrane domains S5 and S6. The P-loop domain forms a channel pore, containing a potassium ion-selective filter, whose function is eliminated by mutations in the pore region [5]. To date, 20 mutations in *KCNQ4* have been reported (Table 1) and it is identified as a common gene with a frequency up to 6.62% in ADNSHL in Japan, predicted to be the most prevalent gene responsible for Japanese ADNSHL patients [6]. However, these mutations have not been found in Chinese mainland populations before this study. Almost all reported cases showed a similar phenotype characterized by post-lingual, progressive, high-frequency hearing impairment (one mid-frequency predominant hearing loss caused by the p.V230E mutation was reported) [6].

Recently, we performed targeted capture and NGS to analyze a cohort of 30 hearing loss probands from Chinese families with ADNSHL (data not shown). Among these families, we identified a novel *KCNQ4* mutation p.W275R in exon 5 in family 025 and a known *KCNQ4* mutation p.G285S in exon 6 in family 727.

Materials and Methods

Ethics Statement

The study was approved by the Committee of Medical Ethics of Chinese People's Liberation Army (PLA) General Hospital. We obtained written informed consents from all the participants in this study. Written informed consents were obtained from the next of kin on the behalf of the minors/children participants involved in this study.

Family Recruitment and Clinical Evaluations

A six-generation family (025) with 66 members segregating ADNSHL and a five-generation family (727) with 84 members segregating ADNSHL were ascertained from the Department of Otolaryngology, Head and Neck Surgery, at the Institute of Otolaryngology of PLA, Chinese PLA General Hospital (Figure 1A, 1B). Either personal or family medical evidence of hearing loss, tinnitus, vestibular symptoms, use of aminoglycosides, and other clinical abnormalities of the participants were identified by a team of experienced doctors and audiologists. Audiometric evaluations included pure tone audiometry, auditory brainstem responses (ABR) and distortion product otoacoustic emissions (DPOAE). High resolution computed tomography (HRCT) was also performed on some subjects to verify whether the family members had other complications other than hearing disorders.

Targeted capture and NGS

Genomic DNA (gDNA) was extracted from the whole blood samples using the Blood DNA kit (TIANGEN BIOTECH, Beijing, China), and 1 ug of purified gDNA fragmented to 200–300 base pairs using an ultrasonoscope (Covaris S2, Massachusetts, USA). End-repair, adenylation and adapter ligation were performed for library preparation following the Illumina's protocol. The same amount of library were pooled then hybridized to the customized capture array (NimbleGen, Roche) including exons, splicing sites and immediate flanking intron sequences of 29 genes for non-syndromic autosomal dominant hearing loss and TNC, a novel causative gene for ADNSHL identified in our previous research (Table S1). Sequencing was carried out on Illumina HiSeq2000 to generate paired end reads (90 bps at each end) [7].

Raw image files were processed by Illumina Pipeline (version 1.3.4) for base-calling with default parameters. Reads were aligned

Table 1. Overview of all *KCNQ4* mutations identified to date.

Mutation DNA	Protein	Exon	Origin	reference
c.211_223del13	p.Q71fs	1	Belguim	Coucke et al. (1999)
c.211delC	p.Q71fs	1	Japan	Kamada et al. (2006)
c.229_230insGC	P.H77fs	1	Japan	Naito, et al. (2013)
c.546C>G	p.F182L	4	Taiwan,	Su, et al. (2007);
			Japan	Naito, et al. (2013)
c.664_681del18	p.G215_220del6	4	Korea	Beak, et al. (2010)
c.689T>A	p.V230E	4	Japan	Naito, et al. (2013)
c.725G>A	p.W241X	5	USA	Hildebrand, et al. (2008)
c.778G>A	p.E260K	5	USA	Hildebrand, et al. (2008)
c.785A>T	p.D262V	5	USA	Hildebrand, et al. (2008)
c.821T>A	p.L274H	5	Neth	Van Hauwe, et al. (2000); De Heer, et al. (2011)
c.823T>C	**p.W275S**	**5**	**China**	**Present study**
c.827G>C	p.W276S	5	Neth, Japan	Coucke et al. (1999), Akita et al. (2001), Camp, et al. (2002), Topsakal, et al. (2005)
c.842T>C	p.L281S	6	USA	Talebizadeh, ea al. (1999)
c.853G>T	p.G285C	6	USA	Coucke et al. (1999)
c.853G>A	**p.G285S**	**6**	France,	Kubisch, et al. (1999)
			China	**Present study**
c.859G>C	p.G287R	6	USA	Arnett, et al. (2011)
c.871C>T	p.P291S	6	Japan	Naito, et al. (2013)
c.872C>T	p.P291L	6	Japan	Naito, et al. (2013)
c.886G>A	p.G296S	6	Spain	Mencia, et al. (2008)
c.891G>T	p.R297S	6	Japan	Naito, et al. (2013)
c.961G>A	p.G321S	7	Neth	Coucke et al. (1999)

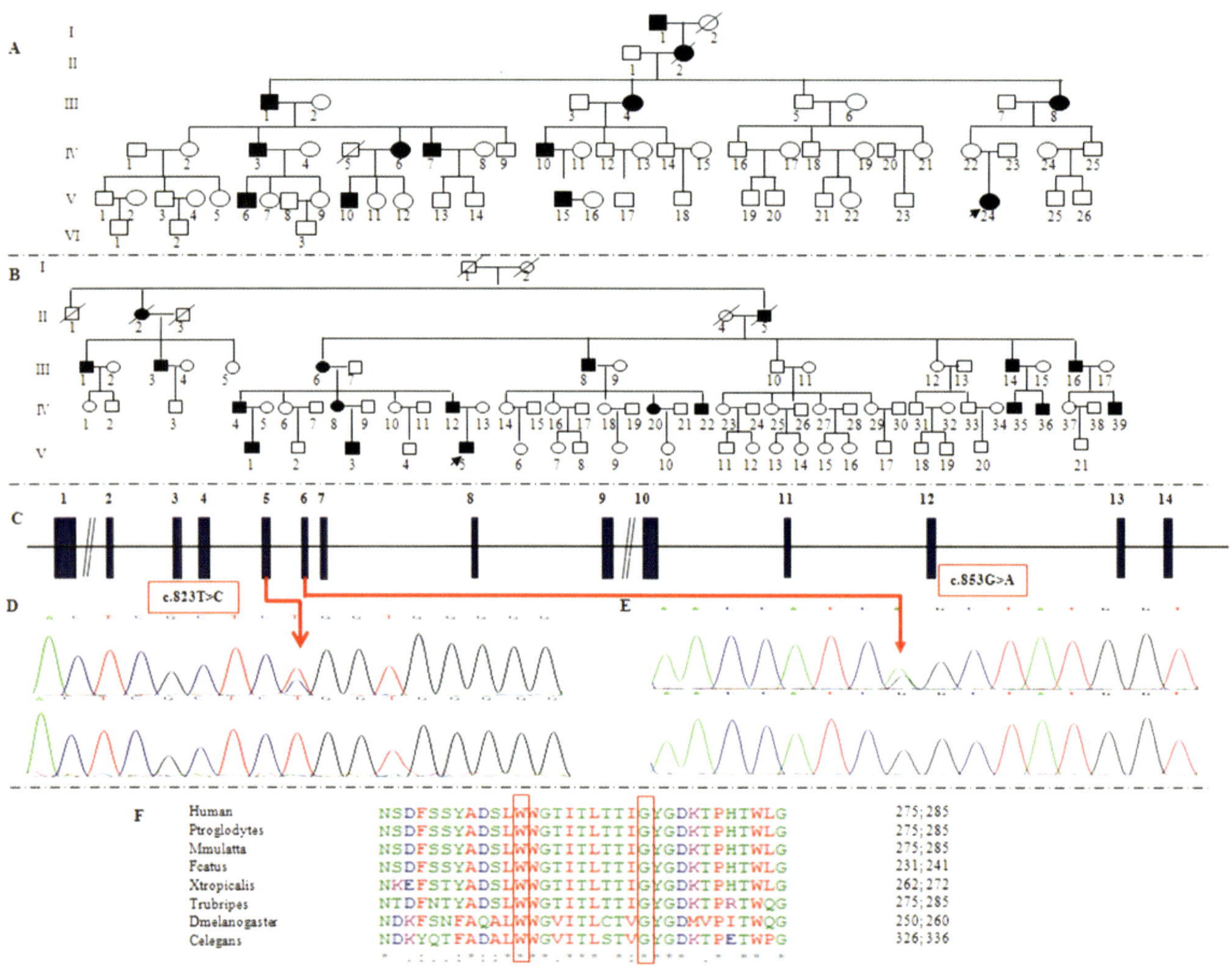

Figure 1. Pedigrees and mutation analysis of the two large Chinese families. (A) & (B) Pedigrees of family 025 and 727. Filled symbols for males (squares) and female (circles) represent affected individuals, and empty, unaffected individuals. (C) Structure of *KCNQ4* gene. *KCNQ4* gene has 14 exons. Mutations of c.823T>C (p.W275R) and c.853G>A (p.G285S) identified in *KCNQ4* are located in exon5 and exon6 respectively. (D) DNA sequence chromatograms showing the two heterozygous missense mutations c.823T>C and c.853G>A in affected individuals (upper panel) compared with the wild type controls (lower panel). (F) Conservation analysis shows that the Trp residue at 275 and the Gly residue at 285 in *KCNQ4* is conserved across human, Ptroglodytes, Mmulatta, Fcatus, Trubripes, Dmelanogaster, Celegans, Xtropicalis.

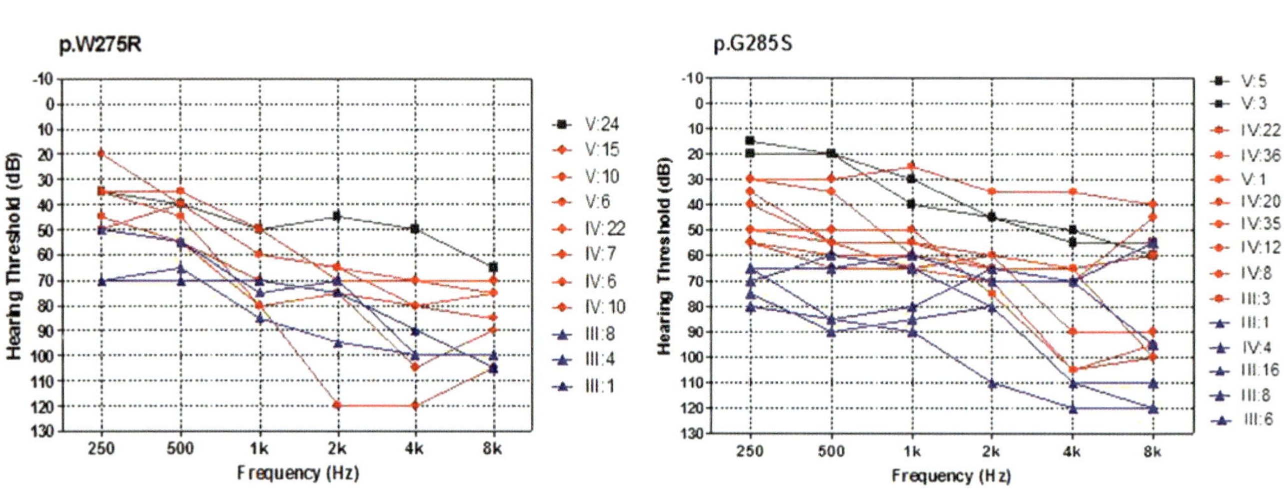

Figure 2. Overlapping audiograms from the better ear for each genotype. In the two cases of p.W275R and p.G285S, black colored audiograms were from the patients aged less than 20 years old, red colored audiograms were from individuals aged 20–49 years old and the blue audiograms were from the patients in their 50 s and over.

Table 2. Summary of clinical data for hearing impaired members in family 727.

Subject	Gender[a]	Age of test (year)	Age of onset (year)	PTA (dB HL)[b]	Hearing impairment[c]	Audiogram	Tinnitus
III:1	M	50	6	78.75	severe	downslope	+
III:3	M	44	10	72.50	severe	downslope	−
III:6	F	68	N/A	91.25	profound	flat	+
III:8	M	67	20	100.00	profound	downslope	+
III:16	M	54	15	66.25	moderately severe	flat	−
IV:4	M	50	30	75.00	severe	flat	+
IV:8	F	41	24	58.75	moderately severe	downslope	+
IV:12	M	34	17	57.50	moderately severe	flat	+
IV:20	F	25	5	70.00	moderately severe	flat	−
IV:22	M	21	6	61.25	moderately severe	flat	+
IV:35	M	25	10	73.75	severe	downslope	−
IV:36	M	22	10	62.50	moderately severe	flat	−
V:1	M	23	N/A	31.25	mild	downslope	N/A
V:3	M	13	11	38.75	mild	downslope	+
V:5	F	8	6	37.50	mild	downslope	+

[a]M, male; F, female.
[b]PTA, pure-tone air-conduction averages (0.5, 1, 2 and 4 kHz) for the better-hearing ear of affected subjects in family 727.
[c]Diagnosed at the time of test. The severity of hearing impairment was defined as mild (26–40 dB HL), moderate (41–55 dB HL), moderately severe (56–70 dB HL), severe (71–90 dB HL) and profound (>90 dB HL).
N/A, not available; +, positive finding; −, negative finding.

Table 3. Summary of clinical data for hearing impaired members in family 025.

Subject	Gender[a]	Age of test (year)	Age of onset (year)	PTA (dB HL)[b]	Hearing impairment[c]	Audiogram	Tinnitus[d]
III:1	M	76	15	76.25	severe	flat	+
III:4	F	72	20	86.25	severe	downslope	−
III:8	F	57	20	75	severe	downslope	+
IV:3	M	52	16	70	moderately severe	flat	+
IV:6	F	46	30	70	moderately severe	downslope	+
IV:7	M	39	25	66.25	moderately severe	downslope	−
IV:10	M	49	20	56.25	moderately severe	flat	−
V:6	M	25	17	61.25	moderately severe	downslope	−
V:10	M	25	15	56.25	moderately severe	downslope	−
V:15	M	24	10	58.75	moderately severe	flat	N/A
V:24	F	9	2	46.25	moderate	downslope	N/A

[a]M, male; F, female.
[b]PTA, pure-tone air-conduction averages (0.5, 1, 2 and 4 kHz) for the better-hearing ear of affected subjects in family 727.
[c]Diagnosed at the time of test. The severity of hearing impairment was defined as mild (26–40 dB HL), moderate (41–55 dB HL), moderately severe (56–70 dB HL), severe (71–90 dB HL) and profound (>90 dB HL).
[d]N/A, not available; +, positive finding; −, negative finding.

Table 4. Target region capture sequencing results.

Proband	Length of target region (bp)	Target Region Map Bases (Mbp)	Coverage (%)	Coverage at least 20× (%)	Mean Depth
025	132,789	54.21	99.71	99.49	408.23
727	132,789	56.11	99.71	99.38	422.59
Average	**132,789**	**55.16**	**99.71**	**99.44**	**415.41**

to NCBI37/hg19 assembly using the BWA (Burrows Wheeler Aligner). SNPs and indels (inserts and deletions) were detected using the GATK software [8].

Sanger sequencing

After filtering against multiple databases, sanger sequencing was used in all available members from family 025 and 727 to determine whether the potential mutations in causative genes co-segregated with the disease phenotype in these families or not. Direct PCR products were sequenced using Bigdye terminator v3.1 cycle sequencing kits (Applied Biosystems. Foster City, CA) and analyzed using a ABI 3700XL Genetic Analyzer.

Results

Clinical description

For family 727, a total of 41 family members, composed of 15 clinical affected and 26 unaffected individuals were ascertained in this study. While in family 025, 11 patients and 26 control individuals were ascertained. Age of onset in family 727 ranged from 5 to 30 years old, with average onset age 13.08 years old, while in 025 the onset age ranged from 2 to 30 years old, with average onset age 16.45 years old. For both two autosomal families, affected members showed a post-lingual, symmetrical, and bilateral non-syndromic sensorineural hearing loss. The hearing loss was initially presented as high frequencies with subsequent gradual progression to severe level involving all frequencies at later ages. Some patients had associated tinnitus, but no vestibular symptoms or signs were reported (Table 2, Table 3, Figure 1A, 1B, Figure 2). High resolution computed tomography (HRCT) of the temporal bone in the probands showed normal middle ears structure, including normal vestibular aqueduct and internal auditory canal. None of the affected members had a history of exposure to aminoglycosides, noise, or other causes that may account for the hearing impairment.

Targeted high-throughput sequencing

Approximately 133K bp of exons and adjacent intronic regions of the 30 genes known to be responsible for ADNSHL were captured and sequenced. The average sequencing depth for target region is about 415×, and 99.44% of the average coverage for targeted region is more than 20×, which is satisfied with the requirements for calling SNPs and InDels (Table 4). For the proband of family 025, a total of 484 variants were identified, 47 of which were nonsynonymous variants, splice acceptor and donor site mutations and coding indels that were more likely to be pathogenic mutations; only 3 of the 47 variants were with the allele frequency which were less than 0.01 in dbSNP137, HapMap, 1000 human genome and local dataset; and a missense variant, c.823T>C (p.W275R) in exon5 of *KCNQ4* (NM_004700), predicted to be "Damaging", "Probably Damaging", "Deleterious", "Disease_causing", "Conserved" and "Conserved" by SIFT, Polyphen2, LRT, Mutation Taster, GERP++, and PhyloP respectively (Tables 5 and 6). For this site, 45% (114/254) reads supported for C vs. 55% (140/254) reads supported for T, which means it is a heterozygote (Het) (Figure S1). This indicated that this novel mutation may be the cause of the hearing loss in this Chinese family. In the proband of family 727, another missense mutation, c.853G>A (p.G285S) in *KCNQ4*, a previously reported mutation (rs28937588) was identified (Figure S2).

Mutation detection and analysis

Sanger sequencing confirmed the co-segregation of p.W275R and p.G285S with the disease phenotype in Family 025 and 727 respectively (Figure 1C and D and E). The two mutations were not detected in other 28 probands from Chinese families with ADNSHL. Both of the mutations occurred at highly conserved amino acids (Figure 1F), and are predicted to be deleterious by the SIFT, Polyphen2, LRT, Mutation Taster, GERP++, and PhyloP programs (IS IT NOT IDENTICAL TO WHAT HAVE MENTIONNED JUST ABOVE (Table 6). Based on these results and the phenotypes of these two families, we concluded that these

Table 5. Candidate genetic variants identified for the proband of family 025.

Filter process	NO. of Variants
All SNPs/InDels	484
Functional_variations	47
Genotype frequency in dbSNP137, HapMap, 1000 human genome dataset ≤0.01	8
Genotype frequency in local dataset≤0.01	3
Predicted to be deleterious by SIFT, Polyphen2, LRT and MutationTaster	1

Table 6. A novel variant in the proband of family 025.

Gene	NM No.	Nucleotide	Amino Acid	Zygosity	Prediction information					
					SIFT	Polyphen2	LRT	MutationTaster	GERP++	PhyloP
KCNQ4	NM_004700	c.823T>C	p.W275R	Het	Damaging	Probably Damaging	Deleterious	Disease_causing	Conserved	Conserved

two mutations in the *KCNQ4* are responsible for the hearing loss in the family 025 and 727.

Discussion

As is known, mutations in gene *KCNQ4* have been associated with ADNSHL, recognized as one of the most frequent causes of ADNSHL, is characterized by post-lingual autosomal dominant non-syndromic progressive sensorineural hearing loss, first affected the high frequencies according to GeneReviews. In this present study, we identified a known mutation and a novel mutation in the P-loop region of the *KCNQ4* potassium channel which yielded dominant non-syndromic hearing loss by high-throughput sequencing as well as conventional genetic testing. It is noteworthy that this is the first report of heterozygous mutations in the *KCNQ4* genes as a cause of ADNSHL in Chinese mainland families. In family 727, the G285S mutation in exon6 affects the first glycine in the GYG signature sequence of K+ channel pores, which has been identified in three affected members of a small French family with DFNA2. This mutation exert a strong dominant-negative effect on the wild type and render heteromeric channels nonfunctional [5]. By using adenoviral delivery of *KCNQ4* channels carrying G285S, Holt JR and colleagues demonstrated that *KCNQ4* channels contributed to the M-like conductances: $G_{K,n}$ of the cochlear outer hair cells and $G_{K,L}$ of the vestibular type I hair cells [9]. As far as we know, this is the second report about this mutation. Recurrent mutations in *KCNQ4* also include c.211delC (p.Q71fs), c.821T>A (p.L274H), c.827G>C (p.W276S), having been reported in more than one family. Among these recurrent mutations, mutation W276S is a hot spot mutation in Belgian, Dutch and Japanese families [10]. Together with specific audiogram configuration, recurrent mutations may promote genetic testing for ADNSHL with a particular phenotype [6]. In family 025, we found a novel missense mutation W275R in exon 5 of KCNQ4. The mutation c.823T>C (W275R) is immediately adjacent to the previously reported mutation c.827G>C (W276S). These two adjacent tryptophan residues, located with the pore helix, are highly conserved across different potassium channel families and play a important role in K^+ channel function, presumably holding the pore open at a correct diameter [11]. Mutations in these conserved tryptophan residues result in a complete loss of function of K^+ channel [12]. Previous studies have demonstrated that the W276S mutation lead to a dramatic decrease in *KCNQ4* surface expression with strong dominant-negative effects on the wild type (WT) *KCNQ4* subunit. We presume that the W275R mutation may have the similar functional mechanism [13,14].

It is noteworthy that this is the first report of *KCNQ4* mutation in Chinese mainland families. Before this report, there was a report of *KCNQ4* missense mutation P182L in a Taiwan family. The mutation locates in the S3 domain of *KCNQ4*. However, it is not conserved in all KCNQ family and unlikely to be pathogenic according to some prediction program, such as SIFT, Polyphen Phylop, LRT, etc. In this study, we found a P182L mutation in one of the 30 probands from ADNSHL families which did not co-segregate with the disease phenotype in the family members. It was also found in a Japanese control sample with normal hearing [4,15].

To date, 16 missense mutations and 4 indels in *KCNQ4* have been reported (Table 1). Phenotype-genotype correlation of *KCNQ4* has been summarized, most of the patients with missense mutation are younger-onset and pure all-frequency hearing loss, while patients with deletion mutations are later-onset and pure high-frequency hearing loss, so the two families in this study are

[16,17]. *KCNQ4* is also predicted to be a candidate gene for age-related hearing loss (ARHI) since *KCNQ4* mutation families have similar pattern of hearing loss with ARHI, especially a unique pattern of hearing loss with striking resemblance to ARHI, in which only the high frequencies were progressively affected while the lower frequencies remained intact until an older age [18]. To investigate the association of *KCNQ4* with ARHI, Van Eyken et al. examined *KCNQ4* and detected a significant association between *KCNQ4* and ARHI in two independent Caucasian populations. All SNPs are located in the same 13-kb region in the middle of the *KCNQ4* gene, indicating that the pathogenic variants for ARHI may locate in this region [19].

KCNQ4 is likely to be a common gene in Chinese ADNSHL: i) *KCNQ4* is one of the more frequent genes in ADNSHL in comparison to the other reported genes [4]; ii) In a large Japanese cohort, *KCNQ4* is found to be the most prevalent gene responsible for Japanese ADNSHL. In their study, 19 families with 7 different mutations were identified in 287 probands from ADNSHL families [6]. Mutations of *KCNQ4* were also found in other east Asian region, such as Korea and other Japanese population (Table 1). iii) Our group found a copy variation of 47 base pairs insertion or deletion in the exon2 and exon3 intron sequence, supposing to be a specific marker for the hearing loss of the pedigree [20]. Then we performed mutation screening of *KCNQ4* in 71 patients with high frequency hearing loss and 40 unaffected individuals of matched geographical ancestry, and found the deletion of the second intron 47 bp in 5 patients as well as 2 males with normal hearing, the insertion of 47 bp in 11 patients [21].

Despite an increasing number of pathogenic *KCNQ4* mutations have been identified, the molecular aetiology of DFNA2 still unknown. The missense mutations are believed to exert a dominant-negative effect by interfering with the normal channel subunit. The two deletions, c.211delC and c.211_223del13, are proposed to exert a pathogenic effect through haploinsufficiency [3]. In the mouse models, loss of *KCNQ4* function leads to progressive sensorineural hearing loss, paralleled by selective degeneration of outer hair cells and spiral ganglion neurons [22]. Among the missense mutations, L274H, W276S, L281S, G285S, G296S and G321S are loss of function mutations and eletrophysiological studies have shown that these mutations lead to loss of *KCNQ4* currents [5,13,22,23,24]. However, the molecular mechanisms about how these mutations lead the loss of *KCNQ4* currents remain unknown. Recently Gao YH et al. reported two mechanisms underlying DFNA2, the decreased cell surface expression detected by immunofluorescent microscopy and Western blot and the impaired conductance of *KCNQ4* demonstrated by electrophysiological studies [14]. Because of the restriction of the lack of the understanding of the molecular aetiology, no therapeutic methods to prevent progressive hearing loss are available for now. Further functional studies regarding mutations in these residues in *KCNQ4* may help clarify the molecular mechanism, which in turn, will facilitate informative genetic counseling, early diagnosis and even treatment of hearing impairment [25]. It is anticipated that future management of these genetic hearing disorders will be more targeted to the cellular processes involved and improve the likelihood of hearing recovery.

In conclusion, we have shown two mutations in Chinese ADNSHL families using targeted high-throughput sequencing. This is the first report of *KCNQ4* mutation in Chinese mainland families, providing more information for discovering the molecular mechanism of KCNQ4 mutation-induced hearing loss. The results also support that the combination of targeted capture and NGS is a valuable molecular diagnostic tool for autosomal dominant hereditary deafness.

Supporting Information

Figure S1 Reads of proband from family 025 (chr1 41285133).

Figure S2 Reads of proband from family 727 (chr1 41285565).

Table S1 The non-syndromic autosomal dominant genes captured.

File S1 Data S1–S4. Data S1. Next generation sequencing results of proband of family 025 (including all SNP and INDEL results). Data S2. Next generation sequencing results of proband of family 727 (including all SNP and INDEL results). Data S3. Sanger sequencing results of family 025. This file shows the sanger sequencing results of 36 members ascertained in this study. Data S4. Sanger sequencing results of family 727. This file shows the sanger sequencing results of 41 members ascertained in this study.

Acknowledgments

We thank the families for their invaluable cooperation and participation in this work.

Author Contributions

Conceived and designed the experiments: QW HW. Performed the experiments: HW YZ YY. Analyzed the data: HW YZ YY LS YG. Contributed reagents/materials/analysis tools: Q. Liu LL NL ZY WX LY. Contributed to the writing of the manuscript: HW YZ YY. Critical reading and discussion of manuscript: DW Q. Li JG BH FZ LZ XY LY CP QW.

References

1. Gao X, Su Y, Guan LP, Yuan YY, Huang SS, et al. (2013) Novel compound heterozygous TMC1 mutations associated with autosomal recessive hearing loss in a Chinese family. PLoS One 8: e63026.
2. Yan D, Zhu Y, Walsh T, Xie DH, Yuan HJ, et al. (2013) Mutation of the ATP-gated $P2X_2$ receptor leads to progressive hearing loss and increased susceptibility to noise. Proc Natl Acad Sci 110: 2228–2233.
3. Zhao YL, Zhao FF, Zong L, Zhang P, Guan LP, et al. (2013) Exome sequencing and linkage analysis identified tenascin-C (TNC) as a novel causative gene in nonsyndromic hearing loss. PLoS One 8: e69549.
4. Hilgert N, Smith RJ, Van Camp G (2009) Forty-six genes causing nonsyndromic hearing impairment: which ones should be analyzed in DNA diagnostics? Mutat Res 681: 189–196.
5. Kubisch C, Schroeder BC, Friedrich T, Lutjohann B, El-Amraoui A, et al. (1999) KCNQ4, a novel potassium channel expressed in sensory outer hair cells, is mutated in dominant deafness. Cell 96: 437–446.
6. Naito T, Nishio SY, Iwasa Y, Yano T, Kumakawa K, et al. (2013) Comprehensive genetic screening of KCNQ4 in a large autosomal dominant nonsyndromic hearing loss cohort: genotype-phenotype correlations and a founder mutation. PLoS One 8: e63231.
7. Wei XM, Ju XC, Yi X, Zhu Q, Qu N, et al. (2011) Identification of sequence variants in genetic disease-causing genes using targeted next-generation sequencing. PLoS One 6: e29500.
8. Wei XM, Sun Y, Xie JS, Shi Q, Qu N, et al. (2012) Next-generation sequencing identifies a novel compound heterozygous mutation in MYO7A in a Chinese patient with Usher Syndrome 1B. Clin Chim Acta 413: 1866–1871.
9. Holt JR, Stauffer EA, Abraham D, Geleoc GS (2007) Dominant-negative inhibition of M-like potassium conductances in hair cells of the mouse inner ear. J Neurosci 27: 8940–8951.
10. Van Camp G, Coucke PJ, Akita J, Fransen E, Abe S, et al. (2002) A mutational hot spot in the KCNQ4 gene responsible for autosomal dominant hearing impairment. Hum Mutat 20: 15–19.

11. Doyle DA, Cabral JM, Pfuetzner RA, Kuo A, Gulbis JM, et al. (1998). The Structure of the Potassium Channel: Molecular Basis of K+ Conduction and Selectivity. Science 280: 69–77.
12. Perozo E, MacKinnon R, Bezanilla F, Stefani E (1993) Gating currents from a nonconducting mutant reveal open-closed conformations in Shaker K+ channels. Neuron 11: 353–358.
13. Kim HJ, Lv P, Sihn CR, Yamoah EN (2011) Cellular and molecular mechanisms of autosomal dominant form of progressive hearing loss, DFNA2. J Biol Chem 286: 1517–1527.
14. Gao YH, Yechikov S, Vazquez AE, Chen DY, Nie LP (2013) Impaired surface expression and conductance of the KCNQ4 channel lead to sensorineural hearing loss. J Cell Mol Med 17: 889–900.
15. Su CC, Yang JJ, Shieh JC, Su MC, Li SY (2007) Identification of novel mutations in the KCNQ4 gene of patients with nonsyndromic deafness from Taiwan. Audiol Neurotol 12: 20–26.
16. Topsakal V, Pennings RJ, te Brinke H, Hamel B, Huygen PL, et al. (2005) Phenotype determination guides swift genotyping of a DFNA2/KCNQ4 family with a hot spot mutation (W276S). Otol Neurotol 26: 52–58.
17. Kamada F, Kure S, Kudo T, Suzuki Y, Oshima T, et al. (2006). A novel KCNQ4 one-base deletion in a large pedigree with hearing loss: implication for the genotype-phenotype correlation. J Hum Genet 51: 455–460.
18. Coucke PJ, Van Hauwe P, Kelley PM, Kunst H, Schatteman I, et al. (1999) Mutations in the KCNQ4 gene are responsible for autosomal dominant deafness in four DFNA2 families. Hum Mol Genet 8: 1321–1328.
19. Van Eyken E, Van Laer L, Fransen E, Topsakal V, Lemkens N, et al. (2006) KCNQ4: a gene for age-related hearing impairment? Hum Mutat 27: 1007–1016.
20. Wang QJ, Cao JY, Li N, Yang Y, Wang QG, et al. (2002) KCNQ4 gene mutations affected pedigree with autosomal dominant hereditary hearing loss. Chin J Otorhinolaryngol 37: 343–347.
21. Li LN, Li QZ, Wu WM, Wang QJ (2007). Screening the mutation of KCNQ4 in patients with high frequency hearing impairment. J of audio and speech pathol 15: 25–27.
22. Kharkovets T, Dedek K, Maier H, Schweizer M, Khimich D, et al. (2006). Mice with altered KCNQ4 K+ channels implicate sensory outer hair cells in human progressive deafness. EMBO J 25: 642–652.
23. Baek JI, Park HJ, Park K, Choi SJ, Lee KY, et al. (2011) Pathogenic effects of a novel mutation (c.664_681del) in KCNQ4 channels associated with auditory pathology. Biochim Biophys Acta 1812: 536–543.
24. Mencia A, Gonzalez-Nieto D, Modamio-Hoybjor S, Etxeberria A, Aranguez G, et al. (2008). A novel KCNQ4 pore-region mutation (p.G296S) causes deafness by impairing cell-surface channel expression. Hum Genet 123: 41–53.
25. Trune DR (2010) Ion homeostasis in the ear: mechanisms, maladies, and management. Current Opinion in Otolaryngology & Head and Neck Surgery 18: 413–419.

Abnormal Pitch Perception Produced by Cochlear Implant Stimulation

Fan-Gang Zeng*, Qing Tang, Thomas Lu

Center for Hearing Research, Departments of Anatomy and Neurobiology, Biomedical Engineering, Cognitive Sciences, and Otolaryngology – Head and Neck Surgery, University of California Irvine, Irvine, California, United States of America

Abstract

Contemporary cochlear implants with multiple electrode stimulation can produce good speech perception but poor music perception. Hindered by the lack of a gold standard to quantify electric pitch, relatively little is known about the nature and extent of the electric pitch abnormalities and their impact on cochlear implant performance. Here we overcame this obstacle by comparing acoustic and electric pitch perception in 3 unilateral cochlear-implant subjects who had functionally usable acoustic hearing throughout the audiometric frequency range in the non-implant ear. First, to establish a baseline, we measured and found slightly impaired pure tone frequency discrimination and nearly perfect melody recognition in all 3 subjects' acoustic ear. Second, using pure tones in the acoustic ear to match electric pitch induced by an intra-cochlear electrode, we found that the frequency-electrode function was not only 1–2 octaves lower, but also 2 times more compressed in frequency range than the normal cochlear frequency-place function. Third, we derived frequency difference limens in electric pitch and found that the equivalent electric frequency discrimination was 24 times worse than normal-hearing controls. These 3 abnormalities are likely a result of a combination of broad electric field, distant intra-cochlear electrode placement, and non-uniform spiral ganglion cell distribution and survival, all of which are inherent to the electrode-nerve interface in contemporary cochlear implants. Previous studies emphasized on the "mean" shape of the frequency-electrode function, but the present study indicates that the large "variance" of this function, reflecting poor electric pitch discriminability, is the main factor limiting contemporary cochlear implant performance.

Editor: Sliman J. Bensmaia, University of Chicago, United States of America

Funding: This work was supported by the National Institutes of Health (RO1-DC008858 and P30-DC008369). The funders had no role in study design, data collection and analysis, decision to publish, or preparation of the manuscript.

Competing Interests: The authors have declared that no competing interests exist.

* E-mail: fzeng@uci.edu

Introduction

Pitch is a fundamental auditory percept that carries not only melodic information in music perception, but also speaker, prosodic or even lexical information in language processing. Pitch may be affected by sound pressure and waveform, but it primarily depends upon sound frequency [1]. Sound frequency is tonotopically organized as spatial location in the entire auditory pathway [2,3,4]. In the human cochlea, frequency from 20 Hz to 20,000 Hz is exponentially mapped to the 35-mm cochlear length, known as the Greenwood function [5]. Over this cochlear length, 3,500 inner hair cells are spatially arranged from apex to base and systematically tuned to different frequencies from low to high. As a result, a normal listener can detect approximately 1,400 steps of frequency differences for medium-loud sounds [6]. Although the detailed mechanisms are not clear, this tonotopic organization and sharp frequency selectivity are needed to support exquisite pitch perception. One example is the pitch of a harmonic sound, whose frequency spectrum (f) consists of integer multiples of a fundamental frequency ($f = nF0$, where $n = 1, 2, 3, \ldots$ and $F0$ = fundamental). A harmonic sound produces pitch at the fundamental, even if the fundamental itself is missing [7].

One design goal for a cochlear implant is to replicate this tonotopic organization and sharp frequency selectivity in a deafened ear. Contemporary multi-electrode cochlear implants have been successful in producing good speech perception in quiet, but fail to produce normal pitch perception [8]. In fact, most cochlear implant users cannot even recognize simple melodies [9,10,11,12]. Several factors have been implicated in poor cochlear implant pitch perception. Vermeire et al. [13] studied 14 cochlear implant subjects who had unilateral implants but significant residual acoustic hearing in the non-implant ear. Using a high-resolution X-ray to identify electrode position in the cochlea and a pitch scaling method to identify the relationship of stimulation of a single electrode to pure tone frequency in the non-implant ear, they found a frequency-electrode function consistent with the Greenwood function for 9 of the 14 subjects. The remaining 5 subjects showed severe departure from the Greenwood function with either non-monotonic or flat functions. On the contrary, several similar studies found a frequency-electrode function that was consistently 1-2 octaves lower than the Greenwood function [14,15,16,17,18]. One reason for this inconsistency could be methodological differences [19]. The other reason was the lack of a gold standard in the non-implant ear, as reasonably good frequency selectivity above 500 Hz may be required for consistent pitch matches to electric stimulation [20]. Nevertheless, the misaligned frequency-electrode function has been assumed to be responsible for poor pitch perception in cochlear implants [13,21,22]. Hypothetically, this misalignment could be relatively easy to correct by individually changing the frequency to electrode map in the speech processor. The present study will directly test this hypothesis.

Relatively little is known about the discriminability of electric pitch. At best, the implant users could use pulse rates (up to several hundred Hz) to judge or produce music intervals [23,24]. However, rate discrimination is an order of magnitude poorer than normal pure tone frequency discrimination [24,25]. At the worst, 22 discriminable electrode steps [26] are 2 orders of magnitude less than 1400 discriminable frequency steps in acoustic hearing [6,27]. The present study also aims to quantify electric pitch discriminability by comparing electric pitch to an established gold standard of pure tone pitch in acoustic hearing.

Methods

Subjects

Three cochlear-implant subjects who had significant acoustic hearing in the non-implanted ear participated in the present study. All procedures in this study were approved by the University of California Irvine Institutional Review Board. Subjects gave written informed consent before data collection. Table 1 shows their demographic information. Figure 1A shows their audiograms. S1 was a musician and audio engineer and suddenly lost hearing on one side for unknown reasons. He received a HiRes90k device from Advanced Bionics Corporation (Valencia, CA) to treat his debilitating tinnitus [28]. In his clinical processor, the pulse rate was 2900 Hz per electrode and the pulse duration was 10.8 µs/phase. He had used the implant regularly and achieved 73% correct sentence recognition score that was typical of an implant user. In the non-implant ear, he had normal hearing (≤20 dB HL) at all tested frequencies except for 4000 Hz at which he had a mild loss of 30 dB HL.

S2 was a veteran and had fluctuating hearing loss most likely due to Meniere's disease. He received a Med El implant (Innsbruck, Austria) and was the subject who had been thoroughly studied by Dorman et al. [18]. Except for his X-ray data, all data were collected independently in Irvine CA. In his clinical processor, the pulse rate was 1652 Hz per electrode and the pulse duration was 25.42 µs/phase. He used his implant on a daily basis and was considered a star user with 97% correct sentence recognition. In the non-implant ear, he had mild hearing loss

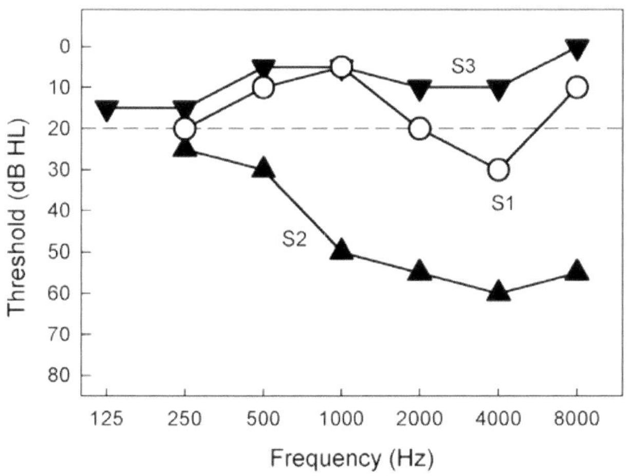

Figure 1. Audiograms for the non-implant ears. Hearing thresholds are plotted as a function of frequency for S1 (open circles), S2 (triangles), and S3 (inverted triangles). The dashed line indicates the conventional limit of normal hearing at 20 dB HL.

Table 1. Subject information.

Subject	Age (years)	Duration of deaf (years)	Implant ear	Implant type	Duration of implant use (years)	Implant speech	Acoustic PTA (dB HL)	Acoustic melody
S1	46	1	Right	HiRes90K (1J)	1	HiRes-S (73%)	12 dB	100%
S2	59	12	Right	Combi40+ (medium)	5	HDCIS (97%)	45 dB	96%
S3	43	1	Left	PULSAR ci100 (medium)	1	HDCIS (43%)	7 dB	92%

Age is reported at the time of test. HiRes90k is a product of Advanced Bionics Corporation (Valencia, CA) and Combi 40+ and PULSAR ci100 are products of Med El (Innsbruck, Austria). Implant speech is specified as the type of speech processing and keyword percent correct for HINT sentences in quiet (all via direct connection to prevent acoustic leakage). PTA (pure tone average) is the average of thresholds in dB HL at 500, 1000 and 2000 Hz for the non-implant ear. Acoustic melody indicates percent correct recognition of 12 familiar melodies delivered to the non-implant ear.

(25 μ30 dB HL) below 1000 Hz and moderate hearing loss (50 μ60 dB) at 1000 Hz and above.

S3, who worked in finance, suddenly lost her hearing on one side and developed debilitating tinnitus on the same side for unknown reasons. She received a Med El implant to control her tinnitus. In her clinical processor, the pulse rate was 1587 Hz per electrode and the pulse duration was 25.42 μs/phase. She did not use the implant on a daily basis and scored 43% correct, which is a below-average sentence recognition score. She had normal hearing (≤15 dB HL) at all test frequencies.

Stimuli

Frequency discrimination. Pure tones were used to measure frequency difference limens. The standard frequencies ranged from 125 to 8000 Hz in octave steps. The duration of each tone was 500 ms with 50-ms cosine-squared ramps. The level of each tone was presented at the individual's most comfortable loudness. All pure tones were generated digitally and presented monaurally to the subject through a Sennheiser headphone (HDA200, Wedemark, Germany).

Frequency-electrode function. Pure tones used to match electric pitch were generated and presented in the same way as for measurement of frequency discrimination in the non-implant ear. All electric stimuli were generated and controlled by a research interface. For S1, electric stimuli were generated by the Bionic Ear Data Collection System software (BEDCS v1.17.208, 2006, Advanced Bionics Corporation, Valencia, California). The stimuli were 500-ms, charge-balanced biphasic pulse trains. The pulse duration was 107.8 μs/phase for the 100-Hz and 200-Hz pulse rates, and 53.9 μs/phase for the 2900-Hz pulse rate. For S2 and S3, electric stimuli were generated by a diagnostic interface box (CI STUDIO+ 2.02 software, Med El, Innsbruck, Austria). The stimuli were 500-ms, charge-balanced biphasic pulse trains. The pulse duration was 240.8 μs/phase for the 200-Hz pulse rate, and 24.2 μs/phase for the 1652-Hz and 2941-Hz pulse rates. Except for S1, pulse duration for relatively high rate (>1000 Hz) stimulation was similar to that used in the clinical processor. A much longer pulse duration was needed for low rate (100 or 200 Hz) stimulation to reach sufficient loudness in all subjects. This difference in pulse duration could affect perception between low- and high-rate electric stimulation, but would not affect pitch matching between acoustic and electric stimulation because pulse duration was held constant in each individual comparison. In all cases, the pulse trains were presented at the most comfortable loudness to each electrode in monopolar stimulation mode. Neither acoustic nor electric level was roved.

Melody recognition. Twelve familiar melodies were used to assess functional pitch performance [11]. The melodies consisted of 12 μ14 notes, with each note having the same rms level and 350-ms duration and a 150-ms silent interval between successive notes. The melodies were presented at the most comfortable loudness through either a Sennheiser headphone in the non-implant ear or a speech processor via direct electric connection in the implant ear.

Procedures

Intra-cochlear electrode position. The same method as previously described [14,29] was used to determine electrode position in the cochlea. Briefly, the modified Stenver's view was used to identify the top of the semi-circular canal arch and the center of vestibule, producing a straight line connecting the top and the center; the round window position was then estimated as the intersection between this straight line and the electrode array. Each electrode position was determined relative to the round window. The estimation of the electrode position was corroborated by the surgeon's visual report and subject's perception of electric stimulation. For example, S3's radiography showed that only 10 electrodes were inserted in the cochlea, which was consistent with the surgeon's report and the subject's dizzy or vestibular responses to stimulation of electrodes 11 and 12.

Frequency discrimination. A 2-alternative, forced-choice (2AFC) adaptive procedure [30] was used to estimate the difference limen. In each trial, the subject had to determine whether the first or the second sound had a higher frequency. Trial-by-trial feedback was provided. The initial frequency difference was large so that the subject could produce a correct response. Two consecutive correct responses led to a decrease in the frequency difference while any incorrect response led to an increase. The increasing or decreasing step size was logarithmically determined. A reversal was defined when an incorrect response occurred after consecutive correct responses or vice versa. The difference limen was the geometric mean of the 8 frequency values from 5 to 12 reversals, representing a 70.7% correct response level. Weber fraction, namely, the ratio of the difference limen over the standard frequency, was obtained as the measure of frequency discrimination.

Frequency-electrode function. For S1 and S2, a modified 2AFC double-staircase adaptive procedure [31,32] was used to find pitch matches between electric stimuli in the implant ear and pure tones in the non-implant ear. For each electric stimulus, there were two randomly interleaved pure-tone sequences, one having an initial frequency that was deemed by the subject to evoke a clearly higher pitch than the electric stimulus and the other having a clearly lower pitch. In each trial, the subject first heard the electric stimulus, then the pure tone, and after that had to judge which sound had the higher pitch. In the first sequence, the pure tone frequency was decreased after the subject judged the pure tone to have the higher pitch than the electric stimulus two consecutive times but increased after the subject judged the pure tone to have the lower pitch any time. In the second sequence, the opposite decision rule was used. Different from the frequency discrimination procedure, the subject received no feedback regarding the correct response. Similar to the frequency discrimination procedure, reversal in the subject's judgment direction was tracked in each sequence and the procedure terminated after at least 12 reversals were obtained for both sequences. The average of the last 8 reversals from the first sequence produced a pure tone frequency value that was judged higher in pitch 70.7% of the time compared to the electric stimulus, while that from the second sequence was judged higher in pitch 29.3% of the time. Mathematically, the average of these two values produced the pure tone frequency that was judged higher in pitch than the electric stimulus for 50% of the trials, or the point of subjective equality between electric and acoustic stimuli. Half of the difference between these two values estimated the difference limen in Hz for the electric stimulus, as it represented the distance between 50% and 70.7% points on the psychometric function.

For S3, the double-staircase adaptive procedure was not used due to time limitation. Instead, the subject was instructed to adjust the pure-tone frequency so that the pure tone was just higher in pitch than the electric stimulus, and then again so that it was just lower in pitch. The pure-tone frequency was adjusted on an unmarked scale from 20 to 20000 Hz. The point of subjective equality in pitch was the average of the just higher and just lower frequency values. The difference limen was half of the difference between these two values. Despite using a different method, S3 produced results similar to those for S1 and S2.

Melody recognition. A 12-alternative, forced-choice method was used to obtain percent correct scores using both the clinical map and the adjusted frequency-electrode function. To produce the adjusted frequency-electrode function, the cut-off frequencies for the bandpass filter in each channel were set to the just lower and just higher pitch matches for the corresponding electrode. The adjusted frequency-electrode function would correct electrode-pitch reversals (e.g., an apical electrode judged to have a higher pitch than an basal electrode), but would not eliminate redundant electrodes (i.e., two different electrodes judged to have overlapping pitches). Each melody was presented 3 times and the order of presentation was randomized. Melodies consist of well-known tunes such as "Twinkle Twinkle Little Star" and "Old Macdonald" [11].

Results

Frequency discrimination and melody recognition in the non-implant ear

Figure 2 shows Weber fraction values as a function of standard frequency. The mean of the Weber fraction over all standard frequencies for normal-hearing subjects was 0.013 (±0.010 SD). This normal control value was not significantly different from the mean of the Weber fraction for the non-implant ear of S1 (0.015±0.005 SD, $p>0.05$) or S3 (0.016±0.008 SD, $p>0.05$), but was significantly better than that of S2 (0.053±0.021 SD; 2-tailed, two-sample unequal variance t-test, $p<0.05$). S2's Weber fraction value was similar to previous results obtained from subjects with cochlear damage [33]. Nevertheless, all 3 subjects produced nearly perfect melody recognition with their non-implant ears, namely, 100%, 96% and 92% for S1, S2 and S3 respectively (Table 1). These nearly normal results from the subjects' non-implant ears validated their use as a "gold standard" for comparing electric pitch in their implant ears.

Frequency-electrode function

Figure 3 shows pure tone frequencies matched to electric pitch as a function of electrode position. In each panel, the upper dashed line depicts the Greenwood function, and the lower dashed line depicts 2 octaves below the Greenwood function; the solid line depicts the clinical map that was used in the subject's speech processor. The symbols represent the point of subjective equality obtained between acoustic and electric stimulation. The error bars represent the difference limen in Hz for electric pitch at its matched pure tone frequency, as defined in the Methods section and will be discussed in the next section.

There was great individual variability, but several trends were apparent in the data. First, there was a roughly monotonic trend between frequency and electrode position, with higher frequencies being matched to more basal electrodes. Second, there was a clear effect of pulse rate on the frequency-electrode function. The lower rates (≤200 Hz) produced lower pitches than the higher rates (>

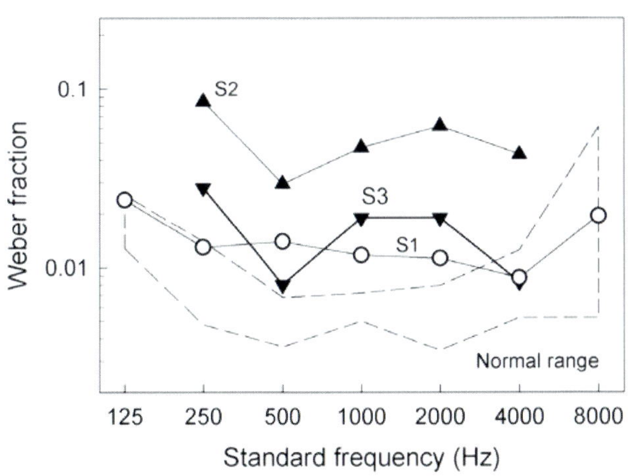

Figure 2. Frequency discrimination for the non-implant ears. The Weber fraction is plotted as a function of standard frequency for S1 (open circles), S2 (triangles), and S3 (inverted triangles). The normal range (mean±2 SDs) is shown as the dashed outlined box, which was obtained using a similar paradigm in a previous study [34].

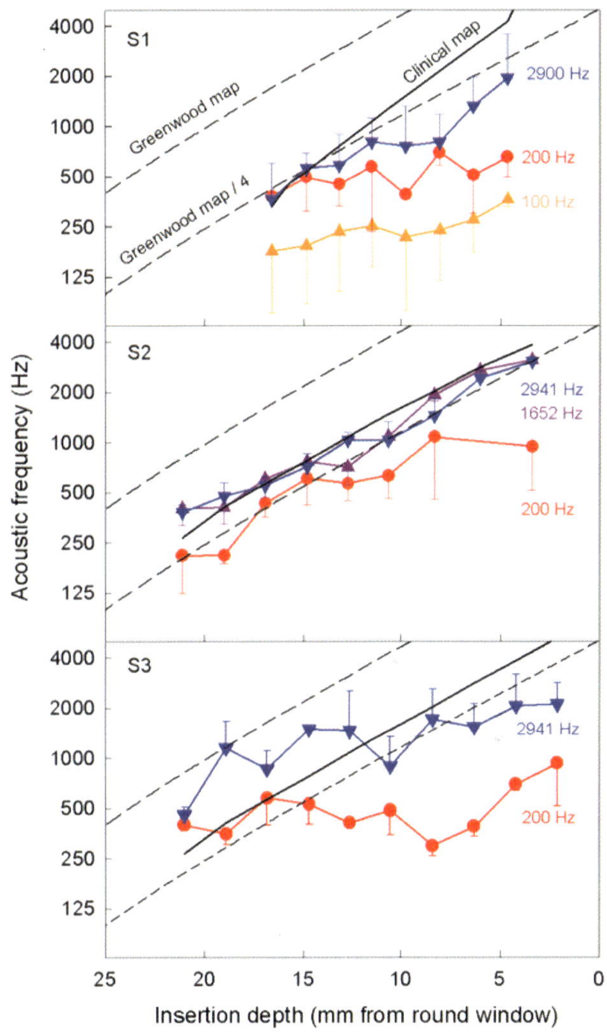

Figure 3. Frequency-electrode functions. The panel shows pure tone frequency matched to an electrode position for each of the 3 cochlear implant subjects with significant contralateral acoustic hearing. The x-axis is the electrode insertion depth from the round window. The y-axis is the pure-tone frequency matched to an electric stimulus delivered to a single electrode at a fixed stimulation rate (different symbols representing different rates). Error bars represent the frequency difference of two pure tones that were judged higher in pitch than the electric stimulus 50% and 70.7% of times (see text in the methods section). The upper dashed line represents the Greenwood function and the lower dashed line represents two octaves below the Greenwood function. The solid line represents the clinical frequency-electrode map used in the speech processor (Advanced Bionics for S1; Med El for S2 and S3).

1600 Hz) at the same electrode position. Third, all frequency-electrode functions were much lower than the Greenwood function. S1 produced functions that were about 2 octaves below the Greenwood function for high-rate stimulation and even more for low-rate stimulation. The high-rate function also departed from the clinical map for basal electrodes (4 µ15 mm from round window). For S2, high-rate stimulation produced a function that was about 1 octave below the Greenwood function for the most apical electrode and about 2 octaves below for the most basal electrode. The measured function was reasonably close to the clinical map, with the former being slightly higher for apical electrodes and lower for basal electrodes. This high-rate result was similar to the result obtained by Dorman et al. from the same subject [18]. The additional 200-Hz rate stimulation for S2 produced a function that was at least 2 octaves lower than both the Greenwood function and the clinical map. For S3, both low and high rate stimulations produced a function that was mostly well below the Greenwood function, particularly for the basal electrodes. Finally, despite the 5-mm insertion difference between the Advanced Bionics (S1) and Med El (S2 and S3) implants, all 3 subjects matched their most apical electrodes to an acoustic pitch range between 200 and 400 Hz, reflecting possibly acclimation to the about 300 Hz lowest cutoff frequency in their speech processors (Table 1).

The slope of all measured frequency-electrode functions was calculated on a logarithmic frequency vs. linear distance scale. The mean slope of the measured functions was −0.075 (±0.047 SD; range = 0.001 to −0.127), which was much shallower than the −0.154 slope for the Greenwood function. On average, the measured frequency-electrode function was 2 times more compressed in frequency range than the Greenwood function.

Frequency discrimination

Figure 4 shows the Weber fraction as a function of standard frequency from a number of experimental and control conditions. Compared with normal-hearing controls [34], the average Weber fraction for the 3 implant ears was 24 times worse (0.302 vs. 0.013, $p<0.05$). Compared with their non-implanted ears, it was 11 times worse (0.302 vs. 0.028). Individually, the Weber fraction in the implant ear was 29 times worse than that in the non-implant ear for S1 (0.422 vs. 0.015), 4 times for S2 (0.197 vs. 0.053), and 17 times for S3 (0.287 vs. 0.016; $p<0.05$ for all subjects). In fact, among all 70 experimental conditions from the 3 subjects involving electric stimulation, only 1 condition from S1 produced a borderline normal value (Weber fraction = 0.009, the lowest red circle touching the dashed line). This lone electric stimulus was a 200-Hz pulse train delivered to the most apical electrode.

The bottom panel (labeled S3) shows 6 additional data sets for comparison. Like the present result, 5 previous studies involving 7 similar unilateral cochlear-implant subjects who had contralateral residual acoustic hearing [14,17,19,21,35] all produced abnormally large Weber fraction values. Because sinusoidally-amplitude-modulated noise is often suggested as an acoustic simulation of a cochlear implant [36], Weber fraction for modulation frequency discrimination of the same sinusoidally-amplitude-modulated noise was obtained in the same group of normal-hearing subjects as in the pure-tone frequency discrimination experiment. Indeed, the Weber fraction was abnormally large: 0.10 for 125-Hz and 0.12 for 250-Hz modulation frequency (open circles).

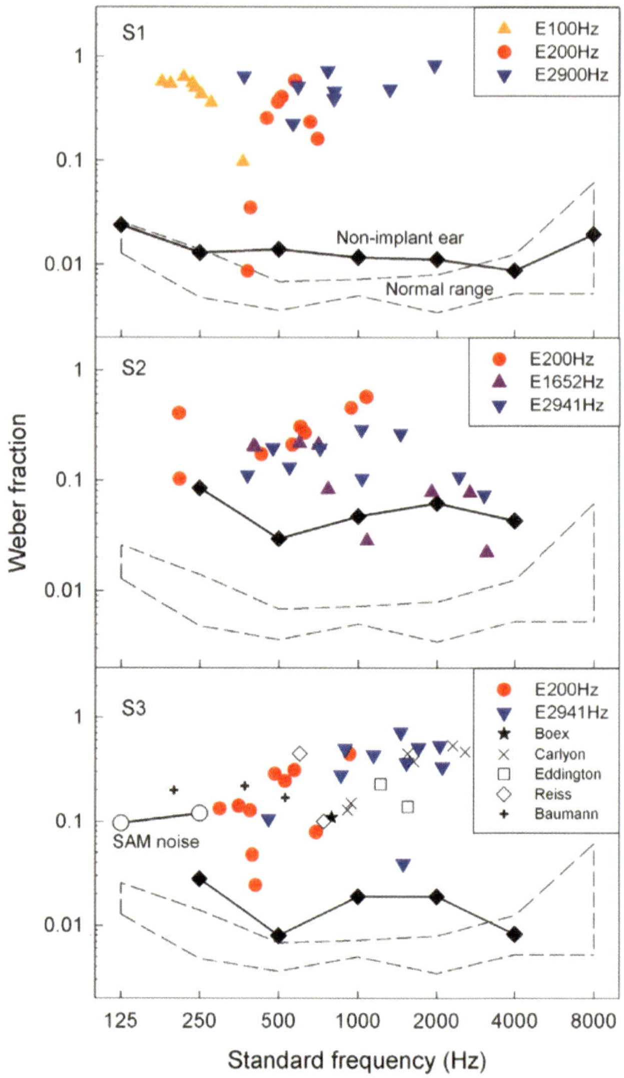

Figure 4. Weber fractions for acoustic and electric hearing. Normal-hearing subjects show relatively constant values (the dashed outlined box in each panel). The individual panels represent Weber fractions for 3 unilaterally implanted subjects: The filled diamonds represent the data for the non-implant ear while triangles and circles represent that for the implant ear. In panel S3 (bottom), comparable data from previously published other studies are also plotted: The two open circles represent Weber fractions for modulation frequency discrimination of sinusoidally-amplitude-modulated noise for a group of normal-hearing subjects [34]; the star represents the datum for a single implant subject from Fig. 4 of Boex et al. [14]; the six crosses represent the data for two subjects from Fig. 2 of Carlyon et al. [19]; the two open squares represent the data for a single subject from Fig. 22 of Eddington et al. [35]; the two open diamonds represent the data for two subjects from Fig. 1 of Reiss et al., in which the Weber fraction was estimated from the monotonic part of the psychometric function in S10 [21]; the three plus symbols represent the data from S1's second estimates in Fig. 7 of Baumann and Nobbe [17].

Melody recognition

Figure 5 shows melody recognition for the 3 subjects using either their clinical (open bars) or adjusted (slanted bars) maps. Despite more closely matched pitch between acoustic frequency and electrode position, none of the adjusted maps improved melody recognition over the standard clinical map. Because the band-pass filter cutoff frequencies were not systemically manipulated in the speech processor, it remained to be seen whether these cutoff frequencies could improve melody recognition. S1 had the highest melody recognition, perhaps as a result of his music training and experience. The other 2 subjects scored barely above

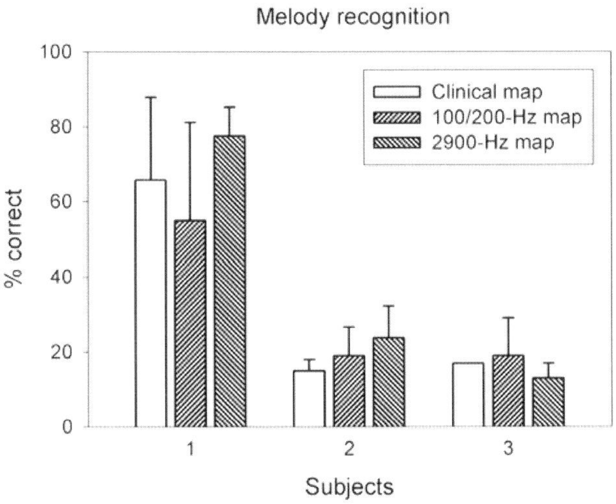

Figure 5. Melody recognition with the clinical map and the adjusted frequency-electrode functions. The results using the clinical map are shown as open bars, those using the low-rate adjusted function as upward-slanted bars, and those using the high-rate adjusted function as downward-slanted bars. Error bars represent one SD of the 3 repeated measurements.

chance. Note also that implant melody recognition was not related to implant speech recognition [37], as S1 produced modest, S2 nearly perfect, and S3 the lowest speech recognition (see Table 1).

Discussion

Poor electric pitch

Previous studies [13,14,15,16,17,18,19,20] have emphasized on the mean values of the frequency-electrode function such as its shape, slope and range in relation to the hair cell or ganglion cell based cochlear frequency map [5,22]. In the majority of cases, the obtained frequency-electrode function deviated from the normal cochlear frequency map. There is also evidence that both stimulation and experience can alter the mean frequency-electrode function in actual cochlear implant users. For example, the present study shows that low-rate stimulation produces shallower frequency-electrode function than high-rate stimulation. Reiss et al. [21] showed that the electrode pitch changed with time, "sometimes by as much as two octaves, during the first few years of implant use." However, various studies including the present one attempting to adjust the frequency-electrode map did not fundamentally improve performance in actual cochlear implant users. The bottleneck must be somewhere else.

The present study suggests that the poor quality of electric pitch perception is mainly responsible for the limited cochlear implant performance. In fact, the 24 times larger Weber fraction for electric stimulation than acoustic stimulation likely represents the best-case scenario. The actual Weber fraction for electric stimulation could be worse than the present estimation because the cochlear implant user could have made lower or higher pitch judgment based on some other subjective quality (e.g., loudness, roughness, intermittency, timbre, or rattle rate). Previous studies using a multi-scaling approach came to a similar conclusion that electric stimulation, with either single- or dual-electrode stimulation, produces multi-dimensional percepts that are incompatible with the salient pitch evoked by a pure tone [38,39,40]. Also consistent with the present finding that adjusting the frequency-electrode function did not improve melody recognition, Spahr et al. [41] concluded that cochlear implant listeners "could likely identify an appropriate frequency-to-electrode map, but only in cases where the pitch strength of the electrically produced notes is very high." Taken together, the previous and present results reinforce the notion that contemporary cochlear implants do not even remotely reproduce pitch sensation of a pure tone, let alone harmonic pitch [42].

Implication for pitch models

Electric stimulation via contemporary intra-cochlear electrodes can produce a temporally precise neural firing pattern that is phase locked to stimulation at rates well above 1000 Hz [43,44], but evokes a much broader than normal spatial excitation pattern [45,46,47]. The present results show that this temporally precise but spatially broad excitation pattern still produces a poor pitch percept. The poor electric pitch result is inconsistent with a large class of temporally-based pitch models, including the Licklider auto-correlation model [48] and its modern variations [49,50,51]. The present result is compatible with the suggestion that, in addition to precise temporal firing, a sharp spatial excitation that is located in a proper tonotopic place is required to produce a salient pitch percept like a pure tone or harmonics [25,52].

Ways to improve electric pitch quality

Although a cochlear spiral ganglion based map can potentially improve the frequency-electrode function [22], the present data suggest that adjustment of the frequency-electrode function is unlikely to improve cochlear implant pitch performance. The key is to develop a means of producing a spatially sharp excitation pattern, which can then be combined with a stimulation rate that is tonotopically appropriate. Two incremental approaches are worth exploring. First, current focusing with multiple electrode stimulation might be able to sharpen local excitation peak [53], but its effect on electric pitch quality has not been systematically explored. The present result suggests that it is important to identify proper stimulation rates for current focusing to improve electric pitch quality. Second, although implant subjects with residual acoustic hearing typically have hearing loss and poorer than normal frequency discrimination, the pitch quality from the residual acoustic hearing is still better than electric pitch (see Fig. 3). As a result, residual low-frequency acoustic hearing has been shown to enhance cochlear-implant melody recognition [54].

Two other approaches using novel stimulation might be considered as true disruptive technology. Different from diffuse electric stimulation, optical stimulation is focused and can produce a highly selective spatial excitation pattern [55]. Still using electric stimulation but with a penetrating electrode array, Middlebrooks et al. [56] found that intra-neural stimulation can also produce a highly selective spatial excitation pattern similar to that produced acoustically by pure tones. Moreover, the penetrating electrodes can access those low-frequency nerve fibers that reside in the middle of the auditory nerve trunk and are not normally accessible to traditional intra-cochlear electric stimulation [57]. Although these novel approaches are likely years away from human trials, they offer the hope of reproducing a salient pure tone sensation, and possibly normal harmonic and music perception in future users of auditory prostheses.

Conclusions

The present study measured frequency-electrode functions and evaluated their effects on melody recognition for 3 unilateral cochlear implant subjects who had significant acoustic hearing over the entire audiometric frequency range in the non-implant ear. Compared with the Greenwood function, the averaged frequency-electrode function was lower in pitch and compressed in frequency range, particularly at low stimulation rates. Adjusted frequency-electrode functions did not improve cochlear implant melody recognition. The derived Weber fraction for electric pitch was 24 times worse than that for acoustic pitch, indicating that the large variance in electric pitch is the main cause for poor cochlear implant melody recognition.

Acknowledgments

We thank the three subjects for their participation and inspiration. We also thank Myles McLaughlin, Carol Q. Pham, Sahara George, Brian Moore, Sliman Bensmaia, and two anonymous reviewers for their comments on the manuscript.

Author Contributions

Conceived and designed the experiments: FZ QT TL. Performed the experiments: FZ QT TL. Analyzed the data: FZ QT TL. Wrote the paper: FZ.

References

1. ASA (1994) ANSI S1.1-1994 (R2004) Acoustical Terminology. American National Standards Institute, Inc.
2. Bekesy G (1952) Direct observation of the vibrations of the cochlear partition under a microscope. Acta Otolaryngol 42: 197–201.
3. Woolsey CN, Walzl EM (1942) Topical projection of nerve fibers from local regions of the cochlea to the cerebral cortex of the cat. Bull Johns Hopkins Hosp 71: 315–344.
4. Zwicker E (1961) Subdivision of Audible Frequency Range into Critical Bands (Frequenzgruppen). J Acoust Soc Am 33: 248.
5. Greenwood D (1990) A cochlear frequency-position function for several species - 29 years later. J Acoust Soc Am 87: 2592–2605.
6. Shower EG, Biddulph R (1931) Differential Pitch Sensitivity of the Ear J Acoust Soc Am 3: 275–287.
7. Schouten JF, Ritsma RJ, Cardozo BL (1962) Pitch of the Residue. J Acoust Soc Am 34: 1418–1424.
8. Zeng FG, Rebscher S, Harrison W, Sun X, Feng HH (2008) Cochlear Implants: System Design, Integration and Evaluation. IEEE Rev Biomed Eng 1: 115–142.
9. Kang R, Nimmons GL, Drennan W, Longnion J, Ruffin C, et al. (2009) Development and validation of the University of Washington Clinical Assessment of Music Perception test. Ear Hear 30: 411–418.
10. Galvin JJ 3rd, Fu QJ, Nogaki G (2007) Melodic contour identification by cochlear implant listeners. Ear Hear 28: 302–319.
11. Kong YY, Cruz R, Jones JA, Zeng FG (2004) Music perception with temporal cues in acoustic and electric hearing. Ear Hear 25: 173–185.
12. McDermott HJ (2004) Music perception with cochlear implants: a review. Trends Amplif 8: 49–82.
13. Vermeire K, Nobbe A, Schleich P, Nopp P, Voormolen MH, et al. (2008) Neural tonotopy in cochlear implants: an evaluation in unilateral cochlear implant patients with unilateral deafness and tinnitus. Hear Res 245: 98–106.
14. Boex C, Baud L, Cosendai G, Sigrist A, Kos MI, et al. (2006) Acoustic to electric pitch comparisons in cochlear implant subjects with residual hearing. J Assoc Res Otolaryngol 7: 110–124.
15. McDermott H, Sucher C, Simpson A (2009) Electro-acoustic stimulation. Acoustic and electric pitch comparisons. Audiol Neuro-Otol 14 Suppl 1: 2–7.
16. Blamey PJ, Dooley GJ, Parisi ES, Clark GM (1996) Pitch comparisons of acoustically and electrically evoked auditory sensations. Hear Res 99: 139–150.
17. Baumann U, Nobbe A (2006) The cochlear implant electrode-pitch function. Hear Res 213: 34–42.
18. Dorman MF, Spahr T, Gifford R, Loiselle L, McKarns S, et al. (2007) An electric frequency-to-place map for a cochlear implant patient with hearing in the nonimplanted ear. J Assoc Res Otolaryngol 8: 234–240.
19. Carlyon RP, Macherey O, Frijns JH, Axon PR, Kalkman RK, et al. (2010) Pitch comparisons between electrical stimulation of a cochlear implant and acoustic stimuli presented to a normal-hearing contralateral ear. J Assoc Res Otolaryngol 11: 625–640.
20. Green T, Faulkner A, Rosen S (2011) Frequency selectivity of contralateral residual acoustic hearing in bimodal cochlear implant users, and limitations on the ability to match the pitch of electric and acoustic stimuli. Int J Audiol 51: 389–398.
21. Reiss LA, Turner CW, Erenberg SR, Gantz BJ (2007) Changes in pitch with a cochlear implant over time. J Assoc Res Otolaryngol 8: 241–257.
22. Stakhovskaya O, Sridhar D, Bonham BH, Leake PA (2007) Frequency map for the human cochlear spiral ganglion: implications for cochlear implants. J Assoc Res Otolaryngol 8: 220–233.
23. Pijl S, Schwarz DW (1995) Intonation of musical intervals by musical intervals by deaf subjects stimulated with single bipolar cochlear implant electrodes. Hear Res 89: 203–211.
24. McDermott HJ, McKay CM (1997) Musical pitch perception with electrical stimulation of the cochlea. J Acoust Soc Am 101: 1622–1631.
25. Zeng F-G (2002) Temporal pitch in electric hearing. Hear Res 174: 101–106.
26. Nelson DA, Van Tasell DJ, Schroder AC, Soli S, Levine S (1995) Electrode ranking of "place pitch" and speech recognition in electrical hearing. J Acoust Soc Am 98: 1987–1999.
27. Wier CC, Jesteadt W, Green DM (1977) Frequency discrimination as a function of frequency and sensation level. J Acoust Soc Am 61: 178–184.
28. Zeng FG, Tang Q, Dimitrijevic A, Starr A, Larky J, et al. (2011) Tinnitus suppression by low-rate electric stimulation and its electrophysiological mechanisms. Hear Res 277: 61–66.
29. Xu J, Xu SA, Cohen LT, Clark GM (2000) Cochlear view: postoperative radiography for cochlear implantation. Am J Otol 21: 49–56.
30. Levitt H (1971) Transformed up-down methods in psychoacoustics. J Acoust Soc Am 49: 467–477.
31. Jesteadt W (1980) An adaptive procedure for subjective judgments. Percept Psychophys 28: 85–88.
32. Zeng FG, Turner CW (1991) Binaural loudness matches in unilaterally impaired listeners. Q J Exp Psych A, Human Exp Psych 43: 565–583.
33. Freyman RL, Nelson DA (1991) Frequency discrimination as a function of signal frequency and level in normal-hearing and hearing-impaired listeners. J Speech Hear Res 34: 1371–1386.
34. Zeng FG, Kong YY, Michalewski HJ, Starr A (2005) Perceptual consequences of disrupted auditory nerve activity. J Neurophysiol 93: 3050–3063.
35. Eddington DK, Dobelle WH, Brackmann DE, Mladevosky MG, Parkin JL (1978) Auditory prosthesis research with multiple channel intracochlear stimulation in man. Ann Otol Rhinol Laryngol 87: 1–39.
36. Shannon RV, Zeng FG, Kamath V, Wygonski J, Ekelid M (1995) Speech recognition with primarily temporal cues. Science 270: 303–304.
37. Singh S, Kong YY, Zeng FG (2009) Cochlear implant melody recognition as a function of melody frequency range, harmonicity, and number of electrodes. Ear Hear 30: 160–168.
38. Collins LM, Zwolan TA, Wakefield GH (1997) Comparison of electrode discrimination, pitch ranking, and pitch scaling data in postlingually deafened adult cochlear implant subjects. J Acoust Soc Am 101: 440–455.
39. McKay CM, McDermott HJ, Clark GM (1996) The perceptual dimensions of single-electrode and nonsimultaneous dual-electrode stimuli in cochlear implantees. J Acoust Soc Am 99: 1079–1090.
40. Vermeire K, Landsberger DM, Schleich P, Van de Heyning PH (2013) Multidimensional scaling between acoustic and electric stimuli in cochlear implant users with contralateral hearing. Hear Res 306: 29–36.
41. Spahr AJ, Litvak LM, Dorman MF, Bohanan AR, Mishra LN (2008) Simulating the effects of spread of electric excitation on musical tuning and melody identification with a cochlear implant. J Speech Lang Hear Res 51: 1599–1606.
42. Zeng FG, Popper AN, Fay RR (2004) Cochlear implants: Auditory prostheses and electric hearing; Popper AN, Fay RR, editors. New York: Springer. 1–437 p.
43. Dynes SB, Delgutte B (1992) Phase-locking of auditory-nerve discharges to sinusoidal electric stimulation of the cochlea. Hear Res 58: 79–90.
44. Hartmann R, Klinke R (1990) Impulse patterns of auditory nerve fibres to extra- and intracochlear electrical stimulation. Acta Otolaryngol Suppl 469: 128–134.
45. Vollmer M, Beitel RE, Snyder RL, Leake PA (2007) Spatial selectivity to intracochlear electrical stimulation in the inferior colliculus is degraded after long-term deafness in cats. J Neurophysiol 98: 2588–2603.
46. van den Honert C, Stypulkowski PH (1987) Single fiber mapping of spatial excitation patterns in the electrically stimulated auditory nerve. Hear Res 29: 195–206.
47. Tang Q, Benitez R, Zeng FG (2011) Spatial channel interactions in cochlear implants. J Neural Eng 8: 046029.
48. Licklider JCR (1951) A Duplex Theory of Pitch Perception. Experientia 7: 128–134.
49. Meddis R, O'Mard L (1997) A unitary model of pitch perception. J Acoust Soc Am 102: 1811–1820.
50. Patterson RD, Allerhand MH, Giguere C (1995) Time-domain modeling of peripheral auditory processing: a modular architecture and a software platform. J Acoust Soc Am 98: 1890–1894.
51. de Cheveigne A (1998) Cancellation model of pitch perception. J Acoust Soc Am 103: 1261–1271.
52. Oxenham AJ, Bernstein JG, Penagos H (2004) Correct tonotopic representation is necessary for complex pitch perception. Proc Natl Acad Sci U S A 101: 1421–1425.
53. Bonham BH, Litvak LM (2008) Current focusing and steering: modeling, physiology, and psychophysics. Hear Res 242: 141–153.

54. Gfeller K, Turner C, Oleson J, Zhang X, Gantz B, et al. (2007) Accuracy of cochlear implant recipients on pitch perception, melody recognition, and speech reception in noise. Ear Hear 28: 412–423.
55. Izzo AD, Suh E, Pathria J, Walsh JT, Whitlon DS, et al. (2007) Selectivity of neural stimulation in the auditory system: a comparison of optic and electric stimuli. J Biomed Opt 12: 021008.
56. Middlebrooks JC, Snyder RL (2008) Intraneural stimulation for auditory prosthesis: modiolar trunk and intracranial stimulation sites. Hear Res 242: 52–63.
57. Middlebrooks JC, Snyder RL (2010) Selective electrical stimulation of the auditory nerve activates a pathway specialized for high temporal acuity. J Neurosci 30: 1937–1946.

Predicting the Perceived Sound Quality of Frequency-Compressed Speech

Rainer Huber[1,2]*, Vijay Parsa[3], Susan Scollie[3]

1 Centre of Competence HörTech gGmbH, Oldenburg, Germany, 2 Cluster of Excellence Hearing4All, Oldenburg and Hannover, Germany, 3 National Centre for Audiology, Western University, London, Canada

Abstract

The performance of objective speech and audio quality measures for the prediction of the perceived quality of frequency-compressed speech in hearing aids is investigated in this paper. A number of existing quality measures have been applied to speech signals processed by a hearing aid, which compresses speech spectra along frequency in order to make information contained in higher frequencies audible for listeners with severe high-frequency hearing loss. Quality measures were compared with subjective ratings obtained from normal hearing and hearing impaired children and adults in an earlier study. High correlations were achieved with quality measures computed by quality models that are based on the auditory model of Dau et al., namely, the measure PSM, computed by the quality model PEMO-Q; the measure qc, computed by the quality model proposed by Hansen and Kollmeier; and the linear subcomponent of the HASQI. For the prediction of quality ratings by hearing impaired listeners, extensions of some models incorporating hearing loss were implemented and shown to achieve improved prediction accuracy. Results indicate that these objective quality measures can potentially serve as tools for assisting in initial setting of frequency compression parameters.

Editor: Bernd Sokolowski, University of South Florida, United States of America

Funding: The work was supported by the following: Deutsche Forschungsgemeinschaft (Research Unit "Individualized Hearing Acoustics"; For-1732) (to Dr. Huber), http://www.dfg.de/en/research_funding/programmes/coordinated_programmes/research_units/index.html; NSERC Discovery grant (to Dr. Vijay Parsa), http://www.nserc-crsng.gc.ca/professors-professeurs/grants-subs/dgigp-psigp_eng.asp; and NSERC Collaborative Health Research grant (to Dr. Scollie), http://www.nserc-crsng.gc.ca/Professors-Professeurs/grants-subs/CHRP-PRCS_eng.asp. The funders had no role in study design, data collection and analysis, decision to publish, or preparation of the manuscript.

Competing Interests: The authors have declared that no competing interests exist.

* Email: Rainer.Huber@HoerTech.de

Introduction

Nonlinear frequency compression

Frequency lowering techniques are now common in digital hearing aids as an alternative amplification strategy for hearing impaired listeners with severe to profound high frequency hearing loss. For this group of listeners, conventional amplification strategies may result in less than optimal performance due to a combination of inadequate gain at higher frequencies, limited bandwidth of the hearing instruments, and/or the potential presence of high frequency cochlear dead regions [1], [2], among other factors. Frequency lowering techniques aim to transfer high frequency information to lower frequency regions. These techniques can improve speech recognition, but may also affect perceived sound quality. In this paper, we investigate a broad range of objective indices of sound quality against a database of sound quality ratings for frequency-lowered speech. This work not only evaluates which models may be effective predictors of the impact of one form of frequency lowering on sound quality, but also develops insights as to the key features of a successful model by varying key modelling parameters and evaluating their impact on successful predictions.

Historically, frequency lowering has been achieved in many ways including slow playback, channel vocoding, frequency transposition, and frequency compression, as well as a combination of these alternative strategies [3]. As described in ([3] - Section 8.3), a frequency transposing hearing aid will shift a portion of high frequency spectrum to lower frequencies by a fixed amount (in Hz). Frequency compression can be linear or nonlinear; in linear frequency compression, all frequencies are proportionally reduced by the same factor (i.e., the output frequency is a fixed fraction of the input frequency), while in nonlinear frequency compression, only frequencies above a certain threshold are compressed.

Currently, frequency lowering is available as an option in commercial hearing aids as frequency transposition (termed "Audibility Extender") in Widex hearing aids [4], as nonlinear frequency compression (termed "SoundRecover") in Phonak and Unitron hearing aids and as "frequency compression" in Siemens hearing aids, as spectral warping (termed "SpectralIQ") in Starkey hearing aids, and as "Frequency Composition", another type of frequency transposition [5], in Bernafon hearing aids.

The differences in frequency lowering implementations can be expected to result in considerably different perceptual effects, even when they are fitted for the same audiometric configuration. For example, McDermott [6] conducted an electroacoustic comparison of Widex's Audibility Extender and Phonak's Sound Recover technologies. Spectrographic analyses with different speech and music samples showed that while both schemes were effective in lowering high frequency content, they also introduced distortion that may affect perception. It is therefore imperative to investigate the perceptual effects of frequency lowering technologies, and to develop electroacoustic tools and computational models that can predict these perceptual effects.

Since this paper focuses on a particular frequency lowering strategy, *viz.* the nonlinear frequency compression (NFC), a brief description of the NFC processing and the evidence surrounding its effectiveness is presented below.

The NFC processing in today's commercial hearing aids uses compression only for frequencies above a cutoff value. Mathematically, the relationship between input and output frequencies is given by

$$F_{out} = \begin{cases} F_{in}, & F_{in} < F_c \\ F_c^{1-p} \times F_{in}^{p}, & F_{in} \geq F_c \end{cases} \quad (1)$$

where F_{in} is the input frequency in Hz, F_{out} is the corresponding output frequency, F_c is the cutoff frequency, p is the compression exponent, and $1/p$ is the compression ratio (CR). Figure 1 illustrates the concept showing short time spectra of speech before and after nonlinear frequency compression.

The specification of the F_c ensures that the lower frequency information is unadulterated while the spectral content beyond the F_c is compressed into a narrower bandwidth. The NFC scheme has been evaluated with both adults and children. Simpson *et al.* [7] investigated the performance of prototype NFC with 17 hearing impaired adults with moderate to profound sensorineural hearing loss and found that the phoneme recognition scores for the group improved by 6%. Glista *et al.* [8] evaluated NFC processing with 13 adults and 11 children with moderately severe to profound sloping high-frequency hearing losses. On average, recognition scores for plurals and consonants improved significantly for the NFC scheme when compared with conventional amplification. Individual variability was present in the results and children derived greater plural recognition benefit from NFC as well as indicated preference for NFC over conventional amplification when compared to the adults [8]. Benefit was also related to audiogram: Those with greater high frequency hearing loss were most likely to demonstrate benefits. More recent studies have evaluated outcomes for those with moderate hearing losses [9], the time course of acclimatization [10] and effects on sound quality [11], [12]. Previous work indicated that sound quality is correlated with the strength of the frequency compressor, with stronger settings having poorer sound quality. This underscores the need for formal evaluation of sound quality of the NFC processor. In

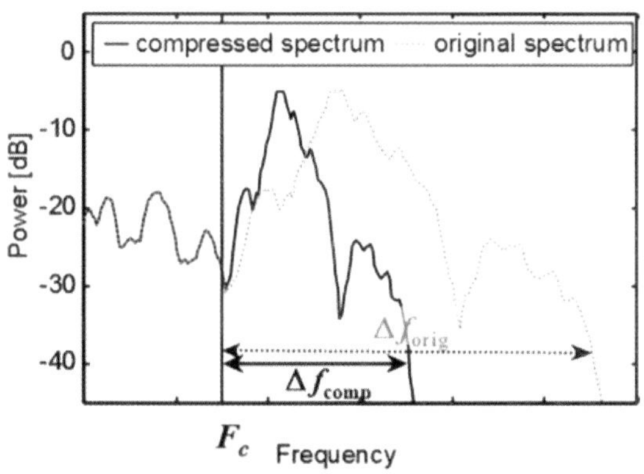

Figure 1. Illustration of nonlinear frequency compression. Dotted, grey line: Power spectrum of unprocessed speech. Solid, black line: spectrum after nonlinear frequency compression. Above a cutoff frequency F_c, the spectrum is compressed by a ratio CR = $\Delta f_{orig}/\Delta f_{comp}$.

particular, computational metrics which can effectively predict speech quality perception by hearing impaired listeners could be of use in determining an initial set of NFC parameters that have acceptable sound quality, potentially improving the acceptability of initial fittings.

Objective sound quality evaluation

The perceived quality of frequency-compressed sounds will depend on a number of variables, including the parameter settings, hearing loss, the type of sound, as well as highly individual, subjective factors like personal experiences, expectations and preferences. In order to estimate the expected sound quality for a given algorithm setting, sound, and listener, one could either follow a data-driven, i.e. statistical model approach (e.g, the E-model [13]), or a perception model approach (e.g. PESQ [14]). A data-driven approach would require a large base of empirical data containing subjective quality ratings of different types of sounds, processed with a variety of algorithm settings, obtained from many listeners with different hearing losses. A perception-model-driven approach would possibly require similar amounts of data if it was developed, trained or optimized, and validated particularly for this application.

Alternatively, existing quality models already validated for similar applications could be tested with a smaller amount of data. However, most of the existing quality models were designed, optimized and validated in the context of telecommunication applications and audio coding for normal-hearing listeners (see [15] for an overview). At present, very few sound quality models for hearing impaired listeners with application for hearing aid (algorithm) quality evaluations have been reported [16–19]. Most of the sound quality models, including current ITU standard methods for speech and audio quality, have in common that they follow the concept of comparing "internal representations", computed by a psychoacoustic model, of a test and a reference sound signal [20], [14]. Detected differences between internal representations are interpreted as quality degradations of the test signal with respect to the reference signal. Hence, these comparison-based models depend on the availability of a reference signal that represents the optimum, or desired, sound quality. This requirement is met in the evaluation of lossy signal processing systems, such as low-bitrate speech and audio codecs, where the unprocessed, original signal serves as a reference.

However, there is no known ideal reference for the evaluation of hearing aids (algorithms) in general. In contrast to audio codecs, whose aim is to produce output signals that are perceptually indistinguishable from the original input, hearing aids aim to alter the input sound in a way that it compensates for the listeners' hearing loss. This intentional alternation could result in the processed sound having higher sound quality than the original signal. Therefore, one would need a "perfect" hearing aid to produce the reference signal for sound quality evaluations. Unfortunately, the perfect hearing aid does not exist.

However, many hearing aid algorithms can be evaluated with comparison-based quality models. Examples include speech enhancement algorithms that operate on already distorted input signals, like noisy and/or reverberant speech. In these evaluations, the original, clean speech recording can serve as a reference signal, and comparison signals are generated by adding noise or reverberation. Such a comparison-based method may also be applicable in the case of frequency-lowering algorithms. Frequency-lowering will always degrade the naturalness of the input sounds. If subjective sound quality ratings are dominated by the perceived naturalness and not influenced by the possibly improved speech intelligibility or other positive effects of the frequency compression, comparison-based quality models using the unprocessed input signal as a reference appear potentially qualified as predictors of sound quality also for this class of hearing aid algorithms.

Objective evaluation of frequency-compressed speech

NFC is a viable choice as an amplification solution for hearing impaired listeners with severe to profound high-frequency hearing loss. Since sound quality is one of the most important factors determining the overall satisfaction and acceptance of hearing aid users [21–24], the negative impact on sound quality by NFC must remain small enough to be overshadowed by the positive effects such as improved intelligibility in order to achieve acceptance and overall preference over conventional processing. Objective sound quality models are useful in this context as they can assist in the initial specification of NFC parameters that achieve a balance between intelligibility enhancement and quality degradation. In the present study, a number of established as well as rather new, mostly perceptual speech and audio quality models, including yet unpublished extended versions, have been applied to predict subjective sound quality ratings of nonlinear frequency-compressed speech [11]. It should be noted that none of the applied models was designed for the present application and some of them were particularly optimized for different experimental conditions, like (monaural) headphone presentation instead of loudspeaker presentation as used in the present study. In spite of this caveat, promising predictor candidates will be identified below.

Subjective Speech Quality Measurement

Speech signals and subjective quality ratings used to test the quality models were obtained from an earlier study [11] and shall be described only briefly here. See [11] for a more detailed description.

Speech quality ratings were obtained from a group of 12 normal hearing adults (ages 21–27 years, mean = 24 years), 12 normal hearing children (ages 8–18 years, mean = 12 years), 12 hearing impaired adults (ages 50–81 years, mean = 69 years), and 9 hearing impaired children (ages 8–17 years, mean = 12 years). The listeners with hearing impairment also participated in a field study with NFC hearing aids [8]. All normal hearing listeners had pure tone thresholds of 20 dB HL or better across the audiometric frequency range. Figure 2 depicts the mean and standard deviation of the pure tone thresholds for hearing impaired adults and children. While the children had higher absolute thresholds than adults, statistical analysis revealed there was no significant interaction between frequency-specific thresholds and age [8], [11].

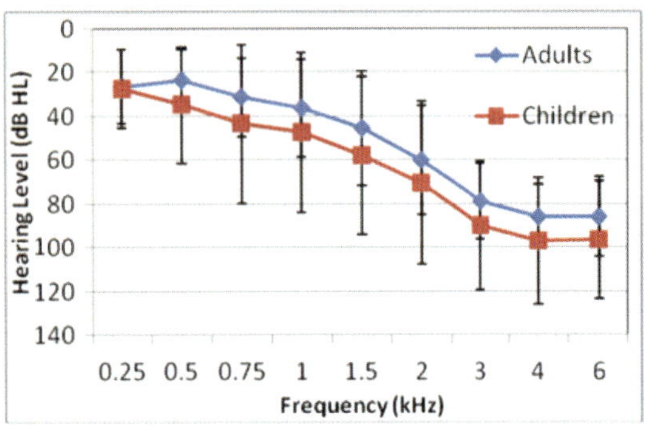

Figure 2. Mean and standard deviations of the pure-tone air conduction thresholds for hearing impaired adults and children.

A database of frequency-compressed speech samples was created to obtain the subjective quality ratings. The database was constructed by first programming a prototype NFC hearing aid with specific cutoff frequency (F_c) and compression ratio (CR) parameters, placing this hearing aid in a Brüel and Kjær portable anechoic test box, and recording the output of the hearing aid separately in response to two male speech samples and two female speech samples. A total of five different NFC settings were investigated: (1) $F_c = 4000$ Hz, CR = 2:1; (2) $F_c = 3000$ Hz, CR = 2:1; (3) $F_c = 3000$ Hz, CR = 6:1; (4) $F_c = 3000$ Hz, CR = 10:1; and (5) $F_c = 2000$ Hz, CR = 2:1.

Hearing aid recordings were later played back to the bilaterally aided study participants in a sound booth through a loudspeaker positioned at 0° azimuth and at a distance of 1.5 m. The playback level was initially presented at 65 dB SPL and then individually adjusted, if needed, to the subject's most comfortable level (MCL) [11]. Calibration was performed using the Brüel & Kjær Sound Level Meter (SLM), Type 2270. Speech quality ratings were obtained using the ITU standard MUltiple Stimulus with Hidden Reference and Anchors (MUSHRA, [25]) protocol mediated by custom software. The MUSHRA protocol uses a numerical quality rating scale from 0 to 100 together with five verbal categories from "bad" to "excellent" as anchors for orientation. In this method, a "reference stimulus" was presented, which was the unprocessed male or female speech sample, while eight "test stimuli" were randomly associated with the five NFC-processed stimuli, the original signal itself ("hidden reference"), and a low-pass version and a peak-clipped version of the original signal, respectively. The low-pass version was obtained by passing the original signal through a 10th order Butterworth filter with a cutoff frequency of 2000 Hz, while the peak-clipped version was obtained through hard-clipping the original stimulus at 25% of its peak value. These stimuli served as "anchor" stimuli that represent sound with poor quality, as recommended by [25]. In the MUSHRA method, all stimuli are rated simultaneously using graphical slider buttons. Participants were instructed to listen to each of these stimuli in comparison to the reference, by clicking on the corresponding icons of the software's GUI and adjust the rating sliders such that a satisfactory quality rating of all eight stimuli was achieved. Participants were allowed to re-listen to any stimulus and re-adjust their quality ratings until they were satisfied with the final set of ratings.

Parsa *et al.* [11] have conducted a detailed statistical analysis of the subjective data collected through this procedure. A high degree of intra- and inter-rater reliability was observed with the speech quality ratings across both normal and hearing impaired groups. As such, this database was used to benchmark the performance of different objective speech quality estimators in predicting the quality of frequency-compressed speech.

Objective Speech Quality Measurement

This paper evaluated twenty-nine objective quality measures including sub-variants in order to benchmark model performance for prediction of sound quality with NFC processing. Table 1 provides a summary of the models/measures tested, and technical information on the nature of each model is provided below.

The objective models investigated in this paper are considered to be "double-ended" or "intrusive" in their operation. Double-ended models compare features extracted from the signal under test to those extracted from an undistorted reference version of the same signal. The comparisons quantify the degree of perceptual

Table 1. Quality models and measures used in this study.

Model/measure name	acronym	authors	ref.	measure(s)	HI?	no.
Hansen model		M. Hansen & Kollmeier	[37]	qc+W+B	–	M1
				qc+W-B	–	M2
				qc-W+B	–	M3
				qc-W-B	–	M4
Hansen model extended for hearing impaired		Huber	unpub.	qc+W+B (HI)	✓	M5
				qc+W-B (HI)	✓	M6
				qc-W+B (HI)	✓	M7
				qc-W-B (HI)	✓	M8
PEMO-Q	PEMO-Q	Huber & Kollmeier	[39]	PSM_fb+B	–	M9
				PSM_fb-B	–	M10
				PSM_lp+B	–	M11
				PSM_lp-B	–	M12
PEMO-Q extended for hearing impaired	PEMO-Q-HI	Huber	unpub.	PSM_fb+B (HI)	✓	M13
				PSM_fb-B (HI)	✓	M14
				PSM_lp+B (HI)	✓	M15
				PSM_lp-B (HI)	✓	M16
Hearing Aid Speech Quality Index	HASQI	Kates & Arehart	[19]	$HASQI_{lin}$	✓	M17
				$HASQI_{nonlin}$	✓	M18
				$HASQI_{comb}$	✓	M19
Perceptual Evaluation of Speech Quality (ITU-T Rec. P.862-2)	PESQ	ITU-T/Beerends et al.	[14], [31]	PESQ-LQO	–	M20
				PESQ-LQO (WB)	–	M21
Loudness Pattern Distortion	LPD	Guo & Parsa	[36]	LPD	–	M22
Moore quality model		Moore & Tan	[33–35]	D	–	M23
				R_{nonlin}	–	M24
				$S_{overall}$	–	M25
Itakura-Saito Distance	ISD	Itakura & Saito	[26]	ISD	–	M26
Log-Area Ratio	LAR	Quackenbush et al.	[28]	LAR	–	M27
Log-Likelihood Ratio	LLR	Itakura	[27]	LLR	–	M28
Weighted Spectral Slope Distance	WSSD	Klatt	[30]	WSSD	–	M29

("ref".: reference; "HI?": Does model account for hearing impairment? Yes: ✓; no: –) Quality measure suffixes: fb/lp: modulation filterbank/lowpass model version; +/– W: with/without frequency band weighting; +/–B: with/without asymmetric weighting of differences ("Beerends weighting").

overall difference or similarity. In contrast, single-ended models do not require a reference signal. The models in Table 1 can be broadly grouped into: (1) metrics based on speech production model parameters, and (2) metrics based on the comparison of "internal representations" obtained with computational models of auditory processing. Double-ended models were chosen for this work, because the subjective quality ratings were obtained using reference signals as well, according to the MUSHRA protocol.

Examples of objective models in the speech production model parameters include the Itakura-Saito Distance (ISD) [26] and the Log-Likelihood Ratio (LLR) [27], which calculate the weighted similarity between the linear prediction coefficients extracted from the distorted and reference speech signals, and the Log-Area Ratio (LAR) [28] measure, which computes the distance between the area ratio coefficients. Software implementations of ISD, LAR, and LLR were taken from a toolbox provided by Hansen and Pellom [29].

A basic objective measure that uses an auditory model is the Weighted Spectral Slope Distance (WSSD) [30] measure. It uses a psychoacoustically motivated bank of critical-band filters to decompose the speech signals, and weights the differences between the slopes of the log magnitudes in each band to produce the final quality measure. Again, the software implementation of the WSSD measure was taken from the Hansen and Pellom toolbox.

The method for the Perceptual Evaluation of Speech Quality (PESQ; ITU-T Recommendation P.862 [14]) and its wide band extension (PESQ-WB; ITU-T P.862.2 [31]) are perhaps the most popularly used objective quality assessment methods incorporating an auditory model. Conceptually, the PESQ technique computes the frame-by-frame internal representations of test and reference signals by first computing the power spectra, and then applying frequency and intensity warping functions based on Zwicker's loudness model [14].

Moore & Glasberg have developed a different loudness model [32], characterized by the computation of excitation patterns at the output of each auditory filter and the subsequent computation of the specific loudness pattern. Moore *et al.* [33–35] applied the Moore & Glasberg model and derived an objective quality metric based on comparisons of the excitation patterns of original and distorted signals. Two intermediate measures of linear (spectral) and nonlinear distortions (D and R_{nonlin}, respectively) are computed separately and combined to an overall subjective score predictor $S_{overall}$ in the end. For the Moore quality model, a custom software implementation was developed. Correlations between model output measures and mean subjective quality ratings will be reported for D, R_{nonlin} and $S_{overall}$.

Chen *et al.* [36] devised an objective measure based on the Moore & Glasberg loudness pattern differences between the reference and degraded speech samples. These differences were used to estimate sound quality in the degraded sample versus the reference sample. This measure was computed using custom software.

The speech quality model of Hansen & Kollmeier [37] (referred to as the "Hansen model" below) employs the auditory processing model of Dau *et al.* [38], "PEMO" (for "PErception MOdel"), for the computation of internal representations of test and reference signals. The bandwidth of the PEMO peripheral (gammatone) filterbank was adapted to telephone-bandpass-filtered speech. A "band importance weighting" function is applied to the frequency channels of the internal representations to emphasize higher frequency channels. The overall correlation between the weighted internal representations determines the quality measure qc.

The audio quality model PEMO-Q of Huber and Kollmeier [39] extends the Hansen model to include quality assessment of general, wideband audio signals (including speech) with low to very high audio qualities. By default, it uses the more recent version of the Dau model [40], with the option of selecting the earlier (much faster) version. The two model versions differ with respect to the processing of amplitude modulations: In [38], the final step of auditory preprocessing (i.e. before the decision stage) is an 8 Hz-lowpass filter, whereas in [40], this lowpass filter is replaced by a filter bank. The band importance weighting function used in the Hansen model was not adopted for PEMO-Q.

PEMO-Q outputs two quality measures: The Perceptual Similarity Measures PSM and PSM_t. The second variant evaluates the temporal course of the instantaneous audio quality, derived from a frame-wise correlation of internal representations, non-linearly mapped to the overall quality estimator PSM_t. In contrast, the PSM is the overall correlation of the complete internal representations. The PSM_t is more sensitive to small distortions and more independent of the type of input audio signal [39]. On the other hand, the "simpler" PSM seems to be more "robust" and more generally applicable, especially for low-to intermediate audio quality. For example, speech enhancement algorithms have been evaluated with this measure and showed good correlations with subjective quality ratings [41–43]. Since speech samples with rather strong quality differences are considered in this study, only the PSM was included here.

By default, PESQ and PEMO-Q apply an asymmetric weighting of differences between internal representations, putting more weight on "added" or increased elements of the internal representation of the distorted signal than on "missing" or attenuated ones [44]. This step is handled as an option for the Hansen model and PEMO-Q and has been switched on and off in this study. The second binary setting option of PEMO-Q that has been varied is the manner of amplitude processing in the auditory processing model (modulation lowpass vs. filterbank). This leads to four PEMO-Q output measure variants that have been tested in total. Since a benefit of the band importance function used in the Hansen model could only be found in the prediction of speech quality in the context of telecommunication, the Hansen model was also tested with the weighting function deactivated in this study. Hence, four versions of the Hansen model have been tested in total: with and without asymmetry weighting of internal representations, and with and without applying the band importance weighting function.

Finally, the Hearing Aid Speech Quality Index (HASQI) by Kates and Arehart [19] was employed. In the computation of the HASQI, a relatively simple auditory processing model is applied to provide internal representations in terms of neural firing rates. Effects of possible sensorineural hearing losses are modeled by estimating the contributions of inner hair cell (IHC) and outer hair cell (OHC) losses to a total hearing loss given by the audiogram. Auditory filter bandwidths are increased and compression ratios are reduced depending on the OHC loss estimate. The effect of IHC loss is modeled by linear signal attenuation in each auditory filter before compression. From the comparison of internal representations of test and reference signals, two intermediate quality metrics are computed, quantifying the amount of linear and non-linear distortions, respectively. The final overall quality index is the product of the linear and the nonlinear distortion metrics. Again, correlations with subjective quality ratings will be reported for linear and nonlinear metrics and overall quality index, referred to as $HASQI_{lin}$, $HASQI_{nonlin}$ and $HASQI_{comb}$, respectively.

In summary, the models and measures for speech and audio quality listed in Table 1 have been applied to the signals of the database.

The versions of PEMO-Q and the Hansen model with extensions for hearing impaired data have not been published before and will therefore be discussed in the next section.

Extended versions of PEMO-Q and the Hansen model for hearing impaired

Modifications of the underlying auditory model of the audio quality prediction methods PEMO-Q and its predecessor, the speech quality model of Hansen and Kollmeier, for describing sensorineural hearing losses have been suggested by Derleth *et al.* [45]. One of their suggestions was to insert an instantaneous expansion and attenuation stage before the adaptation and compression stage in the PEMO (Figure 3), to account for a loss of sensitivity and reduced dynamic compression. This suggestion has been adopted and implemented in the extended version of PEMO-Q and the Hansen model. Given an audiogram as the input, the hearing thresholds in dB HL at audiometric frequencies are interpolated internally to the center frequencies of the model's peripheral filterbank. The inserted processing stage operates on the output of each of these filters, after envelope extraction. The total hearing loss in the respective channel is decomposed into contributions attributed to losses of inner (IHCL) and outer hair cells (OHCL), respectively, as shown in the equation below [32]:

$$\mathrm{OHCL} = \begin{cases} \min\{65\,\mathrm{dB}, 0.8\cdot\mathrm{THL}\}, f > 2000\,\mathrm{Hz} \\ \min\{55\,\mathrm{dB}, 0.8\cdot\mathrm{THL}\}, f \leq 2000\,\mathrm{Hz} \end{cases} \qquad (2)$$

$$\mathrm{IHCL} = \mathrm{THL\text{-}OHCL}$$

In the model stage, the signal amplitude is attenuated by the amount of IHCL. Then, it is raised to the power k, which itself is a function of the input signal amplitude I and OHCL. The attenuation and expansion operations are performed instantaneously (i.e. sample-by-sample). For simulating normal hearing, k equals 1 for any I. For simulating impaired hearing, $k(I)$ becomes larger than 1 and increases with OHCL. The input/output

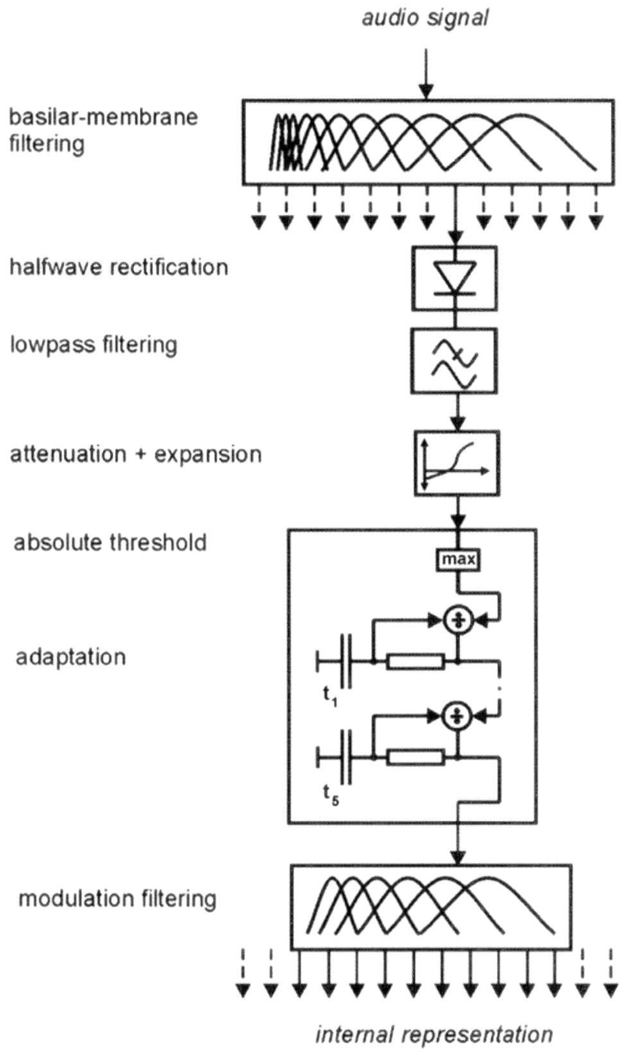

Figure 3. Schematic plot of the auditory processing model PEMO, modified to simulate normal and impaired hearing (after [40] **and** [45]**).**

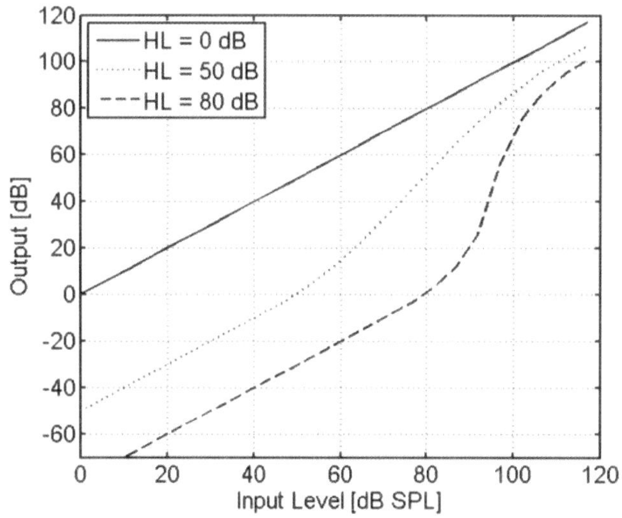

Figure 4. Input/output functions of the expansion and attenuation model stage for normal hearing (solid line) and impaired hearing with an assumed total hearing loss of 50 dB (dotted line) and 80 dB (dashed line).

function of this stage is shown in Figure 4 for normal hearing and two hearing losses. The parameters of the input/function were chosen such that its shape matches the inverse function of the assumed input/output function of the unimpaired cochlea proposed by Moore [46]. Again, model parameters were not adjusted in the present study.

Results

The performance of the objective measures was characterized by their correlations with averaged subjective quality ratings of all processing conditions (including hidden reference and anchors), quantified by Pearson's linear correlation coefficient r and Spearman's rank correlation coefficient rs. Quality measure values were taken directly as output by the models and not transformed by, e.g., nonlinear regression functions.

As there were no systematic differences between the quality ratings of normal hearing adults and children, quality ratings were averaged across the complete group of normal hearing subjects. Consequently, results are stated for three groups of subjects separately: (1) normal hearing (adults and children), (2) hearing impaired children, and (3) hearing impaired adults. In addition to averaging across subjects, quality ratings were also averaged across different talkers per processing condition. Results will be stated for both levels of averaging. For clarity, results per subject group will be presented separately in succession and only for a selection of measures. The complete results are reported in the Appendix S1. The relation between subjective ratings and corresponding model predictions will be illustrated by scatter plots for the best performing quality measures.

Results for normal hearing

Table 2 shows linear and rank correlations between selected model predictions and mean subjective ratings obtained from normal hearing subjects. (The complete correlation table is given in the Appendix S1) In this table, the suffixes of the PSM and qc measures have the following meaning: fb/lp indicate the modulation filterbank/lowpass version of PEMO-Q respectively, +/−W indicate the activation/deactivation of the frequency-band weighting, and +/−B denote activation/deactivation of the asymmetric weighting of internal representation differences ("Beerends weighting"). When frequency weighting is deactivated in the Hansen model, and the modulation lowpass version is used in PEMO-Q, these models become very similar. They mainly differ in the bandwidth of the peripheral filterbank. It must be noted that because the results obtained with the −B option tended to be better than with option +B, the latter are only reported in the complete set of results given in the Appendix S1.

It can be seen from Table 2 that the correlation coefficients are reasonable for several of the objective quality metrics, especially when averaged across different talkers per processing condition (right column "av.") Four of the five measures with highest correlations are PEMO-Q and related measures (PSM..., qc...), complemented by the LAR (M27 of Table 1) measure. The latter, however, shows only a rather poor rank correlation with the subjective ratings. Good correlations, especially rank correlations, are achieved when ratings are averaged across different talkers per processing condition because averaging reduces the statistical noise of the ratings and thus increases the reliability of the data. On the

Table 2. Results of the quality predictions (including anchor conditions) for the normal hearing subjects, expressed by linear correlation coefficients and rank correlation coefficients (*italic*).

measure	ind.	av.
qc+W-B (M2)	0.84	0.86
	0.89	*0.93*
qc-W-B (M4)	0.84	0.87
	0.84	*0.95*
PSM_lp-B (M12)	0.85	0.88
	0.84	*0.91*
PSM_fb-B (M10)	0.88	0.89
	0.92	*0.98*
$HASQ_{comb}$ (M19)	0.54	0.54
	0.24	*0.19*
PESQ (M21)	0.64	0.64
	0.41	*0.45*
S_{overal} (M25)$_l$	0.76	0.76
	0.63	*0.64*
LPD (M22)	−0.75	−0.77
	−0.64	*−0.62*
LAR (M27)	−0.83	−0.84
	−0.74	*−0.71*

Subjective ratings were averaged across subjects. Middle column: correlations based on ratings for individual talkers (ind.); right column: ratings averaged across talkers (av.). Quality measure suffixes: fb/lp: modulation filterbank/lowpass model version; +/−W: with/without frequency band weighting; +/−B: with/without asymmetric weighting of differences ("Beerends weighting").

other hand, the significance of the correlation coefficients gets lower as the number of data points is reduced to only eight.

Figure 5 shows a scatter plot of the results obtained with the measure PSM_fb-B (M10). It must be noted that the results for two of the four talkers processed by the NFC condition cr2_fc3k were not available due to a labelling error and a processing error of the concerned test files. It can be observed from this figure that the quality ratings for the NFC test conditions are bordered by the ratings of the high quality (hidden) reference and the low quality anchor stimuli (lowpass-filtered and clipped speech, respectively). The scatter plot reveals that the model underestimates the perceived quality of the clipped speech samples whose predicted quality was lower than that of the lowpass-filtered samples, whereas the subjects ranked the qualities of these conditions in an opposite manner. Another noteworthy difference between model predictions and the subjective ratings is the larger predicted quality difference between the reference condition and the processed conditions compared to the differences among processed conditions.

Both subjects and model rate the frequency-compressed signals with the lowest cutoff frequency 2 kHz (condition cr2-fc2k) very poorly compared to the other frequency compression conditions. A possible cause for this non-linear relation between compression cutoff frequency and perceptual effect could be the alteration of speech formant frequencies and/or the interference of down-shifted higher frequency contents with these formants. Vowel formants have significant energy in the second and third formants in approximately the 1000–4000 Hz region for female speech and approximately 750–3000 Hz for male speech, depending on the specific vowel and talker. Recalling that both male and female speech samples were used, it is reasonable to conclude that the cr2-fc2k setting was strong enough to lower significantly the upper formants of many vowels for both male and female speech and was therefore much more noticeable than settings that likely did not disrupt the harmonic relationships within vowels, such as those that used a 4000 Hz cutoff frequency.

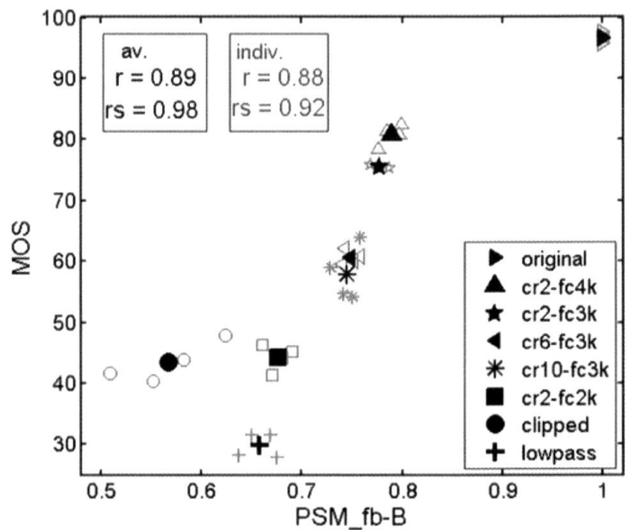

Figure 5. Scatter plot of the results obtained with the PEMO-Q measure PSM_fb-B for the normal hearing subjects. Subjective ratings (Mean Opinion Scores – MOS) are plotted versus corresponding model predictions. r: linear correlation, rs: rank correlation.

Figure 5 shows that in general, the influence of the talker on the measured and predicted quality ratings is very small, except for the clipping condition. Here, the influence of the talker is overestimated by the PSM measure.

Results for hearing impaired children

The results obtained for the hearing impaired children are shown in Table 3 and Figure 6. According to the correlations with subjective ratings (Table 3), the prediction accuracy of the models for hearing impaired listeners for separate talkers was very good (r up to 0.94), and even higher when averaged across talkers (r up to 0.99). The slightly better performance of the modulation filterbank version of PEMO-Q in the prediction of normal hearing subjects' ratings (Table 2) was not confirmed by the results obtained with hearing impaired children (Table 3).

Figure 6 depicts a scatter plot for PSM_lp-B, hearing impaired (HI) version (M16) and subjective ratings from hearing impaired children. In contrast to Figure 5, a greater variation of quality ratings and predictions for different talkers can be seen in this figure. Note that the predicted quality of the original, unprocessed condition is always maximal, since this condition is used as the reference by the comparison-based quality models. Hence, possible influences of different talkers cannot be modeled for this condition. Another difference from the normal hearing data concerns the rank order of the three processing conditions with the lowest ratings, i.e. lowpass filtering (LP), clipping (CL) and frequency compression with the lowest cutoff frequency, 2 kHz (cr2-fc2k). Normal hearing subjects ranked LP< CL ≈ cr2-fc2k. The model, in contrast, ranked CL<LP< cr2-fc2k. Hearing impaired children, however, ranked these conditions clearly differently: cr2-fc2k<CL<LP. This rank order was correctly predicted by the quality measure PSM_lp-B (HI) (M16). As a consequence, a very high linear correlation ($r = 0.99$) and a perfect rank correlation ($rs = 1$) between PSM_lp-B and subjective ratings were achieved when averaged across talkers. Finally, the range of PSM_lp-B (HI) (M16) values is smaller compared to PSM_fb-B (M10) values used for normal hearing subjects, while the range of subjective ratings is about the same in both cases. This difference is due to the greater sensitivity of the modulation filterbank version of the auditory model PEMO used for the computation of

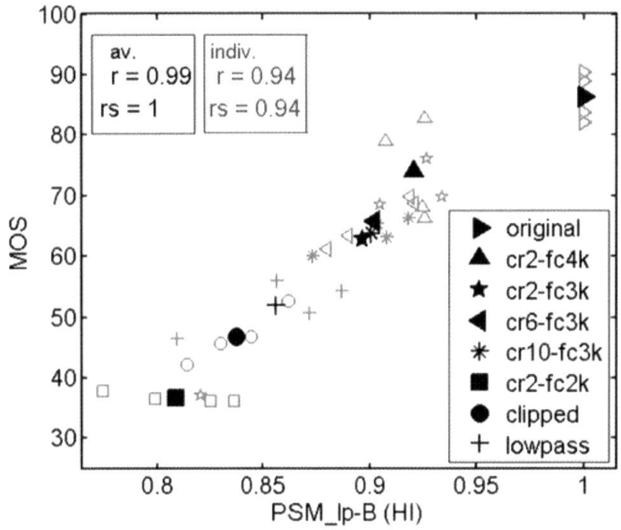

Figure 6. Same as Figure 5, but for hearing impaired children.

Table 3. Quality prediction results (linear and rank correlation (*italic*) coefficients) for the hearing impaired children group.

measure	NH models		HI models	
	ind.	**av.**	**ind.**	**av.**
qc+W-B (M2, M6)	0.58	0.59	0.87	0.90
	0.78	*0.88*	*0.89*	*0.93*
qc-W-B (M4, M8)	0.82	0.87	0.90	0.95
	0.80	*0.91*	*0.91*	*0.93*
PSM_lp-B (M12, M16)	0.87	0.91	0.94	0.99
	0.86	*0.95*	*0.94*	*1.00*
PSM_fb-B (M10, M14)	0.84	0.87	0.94	0.97
	0.87	*0.93*	*0.95*	*0.95*
$HASQ_{comb}$ (M19)	*0.73*	*0.76*	*0.81*	*0.85*
	0.80	*0.69*	*0.87*	*0.88*
PESQ (M20)	0.90	0.92		
	0.90	*0.83*		
$S_{overall}$ (M25)	0.83	0.85		
	0.90	*0.88*		
LPD (M22)	−0.51	−0.55		
	−0.53	*−0.57*		
LAR (M27)	−0.61	−0.63		
	−0.65	*−0.67*		

Results for the PEMO-Q measure PSM and the related measure qc are given for normal hearing (NH) and hearing impaired (HI) model versions. Quality measure suffixes: fb/lp: modulation filterbank/lowpass model version; +/−W: with/without frequency band weighting; +/−B: with/without asymmetric weighting of differences ("Beerends weighting").

PSM_fb-B (M10), compared to the modulation lowpass filter version used for computing PSM_lp-B (HI) (M16).

Results for hearing impaired adults

Hearing impaired adults exhibited a different rating behavior than hearing impaired children on average, although there were no significant differences between the distributions of hearing losses in these two groups (children's hearing losses were somewhat higher than adults' hearing losses on average). Adults rated NFC conditions generally higher, except for condition cr2-fc2k, whereas their ratings of the anchor condition (LP, CL) were similar to children's ratings (compare Figure 7 with Figure 6). As a result, adults' average ratings of cr2-fc2k, LP and CL conditions were very similar, whereas the quality measure PSM_lp-B (HI) (M16) clearly rated cr2-fc2k<LP< CL, which led to a lower correlation between measured and predicted mean quality ratings ($r = 0.88$) compared to the results obtained for the children ($r = 0.99$). In contrast, a very high correlation was achieved by the related quality measure qc-W-B (HI) (M8) ($r = 0.96$). As described earlier, qc-W-B (HI) (M4, M8) mainly differs from PSM_lp-B (HI) (M12, M16) in the lower cutoff frequency of the peripheral filterbank. Looking at Figure 8, the higher correlation obtained with qc-W-B (HI) (M8) is mainly due to a shift of quality ratings of NFC conditions towards higher values compared to the PSM_lp-B (HI) (M16) values, whereas ratings of the anchor conditions LP and CL basically correspond to the PSM_lp-B (HI) (M16) values. This agrees well with the observed difference in subjective ratings between hearing impaired children and adults. Table 4 summarizes the prediction performances of the different quality measures. Amongst others, it clearly shows the advantage of using models that account for hearing impairment, as evidenced by the higher correlations with subjective quality ratings for most of the evaluations.

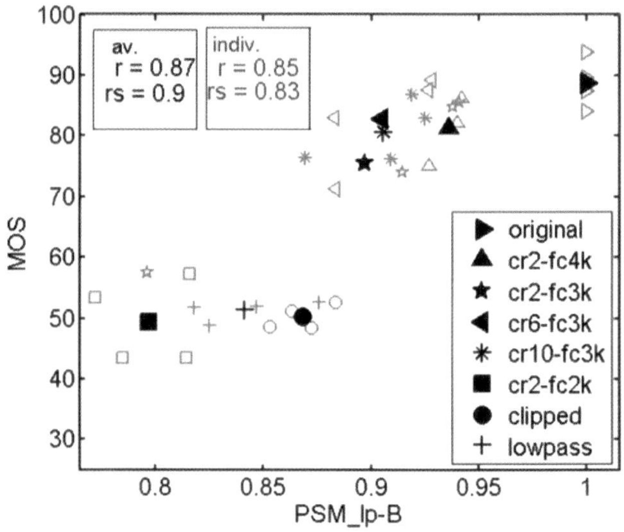

Figure 7. Same as Figure 5, but for hearing impaired adults.

Discussion

The obtained results show that predicting the perceived sound quality of nonlinearly frequency-compressed speech by means of objective, perceptual speech/audio quality models is possible. From the models tested, the PEMO-Q (related) measures, in

Table 4. Quality prediction results (linear and rank correlation (*italic*) coefficients) for the hearing impaired adults group.

measure	NH models		HI models	
	ind.	av.	ind.	av.
qc+W-B (M2, M6)	0.65	0.67	0.77	0.79
	0.68	*0.74*	*0.75*	*0.74*
qc-W-B (M4, M8)	0.85	0.88	0.91	0.96
	0.86	*0.76*	*0.87*	*0.81*
PSM_lp-B (M12, M16)	0.85	0.88	0.86	0.88
	0.86	*0.81*	*0.84*	*0.81*
PSM_fb-B (M10, M14)	0.78	0.81	0.82	0.85
	0.79	*0.81*	*0.79*	*0.86*
$HASQ_{comb}$ (M19)	*0.50*	*0.51*	*0.78*	0.79
	0.53	*0.62*	*0.86*	0.95
PESQ (M20)	0.62	0.63		
	0.79	*0.81*		
$S_{overall}$ (M25)	0.50	0.51		
	0.42	*0.48*		
LPD (M22)	−0.52	−0.57		
	−0.37	*−0.43*		
LAR (M27)	−0.62	−0.65		
	−0.49	*−0.48*		

Quality measure suffixes: fb/lp: modulation filterbank/lowpass model version; +/−W: with/without frequency band weighting; +/−B: with/without asymmetric weighting of differences ("Beerends weighting").

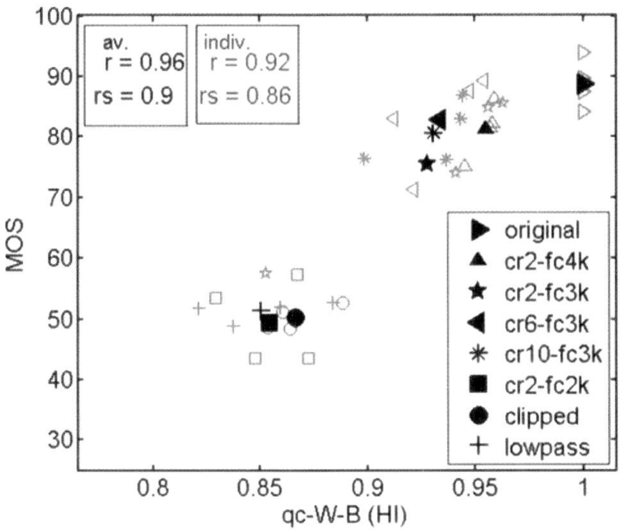

Figure 8. Quality prediction results for the hearing impaired adults group, obtained with quality measure qc-W-B (version for hearing impaired). r: linear correlation, rs: rank correlation.

particular, the Perceptual Similarity Measure (PSM) and the speech quality measure qc of the Hansen model (with deactivated frequency weighting function), showed the highest correlations with mean subjective ratings. These measures represent the most "basic" PEMO-based quality measures with the lowest degree of optimization for a specific task and hence the highest generality and robustness. This is in line with results of other studies where different quality measures have been applied for tasks other than those for which they were originally developed (e.g. [41–43]). Through the results of the present study, the generality of abovementioned measures is further proven given that the predicted quality degradations caused by very different kinds of distortions (i.e. frequency compression, amplitude clipping and lowpass filtering) correlated highly with subjective ratings.

A number of objective measures that were previously either applied to speech or audio quality estimation were evaluated in this paper. Of the objective measures based on speech production model parameters (viz. ISD (M26), LAR (M27), LLR (M28)), LAR (M27) performed the best. In the past, these metrics were primarily used for estimating narrowband (0–4 kHz bandwidth) speech quality (e.g. [28], [29]). Since some of the PEMO-based quality measures employed a wider bandwidth, experiments were conducted with implementations of ISD (M26), LAR (M27) and LLR (M28) metrics using an extended 8 kHz bandwidth. Results, however, showed a degradation in the correlation coefficients with subjective ratings for LAR (M27) and LLR (M28) metrics compared to the original versions with 4 kHz bandwidth. Similarly, the LPD (M22) metric was developed and validated for narrowband speech applications [36], and its performance with an extended bandwidth is not investigated in this work and is a worthwhile topic for future study.

Speech quality measures (M22, M25) based on the Moore & Glasberg model ([33–36]) performed decently with normal hearing data, but were inferior with the hearing impaired data. A revised model of loudness perception incorporating cochlear hearing loss was proposed by Moore and Glasberg [47], and further investigation would be interesting to determine whether the incorporation of this revised model would lead to an improvement in correlations with hearing impaired subjective data.

The Hearing Aid Speech Quality Index (HASQI, M17–M19) showed good rank correlations and moderate linear correlations with hearing impaired data, but only low correlations with normal hearing data. This is in clear contrast to the results reported in a recent publication on an updated version of the HASQI [48], which was also tested successfully on frequency-compressed speech. The main reason for the lower correlations observed in the present study was found to be a significant quality overestimation of the lowpass condition. The clipping condition was overestimated as well, although to a lesser extent. Without these anchor conditions, linear correlations of the $HASQI_{comb}$ (M19) with subjective ratings increase to 0.83 for normal hearing data (0.85 when ratings are averaged across different talkers per condition), 0.75 (0.78) for hearing impaired adults' data, and 0.78 (0.82) for hearing impaired children's data. The HASQI submeasure for linear distortions (M17) achieves very high correlations in this case: 0.93 (0.95), 0.89 (0.95) and 0.95 (0.996) for normal hearing subjects', hearing impaired adults' and hearing impaired children's data, respectively.

In the present application, PESQ (M20, M21) surprisingly achieved poor correlations with subjective ratings from normal hearing listeners, but moderate and even high correlations with ratings from hearing impaired adults and children, respectively. The main reason for the poor results regarding normal hearing listeners was found to be a quality overestimation of the lowpass-filtered items by PESQ. Without this processing condition, the linear correlation obtained with the narrow-band version of PESQ increases to 0.89 (0.92) for normal hearing subjects. Correlations obtained with the wideband version of PESQ are lower in this case.

The successful "basic" PEMO-Q measures required minimal optimization during development, and use a very simple back-end of the underlying quality model. This result is interpreted as a reflection of the validity of the auditory model originally derived by Dau *et al.* [38], [40]. It represents a well-founded model of the "effective" signal processing in the auditory system and has been validated in a wide variety of psychoacoustical experiments [40], [49–55]. Its free parameters were adopted from psychoacoustical modeling and kept fixed in the development of the Hansen model and PEMO-Q as well as in the present study. When applied as a front-end for speech and audio quality prediction, only the bandwidth of the peripheral filterbank (i.e. the range of center frequencies) and the modulation filterbank were set appropriately. The bandwidth used in PEMO-Q appears to have been appropriate for use with the NFC data modeled in this study, too, although we did not evaluate impacts of any adjustments to these original settings. In the hearing-impaired adults group, however, better results were obtained with the quality measure qc with its smaller filterbank bandwidth compared to PSM. This suggests that the bandwidth could still be optimized for the present task and possibly lead to a further improvement of the quality prediction accuracy.

As already pointed out before, the higher correlation with the adults' quality ratings obtained with the measure qc-W-B (HI) (M8) compared to PSM_lp-B (HI) (M16) is mainly due to an upward shift of quality predictions for the 2 kHz-lowpass condition and the frequency-compressed condition with the lowest cutoff frequency of 2 kHz, which is in line with the adults' rating behavior. The upper cutoff frequency of the peripheral filterbank used in the computation of qc-W-B (HI) (M8) is 4 kHz, whereas it is 15.3 kHz for PSM. The two processing conditions of concern cancel (most of) the energy at frequencies higher than 4 kHz. The measure qc-W-B (HI) (M8) does not "notice" the missing energy above 4 kHz, in contrast to PSM_lp-B (HI) (M16). As a consequence, PSM_lp-B (HI) (M16) detects a larger overall difference between original and processed signals which leads to a lower quality estimate. A possible reason for the better correspondence between hearing impaired adults' ratings and the qc-W-B (HI) (M8) predictions could be a reduced sensitivity of these subjects for missing energy at frequencies above 4 kHz, or/ and a lower perceptual weighting of this degradation component when rating the overall quality. Apparently, the hearing impaired children of this study were more sensitive or less tolerant towards the quality degrading effects of frequency compression than the hearing impaired adults. They rated the quality of frequency-compressed speech samples clearly lower than the adults did, although the distributions of hearing losses as described by audiograms are similar in these two groups; the children's hearing losses are in fact somewhat higher on average than the adults' hearing losses. There are two factors that may be related to this difference between age groups. First, age-related auditory and/or cognitive declines not revealed by the audiogram, but influencing quality perception might be factors related to this result. Moreover, age-dependent different experiences with and expectations on the quality of sound reproducing systems might play a role and have been speculated before [56]. However, to the knowledge of the authors, there is no data yet that would support such hypotheses, so these considerations remain speculative. Second, as is clinically typical, we provided the children with a higher level of gain and output in their hearing aids than was provided to adults [57]. For this reason, the children in this study may have had enhanced access to low-level effects in the processed signals and may have responded accordingly in their perceptual ratings. Again, this is a speculation and further study would be required to clarify whether this is a factor.

The fact that similar quality rating scores were obtained from normal hearing adults and children does not contradict the hypothesis of an age-related effect, because normal hearing adults in this study were much younger (mean = 24 years) than hearing impaired adults (mean = 69 years). However, in the present data, not all kinds of distortions were rated differently by older listeners, but mainly the frequency-compressed items. Lowpass-filtered and clipped samples received similar quality ratings from children and adults. The same is observed with the quality measure qc-W-B (HI) (M8), in contrast to PSM_lp-B (HI) (M16) for reasons explained above. As a result, qc-W-B (HI) (M8) correlates better with hearing impaired adults' quality rating scores, whereas PSM_lp-B (HI) (M16) is better suited to predict the hearing impaired children's ratings. However, the results obtained from hearing impaired adults and corresponding quality predictions obtained with the measure qc-W-B (HI) (M8) might represent a rather special data subset. In contrast, the measure PSM_lp-B (HI) (M16) appears to have a higher degree of generality and is thus recommended for general application.

Effect of PEMO-Q options

Modulation processing. A clear, consistent effect of the kind of modulation processing stage in PEMO-Q on the prediction accuracy could not be found in the results of the present study. Correlations achieved with the modulation lowpass and modulation filterbank versions of the PEMO-Q quality measure PSM, i.e. PSM_lp and PSM_fb, respectively, were mostly comparable and not consistently ranked with regard to subject group, individual vs. averaged talkers, and linear vs. rank correlation coefficients. Since the computational effort required for PSM_fb is about ten times higher than for PSM_lp, the latter might be preferred for practical applications.

Asymmetric weighting of internal representation differences. The first application for which PEMO-Q was originally developed and optimized was the evaluation of audio codecs. For that purpose, a partial, asymmetric assimilation of internal representations of test and reference signals, equivalent to Beerends' asymmetry weighting of internal representation differences [44], was introduced into the quality model (option +B). In this procedure, negative deviations of the internal representation of the test signal from the reference are partially compensated (differences are halved), whereas positive deviations remain unchanged. This approach follows the hypothesis that "missing" components in a distorted signal are perceptually less disturbing than "additional" ones. This processing step was found to improve the quality prediction accuracy of PEMO-Q for audio codecs [58]. In the present application, however, better results were obtained without this processing step. The reason for this result is that the negative effect of strong frequency compression and lowpass filtering on sound quality by cancelling energy at medium to high frequencies (>3 kHz) is over-compensated by the assimilation procedure. Consequently, quality estimates are shifted towards higher values disproportionately with increasing frequency compression (i.e., increasing compression ratio and decreasing cutoff frequency) and for the 2 kHz-lowpass filter condition. Figure 9 illustrates this effect with the example of quality prediction results obtained with the quality measure PSM_fb (M9, M10) for the normal hearing subject group with and without assimilation of internal representations (+/−B).

Summary and Conclusions

In this paper, we presented results from a study on quality prediction of frequency-compressed speech in hearing aids by different objective speech and audio quality measures. Objective measures based on the audio quality model PEMO-Q and the related speech quality measure qc of the Hansen model achieved

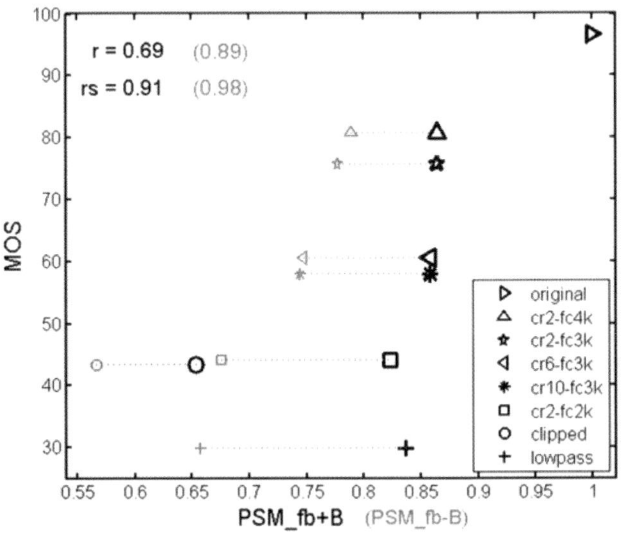

Figure 9. Effect of PEMO-Q model option +B (partial compensation of differences between test and reference internal representations) on quality estimates for the normal hearing subject group. Gray, small symbols: Results obtained with option −B (i.e. without partial compensation); black, large symbols: results obtained with option +B.

good correlations with averaged subjective ratings. The extension of these models incorporated hearing impairment, and improved prediction accuracy for quality ratings from hearing impaired subjects. Hearing impaired adults and children rated the quality of frequency-compressed speech differently. Best prediction results were achieved with different quality measures per subject group; adults' ratings were predicted better with a model that analyzes a smaller frequency bandwidth. Optimizations of bandwidth and possibly further model parameters were not carried out in the present study, but are considered to bear significant potential for further improvements. The HASQI model was also evaluated, and revealed consistently high results across subject groups for the linear submeasure of this index. Again, further evaluation could reveal optimization to the main HASQI model to further improve its performance.

In summary, the present study reports first-of-a-kind results on a broad range of objective sound quality evaluation models of frequency-compressed speech. Further studies are needed to validate the performance of the PEMO-Q quality measures for this application with a larger group of hearing impaired listeners and across more NFC parameter settings. Moreover, the predictability of perceived quality of other sound stimuli than speech, such as music, should be investigated. In addition, the objective modeling of sound quality for frequency lowering schemes other than the NFC scheme evaluated here would require further investigation. In addition, possible influences of age and acclimatization to frequency-compressed sound will have to be investigated and modeled. Research on this topic is driven by the fact that a successful objective speech quality model will have the potential to serve as a valuable supplemental tool for the fitting and evaluation of frequency lowering algorithms in hearing instruments.

Acknowledgments

We thank Andreas Seelisch and Danielle Glista for sharing their data and Prof. James Kates for sharing his HASQI code, and Phonak AG for providing hearing instruments for this work. We also thank four anonymous reviewers for their helpful comments on earlier versions of this article.

Author Contributions

Conceived and designed the experiments: RH VP SS. Performed the experiments: RH. Analyzed the data: RH VP SS. Contributed reagents/materials/analysis tools: RH VP SS. Wrote the paper: RH VP SS.

References

1. Moore BCJ (2010) Dead regions in the cochlea: conceptual foundations, diagnosis, and clinical applications. Ear and Hearing, 25(2): 98–116.
2. Stelmachowicz PG, Lewis DE, Choi S, Hoover B (2007) Effect of stimulus bandwidth on auditory skills in normal-hearing and hearing-impaired children. Ear and Hearing, 28: 483–494.
3. Dillon H (2012) Hearing Aids. Thieme Medical Publishers, 2nd edition.
4. Kuk P, Korhonen H, Peeters D, Keenan A, Jessen H et al. (2006) Linear frequency transposition: extending the audibility of high-frequency energy. Hearing Review, 13(10): 42–48.
5. www.bernafon.com/Professionals/Downloads/~/media/PDF/English/Global/Bernafon/WhitePaper/BF_WP_Frequency_Composition_UK.ashx.
6. McDermott HJ (2011) A Technical Comparison of Digital Frequency-Lowering Algorithms Available in Two Current Hearing Aids. PLoS ONE 6(7): e22358. doi:10.1371/journal.pone.0022358.
7. Simpson A, Hersbach AA, McDermott HJ (2005) Improvements in speech perception with an experimental nonlinear frequency compression hearing device. Int J Audiol, 44: 281–292.
8. Glista D, Scollie S, Bagatto M, Seewald R, Parsa V et al. (2009) Evaluation of nonlinear frequency compression: Clinical outcomes. Int J Audiol, 48: 632–644.
9. Wolfe J, John AB, Schafer E, Nyffeler M, Boretzki M et al. (2010) Evaluation of non-linear frequency compression for school-age children with moderate to moderately-severe hearing loss. J Amer Acad Audiol, 21(10), 618–628.
10. Glista D, Scollie S, Sulkers J (2012) Perceptual Acclimatization Post Nonlinear Frequency Compression Hearing Aid Fitting in Older Children. J Speech Lang Hear Res, 55(6): 1765–87. Doi: 10.1044/1092-4388(2012/11-0163).
11. Parsa V, Scollie S, Glista D, Seelisch A (2013) Nonlinear frequency compression: Effects on sound quality ratings of speech and music. Trends Amplif, 17(1): 54–88.
12. Souza PE, Arehart KH, Kates JM, Croghan NB, Gehani N. (2013) Exploring the limits of frequency lowering. J Speech Lang Hear Res., 56(5): 1349–63.
13. ITU-T Rec. G.107 (2002). The E-Model, a Computational Model for Use in Transmission Planning. International Telecommunication Union, CH-Geneva.
14. ITU-T (2001) Perceptual evaluation of speech quality (PESQ), an objective method for end-to-end speech quality assessment of narrow-band telephone networks and speech codecs. ITU-T Recommendation P.862, International Telecommunications Union, Geneva, Switzerland.
15. Rix AW, Beerends JG, Kim DS, Kroon P, Ghitza O (2006) Objective Assessment of Speech and Audio Quality - Technology and Applications. IEEE Trans Audio Speech Lang Processing, 14 (6): 1890–1901.
16. Beerends JG, Krebber J, Huber R, Eneman K, Luts H (2008) Speech quality measurement for the hearing impaired on the basis of PESQ. Proc. of the 124th AES Convention, Amsterdam, The Netherlands.
17. Nielsen LB (1993) Objective Scaling of Sound Quality for Normal-Hearing and Hearing-Impaired Listeners. The Acoustics Laboratory, Technical University of Denmark, Lyngby, Denmark.
18. Schmalfuß G (2004) Anwendung psychoakustischer Methoden und Modelle zur Feinanpassung von Hörgeräten mit natürlichen Schallen [Application of psychoacoustic methods and models for fine-fitting of hearing aids using natural sounds. Ph.D. thesis, Technical University of Munich, Germany, 2004.
19. Kates JM, Arehart KH (2010) The Hearing-Aid Speech Quality Index (HASQI). J Audio Eng Soc, 58(5): 363–381.
20. ITU-R (1998) Method for objective measurement of perceived audio quality. ITU-R Recommendation BS.1387, International Telecommunications Union, Geneva, Switzerland.
21. Hagerman B, Gabrielsson A (1985) Questionnaires on desirable properties of hearing aids. Scand Audiol, 14(2): 109–111.
22. Kochkin S (2002) Marketrak VI: 10-year customer satisfaction trends in the US hearing instrument market. Hearing Review, 9 (10): 14–25.
23. Ovegård A, Lundberg G, Hagerman B, Gabrielsson A, Bengtsson M et al. (1997) Sound quality judgment during acclimatization of hearing aid. Scand Audiol, 26: 43–51.
24. Wong LLN, Hickson L, McPherson B (2003) Hearing aid satisfaction: what does research from the past 20 years say? Trends Amplif, 7(4): 117–161.
25. ITU-R (2003) Method for the subjective assessment of intermediate quality levels of coding systems. ITU-R Recommendation BS.1534, International Telecommunications Union, Geneva, Switzerland.
26. Itakura F, Saito S (1997) A Statistical Method for Estimation of Speech Spectral Density and Formant Frequencies. In: Schafer RW, Markel, JD, editors. Speech Analysis. IEEE Press. New York.
27. Itakura F (1975) Minimum prediction residual principle applied to speech recognition. IEEE Trans Acoust, 23(1): 67–72.
28. Quackenbush S, Barnwell T, Clements M, (1998) Objective Measures of Speech Quality. Prentice Hall, Englewood Cliffs/New Jersey.
29. Hansen J, Pellom B (1998) An effective quality evaluation protocol for speech enhancement algorithms. Proc. ICSLP '98, Sydney, Australia.
30. Klatt D (1998) Prediction of perceived phonetic distance from critical-band spectra: A first step. Proc. IEEE ICASSP 1982: 1278–1281.
31. ITU-T (2005) Wideband extension to Recommendation P.862 for the assessment of wideband telephone networks and speech codecs. ITU-T Recommendation P.862.2 International Telecommunications Union. Geneva, Switzerland.
32. Moore BCJ, Glasberg BR (1997) A Model of Loudness Perception Applied to Cochlear Hearing Loss. Aud Neurosci, 3: 289–311.
33. Moore BCJ, Tan CT, Zacharov N, Matilla VV (2004) Measuring and predicting the perceived quality of music and speech subjected to combined linear and nonlinear distortion. J Audio Eng Soc, 52: 1228–1244.
34. Tan CT, Moore BCJ, Zacharov N, Matilla VV (2004) Predicting the perceived quality of nonlinearly distorted music and speech signals. J Audio Eng Soc, 52: 699–711.
35. Moore BCJ, Tan CT (2004) Development and Validation of a Method for Predicting the Perceived Naturalness of Sounds Subjected to Spectral Distortion. J Audio Eng Soc, 52: 900–914.
36. Chen G, Parsa V, Scollie S (2006) An ERB Loudness Pattern Based Objective Speech Quality Measure. Proc. Int. Conf. on Spoken Language Processing, Pittsburgh, USA, 2174–2177.

37. Hansen M, Kollmeier B (2000) Objective modelling of speech quality with a psychoacoustically validated auditory model. J Audio Eng Soc, 48: 395–409.
38. Dau T, Püschel D, Kohlrausch A (1996) A quantitative model of the 'effective' signal processing in the auditory system: I. Model structure. J Acoust Soc Am, 99: 3615–3622.
39. Huber R, Kollmeier B (2006) PEMO-Q - A New Method for Objective Audio Quality Assessment Using a Model of Auditory Perception. IEEE Trans Audio Speech Lang Processing, 14(6): 1902–1911.
40. Dau T, Kollmeier B, Kohlrausch A (1997) Modeling auditory processing of amplitude modulation: I. Modulation Detection and masking with narrowband carriers. J Acoust Soc Am, 102(5): 2892–2905.
41. Rohdenburg T, Hohmann V, Kollmeier B (2005) Objective Measures for the Evaluation of Noise Reduction Schemes. Proc. Int. Workshop on Acoustic Echo and Noise Control (IWAENC), Eindhoven, The Netherlands.
42. Goetze S, Albertin E, Kallinger M, Mertins A, Kammeyer KD (2010) Quality Assessment for Listening-Room Compensation Algorithms. Proc. ICASSP, Dallas, USA.
43. Huber R, Schulte M, Vormann M, Chalupper J (2010) Objective measures of speech quality in hearing aids: Prediction of listening effort reduction by noise reduction algorithms. Presented at the 2nd Workshop on Speech in Noise: Intelligibility and Quality, Amsterdam, The Netherlands Available: http://www.phon.ucl.ac.uk/events/quality2010/talks/RainerHuber.pdf.
44. Beerends JG (1994) Modelling cognitive effects that play a role in the perception of speech quality. Presented at the Workshop on Speech quality assessment at the Ruhr-Universität Bochum, Germany.
45. Derleth RP, Dau T, Kollmeier B (2001) Modelling temporal and compressive properties of the normal and impaired auditory system. Hearing Research, 159: 132–149.
46. Moore BCJ (1997) Psychoacoustic consequences of compression in the peripheral auditory system. In: Schick A, Klatte M, editors. Contributions to Psychological Acoustics. BIS Oldenburg, Germany.
47. Moore BCJ, Glasberg BR (2004) A revised model of loudness perception applied to cochlear hearing loss. Hearing Research, 188: 70–88.
48. Kates JM, Arehart KH (2014). The hearing-aid speech quality index (HASQI) version 2/J. Audio Eng. Soc. 62, 99–117.
49. Münkner S (1993) A psychoacoustical model for the perception of non-stationary sounds. In: Schick A, editor. Contributions to Psychological Acoustics. BIS Oldenburg, 121–134.
50. Fassel R (1994) Experimente und Simulationsrechnungen zur Wahrnehmung von Amplitudenmodulationen im menschlichen Gehör. [Experiments and simulations on the perception of amplitude modulations in the human auditory system.] PhD thesis, University of Göttingen, Germany.
51. Sander A (1994) Psychoakustische Aspekte der subjektiven Trennbarkeit von Klängen. [Psychoacoustic aspects of the subjective separability of sounds.] PhD thesis, University of Oldenburg, Germany.
52. Dau T, Püschel D, Kohlrausch A (1996) A quantitative model of the 'effective' signal processing in the auditory system: II. Simulations and measurements. J Acoust Soc Am, 99: 3623–3631.
53. Dau T, Kollmeier B, Kohlrausch A (1997) Modeling auditory processing of amplitude modulation. II. Spectral and temporal integration in modulation detection. J Acoust Soc Am, 102(5), 2906–2919.
54. Verhey JL (1998) Psychoacoustics of spectro-temporal effects in masking and loudness patterns. BIS, Oldenburg. ISBN 3-8142-0622-2.
55. Derleth RP, Dau T (2000) On the role of envelope fluctuation processing in spectral masking. J Acoust Soc Am, 108(1): 285–96.
56. Krebber J, Eneman K, Huber R (2007) Report on Experiments on the Performance of Normal and Non-normal-hearing Listeners for a Range of (Simulated) Transmission Conditions with Combined Technical Disturbances. HearCom Deliverable D-4-3 Available: http://hearcom.eu/about/DisseminationandExploitation/deliverables.html.
57. Scollie S, Seewald R, Cornelisse L, Moodie ST, Bagatto M et al., 2005. The desired sensation level multistage input/output algorithm. Trends Amplif, 9, 159–197.
58. Huber R (2003) Objective assessment of audio quality using an auditory processing model. PhD thesis, University of Oldenburg, Germany Available: http://docserver.bis.uni-oldenburg.de/publikationen/dissertation/2004/hubobj03/hubobj03.html.

24

Tinnitus and Other Auditory Problems – Occupational Noise Exposure below Risk Limits May Cause Inner Ear Dysfunction

Ann-Cathrine Lindblad[1]*, Ulf Rosenhall[2], Åke Olofsson[1], Björn Hagerman[1]

1 Department of Clinical Science, Intervention and Technology, Division of Ear, Nose and Throat Diseases, Unit of Technical and Experimental Audiology, Karolinska Institutet, Stockholm, Sweden, **2** Department of Clinical Science, Intervention and Technology, Division of Ear, Nose and Throat Diseases, Karolinska Institutet; and Department of Audiology and Neurotology, Karolinska University Hospital, Stockholm, Sweden

Abstract

The aim of the investigation was to study if dysfunctions associated to the cochlea or its regulatory system can be found, and possibly explain hearing problems in subjects with normal or near-normal audiograms. The design was a prospective study of subjects recruited from the general population. The included subjects were persons with auditory problems who had normal, or near-normal, pure tone hearing thresholds, who could be included in one of three subgroups: teachers, *Education*; people working with music, *Music*; and people with moderate or negligible noise exposure, *Other*. A fourth group included people with poorer pure tone hearing thresholds and a history of severe occupational noise, *Industry*. $N_{total} = 193$. The following hearing tests were used: – pure tone audiometry with Békésy technique, – transient evoked otoacoustic emissions and distortion product otoacoustic emissions, without and with contralateral noise; – psychoacoustical modulation transfer function, – forward masking, – speech recognition in noise, – tinnitus matching. A questionnaire about occupations, noise exposure, stress/anxiety, muscular problems, medication, and heredity, was addressed to the participants. Forward masking results were significantly worse for *Education* and *Industry* than for the other groups, possibly associated to the inner hair cell area. Forward masking results were significantly correlated to louder matched tinnitus. For many subjects speech recognition in noise, left ear, did not increase in a normal way when the listening level was increased. Subjects hypersensitive to loud sound had significantly better speech recognition in noise at the lower test level than subjects not hypersensitive. Self-reported stress/anxiety was similar for all groups. In conclusion, hearing dysfunctions were found in subjects with tinnitus and other auditory problems, combined with normal or near-normal pure tone thresholds. The teachers, mostly regarded as a group exposed to noise below risk levels, had dysfunctions almost identical to those of the more exposed *Industry* group.

Editor: Manuel S. Malmierca, University of Salamanca- Institute for Neuroscience of Castille and Leon and Medical School, Spain

Funding: This project was supported by AFA Insurance, T-50:05, www.afaforsakring.se; and by the Swedish Council for Working Life and Social Research (2003-0154), www.fasarbetsliv.se. The funders had no role in study design, data collection and analysis, decision to publish, or preparation of the manuscript.

* E-mail: anncat.lindblad@ki.se

Introduction

Hearing problems are not just a matter of reduced ability to recognize speech and other sounds, but also of tinnitus, abnormal sensitivity to loud sound and sound distortion. Hearing loss, as measured by pure tone audiometry, is often accompanied by tinnitus. However, tinnitus occurs without concurrent self-reported hearing loss in about 1/3rd of all cases[1] (but bear in mind that self-reported hearing loss is poorly correlated to audiometric status). There are some reasons for this: 1) Tinnitus can be a non-auditory symptom, not involving the peripheral auditory system[2]; 2) Tinnitus can occur in conjuncture with a subclinical dysfunction of the cochlea[3,4], e.g. as a symptom at an early stage of noise-induced hearing loss (NIHL).

In a study of risk factors for tinnitus in a population 55 years and older Sindhusake et al[5] described a number of extrinsic and health factors that could be linked to tinnitus. The factor with the largest attributable risk was self-reported work-related noise exposure (almost 14%). The largest single factor was self-reported tolerable occupational noise exposure (9.3%). This means that a number of occupations with less noise burden than industrial exposure are at risk for noise-induced tinnitus. Teachers/preschool teachers are exposed to sudden slamming of for example lids, doors or toys, and preschool teachers may also suffer sudden screams near to the ear, although the mean noise levels are not excessive[6,7]. In occupations related to music the noise often varies around the sound level above which there is a risk of NIHL according to the international standardisation[8]. However, music sounds can be very loud, and alterations in the audiogram indicative of NIHL have been reported[9,10]. In other studies no relationship between music exposure and hearing loss, in terms of pure tone thresholds, has been found (for a review, see Zhao et al[11]). Tinnitus is common among rock/jazz musicians, also when the audiogram is similar to that of a reference group not exposed to excessive music[12].

These days when tinnitus is being paid so much attention, it may not be provocative to claim that hearing problems can be more than, or different from, having bad pure tone thresholds. Therefore there should be a demand for diagnostic test methods for identifying or excluding dysfunctions associated to the cochlea as the origin(s) of the hearing problems. Results from such tests could form the basis for individual treatment plans.

A test protocol, intended to be sufficiently sensitive to detect dysfunctions associated to minute cochlear lesions that cannot be diagnosed by routine clinical audiological tests, was developed. The protocol now consists of six auditory physiological tests, a Békésy audiogram, and a questionnaire.

In a first study, with fewer tests and test subjects (n = 46), who had tinnitus and normal or near-normal hearing-thresholds, we found that certain results could be associated with certain backgrounds[4]: 1) Persons exposed to impulse noise or other sudden loud sounds showed characteristic results. 2) Irregularities in the regulatory system may be a trustworthy sign of the cause of the tinnitus in persons well below middle-age, and with suspected hereditary tinnitus. 3) Subjects working with music had a variety of dysfunctions, but no features making them stand out from persons with other backgrounds. 4) Persons with suspected non-auditory tinnitus, on the other hand, showed very few dysfunctions.

The aim of the current study was to use the full test protocol to possibly identify dysfunctions associated with cochlear lesions in persons with up to moderate noise levels at work, with hearing problems, and without apparent deteriorations in the audiogram. If we found dysfunctions, would professions with different types of noise show their own characteristics?

The main finding of the current study was that teachers had characteristic results for two measurements not used in the first study. Those results were similar to results from industry workers tested for comparison, although the teachers had about 20 dB better pure tone thresholds. However, there were still no characteristic features to be found for musicians.

Materials and Methods

Ethics statement

The investigation was approved by the Regional ethical review board in Stockholm, no. 04-228/4. All test subjects gave their informed consents (written) to participate in the study.

Test subjects

Altogether 272 subjects of working age with tinnitus or other hearing problems, and not wearing a hearing aid, were tested in the study. About half of them were recruited by announcements in hearing clinics in Stockholm. The other half was recruited by an announcement at the home page of Karolinska University Hospital, and participants came from all over the country. The subjects were recruited and measured during a period of three years. There was no medical examination of the test subjects. The characterization of symptoms and exposure to e.g. noise was entirely based on the questionnaire. As it happened, very few professions were represented among these volunteers. Thus groups were formed to fit the assortment of volunteers regarding the amount and characteristics of noise exposure. It was not possible to match the participants regarding gender and age. Therefore the results should be interpreted with caution. However, some of the results have been compared with results for groups of persons of similar ages, but without hearing problems, or with internationally standardised pure tone thresholds. Reported here are results of subjects, who fulfilled the threshold criterion of having normal or near-normal hearing thresholds and who could be included in one of three groups of professions. Results of a fourth group with industrial noise and worse hearing thresholds are also reported for comparison. This study may have found dysfunctions that are characteristic for these groups before the audiogram is affected, but it will not give us a general overview of the effects of noise on hearing for these groups of professions at later stages of deterioration of the audiogram. Neither can it tell how common the detected dysfunctions are.

The groups were: 1) teachers, with 1/3rd of them preschool teachers, forming the group *Education*; 2) people working professionally with music, the group *Music*; and 3) subjects with low or, in a few cases, moderate occupational noise exposure, mostly medical staff and students, the group *Other*. The group *Other* seemed the least homogenous regarding noise exposure. In these groups (1–3) pure tone thresholds on both ears had to be $\leq$25 dB hearing level (HL) at the frequencies 500, 1000, 1500 and 2000 Hz, and $\leq$ 40 dB HL at 4000 Hz. The average threshold at the frequencies 3000, 4000, and 6000 Hz on both ears had to be $\leq$35 dB HL. The threshold fence defining normality or near-normality was chosen to include the effect of normal aging for all the test subjects. At the higher frequencies it corresponds to the median thresholds of otologically normal 66 year old men with no history of undue noise exposure[13].

For comparison a fourth group was selected 4) constituted of persons with blue-collar occupations, having audiograms with high- (and sometimes mid-) frequency hearing impairments, indicative of noise-induced hearing loss, and also having tinnitus, the group *Industry*.

After omission of data from people not conforming to the threshold criterion or being unsuitable for the chosen groups of professions there was a total of 193 subjects, 102 men and 91 women, 18 to 66 years of age, to be analysed. The groups are presented in Table 1. The proportion of genders in the profession groups seems roughly the same as in working life in our country. Mean audiograms for the four test groups are shown in Figure 1.

Reference groups

"Normal" reference results for our methods and our equipment were used for comparison. These results were meant to be to be used in several projects. A *middle-aged reference group* consisted of fifty-seven 41–60 year old subjects, all without hearing problems and with hearing thresholds no worse than the median for 50-year-old men[13]. (In the 5-year age intervals there were 8 women and 8 men who were 41 to 45 years old, 7 women and 7 men who were 46 to 50, 7 women and 9 men who were 51 to 55, and 8 women and 4 men who were 56 to 60.) Another group consisted of twenty-seven young women, 18–24 years old, considering themselves normal and unexposed, and with normal hearing thresholds (< 20 dB HL 125–8000 Hz except for four individual thresholds exceeding 20 but not 23 dB HL). The mean pure tone thresholds for the group turned out to be 5 dB HL. A comparison to the ISO-standard above tells that 80% of unexposed women at those ages have better thresholds than our group of young women. Several of these young women often went to discos or pop concerts and had tinnitus. Thus they were not an ideal, "normal", "unexposed" group.

Equipment and measurements

A computer-controlled Tucker-Davis Technologies (System III) module system was used with Sennheiser HDA 200 headphones at the psychoacoustical tests, and with amplifiers plus probe systems ER-10C from Etymotic Research on both ears for the measurements of otoacoustic emissions. The HDA 200 headphones were

Table 1. Number, age, and gender of subjects in groups.

Profession	Group name	Number	Mean age (SD)	No. of men	No. of women
Teachers	*Education*	48	45.4 (10.6)	9	39
Musicians	*Music*	32	37.8 (11.5)	20	12
Other	*Other*	97	39.2 (13.5)	57	40
Noisy industry	*Industry*	16	54.4 (9.3)	16	0
TOTAL		193	45.0 (13.0)	102	91

calibrated according to ISO 389-8 and the ER-10C probe systems were calibrated in an ear simulator according to IEC 60711.

The software for all the methods, for the computer and the Tucker-Davis equipment, was written in our laboratory. The TDT system was programmed to produce and present stimuli, for example the OAE stimuli and the contralateral noise, as well as collect and store the responses. However, the speech test used stored sound files for the words and their respective noise stimuli. The adaptive procedure of the speech test was controlled by the computer. All tests were performed in a sound proof audiometric test room.

Basic otoscopy and tympanometry were performed. When necessary, cerumen was removed.

The hearing measurements took about three and a half hours including a coffee break. All the participating subjects performed all the tests. However, individual test subjects were allowed to exclude stimulus levels they considered too high.

Questionnaire. In the intermission between the measurements the subjects were given a questionnaire. Apart from questions about age and profession there were 22 questions with two to eight response alternatives, sometimes also with a possibility of an open response. The questions regarded hearing problems, tinnitus, sensitivity to loud sounds, noise exposure at work and in their leisure time, musical activities, impulse noise incidents, military service, medication (pain relieving and tinnitus medicine), eye and hair colour, smoking, neck problems, headache, stress, and relatives with hearing problems. The questions on tinnitus and

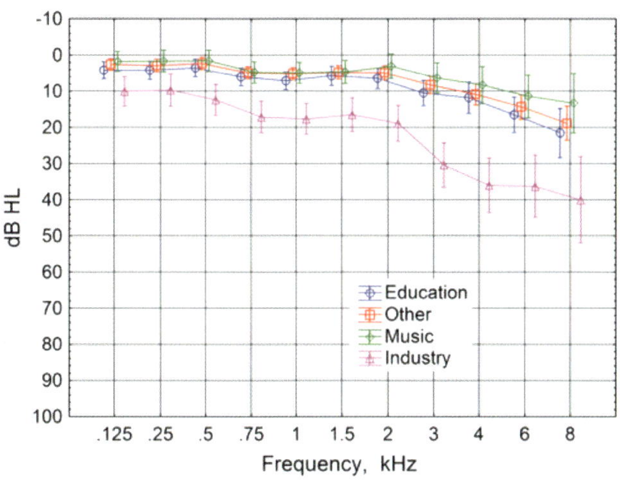

Figure 1. Mean audiograms for the profession groups. Group names as shown in Table 1. Please note that the group *Industry* had no threshold restrictions. The vertical bars represent 95% confidence intervals. The data points are horizontally displaced for clarity.

sensitivity to loud sounds had the response alternatives: never, only after a loud sound, at certain occasions, often, and constantly. The questions on headache and neck problems had only the response alternatives yes and no. The question "Do you feel stressed/ anxious?" had the five response alternatives: never, seldom, sometimes, often and always. A translation of the questionnaire, including number of responses to each alternative, is presented in Appendix S1.

From the responses to the questions about profession, different types of noise exposure and exposure times, figures of noise exposure were estimated. The underlying principles for the judgements are found in Appendix S2. A summary is presented here: The range for 1) work noise exposure was 0 to 4, for 2) leisure time 0 to 3, and for 3) military service 0 to 2. Persons with only marginal noise exposure in compulsory military service, being well protected during a few initial shooting exercises, got the estimate 0, the same as persons not having been in military service. The total noise exposure was calculated as the sum of the three figures, which gave a scale from 0 to 9. However, the highest value for an individual in this study was 4. Within each profession group the figures were fairly equal. 4) Self-reported incidents with impulse noise were treated separately, range 0 to 3.

Békésy audiometry. Pure tone thresholds for left and right ears separately were measured at 125, 250, 500, 750, 1000, 1500, 2000, 3000, 4000, 6000, and 8000 Hz.

A pulsating tone is presented. The duration is 225 ms, including attack and release times, and with a 175 ms long interval between pulses. The level of the tone is increased by 2.8 dB/s until the subject detects the tone and starts pressing the button. The level of the tone decreases with the same speed until the button is released again, etc. Thus a zigzag pattern is formed around the threshold level. The turning-points are registered by the computer. The measurement is concluded after 10 turning points. The first two turning points are not used in the calculation. The threshold is calculated as the mean value of the medians of the remaining upper and lower turning points, and presented with the resolution of 1 dB. These parameters should give high accuracy with a standard deviation of repeated measures not exceeding 1.8 dB[14].

Otoacoustic emissions, TEOAEs. Transient evoked otoacoustic emissions, TEOAEs, were measured at two input levels without or with contralateral noise. Normally the contralateral noise will make the efferent system controlling the outer hair cells, OHCs, reduce, suppress, the response amplitude. We measure the response correlated to the stimulus signal, but also the uncorrelated response.

Clicks with the duration of 80 μs were repeated with a frequency of 50 Hz. The measurement was performed in a nonlinear mode to enhance those components in the response, which have a nonlinear dependence of the stimulus level, and to suppress the linear components. To accomplish this, the polarity of every fourth click is reversed and the sound pressure level is increased by a factor of 3. After removal of the primary click by windowing technique, the acoustical responses from 1000 clicks are averaged. The stimulus level is specified as so called peak equivalent sound pressure level, peSPL. TEOAEs were measured at 70 and 85 dB peSPL with and without contralateral masking consisting of a 70 dB SPL broadband noise. The RMS-values for the correlated and uncorrelated responses, over the interval of measurement, are used as variables in the analyses and so are the RMS-values in three different frequency areas, Low (500–2500 Hz), Mid (2500–5000 Hz), and High (5000–8000 Hz).

Otoacoustic emissions, DPOAEs. When measuring distortion product otoacoustic emissions, DPOAEs, two stimulus tones are given, with frequencies near each other, $f_2/f_1 = 1.25$, and near the measurement frequency. The measurements were performed on both ears at an input level, L, of f_1 of 65 dB SPL, $L_{f1}/L_{f2} = 10$ dB, nominal frequency $\sqrt{f_1}*\sqrt{f_2}$. A weak response is measured at the frequency $2f_1-f_2$. Two measurements were done, the first one at the nominal frequency 1000 Hz and the second one at 2000 Hz. To avoid measuring in a notch of the DPOAE microstructure an automatic procedure measured at a few frequencies between 0.95 and 1.05 times the nominal frequency with an increment of 0.01 times the nominal frequency. The measurements were then performed at the frequency with the largest response. To estimate the background noise from equipment and ear, the level in narrow frequency areas below and above the response tone frequency was measured.

The measurements were made without and with contralateral noise. We made 20 3s long measurements of the response from the two tones without contralateral noise. We calculated the individual standard deviation of these responses to test the stability.

Measurements were also made with on-off noise (12 s on, and 12 s off, 5 times) on the contralateral ear in order to investigate the ability of the ear to regulate the sensitivity of the other ear. The response normally decreases somewhat when the contralateral noise is on. The difference between the medians of the five off-periods and the medians of the five on-periods shows the ability and endurance of the ear to suppress the response when the noise is on.

Psychoacoustical modulation transfer function, PMTF. The active nonlinear process in the cochlea is mediated by the OHCs and facilitates the perception of the complex sound patterns in speech. These patterns are characterized by rapid sound variations combined with slow modulations caused by speech syllables, words and intonation. A measurement termed the psychoacoustical modulation transfer function (PMTF) reflects the functioning of the inner ear when handling slow intensity variations like those of speech. PMTF measures the thresholds of brief tones placed at the peaks or in the valleys of a fully, sinusoidally intensity-modulated, octave-band noise at various sound pressure levels centred at the test tone frequency[15], thus involving simultaneous, forward and backward masking. The measurements were performed with Békésy-technique at various sound pressure levels of the noise. The test has been shown to measure more subtle qualities of hearing, and there is evidence that it reflects hair cell function[15].

PMTF measurements: The measurements were performed with the brief tone, 4 ms with raised cosine flanks, first with the octave-band filtered noise at 2000 Hz, and with a modulation frequency of 2.5 Hz; and then with the octave-band filtered noise at 4000 Hz, and with a modulation frequency of 10 Hz. The noise levels were 35 to 85 dB SPL in steps of 10 dB. Initially, the threshold for the brief tone was measured without noise to familiarize the subject with the brief tone. Both ears were measured, with the left ear first. When the subject expressed tiredness or discomfort, only one ear, mostly the left ear, was measured.

Typical PMTF results: Figure 2 shows a few stylized, but characteristic PMTF curves. The normal PMTF curves are nonlinear, with a maximum in signal-to-noise-ratio, S/N, for the peak threshold, occurring at a noise level around 55 dB SPL (Figure 2A). (The term *peak threshold* is used for the threshold of the brief tone when the tone is placed at the peak of the noise. The term *valley threshold* is used when the tone is placed in the valley of the noise.) For the valley threshold there is a corresponding maximum at about 65 dB SPL (Figure 2A).

For a sensorineural hearing loss of cochlear origin, the nonlinearity is weaker. Both maxima have lower S/N and they occur at higher noise levels (Figure 2B). This type of pattern indicates *reduced nonlinearity*. However, in this study we focused on the effects described in the following paragraphs.

A second type of abnormal PMTF pattern is presented in (Figure 2D). The S/N maxima of the peak and valley threshold curves have markedly increased amplitudes and occur at the same, low noise level (35–45 dB SPL). The peak and valley curves are almost identical, which implicates that the affected ear can hardly take advantage of the silent interval around the brief tone in the valley. The term "hyper-PMTF" was coined for this pattern, which can appear after unprotected exposure to impulse noise or other sudden, loud noise with a rapid onset[4]. We speculate that there are lesions in the inner hair cell, IHC, region, since impulse noise by itself or embedded in continuous noise causes a larger proportion of damage to IHCs than continuous noise[16].

There are also intermediate varieties between normal and hyper-PMTF. A mildly abnormal variety is shown in Figure 2C. Like in the hyper-PMTF the S/N maxima of the peak and valley curves are positioned at the same noise level, but here they occur at a normal noise level (>45 dB SPL), and they are not as high as in the hyper-PMTF. The level dependence for peak and valley curves is the same. At every noise level used the S/N for the peak threshold is a roughly constant number of dB higher than the S/N for the valley threshold.

It is evident from the examples above that there are two main types of abnormal PMTF results: The positions of the maximum peak and valley thresholds can occur at higher (Figure 2B) or lower (Figure 2D) than normal noise levels (horizontal position in graph), and the corresponding S/N maxima are then either lower (Figure 2B) or higher (Figure 2D) than normal (vertical position in graph). Therefore, a practical way of analysis is to use a qualitative method to define certain typical patterns, for example the hyper-PMTF.

Depending on combinations of shapes and positioning of the peak and valley curves (relative each other and regarding the noise levels of the maxima) we divided the PMTF curves into classes depending on the likeness to hyper-PMTF. We called them P-type, and numbered them 0 to 3. A few P-types are exemplified in Figure 2. Curves denoted P-type = 3, called hyper-PMTF, indicate dysfunction, possibly from impulse noise or other sudden, loud noise with a rapid onset, Figure 2D. P-type = 0 means normal, or typical sensorineural loss that is still measurable at fairly low noise levels, Figure 2A and 2B. P-type = 1, seen in Figure 2C, and P-type = 2 fall in between: P-type = 1 looks more like P-type = 0; and P-type = 2 looks more like P-type = 3 by showing curves with maxima at low noise levels but not as high and/or regular as in the typical hyper-PMTF, i.e. "suspected hyper-PMTF". P-type = NM means not measurable, i.e. the peak and valley thresholds for the brief tone are entirely determined by the threshold for the brief

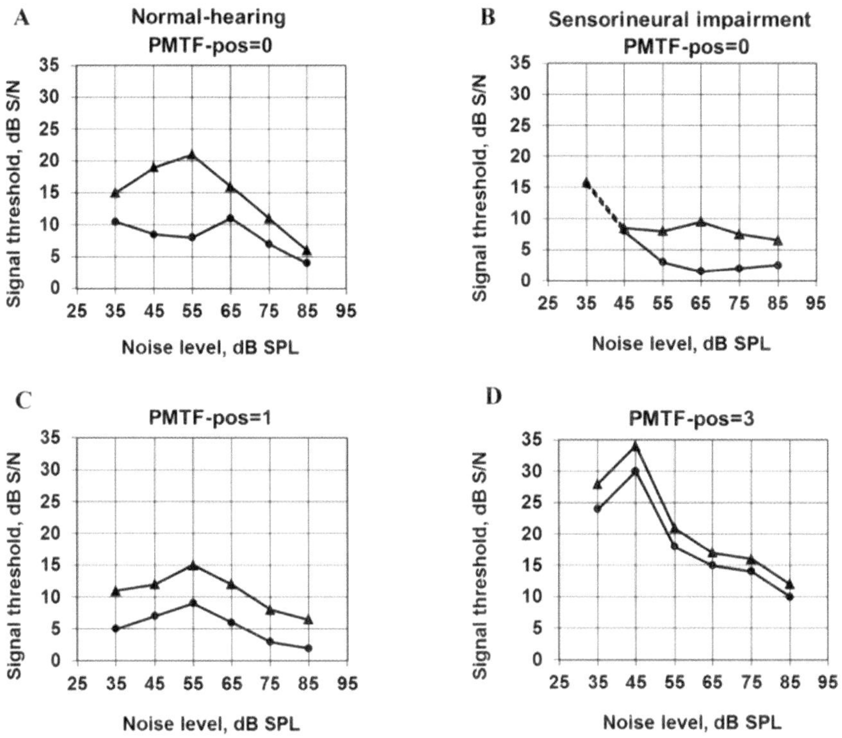

Figure 2. Characteristic PMTF-curves. The PMTF-curves are classified as four different P-types. 0 = normal PMTF-curves (2A) or typical sensorineural loss (2B) that is still measurable; 1 = mildly abnormal (2C), see text; 2 = suspected hyper-PMTF (not shown in the figure); 3 = hyper-PMTF (2D), indicates damage from impulse noise or other sudden, loud noise with a rapid onset; NM = not measurable (not shown in the figure). Triangles indicate peak thresholds. Round markers indicate valley thresholds.

tone without noise at the low noise levels where the characteristics of the hyper-PMTF are seen.

Forward masking. Experiments on mice, using auditory brainstem responses[17], have suggested that forward masking results indicate the status of the IHCs. After the offset of a noise burst the masking effect on a brief tone decreases rapidly in a good ear, but, according to that article, not in an ear with loss of IHCs. In our project a brief tone, 4 ms, at 2000 Hz (the same as used in the PMTF measurements), is presented 5 or 50 ms after the offset of an octave-band noise burst of 400 ms duration and a repetition interval of 800 ms at 65, 75 or 85 dB SPL, and the corresponding thresholds are measured with Békésy technique for one ear at a time, both ears. The difference between the thresholds for 5 and 50 ms interval between noise burst and tone at the same noise level is calculated. A small difference means that the masking effect from the noise burst has not decreased much after 50 ms, which has been attributed to less well-functioning IHCs[17,18]. Our middle-aged reference group showed a threshold difference of 27 ±9 dB. The median was also 27 dB, with lower quartile 22 dB, and a maximum of 49 dB. With results at the lower quartile the speech recognition in noise seemed to start to be degraded. For the group of young women the threshold difference was just 1 dB larger, 28 ±11dB, but the median was 30 dB, and the maximum threshold difference 51 dB.

Speech recognition threshold in modulated noise. The speech recognition threshold in modulated noise was measured on the self-reported worst ear. Hagermans 5-word sentences in noise were used with the original versions of the various words stored in the computer[19]. The noise was modulated to a degree of 100%, i.e. as much as possible without getting overflow[20], and had a long-term average spectrum identical to that of the speech read by a female voice. The modulating signal was a noise with most of its energy between 1 and 5 Hz, and a spectrum similar to the modulation spectrum of normal speech[19]. An adaptive method was used for the threshold measurement, with the change of the speech level after each sentence depending on number of correct words obtained. For a more detailed description see [20]. The threshold is defined as S/N for 40% correct words. The measurements were performed at noise levels 70 and 85 dB SPL. When 85 dB SPL was considered too loud, both ears were measured at 70 dB SPL. For the *middle-aged reference group* the S/N at threshold, over both ears, were −13.6 ±2.1 dB, at 70 dB SPL presentation level, and −15.5 ±2.2 dB, at 85 dB SPL. Corresponding values for the *group of young women*, for the left ear only, were −15.4 ±0.9 and −16.3 ±1.1 dB.

Tinnitus matching. The subjects were asked to compare pure tones from a modified version of the Békésy audiometry program to match the pitch of their tinnitus. The level was changed in steps of 1 dB, and the frequency in steps of 1 Hz. The participants were asked to: "Try to match the frequency of the tone in the earphone with the pitch of your tinnitus. After that, match the level of the tone to that of your tinnitus". The drawback with this method is that it is only applicable to tinnitus with a tonal character. The matching is less accurate for those perceiving their tinnitus as noise or other non-tonal sounds.

Statistical analyses. The program Statistica 9.1 was used for statistical analyses. For the hearing measurements, all of them resulting in continuous variables, analysis of variances was used, often with subsequent Tukey's post hoc tests. To find relations between continuous variables linear regression with age as covariate was used. However, in analyses where age was not significant, results from ANOVAS without age as covariate are presented. For the variables from the questionnaire, with rank order variables, where no information is given in the text, Kruskal-Wallis ANOVA by ranks was used, sometimes with subsequent multiple comparisons. Other statistical tests are mentioned in Results and Discussion.

Results and Discussion

Questionnaire

Hearing problems. Among the 193 subjects analysed, 69% had tinnitus and were also hypersensitive to loud sound, 22% had tinnitus only, 7% were only hypersensitive to loud sound and 2% had neither of these two symptoms, but felt they had difficulties hearing in noise. On a general question about hearing problems 25% answered that their hearing symptoms disturb them always: affect sleep, affect their whole life; 28% that their symptoms affect them in normal sound environments, but their tinnitus is masked by louder sounds; 25% that their symptoms affect them only in a quiet environment; 7% that they have symptoms but no problems (although the criterion for participating was having problems); 13% said they have problems, but did not specify to what extent. There was no statistical difference between the profession groups in this respect. Neither was there any difference between groups regarding hypersensitivity to loud sound.

Noise exposure. Very rough estimates of noise exposure based on the individual responses to the questionnaire indicated that the groups *Education* and *Other* were significantly different from the groups *Music* and *Industry* by being judged less noise exposed ($p<0.05$). This was the result of a Kruskal-Wallis ANOVA by ranks with estimated noise exposure as the dependent variable and with profession group as the between subjects factor. The questions referred to regarded profession, number of years working, leisure activities, and military service.

Regarding self-reported incidents with impulse noise or sudden very loud noise, a corresponding analysis showed that the exposure estimate for the *Industry* group was significantly higher than for the three other groups ($p<0.01$). Another group, which might have reported incidents for example with positive feedback in electronic systems, is the *Music* group. In our study, however, the musicians claimed that they were not using electronic amplification. This should have decreased the risk of unexpected sudden changes of the sound level. And the number of reported incidents did not differ significantly from those of the groups *Education* and *Other*.

The *Other* group included mainly hospital staff, and students. Only few of the participants had been exposed to occupational noise. In those cases, they handled medical devices.

Other data from the questionnaire. Regarding neck problems, *Education* had significantly higher values than *Industry* ($p<0.0005$, Pearson Chi-square). The *Education* group had significantly more self-reported tension headaches than the groups *Other* and *Industry* ($p<0.05$, Pearson Chi-square). The groups *Education* and *Music* had similar, slightly higher values for stress/ anxiety than *Industry* and *Other*, but the differences were not significant. There were no significant differences between groups regarding pain relieving medication, eye and hair colour, smoking, and relatives with hearing problems. Tinnitus medicine was only used by ten subjects. Therefore it was not subjected to analyses. There was no difference in stress problems between the subgroups preschool teachers and other teachers.

Some relations between data from the questionnaire. Self-reported stress seemed to give tension headache and neck problems ($p<0.05$, $p<0.005$; binomial logit model). Headaches and neck problems influenced the use of medication ($p<0.0001$, $p<0.05$, Kruskal-Wallis ANOVA by ranks). The amount of medication was not influenced by age (ordinal logit model), gender or stress.

Békésy audiometry

An ANOVA was performed with hearing threshold as the dependent variable, with profession group as a between subjects factor, and with ear and frequency as within subjects factors. The group *Industry*, the blue-collar group without threshold restrictions, chosen to have worse noise exposure than the other groups, was significantly different from all the other groups for left and right ears combined ($p<0.00001$, Tukey's HSD), Figure 1. For the *Industry* group the right ear was on average 2.8 dB worse than the left ear for all frequencies, but the difference was not significant. This group had worse pure tone thresholds than those of unexposed men of the same age[13].

TEOAES

An ANOVA with the correlated TEOAE response as the dependent variable, with profession group as between subjects factor; and with ear, stimulus level, and frequency area as within subjects independent factors; showed no significant difference between the various professions or between left and right ear. For normal ears the response increases when the stimulus level is increased from 75 to 85 dB peSPL. There was such increases of 4.4 dB for each of the groups *Education*, *Other* and *Music*, and they were highly significant ($p<0.00005$, Tukey's HSD). However, when compensated for age they were not, and the response of the *Industry* group at the higher level was just marginally higher, 1.4 dB, than at the lower level. For the uncorrelated response signal, on the other hand, the *Industry* group showed a 6 dB higher response than *Education*, *Other* and *Music* ($p<0.005$ for all the three comparisons, Tukey's HSD). The TEOAE results of the *Industry* group may be explained by dysfunctional OHCs with reduced ipsilateral restraining regulation.

The contralateral suppression effect was very small, the means for the groups ranging from 0.22 dB to −0.26 dB without significant differences, although age was a significant factor.

DPOAES

An ANOVA with the DPOAE response level without contralateral noise as the dependent variable, with profession group as between subjects factor; with ear and frequency as within subjects factors, and age as covariate, showed that the mean response level was significantly higher at 1000 Hz than at 2000 Hz, 7.5 and 3.7 dB SPL respectively ($p<0.00001$). There was a strongly significant age dependence ($p<0.00001$). From the right ear *Industry* had a very weak mean response over frequencies, −1.9 dB SPL, which was significantly lower than the responses of the other groups ($p<0.005$, Tukey's HSD).

To estimate the background noise from equipment and ear, the level in narrow frequency areas below and above the response tone frequency was measured. A statistical analysis corresponding to the one above was performed, now with this noise level as the dependent variable. In the left ear this noise level was about 3 dB higher than in the right ear ($p<0.00001$). Furthermore, the group *Industry* had an almost 3 dB higher value of that noise in the left ear than the groups *Education*, *Other*, and *Music* ($p<0.05$, Tukey's HSD).

A corresponding statistical analysis was also performed with the individual standard deviation of 20 consecutive measurements as the dependent variable. Also for this standard deviation the group *Industry* had a significantly higher value, 4.0 dB, than the groups *Education*, *Other*, and *Music* (2.0–2.1 dB), when averaged over ears and frequencies ($p<0.00005$). Age had a significant influence, but compensation for age did not change any values. Thus, the group *Industry* differed from the other groups by low DPOAE responses on the right ear, a high noise level around the tone response on the left ear, and a large variation in the 20 measurements without contralateral noise. It looks like the DPOAE response from this group mostly consists of noise. Compare to TEOAE results.

There was no significant influence of any of the factors ear, frequency or profession group on the suppression effect using the contralateral on-off noise. The range of suppression for the groups was 0.4 to 0.6 dB.

OAEs in short. As the *Industry* group was chosen to have a noise induced hearing loss it was a natural finding that *both types of OAEs* for the *Industry* group were marginal, unstable and considerably noisy. There were deteriorations in the contralateral regulatory system for all groups, but considerably more so in the *Industry* group. A few individuals in the other three groups had abnormally high emissions at some frequencies suggesting impaired ipsilateral regulatory function.

As a whole our results regarding OAEs did not give much information, probably because most of our test subjects were middle-aged. One should keep in mind that there is a normal degradation of OAEs and regulatory efferent system with age, which may obscure for example noise induced degradation [21].

PMTF

The stimulus noise levels at which the maximum values of the threshold curves were found, were used as dependent variables in a multivariate ANOVA with profession group as between subjects factor; and with peak/valley curve and frequency as within subjects factors. Those noise levels did not differ significantly between the groups. This was true for both peak and valley curves and both ears.

The corresponding analyses, with the maximum value of the PMTF threshold curve on the left ear as dependent variable, showed that the maximum of the valley curve was significantly higher for the *Education* group than for *Other* and *Music* ($p<0.05$, Tukey's HSD). The same tendency was found on the right ear, but without statistical significance. An analysis for different types of teachers showed a tendency to higher maxima for preschool teachers than for other teachers. In this context it should be noted that a high maximum, especially on the valley curve, is one characteristic of a hyper-PMTF, Figure 2D. Although one cannot be certain that the results of the *Education* group are caused by sudden loud sounds, they definitely indicate a reduced ability to detect short sounds in silent intervals of a complicated signal, poor temporal processing.

Very few subjects with fully developed hyper-PMTFs (P-type = 3), suggesting exposure to impulse noise possibly associated to damage in the inner hair cell area [4,16,22], were found in this study. Although the *Industry* group had more self-reported impulse noise incidents ($p<0.01$) than the other groups, this did not result in significantly more hyper-PMTFs than in the other groups. One reason may be that some of the test subjects, especially in the *Industry* group, could not be measured at the low levels of the modulated noise at which the characteristics of the hyper-PMTF are seen. Measurements closer to the incidents, before the characteristics in our PMTF-measurements had been obscured by further deterioration of pure tone thresholds, would have clarified if there was a hyper-PMTF. Those actually classified with P-type = 3, hyper-PMTF showed fairly flat audiogram curves. See Figure 3. In the figure there is one curve showing the mean pure tone thresholds for the two subjects among the 193 who had P-type = 3 on the left ear. This curve shows thresholds around 10 dB HL. There is also an extra curve for these two subjects plus four

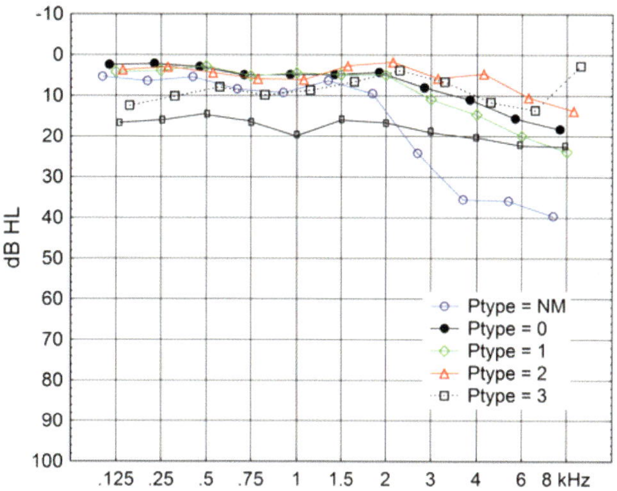

Figure 3. Mean audiograms for subjects with different types of PMTF-curves, 4000 Hz, left ear. See legend of Figure 2 about the PMTF classification. Numbers of subjects for P-types NM, 0, 1, 2, and 3 are 12, 40, 54, 13, and 2, respectively. An extra curve, black continuous line with smaller markers, black boxes, is added, which includes 4 more subjects with hyper-PMTF (P-type = 3), but outside the threshold criterion limiting to 193 subjects. Note that the two curves for hyper-PMTF are fairly flat. The data points are horizontally displaced for clarity.

more subjects with P-type = 3, left ear, from the total of 272 subjects measured. Most thresholds forming this curve are slightly better than 20 dB HL. Also the curve representing the 13 ears with P-type = 2, suspected hyper-PMTF, is fairly flat.

Audiograms with similar hearing thresholds for all frequencies have also been observed in conscripts sent to us for measurements after severe shooting incidents, unpublished data. It is not unusual that all thresholds have positions around 10 dB HL, i.e. totally normal. This may be a warning flag when a person with normal thresholds complains of hearing problems. In experiments on chinchilla, Wang[23] and El-Badry[24] have shown that as much as 70 – 85% of the IHCs could be damaged before threshold levels became abnormal. Another paper[25] shows that at sound levels well above threshold, other hearing functions, including forward masking, were strongly deteriorated before such a degree of degeneration.

Forward masking

An ANOVA was performed with the forward masking threshold difference (difference between the thresholds of the brief tone at 5 ms and at 50 ms after the noise burst) as the dependent variable, with profession group as a between subjects factor, and with ear and level as within subjects factors. The two older groups *Industry*, mean age 54, and *Education*, mean age 45, showed significantly worse forward masking mean results (over ears and levels), 19 and 21 dB threshold difference, than the about five years younger groups *Music* and *Other*, 32 and 30 dB, ($p<0.005$, Tukey's HSD). These results could be compared to the threshold difference, 27 ± 9 dB (median 27 dB, lower quartile 22 dB) for our *middle-aged reference group* without hearing problems. Most notable is that the median of the teachers, the *Education* group, 23 dB, was almost as low as the lower quartile of the *middle-aged reference group*, 22 dB. The lower quartile of *Education* was 12 dB.

On the other hand one may note that the results of *Music* and *Other* are as good as the median result of the (much younger) *group of young women*, 30 dB. Walton[26] found that aging changed forward masking for the worse. This was also the general effect over all our test subjects. The change was 3 dB per decade ($p < 0.00001$ in all six linear regressions, i.e. two ears times three sound levels). However, in our study the significant differences between profession groups became even stronger when compensated for age ($p<0.001$, Tukey's HSD with age as covariate).

Figure 4 shows individual audiograms for six subjects with a threshold difference less than 5 dB for 5 and 50 ms delay between short tone and noise, on the left ear. Three of them came from the *Industry* group, two from *Education* and one from *Other*. Their PMTF results suggested either exposure to impulse noise or other sudden loud noise or they could not be measured at the levels of the modulated noise at which the characteristics of the hyper-PMTF are seen.

If an analogy with research animals is proposed, abnormal forward masking results may indicate IHC dysfunction or radial dendrite damage, independent of OHC status[18]. Later research on animals has found other damage in the IHC area [27–31], from earlier noise exposure not causing permanent threshold shifts, but with supra-threshold effects. If the speculation is true, that the ears of the research animals and humans work in a similar way, the results of this study suggest that some persons with professions considered less noise exposed may have considerable damage in the IHC area – and more such damage than in normal aging. However, this remains a speculation until more research has been carried out in humans.

Speech in noise

In the speech-in-noise test some subjects regarded 85 dB SPL listening level too loud and were measured at the lower level on both ears. Three subjects found even the lower listening level too loud and did not complete any speech test at all. The resulting number of measurements on the left ear was 125 at 70 dB SPL and 83 at 85 dB SPL, and on the right ear 108 and 72, respectively. ANOVAs were performed separately for the left and right ears with the S/N threshold as the dependent variable, with profession group as a between subjects factor, and with sound level as a within subjects factor.

Industry and *Education* were, on the left ear, significantly worse ($p<0.05$, Tukey's HSD) than *Music*, the only group that was normal at both levels. *Industry* was also significantly worse than *Other* ($p<0.05$, Tukey's HSD). However, when age was introduced as a covariate all the significant group differences disappeared. (The change in S/N at threshold per decade was 1 dB.)

More important was that, still on the left ear, *Industry* and *Education* were markedly worse than the *middle-aged reference group* ($p<0.0001$ for both groups at 85 dB SPL, t-tests), see Figure 5, like in the forward masking results. The group *Other* was normal at 70, but not at 85 dB SPL. Note that both the *middle-aged reference group* and the *group of young women* had considerably better results on the speech-in-noise test at the presentation level 85 dB SPL than at 70 dB SPL. Also the test groups in the current study had better results at the higher level, but the improvement was smaller due to larger deteriorations at the higher level than at the lower level.

On the right ear all group means except *Industry*'s were within normal limits compared to the mean over right and left ear of our *middle-aged reference group* without hearing problems. However, only two subjects in *Industry* were tested on the right ear.

Tinnitus matching

An ANOVA was performed with the matched tinnitus level as the dependent variable, with profession group as a between subjects factor and with ear as a within subjects factor. The group *Industry* had significantly louder tinnitus than *Music* and *Other* ($p< 0.05$, Tukey's HSD) according to the matching, but not significantly louder than *Education*. Figure 6 shows a histogram of the matched tinnitus levels for the left ear ($n = 110$). The results of the right ear were similar, as many subjects located their tinnitus in the centre of the head or in both ears. The subjects who did no matching to the test tone ($n = 83$) either had no pitch in their tinnitus or, for most of them; they had no tinnitus to match to at the test moment.

Relations between measurements

Relations between measurements were tested with linear regression. When forward masking was involved it was used as

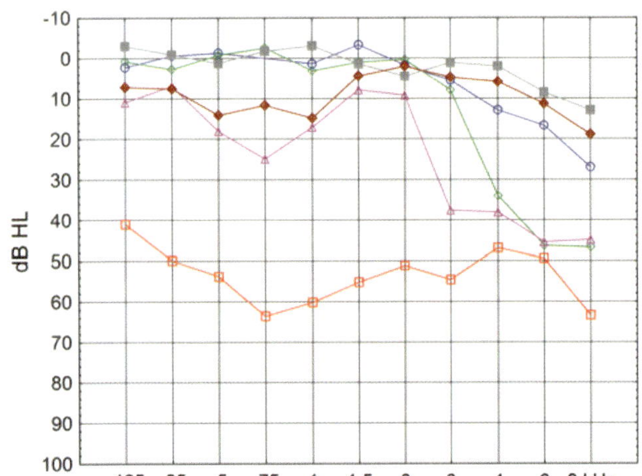

Figure 4. Individual audiograms for subjects with a forward masking threshold difference of less than 5 dB. Left ear, n = 6. The three worst audiograms come from the group *Industry* without restrictions on pure tone thresholds.

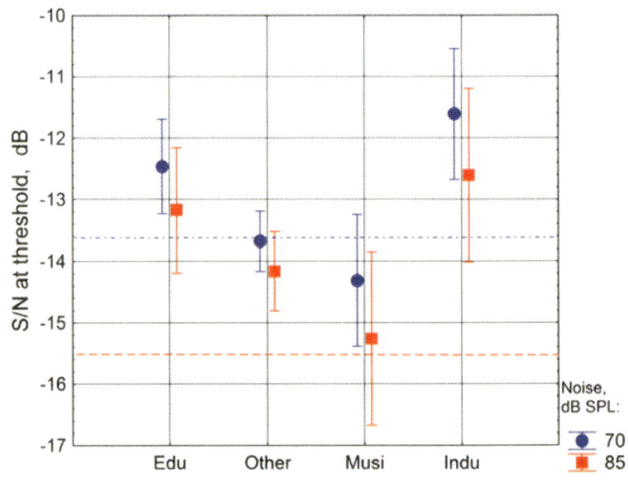

Figure 5. Mean of the speech recognition thresholds in noise. S/N at threshold for the profession groups, two noise levels 70 and 85 dB SPL, left ear. The vertical bars show 95% confidence intervals. Numbers of subjects in the different groups are from left to right 23, 58, 12, and 12. The horizontal lines show values for a *middle-aged reference group* without hearing problems for the noise levels 70 (dashed) and 85 (dotted) dB SPL. (The means and the numbers of measurements were obtained from the ANOVA, which explains the discrepancy from the number of measured ears.)

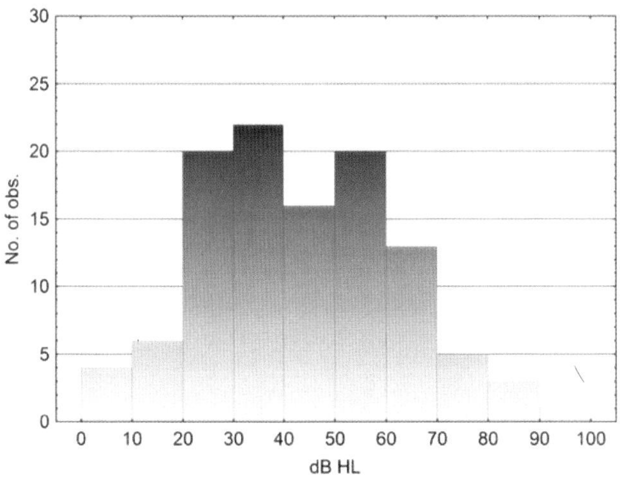

Figure 6. Histogram of matched tinnitus level, left ear, n = 110. Right ear's histogram (n = 89) was similar. Median levels for left and right ears were 40 and 38 dB HL, respectively.

the independent variable. There were significant negative, and similar, correlations between *forward masking* results at each of the three test levels and *matched tinnitus level* for both ears (at best r = −0.36, p<0.001 at 65 dB SPL, right ear). This means that louder tinnitus was correlated to poor forward masking. The two groups with louder tinnitus, *Industry* and *Education*, had significantly worse forward masking results than *Music* and *Other*. That subjects with worse forward masking had louder matched tinnitus is in concordance with reports of increased gain at higher levels in the auditory system following loss of IHCs[32]. This is also in accordance to the assumption that there is an increased risk of tinnitus and abnormal sensitivity to loud sound in case of neural degeneration proximal to intact IHCs[27,28].

There was a significant correlation between the threshold difference in *forward masking* and the *speech recognition threshold in noise*. The groups with the poorest forward masking results (possibly also with the worst IHC status) had the worst speech recognition in noise. The correlation was strongest for both speech-in-noise levels on the right ear, and for the lower noise level on the left ear with correlations between −0.5 and −0.6 (p<0.00001) for relevant level combinations of speech-in-noise and forward masking results (with forward masking level equal to or lower than the noise level in the speech test). For the left ear at the higher speech-in-noise level the correlation was −0.3 to −0.4 (p<0.005).

Unlike the difference between the groups in the forward masking test, the differences between the groups in the speech-in-noise test were not significant when compensated for age. One may speculate that forward masking may be a basic measure of the status of receptor hair cells and a neural degeneration beyond, which has been shown to be a long-term after-effect of noise exposure[27,28,30], whereas speech recognition also has an added age-dependent component of cognition.

There were strongly significant correlations between *forward masking* results, only measured at 2000 Hz, and *PMTF*-results at the same frequency, indicating characteristics of the PMTF-curves concordant with hyper-PMTF (P-type = 3) or suspected hyper-PMTF (P-type = 2): Small forward masking threshold differences were accompanied by high maximum valley thresholds (r = −0.44, p<0.0001 for both ears and forward masking at 65 dB), and by positioning of the maximum valley thresholds at low noise level (r = 0.31, p<0.005 for both ears and forward masking at 65 dB SPL). The bond between forward masking and PMTF regarding incidents with sudden loud sound was further strengthened by the fact that high maximum valley thresholds were accompanied by positioning of the maximum valley thresholds at low noise level (p<0.00001, r = −0.49 for the left ear, r = −0.54 for the right ear), both typical for the hyper-PMTF, Figure 2D. There were also significant correlations between the forward masking variables and the corresponding PMTF variables at 4 kHz on the left ear.

Relations between results of questionnaire and hearing tests

Forward masking proved to be the hearing test that showed the most revealing differences (or similarities) between persons with different professions. Therefore it was considered suitable to investigate if non-auditory factors could influence the forward masking results. Thus ANOVAs were performed with the forward masking threshold difference (difference between the thresholds of the brief tone at 5 ms and at 50 ms after the noise burst) as the dependent variable, and with ear and one non-auditory factor at a time as within subjects factors. The non-auditory factors were self-reported medication, headaches, neck problems, smoking or stress. The only non-auditory factor with a possible influence on forward masking was *medication* (p<0.05, p = 0.05, Kruskal-Wallis). The dose response indicates that this is not a spurious finding: The mean threshold difference for individuals taking more than 50 pain relieving tablets/year was 22 dB. For those taking 1–50 tablets/year the mean was 28 dB, and for those taking 0 tablets/year it was 29 dB. However, we have no explanation to this correlation between medication and forward masking. The fact that the *Education* group had forward masking results similar to the *Industry* group and not to the less noise exposed groups *Music* or *Other* could not be explained by this correlation, since there was no difference whatsoever in use of medication between any of the groups.

Hypersensitivity to loud sound as reported in the questionnaire (no or yes response) was related to *speech recognition in noise* at the lower test level, 70 dB SPL, right ear (p<0.005, simple ANOVA). Persons, who were hypersensitive to loud sound, had a better S/N, −14.1 dB, than persons who were not so sensitive, S/N = −12.4 dB. This effect may be caused by healthy OHCs combined with ipsilateral and contralateral regulatory systems with defective restraining capacity, resulting in higher levels in the cochlea [4,33,34]. OAE data showed such tendencies, but no significances. The hypothesis that persons hypersensitive to loud sound may have worse results on speech recognition in the 85 dB SPL noise than those not so sensitive could not really be tested, since there were too few persons tested at that level. Neither could any differences between the two categories in the amount of improvement with noise level be reliably analysed.

Complementary discussion

The hearing tests in this study show, that individuals with hearing problems in the profession group *Other*, consisting mainly of medical staff and students, have small deviations from results normal for their age, and that the group *Industry*, used for comparison, has substantial deviations in all tests. This might have been suspected from the self-estimated noise exposure including profession and other risk factors.

In our previous study musicians had some dysfunctions associated to damage to OHCs and the regulatory system, and a few of them showed the typical signs of incidents with sudden loud noise[4]. In the present study the group *Music* showed the same indications, but in addition the results were very normal for the two new measurements, forward masking and speech recognition in noise. The forward masking results were even as good as the results of the (much younger) *group of young women*. Thus the *Music*-group, except a few individuals exposed to incidents, had good results regarding measurements associated to IHC-function. Musicians are acknowledged to work at sound levels at which there is a risk of NIHL according to the international standardisation[8], and our estimations of noise exposures suggested that the musicians should have more dysfunctional hearing than the teachers. However, the participating musicians seemed to have come from fairly controlled soundscapes without unexpected loud sounds from electronic systems. The changes in sound level in the music are expected by the musicians.

In contrast the *Education* group showed results similar to those of the *Industry* group, and worse than normal for middle-aged persons, regarding forward masking, and speech recognition in noise. The self-reported tinnitus level was about the same and worse than for the other two groups. There were also PMTF-results that may be associated to exposure to sudden loud sounds. According to animal research, one may speculate that there are lesions in the inner hair cell area as referred to in the result/discussion section. Although there is an uncertainty of the location of the possible lesions, this study has clearly shown that our *Education* group had poor temporal processing. Regarding the location of possible lesions in the hair cell areas and the regulatory system we have based the discussions on the literature. Unfortunately there is hitherto less literature regarding inner hair cells than outer hair cells, because of physiological difficulties to measure. Our findings seem to justify more studies in this area.

Our assumption was that the participants of the *Education* group had been exposed to lower noise levels than the *Industry* and *Music* groups. In the questionnaire, the estimates of self-assessed noise exposure supported that assumption. However, recent results from noise measurements in preschools show that preschool teachers are exposed to considerable noise levels[6]. In the seventeen preschools in that study the mean equivalent sound level over a working day was less than 80 dB(A), but the maximum was 85 dB(A), The mean rating of the noise was between "somewhat troublesome" and "very troublesome". About 80% of the 101 teachers judged unexpected sudden changes of the sound level to occur "several times per day" to "several times per hour". It is reasonable that noise levels and noise characteristics, e.g. the content of sudden, unexpected loud noises, depend on type of school, age of pupils, classroom acoustics and cultural factors. The teachers in our study had not used hearing protection, although it may be used by for example woodwork teachers.

It is possible that many of the teachers may have come from soundscapes like the one described above, with noise described as troublesome but still tolerable, with several unexpected sudden changes of the sound level every working day. Other reasons for the *Education* group having worse results than the *Music* group could not be found in the analyses of answers to the questionnaire. Self-reported neck problems, pain relieving medication, eye and hair colour, smoking, and relatives with hearing problems were about the same in the two groups. The self-reported amounts of stress and tension headaches were slightly higher for these two groups than for the other groups.

In the study of risk factors for tinnitus in a population 55 years and older a number of extrinsic and health factors that could be linked to tinnitus were described[35]. The largest single factor was reported occupational tolerable noise exposure (9.3%), which may correspond to what Sjödin reported for preschools[6]. The conclusion was that a number of occupations with less noise burden than industrial exposure are at risk for noise-induced tinnitus. Another study found poor temporal processing and speech recognition in adverse listening conditions in individuals exposed to occupational noise more than 80 dB(A), but still with pure tone thresholds less than 25 dB HTL[36]. Those skills deteriorated with age, but were worse for exposed groups than for unexposed controls. Also that study seems to have relevance for the tested groups of teachers.

Our results show that persons exposed to moderate noise levels at work may run the risk of hearing dysfunction. Mean results of the 48 teachers in two measurements as well as of individual musicians and hospital staff with moderate noise exposure seem to prove that.

This study may have found dysfunctions that are characteristic for these groups before the audiogram is affected, but it will not give us a general overview of the effects of noise on hearing for these groups of professions at later stages of deterioration of the audiogram. Neither can it tell how common the dysfunctions are.

Conclusions

In this study, individuals having auditory problems and normal or near-normal hearing thresholds were divided into groups of subjects with similar noise exposure, and measured with advanced hearing tests. For each type of measurement there were individuals with abnormal results possibly indicating cochlear dysfunction.

For many of the subjects these dysfunctions caused less improvement than normal when the listening level in the speech in noise test was increased. Subjects sensitive to loud noise had significantly better speech recognition in noise at the lower test level than subjects not sensitive.

There were characteristic results:

Teachers had results suggesting substantial dysfunction in the auditory system reflected in far worse forward masking and speech recognition in noise than a group of middle-aged without hearing problems. These results, suggesting poor temporal processing, were about equally poor as those of a group exposed to industrial noise. The latter group was tested for comparison and had about 20 dB worse pure tone thresholds. The matched tinnitus level was correlated to the forward masking results and those two groups had the loudest matched tinnitus, possibly caused by dysfunction in the inner hair cell area.

Musicians showed some deficits normally associated to outer hair cells and had good results for their age at forward masking, and so did a group mainly consisting of hospital staff and students. The musicians had normal speech recognition in noise at both listening levels.

The study suggests that persons exposed to occupational noise below or around risk levels may risk hearing dysfunction. Several of the teachers in this study are examples of that, possibly because of combinations of unfavourable working environment and individual susceptibility. Medication or other self-reported non-auditory factors could not explain the poor results of the teachers.

Acknowledgments

We want to express our gratitude to Karin Erikson, and Eva B Svensson, who performed the measurements, and to our test subjects.

Author Contributions

Conceived and designed the experiments: ACL UR BH ÅO. Performed the experiments: ACL ÅO. Analyzed the data: ACL BH. Wrote the paper: ACL UR BH ÅO. Designed the software used for hearing tests: ÅO.

References

1. Axelsson A, Ringdahl A (1989) Tinnitus a study of its prevalence and characteristics. Br J Audiol 23: 53–62.
2. Cacace AT (2003) Expanding the biological basis of tinnitus: crossmodal origins and the role of neuroplasticity. Hear Res 175: 112–132.
3. Attias J, Bresloff I, Furman V (1996) The influence of the efferent auditory system on otoacoustic emissions in noise induced tinnitus: clinical relevance. Acta Otolaryngol 116: 534–539.
4. Lindblad AC, Hagerman B, Rosenhall U (2011) Noise-induced tinnitus: a comparison between four clinical groups without apparent hearing loss. Noise Health 13: 423–431.
5. Sindhusake D, Golding M, Newall P, Rubin G, Jakobsen K, et al. (2003) Risk factors for tinnitus in a population of older adults: the blue mountains hearing study. Ear Hear 24: 501–507.
6. Sjödin F, Kjellberg A, Knutsson A, Landström U, Lindberg L (2012) Noise exposure and auditory effects on preschool personnel. Noise Health 14: 72–82.
7. McAllister AM, Granqvist S, Sjölander P, Sundberg J (2009) Child voice and noise: a pilot study of noise in day cares and the effects on 10 children's voice quality according to perceptual evaluation. J Voice 23: 587–593.
8. ISO1999 (1990) Acoustics – Determination of occupational noise exposure and estimation of noise-induced hearing impairment. Geneva: International Organization for Standardization.
9. Jansen EJ, Helleman HW, Dreschler WA, de Laat JA (2009) Noise induced hearing loss and other hearing complaints among musicians of symphony orchestras. Int Arch Occup Environ Health 82: 153–164.
10. Schmuziger N, Patscheke J, Probst R (2006) Hearing in nonprofessional pop/rock musicians. Ear Hear 27: 321–330.
11. Zhao F, Manchaiah VK, French D, Price SM (2010) Music exposure and hearing disorders: an overview. Int J Audiol 49: 54–64.
12. Kähäri K, Zachau G, Eklöf M, Sandsjö L, Möller C (2003) Assessment of hearing and hearing disorders in rock/jazz musicians. Int J Audiol 42: 279–288.
13. ISO7029 (2000) Acoustics - Statistical distribution of hearing thresholds as a function of age. Geneva: International Organization for Standardization.
14. Berninger E, Karlsson KK (1999) Clinical study of Widex Senso on first-time hearing aid users. Scand Audiol 28: 117–125.
15. Lindblad A-C, Hagerman B (1999) Hearing tests for selection of sonar operators. ACUSTICA - Acta acustica 85: 870–876.
16. Davis RI, Qiu W, Hamernik RP (2009) Role of the kurtosis statistic in evaluating complex noise exposures for the protection of hearing. Ear Hear 30: 628–634.
17. Duan ML, Canlon B (1996) Forward masking is dependent on inner hair cell activity. Audiol Neurootol 1: 320–327.
18. Duan ML, Canlon B (1996) Outer hair cell activity is not required for the generation of the forward masking curve. Audiol Neurootol 1: 309–319.
19. Hagerman B (1982) Sentences for testing speech intelligibility in noise. Scand Audiol 11: 79–87.
20. Hagerman B (2002) Speech recognition threshold in slightly and fully modulated noise for hearing-impaired subjects. Int J Audiol 41: 321–329.
21. Jacobson M, Kim S, Romney J, Zhu X, Frisina RD (2003) Contralateral suppression of distortion-product otoacoustic emissions declines with age: a comparison of findings in CBA mice with human listeners. Laryngoscope 113: 1707–1713.
22. Lindblad AC, Rosenhall U, Olofsson A, Hagerman B (2011) The efficacy of N-acetylcysteine to protect the human cochlea from subclinical hearing loss caused by impulse noise: a controlled trial. Noise Health 13: 392–401.
23. Wang J, Powers NL, Hofstetter P, Trautwein P, Ding D, et al. (1997) Effects of selective inner hair cell loss on auditory nerve fiber threshold, tuning and spontaneous and driven discharge rate. Hear Res 107: 67–82.
24. El-Badry MM, McFadden SL (2007) Electrophysiological correlates of progressive sensorineural pathology in carboplatin-treated chinchillas. Brain Res 1134: 122–130.
25. McFadden SL, Kasper C, Ostrowski J, Ding D, Salvi RJ (1998) Effects of inner hair cell loss on inferior colliculus evoked potential thresholds, amplitudes and forward masking functions in chinchillas. Hear Res 120: 121–132.
26. Walton J, Orlando M, Burkard R (1999) Auditory brainstem response forward-masking recovery functions in older humans with normal hearing. Hear Res 127: 86–94.
27. Kujawa SG, Liberman MC (2009) Adding insult to injury: cochlear nerve degeneration after "temporary" noise-induced hearing loss. J Neurosci 29: 14077–14085.
28. Lin HW, Furman AC, Kujawa SG, Liberman MC (2011) Primary neural degeneration in the Guinea pig cochlea after reversible noise-induced threshold shift. J Assoc Res Otolaryngol 12: 605–616.
29. Wang Y, Ren C (2012) Effects of repeated "benign" noise exposures in young CBA mice: shedding light on age-related hearing loss. J Assoc Res Otolaryngol 13: 505–515.
30. Liu L, Wang H, Shi L, Almuklass A, He T, et al. (2012) Silent damage of noise on cochlear afferent innervation in guinea pigs and the impact on temporal processing. PLoS One 7: e49550.
31. Shi L, Liu L, He T, Guo X, Yu Z, et al. (2013) Ribbon synapse plasticity in the cochleae of Guinea pigs after noise-induced silent damage. PLoS One 8: e81566.
32. Qiu C, Salvi R, Ding D, Burkard R (2000) Inner hair cell loss leads to enhanced response amplitudes in auditory cortex of unanesthetized chinchillas: evidence for increased system gain. Hear Res 139: 153–171.
33. El-Badry MM, McFadden SL (2009) Evaluation of inner hair cell and nerve fiber loss as sufficient pathologies underlying auditory neuropathy. Hear Res 255: 84–90.
34. Sztuka A, Pospiech L, Gawron W, Dudek K (2010) DPOAE in estimation of the function of the cochlea in tinnitus patients with normal hearing. Auris Nasus Larynx 37: 55–60.
35. Sindhusake D, Mitchell P, Newall P, Golding M, Rochtchina E, et al. (2003) Prevalence and characteristics of tinnitus in older adults: the Blue Mountains Hearing Study. Int J Audiol 42: 289–294.
36. Kumar UA, Ameenudin S, Sangamanatha AV (2012) Temporal and speech processing skills in normal hearing individuals exposed to occupational noise. Noise Health 14: 100–105.

25

Camera Traps can be Heard and Seen by Animals

Paul D. Meek[1,2,3]*, Guy-Anthony Ballard[1,2,3], Peter J. S. Fleming[1,3,4], Michael Schaefer[3,6], Warwick Williams[7], Greg Falzon[1,5]

1 Invasive Animals CRC, Coffs Harbour, New South Wales, Australia, **2** Vertebrate Pest Research Unit, NSW Department Primary Industries, Armidale, New South Wales, Australia, **3** School of Environmental and Rural Sciences, University of New England, Armidale, New South Wales, Australia, **4** Vertebrate Pest Research Unit, NSW Department Primary Industries, Orange, New South Wales, Australia, **5** School of Science and Technology, University of New England, Armidale, New South Wales, Australia, **6** Marine and Atmospheric Research, CSIRO, Canberra, Australian Capital Territory, Australia, **7** National Acoustic Laboratory, Sydney, New South Wales, Australia

Abstract

Camera traps are electrical instruments that emit sounds and light. In recent decades they have become a tool of choice in wildlife research and monitoring. The variability between camera trap models and the methods used are considerable, and little is known about how animals respond to camera trap emissions. It has been reported that some animals show a response to camera traps, and in research this is often undesirable so it is important to understand why the animals are disturbed. We conducted laboratory based investigations to test the audio and infrared optical outputs of 12 camera trap models. Camera traps were measured for audio outputs in an anechoic chamber; we also measured ultrasonic (n = 5) and infrared illumination outputs (n = 7) of a subset of the camera trap models. We then compared the perceptive hearing range (n = 21) and assessed the vision ranges (n = 3) of mammals species (where data existed) to determine if animals can see and hear camera traps. We report that camera traps produce sounds that are well within the perceptive range of most mammals' hearing and produce illumination that can be seen by many species.

Editor: Zhigang Jiang, Institute of Zoology, China

Funding: These authors have no support or funding to report.

Competing Interests: The authors have declared that no competing interests exist.

* Email: paul.meek@invasiveanimals.com

Introduction

Camera traps are being used widely throughout the world although the limitations and constraints of these devices are rarely considered. The study of animal ecology, biology and behaviour requires thorough planning, robust analysis and an element of good luck. Irrespective of the tools being used, there will always be expected errors, variability, unknowns or biases, described as being similar to the "Observer Effect" or "Heisenberg's Uncertainty Principle" [1]. The study of animals can only provide an insight into their life history; nothing is absolute and understanding the variability is an important component of research investigations. Camera trapping is a survey tool that has improved our capacity to infer the life history of animals, especially where minimising observer effects on animal behaviour is critical [2–4]. Some consider that camera traps are a non-intrusive method of studying animals [5]. However, there is increasing evidence throughout the world that animal behaviour is affected by the presence of camera traps [6–9]. In some circumstances this 'effect' may have little impact on the investigation. In other studies, for example those using indices and mark-recapture estimators (e.g., [1,10,11]), it is paramount that the technology used does not alter animal behaviour during or between monitoring sessions to ensure constancy of detectability [8]. Where bias occurs, it is crucial that this effect is understood and measured when interpreting the results of the observations; "the accuracy of an index is irrelevant; precision is paramount" [11]. Irrespective of the hypothesis being tested, the effect on behaviour can scarcely be considered non-intrusive [8] if animals display behavioural responses to sampling tools.

Observations of responses to mensurative devices strongly imply that learning can occur as a consequence of exposure to the devices. For examples, camera traps could be detected by animals for the following reasons:

1. Auditory – by the emission of sounds from the electronic and mechanical components of the device: these could be in the infra, audible and ultra-sound ranges.
2. Olfactory – metal, plastic and human scents on the device [6,9],
3. Learned association – avoidance of the camera trap through wariness of human presence at a site [6] or attraction to the camera trap through lures and food baits,
4. Visual (day) – neophobia towards foreign objects introduced into their environment; regular-shaped objects (essentially rectangular prisms) attached to trees or posts [12,13],
5. Visual (night) – the flash of xenon light, white LED or infrared LED illumination [7].

The hearing and vision [22] of animals varies depending on their life history, hunting *modis operandi*, body size [23,24] and favoured prey [25]. It is commonly accepted that the combination of hearing and vision is important for animal localisation acuity

[22], for hunting and social interactions and to avoid predators [26].

Auditory ranges

Hearing ranges are broad in mammals, as an example; mice (*Mus domesticus*) have a range from 2.3–92 kHz [29], horses (*Equus cabalus*) hear up to 33.5 kHz, cows (*Bos taurus*) to 35 kHz [32], kangaroo rat (*Dipodomys merriami*) to 74 kHz, while the rabbit (*Oryctologus cuniculus*) can only hear to 49 kHz., cotton rat (*Sugmondon hispidus*) to 72 kHz [29], wood rat (*Neotoma floridana*) to 56 kHz, grasshopper mouse (*Onychomys leucogaster*) 69 KhZ [33], and fox squirrel (*Sciurus niger*) 49 kHz [34]. A small Australian predator, the northern quoll (*Dasyurus hallucatus*) hear best from 8–10 kHz although their hearing range is 0.5–40 kHz [31]. Six Australian Brush-tailed possum (*Trichosurus vulpecula*) were trained to respond to frequencies of 88 kHz [35]. Only bats, dolphins and shrews have been reported to recognise and detect high frequency signals [36], although the authors propose that "it is not impossible that all primitive mammals are capable of echolocation".

Our associated research primarily focuses on the management of introduced predators [1], wild dogs (*Canis lupus ssp*) and European red foxes (*Vulpes vulpes*) and to a lesser extent on feral cats (*Felis catus*). Feral and domestic cats have one of the broadest hearing ranges of all mammals [27], ranging from 48 Hz to 85 kHz, although responses have been reported up to 100 kHz [28]. Dogs show variability in sensitivity to sound depending on breed (6–45 kHz) (https://www.lsu.edu/deafness/HearingRange.html accessed 3 July 2013) and as high as 65 kHz [28], although this has been disputed [30]. Foxes have evolved with a wide ranging hearing capacity (0.9–34 kHz) with optimal hearing at 10–14 kHz and an upper limit of 34 kHz [25] and 65 kHz [28].

Visual ranges

Dogs are known to have dichromatic colour vision with an upper limit of detection around 555 nm [16], while Mustelids have been reported to have the capacity to detect infrared light up to 870 nm [17]. In the case of Australian marsupials there is clear evidence of colour vision [18–20] with taxa variability in regards to spectral sensitivity (dichromatic vs trichromatic) [21].

Camera traps that use xenon white flash to illuminate animals have been widely used in hunting and wildlife research [7] even though there is concern that the bright flash affects the short and long term behaviour of target animals. In a study of Kinkajous (*Potos flavus*) behavioural avoidance of 'canopy-highway' branches where white flash camera traps were placed has been reported [8]. Tiger (*Panthera tigris tigris*) capture rates in Nepal decreased by 50% over 5 nights of camera trapping using xenon flash devices [7] and similar concerns have been raised in studies of grey wolves (*Canis lupus*) [14]. Technological advances have resulted in infrared camera traps dominating the market based on claims that animals can't see the infrared flash [15].

Most of the mammal species being studied using camera traps are nocturnal-crepuscular animals, although not always [19], with some showing a slight preponderance for diurnal activity; so their eye physiology reflects this behaviour. It would not be accurate to state that animals can "see in the dark"; a more accurate description may be that they are able to "see what is in the dark" [37]. Knowledge on the vision capabilities of animals continues to improve despite limitations in fully understanding how they view the world because of the challenges of measuring what they perceive [38]. In fact some believe that the perception of colour vision requires some form of learning, association and consciousness [39]. Moreover, there is uncertainty as to whether animals perceive brightness and hue [39] or if colour vision is in fact important to cats and dogs [40]. Interestingly, apart from *Mustela* spp. [17] very little is known about the detection of infrared signals by animals.

In the three main species of interest to us (dogs, cats and foxes), their night visual acuity as primarily nocturnal predators is high; in the case of the cat, and more than likely foxes and dogs, their superior night vision is adapted for low visual stimuli [41]. Of most interest is the animal's ability to detect near infrared (700–3000 nm) illumination: the part of the light spectrum used in infra-red camera traps.

Objectives

We were interested in two critical questions related to the effect of camera trapping on predator behaviour;

1. Do camera traps produce an audible sound that animals can hear, and infrared flash illumination that they can see, and is there variability between camera trap models and modes?
2. What is the effect of the sound and illumination on animal behaviour?

To answer the first part of this question we tested a range of commonly used camera traps to determine the frequency and loudness of audio outputs and whether they fell within the hearing range of target mammals. We then tested whether the infra-red illumination from a range of models produced outputs that were within the perceptible range of known animal vision. Conducting tests on these camera traps was made possible using sophisticated technology; the challenge was obtaining enough data on vision and hearing in mammals. Our objectives were to determine whether 1) camera traps emit any sounds in the audible, infra or ultrasonic ranges for humans; 2) camera traps emit infrared illumination above the observable range of mammals; 3) mammals see or hear camera traps, 4) if there is variability in sounds and light emissions within and between camera trap models.

Two authors have suggested that human odour on camera traps may have been a deterrent to coyotes (*Canis latrans*) visiting camera trap sites [6,9]; we constrained our investigations here to sound and light emissions. Our investigations achieved all four objectives in comprehensively reporting the sound and visual outputs of and between camera trap models, and how these outputs compare to the known hearing and visual acuity of animals.

Materials and Methods

The main focus of this study was to evaluate the camera trap audio outputs (<20 kHz) in relationship to the known hearing ranges of animals; complementary to this was to quantify potential ultrasound outputs (20–60 kHz) and the infrared illumination spectrums for a range of camera trap models in relation to the known vision spectral data of animals.

Camera Traps, Set-up and Triggering

We tested 12 models of camera traps for audio outputs using still and video functions; 7 models for infrared outputs and 5 models for ultra-sonic outputs (Table 1); the camera trap settings varied between models according to their specifications and functionality (see Table 1 for some details).

For all measurements during the audio and infra-red optical output tests, camera traps were fixed on a tripod, 100 cm above the surface and set so that the front of the camera was 50 cm from the measuring device to optimise signal detection. Every camera

Table 1. The camera trap models and numbers used to evaluate the sound outputs in an anechoic chamber.

Make	Model	Sample	Acoustic	Infra-red	Ultrasonic	Photos/trigger	Video time	Sensitivity
Reconyx	HC600	10	•	•	•	3	NA	H
Scoutguard	550	10	•	•		3	10	H
Scoutguard	SG680 V	8*	•	•		3	10	H
Moultrie	I65	5*	•	•		1	10	H
Moultrie	I60	1		•		3	NA -	H
Cuddeback	Capture	3	•		•	1	NA	H
Picxontroller	DigitalEye	3	•			1	NA	H
Bushnell	119466	1	•	•		3	10	H
Bushnell	119456C	1	•			3	10	H
Moultrie	I40	1	•			1	10	H
Moultrie	D40	1	•	•		1	10	H
Scoutguard	560D	1	•	•	•	3	NA -	H
Uway	NT50	1	•	•	•	3	10	H
Uway	NX50	1	•			3	10	H

*Ten units of this model were tested but some failed to operate and were removed from the analysis. NA = not available.

Table 2. The approximate hearing ranges of 24 animals using data extracted from (https://www.lsu.edu/deafness/HearingRange.html) and additional data from papers cited in this study.

Animal	Scientific name	Approximate Range (Hz)	Upper Range (KHz)
bat	Unknown sp	2,000–110,000	110
cat	*Felis catus*	45–64,000	64
chicken	*Gallus gallus*	125–2,000	2
cow	*Bos taurus*	23–35,000	35
dog	*Canis lupus*	67–45,000	45
elephant	*Loxodonta sp*	16–12,000	12
ferret	*Mustela putorius furo*	16–44,000	44
guinea pig	*Cavia porcellus*	54–50,000	50
hedgehog	*Erinaceinae sp*	250–45,000	45
horse	*Equus caballus*	55–33,500	33
human	*Homo sapien*	64–23,000	23
house mouse	*Mus musculus*	2300–92,000	92
opossum	*Didelphis sp*	500–64,000	64
rabbit	*Oryctolagus cuniculus*	96–49,000	49
raccoon	*Procyon lotor*	100–40,000	40
rat	*Rattus rattus*	200–76,000	76
sheep	*Ovis aries*	100–30,000	30
cotton rat	*Sigmondon hispidusi*	1000–72,000	72
brush tailed possum	*Trichosurus vulpecula*	*??-88,000	88
fox squirrel	*Sciurus niger*	113–49,000	49
northern quoll	*Dasyurus hallucatus*	500–40,000	40
wood rat	*Neotoma floridana*	940–56,000	56
grasshopper mouse	*Onychomys leucogaster*	1850–69,000	69
kangaroo rat	*Dipodomys merriami*	50–62,000	62

*lower hearing range is unknown for this species.

was tested separately and we conducted a countdown to synchronise the measuring devices and to trigger the passive

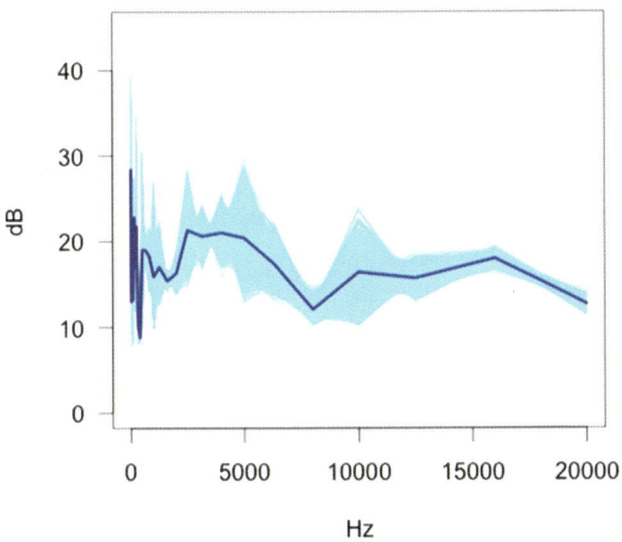

Figure 1. Bootstrap estimates of the functional mean of the anechoic chamber background sound envelope.

infra-red sensor (PIR), resulting in stills and/or videos being taken. To trigger the camera traps, one of the authors stood in front and to one side of the device and waved a hand across the front of the camera four times at the end of the countdown.

Every camera was tested for audio and optical outputs using still photos and where the function existed in a camera trap model, we tested video outputs.

Acoustic Measurements

Auditory outputs (.01–20 kHz). A Briel and Kjoer Type 2250 Hand held analyser was used in an anechoic chamber at the National Acoustics Laboratory in Chatswood, Sydney. The device was placed in front of the camera traps and automatically set to record camera outputs for 15 second periods. The equipment was calibrated to 94 db @1000 Hz using a Type 4230 Sound Level Calibrator.

The data were generated by the analyser using an average amplification value for each of 17 frequencies over the 15 second recording period using five measurements (L_{ZFmax}, L_{ZSmax}, L_{ZFmin}, L_{ZSmin}, L_{Zeq}). Given our objective was to determine the maximum audio outputs of the cameras, we only used L_{ZFmax} values in our analysis. L_{ZFmax} is the maximum un-weighted audio level recorded over the sampling period, so it is the highest level measured irrespective of frequency.

In order to calibrate the equipment to any background sound in the anechoic chamber, we carried out ten 'control' recordings at

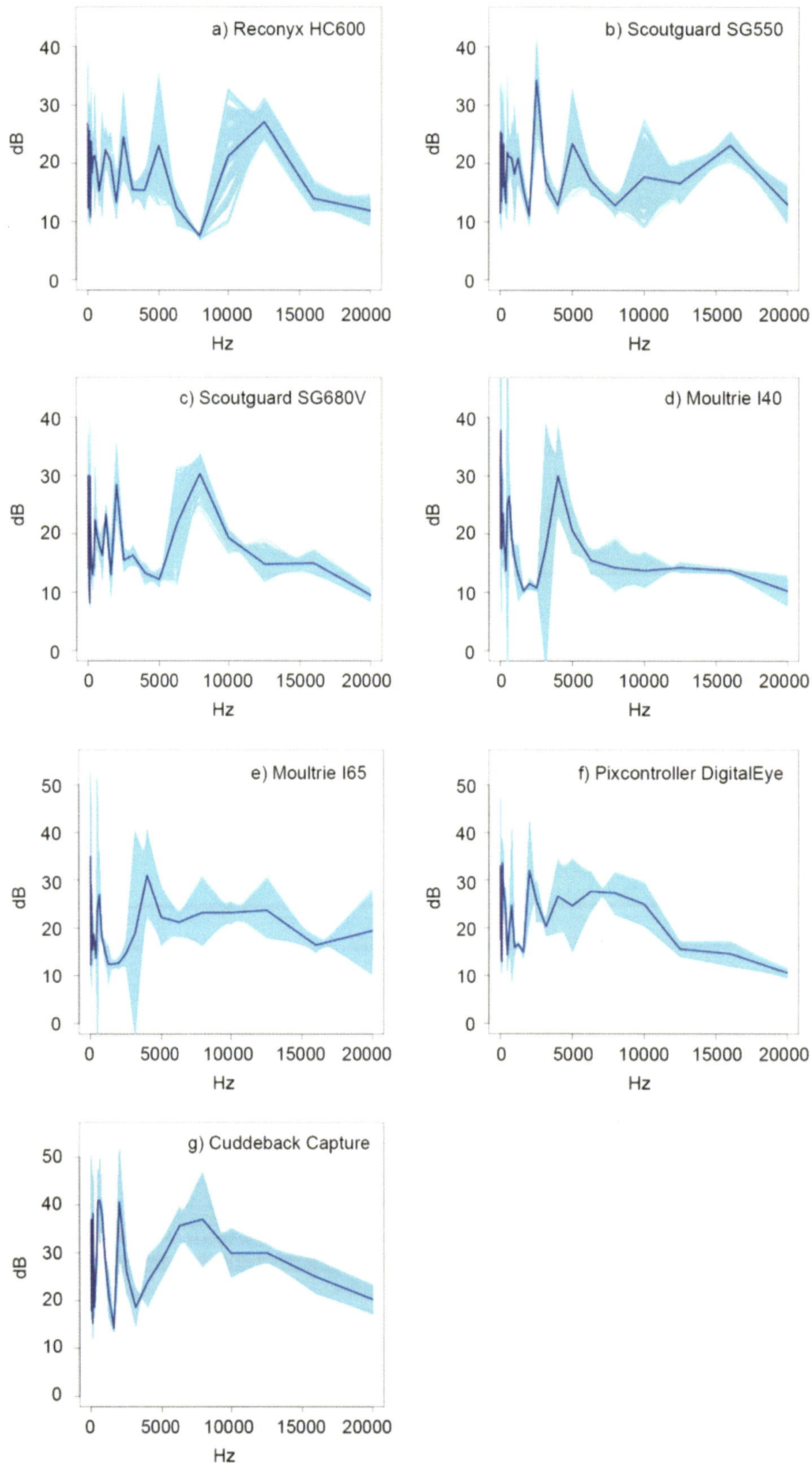

Figure 2. Bootstrap estimates of the functional mean (95% CI) of the sound emissions of the a) Reconyx HC600, b) Scoutguard SG 550, c) Scoutguard SG680 V, d) Moultrie I40, c) Moultrie I65, e) Pixcontroller DigitalEye and f) Cuddeback Capture taking still photos.

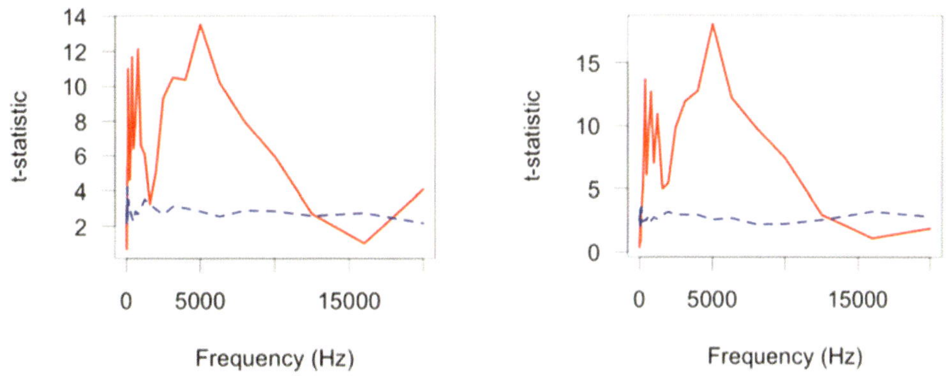

Figure 3. Functional t-test results as a function of frequency for two select contrasts: a) Background sound- Cuddeback and b) HC600-Cuddeback. The red (solid) line indicates the permutation statistic (t_{max}) results for 999 random permutations of the input data sequence whilst the blue (dashed) line indicates the $\alpha = 0.05$ critical level as a function of frequency. When the red (solid) line is equal or above the blue (dashed) line there was a significant difference at that frequency.

each of the 17 frequencies to derive the background sound envelope, with the decibels referenced to 20 micro Pascals (20×10^{-6} Pa).

Table 3. Comparisons between different camera outputs (still) and the background sound envelope.

Model 1	Model 2	Statistic	p-value	Adjusted p-value
Background	HC600	$t_{max} = 5.43$	<0.01*	0.056
Background	SG550	$t_{max} = 2.73$	0.22	1.00
Background	KG680 V	$t_{max} = 4.62$	0.02*	0.53
Background	MI40	$t_{max} = 5.14$	0.02*	0.62
Background	MI65	$t_{max} = 4.47$	0.06	1.00
Background	Pixcontroller	$t_{max} = 4.27$	0.13	1.00
Background	Cuddeback	$t_{max} = 13.53$	<0.01*	0.00 *
HC600	SG550	$t_{max} = 3.44$	0.07	1.00
HC600	KG680 V	$t_{max} = 2.99$	0.20	1.00
HC600	MI40	$t_{max} = 8.70$	<0.01*	0.00*
HC600	MI65	$t_{max} = 3.60$	0.17	1.00
HC600	Pixcontroller	$t_{max} = 5.89$	0.03*	0.76
HC600	Cuddeback	$t_{max} = 18.03$	<0.01*	0.00*
SG550	KG680 V	$t_{max} = 3.10$	0.17	1.00
SG550	MI40	$t_{max} = 6.74$	0.01*	0.17
SG550	MI65	$t_{max} = 3.561835$	0.16	1.00
SG550	Pixcontroller	$t_{max} = 5.09$	0.11	1.00
SG550	Cuddeback	$t_{max} = 15.10$	<0.01*	0.00*
KG680 V	MI40	$t_{max} = 2.40$	0.56	1.00
KG680 V	MI65	$t_{max} = 3.53$	0.17	1.00
KG680 V	Pixcontroller	$t_{max} = 5.01$	0.04*	1.00
KG680 V	Cuddeback	$t_{max} = 15.10$	<0.01*	0.00*
MI40	MI65	$t_{max} = 3.81$	0.12	1.00
MI40	Pixcontroller	$t_{max} = 4.16$	0.21	1.00
MI40	Cuddeback	$t_{max} = 11.00$	0.03*	0.84
MI65	Pixcontroller	$t_{max} = 4.38$	0.08	1.00
MI65	Cuddeback	$t_{max} = 12.99$	<0.01*	0.00*
Pixcontroller	Cuddeback	$t_{max} = 21.97$	<0.01*	0.00*

Test statistics (t_{max}) falling below the critical value are not significant at the particular frequency whilst those at or above were considered significant. (*denotes significance at $p<0.05$).

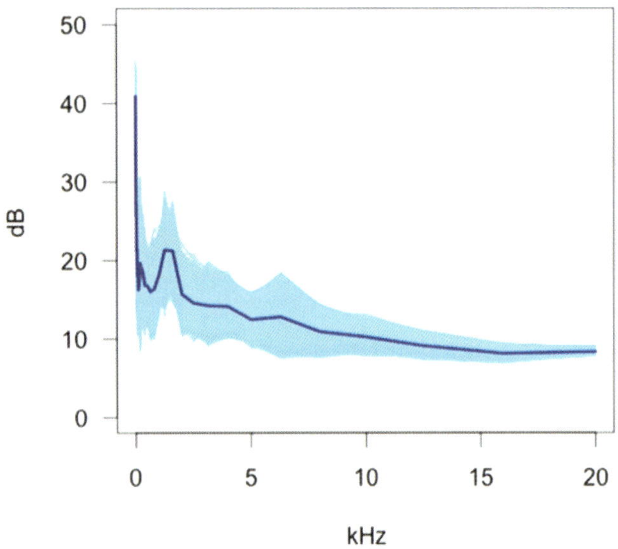

Figure 4. Bootstrap estimates of the functional mean and 95% confidence envelopes for the Scoutguard SG550.

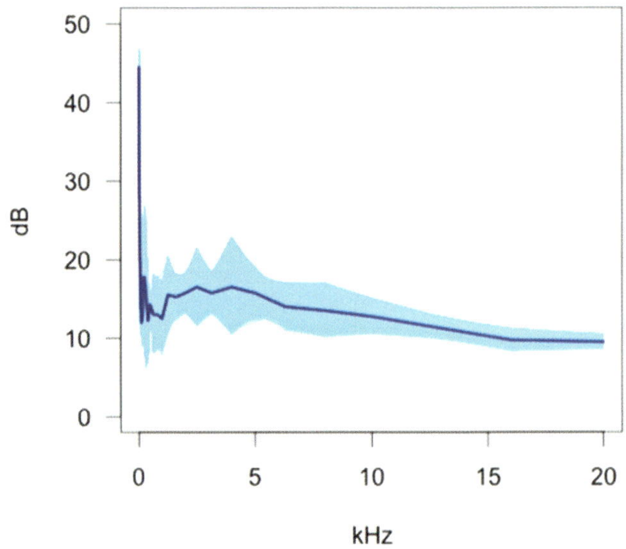

Figure 5. Bootstrap estimates of the functional mean and 95% confidence envelopes for the Scoutguard KG680.

Ultrasonic outputs (4–200 kHz)

To determine if ultrasonic frequencies were emitted by camera traps we used 10 Reconyx Hyperfire HC600, 3 Cuddeback Captures, 3 Pixcontroller DigitalEye, 1 Scoutguard 560D and 1 Uway NT50 camera traps. Control detections were also collected without a camera trap to measure any possible background sound outputs within the laboratory. As before, the camera traps were placed individually on a tripod 50 cm in front of two ANABAT Detectors connected to a ZCAIM unit. One detector was directly in front of the camera and the second at a 45 degree angle from the central axis of the camera. We tested both angles to assess whether signals were different when the devices were directly in front compared to off centre. Cameras were triggered by hand movements across the front of the camera and recordings were for 15 seconds each. Ultrasonic outputs were analysed using the acoustic analyser software, AnalookW.

Light measurements

Tests were conducted on 32 cameras comprising 7 models (Table 1) in a laboratory at the University of New England on April 20th 2011. Each camera was placed 80 cm from a hand-held ASD Field Spectrometer (FS HH 325-1075) connected to a laptop computer to enable automated data storage. Flash outputs were recorded over a 17 millisecond per acquisition period using a 10 degree field of view lens. Ten measurements per camera motion (see above) were recorded.

Analysis

Due to the data collected by the sound analyser at 33 frequencies, we treated the audio spectrums as "functional", thus L_{ZFmax} was a function of frequency. Analysis of the infrared illumination and ultrasonic outputs were constrained to presentation of summary statistics and raw data because the data was constrained by the unequal sample sizes of the camera trap models we had available. Furthermore, the ultrasonic data can only be reported in ANALOOK format as ranges and not as raw data.

Background sound. The L_{ZFmax} variable was used for analysing the audio outputs in our analysis. A background sound 'envelope' and the 95% confidence envelope across a range of frequencies (12.5 Hz–20 kHz) was established for a set of 10 independent observations. Functional bootstrapping was applied to get the estimate of the mean curve and the associated 95% confidence curves [42].

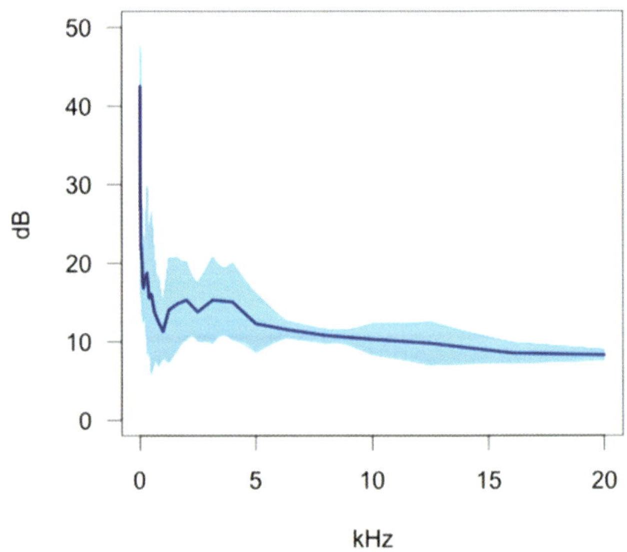

Figure 6. Bootstrap estimates of the functional mean and 95% confidence envelopes for the Moultrie MI40 camera.

Audio Outputs. Functional bootstrapping ($n^{boot} = 9999$) [42] was used to estimate the mean curve and confidence curves (95% CI) using the L_{ZFmax} outputs for each camera trap model (stills and videos or both) where these features were available. Comparisons of still images within camera trap models were undertaken to evaluate variability using the functional mean to estimate average response for each camera trap model, and functional standard deviation to assess variability within the same models.

Intra-and Inter Model Comparisons. Functional *t*-tests [43] were used to compare outputs between camera traps, and between camera trap models and to the background sound

Table 4. Comparisons between different video camera outputs as well as the background (*: denotes statistical significance below the p = 0.05 level).

Model 1	Model 2	Statistic	p-value	Adjusted p-value
Background	MI40	$t_{max} = 4.15$	0.08	0.75
Background	MI65	$t_{max} = 4.89$	0.03*	0.28
Background	SG550	$t_{max} = 3.02$	0.17	1.00
Background	KG680 V	$t_{max} = 2.88$	0.41	1.00
MI40	MI65	$t_{max} = 4.33$	0.13	1.00
MI40	SG550	$t_{max} = 10.24$	<0.01*	0.02*
MI40	KG680 V	$t_{max} = 3.71$	0.21	1.00
MI65	SG550	$t_{max} = 4.32$	0.05	0.52
MI65	KG680 V	$t_{max} = 3.71$	0.12	1.00
SG550	KG680 V	$t_{max} = 3.50$	0.21	1.00

envelope. Given there were 28 comparisons we predicted an increased chance of 'false positives', as such we adjusted the p-values using the '*false discovery rate*' method [44] to account for this situation.

Ultrasonic Outputs. Ultrasonic camera trap outputs were recorded using an ANABAT Detector but this device does not provide raw data points and merely plots the data as a graph displaying the range of signals detected and the patterns. As such we were unable to accurately analyse variability within and between models so the data has been collated to report on the ranges detected.

Infrared Outputs. Summary statistics were generated for the light outputs across the range of infrared camera trap models, these are presented graphically; comparisons between infrared ranges and animal range was not undertaken in detail due to a lack of data on animal infrared vision.

Comparison with known animal hearing range. A mean audio output using ten HC600 Reconyx camera traps (chosen to be representative of the quietest models) was produced and compared to the published frequency hearing range of animals using a Wilcoxon test (non-parametric). We plotted mean frequency and 95% confidence intervals and used the reported hearing frequencies of 24 animals (Table 2) to determine likely relationships between hearing and sound outputs. Data available on the University of Toledo 'Behavioural Audiograms of Mammals website (http://psychology.utoledo.edu/showpage.asp?name=mammal_hearing, accessed 6 June 2014) of known hearing ranges of animals was compared to the audio output of the camera traps. The hearing of one key species, the European Red Fox (*Vulpes vulpes*) has not been recorded in any investigations, so the known hearing range was unavailable. To overcome this constraint we extracted the calling frequencies of red foxes from published research [28,45] using data extraction software (PlotDigitizer http://plotdigitizer.sourceforge.net, accessed 6 June 2014). We then used these data as a baseline hearing range for the red fox based on the assumption that foxes are calling to each other on this frequency and as such should hear these ranges.

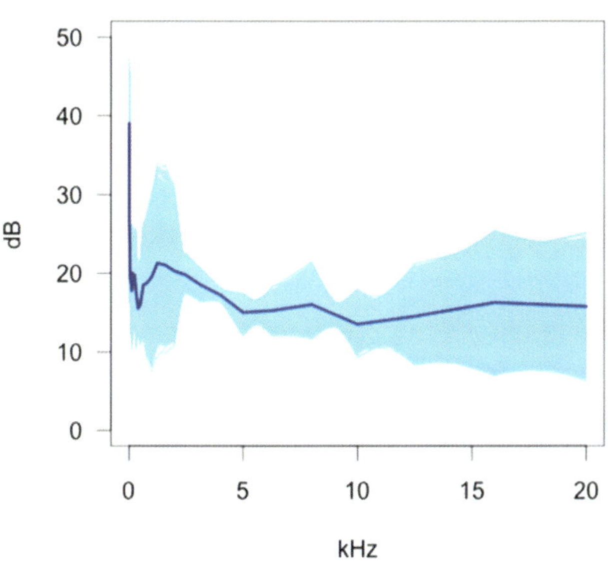

Figure 7. Bootstrap estimates of the functional mean and 95% confidence envelopes for the Moultrie MI65 camera.

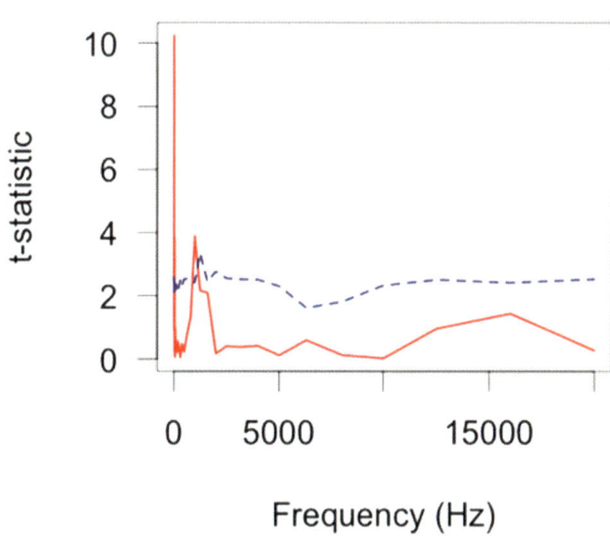

Figure 8. Functional t-statistics as a function of frequency for the MI40-SG550 V contrast in video mode. The test statistic (t_{max}) is displayed as a solid line and the α = 0.05 critical value as a function of frequency is displayed as a dashed line.

Table 5. Still vs Video comparisons using functional t-tests (*: denotes statistical significance below the p = 0.05 level).

Model	Statistic	p-value	Adjusted p-value
MI40	$t_{max} = 2.17$	0.74	1.0
MI65	$t_{max} = 2.99$	0.41	1.0
SG550	$t_{max} = 1.95$	0.73	1.0
KG680 V	$t_{max} = 2.98$	0.35	1.0

Results

We found strong evidence that animals can hear the sound of, and see the infra-red illumination of camera traps.

Audio Outputs of Camera Traps

Background sounds. Our data show that the functional mean and standard deviation magnitudes of the background sounds were highly frequency dependent (Fig. 1). Particular frequencies tended to be associated with a higher level of average background sound (e.g. 12.5 Hz, 160 Hz, 250 Hz) with sound ranging from 8.8 dB to 28.4 dB. The variation in the sound measurements changed considerably as a function of frequency. The three largest standard deviations in sound outputs of camera traps occur at 50 Hz, 12.5 Hz, and 500 Hz, with the total range of the standard deviation estimates across frequency being 0.9–14.3 Hz. The largest mean values and the greatest standard deviation of sound components occurred at the lower frequencies suggesting that the values measured might be related to the frequency dependent accuracy of the measuring equipment.

Intra-camera trap comparisons - Still Images. Both the background sound and the camera models displayed means and standard deviations that were frequency dependent. Each model of camera seemed to have their own unique signature (see Table S1 and Figure S1) with characteristic peaks and oscillations. There was a semi-regular pattern to the uncertainty within a camera model, with particular sets of frequencies specific to camera model although displaying the greatest variation within camera trap models.

In analysing 10 Reconyx HC600 we established that the mean values range from 7.6 dB to 27.1 dB across the frequency range (12.5 to 20,000 Hz) with a standard deviation ranging from 0.8 dB to 17.2 dB (Fig. 2). There was a substantial difference in the magnitude of the camera output with the top three 'loudest' frequencies (12,500 Hz, 12.5 Hz, and 25 Hz) and the three

Table 6. Ultrasonic outputs from five camera trap models including two control recordings, two ANABAT directions were utilised (directly in front and offset 45 degrees to the central axis of the camera).

	directly in front		off-set 45 degrees	
Model and Code	**Lower (kHz)**	**Upper (kHz)**	**Lower (kHz)**	**Upper (kHz)**
HC600–1	3	35	3	40
HC600–2	3	20	3	35
HC600–3	3	50	3	45
HC600–4	3	55	3	50
HC600–5	3	60	3	55
HC600–6	3	55	3	0
HC600–7	0	0	0	0
HC600–8	3	55	3	50
HC600–9	0	0	0	0
HC600–10	3	50	3	45
Cuddeback-1	3	40	3	55
Cuddeback-2	3	40	3	60
Cuddeback-3	3	60	3	40
Pixcontroller-1	0	0	0	0
Pixcontroller-2	0	0	3	45
Pixcontroller-3	3	35	0	0
Scoutguard 560D-1	3	0	0	0
Uway NT50–1	3	35	3	0
Control 1	0	0	0	0
Control 2	0	0	0	0

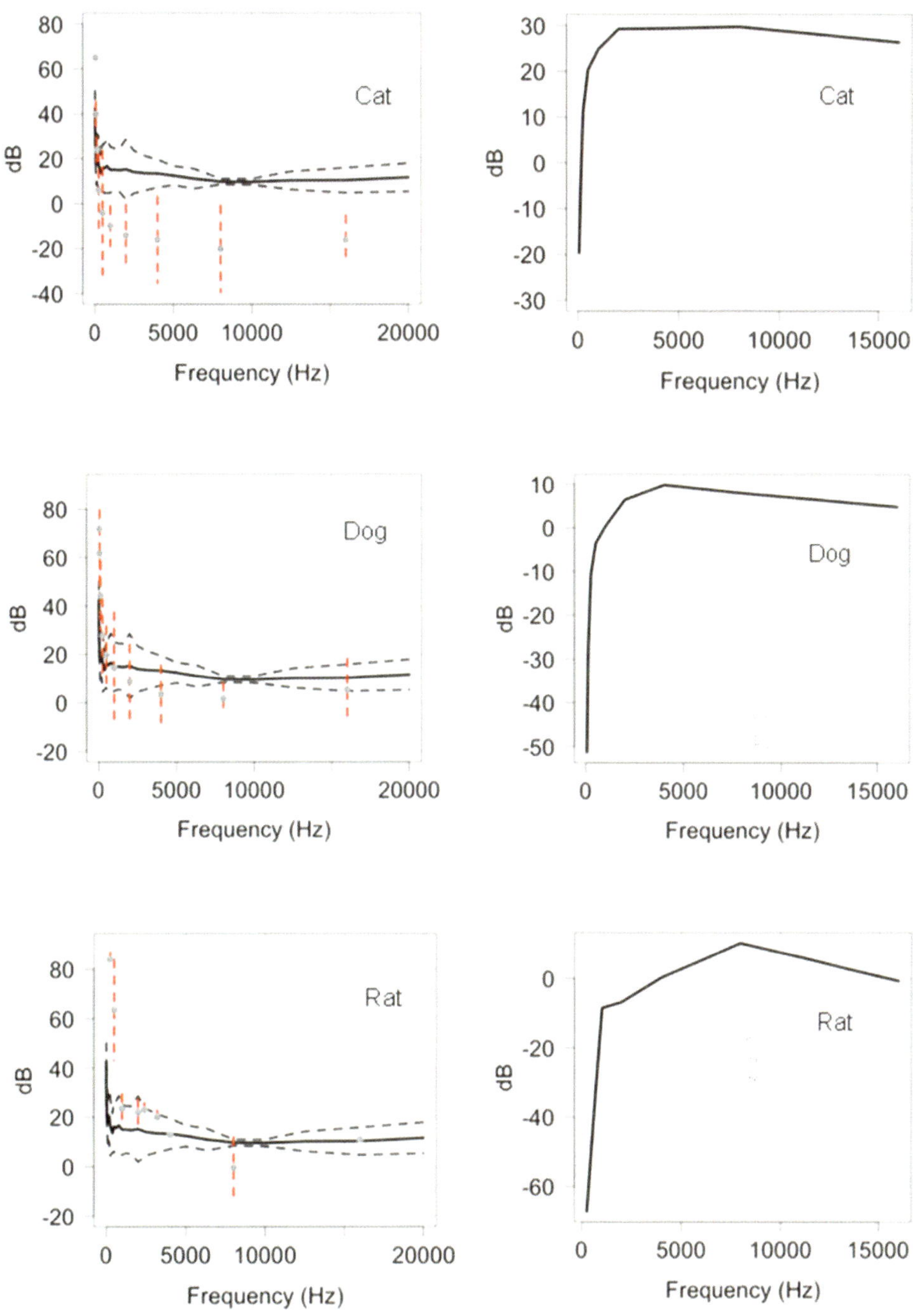

Figure 9. Dog (1), cat (2) and rat (3) hearing ranges in relation to the outputs of HC600 camera traps (1a, 2a, 3a) and as a function of frequency (1b, 2b, 2c). The black line is the mean audio output of the camera trap; the grey dotted lines are the 95% confidence limits. The red dotted lines represent the standard error around the known hearing range of the dog, cat and rat. Where the grey points and red dotted lines (SE) are below and closest to the mean audio output of the camera, the sound can be detected by the animal.

highest standard deviation values 10,000 Hz, 5,000 Hz, and 25 Hz.

The Scoutguard SG 550 (still) functional mean was frequency dependent with spikes at 2500 Hz, 5000 Hz, and 10,000 Hz, although different to the HC600 (stills) and the background sound (Fig. 2). The functional standard deviation was also frequency dependent and similar to the HC600. At 250, 5000 and 10000 Hz the variability in the output (L_{ZFmax}) between cameras was greatest within a model (i.e., Reconyx still, Scoutguard still). The range of the functional mean was from 11.0 dB to 34.3 dB, with the top three highest values occurring at 2,500 Hz, 31.5 Hz, and 125 Hz.

The Scoutguard KG680 V had a unique 'signature' as well as frequency dependent characteristics in the functional mean. The range of the functional mean was 8.1 dB to 30.2 dB with the three highest values occurring at 8,000 Hz, 160 Hz, and 12.5 Hz. These frequencies show the greatest variability within a model and are quite different to the HC600 and SG 550. The functional means of the Moultrie I40 display frequency dependency. The

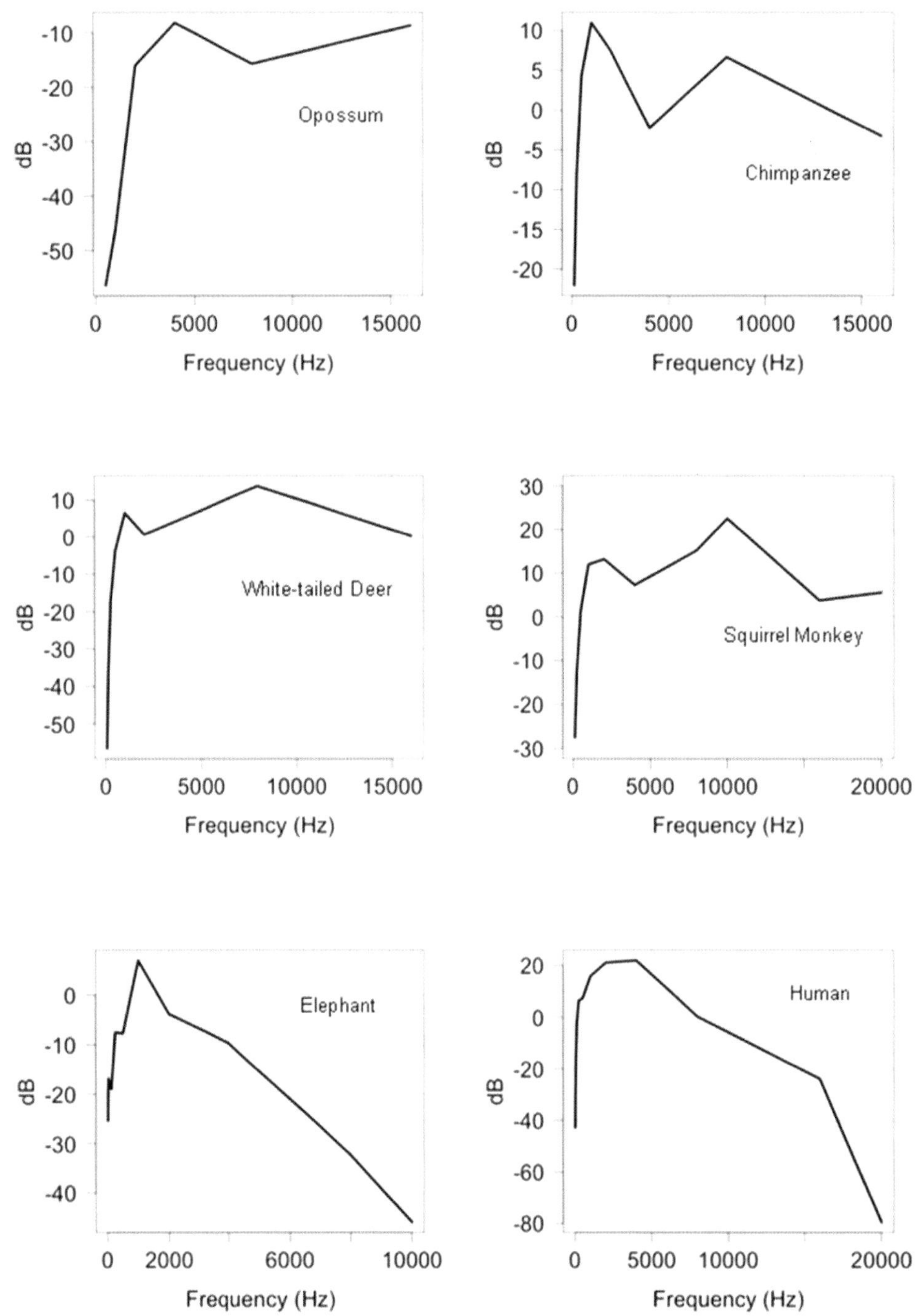

Figure 10. The auditory threshold of 6 mammals represented as a function of frequency.

signature was also unique but due to the very small sample size (n = 4) there is some uncertainty in the estimates.

We found that there were sharp and sudden shifts in the L_{ZFmax} statistic for different frequencies in this model. The range of the functional mean was 10.3 dB to 37.8 dB whilst the functional standard deviation ranged from 0.4 dB to 16.3 dB. The three greatest values of the functional mean occurred at 50 Hz, 40 Hz, and 12.5 Hz. The greatest variability occurred at 3150 Hz, 500 Hz, and 80 Hz in this order. Similarly, there was a frequency dependence and unique sound signature in the Moultrie I65 camera trap The range of the functional mean was from 12.3 dB–35.0 dB with the top three values occurring at 12.5 Hz, 4000 Hz, and 80 Hz.

The Pixcontroller DigitalEye also had a unique sound signature and shared some similarities with the background sound profile. It also exhibited frequency dependent structure in both the functional mean (10.7 dB–33.7 dB, maximal values at 160 Hz, 12.5 Hz, and 2000 Hz.) and standard deviation (0.5 dB–10.3 dB) with the top three values occurring at 800 Hz, 63 Hz, and 12.5 Hz.

Three Cuddeback cameras produced functional mean ranges from 14.3 dB to 41 dB with the top three values occurring at

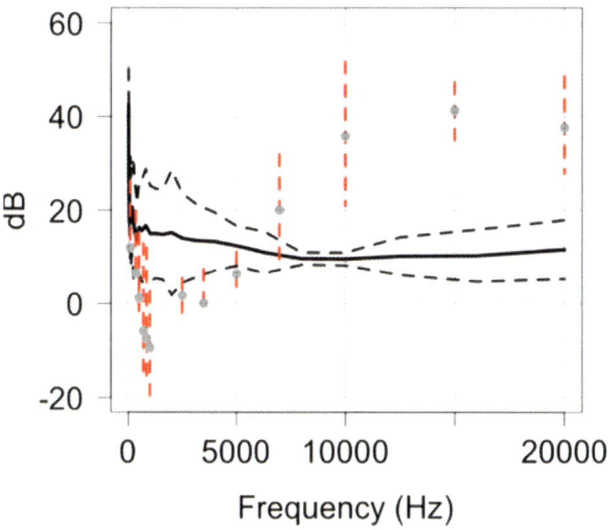

Figure 11. Comparison of the predicted hearing range of the red fox in relation to the outputs of HC600 camera traps and as a function of frequency.

400 Hz, 500 Hz (equal highest), and 2000 Hz (functional standard deviation 0.5 dB–7.9 dB with the three largest values occurring at 12.5 Hz, 2000 Hz, and 8000 Hz.

Comparisons between camera traps in still modes and background sounds

There were several contrasts displaying significant differences between models (Table 3). Specifically, comparisons between the Background-Cuddeback, HC600-MI40, HC600-Cuddeback, SG550-Cuddeback, KG680 V-Cuddeback, MI65-Cuddeback, and Pixcontroller-Cuddeback were statistically significantly different. There were a further seven contrasts that seem to be statistically significant different but they did not pass the multiple comparisons adjustment. There was a significant difference in the background sound and the Cuddeback, which consistently produced louder sound outputs (16 Hz: Background – 15.9 dB Cuddeback- 23.7 dB, 80 Hz: Background- 14.9 dB Cuddeback- 29.0 dB, 400 Hz: Background – 8.8 dB, Cuddeback- 28.0 dB) (Fig. 3). The contrast between Reconyx HC600- Moultrie MI40 could either be a statistical anomaly or could indicate a difference in the operational frequency response for these two cameras, which is so minute that it is within the variation of the background sound envelope. These analyses confirm that different camera models exhibit unique sound profiles but not discernibly different to the variability within models.

We found that for most frequencies, particularly the low to medium frequencies, significant differences exist.

Intra camera trap comparisons - Video

Of the four camera trap models tested, the Scoutguard SG550 (Fig. 4) showed an overall decreasing trend with an occasional minor peak where the operational sound or the uncertainty in the estimate or uncertainty between models was higher. The operational sound characteristics appeared similar to that of the Moultrie MI40 but the functional standard deviation was higher at lower frequencies.

In the Scoutguard KG680, the functional mean exhibited a slow decrease in operational sound level with frequency (Fig. 5). Of note was the relative tight envelope around the estimate of the mean indicating that this curve was estimated with far less uncertainty than the other models.

In the Moultrie MI40 the functional mean of the sound is highly frequency dependent (Figures 6 and Table 4). The operational sound of the camera and the variation between models vary with

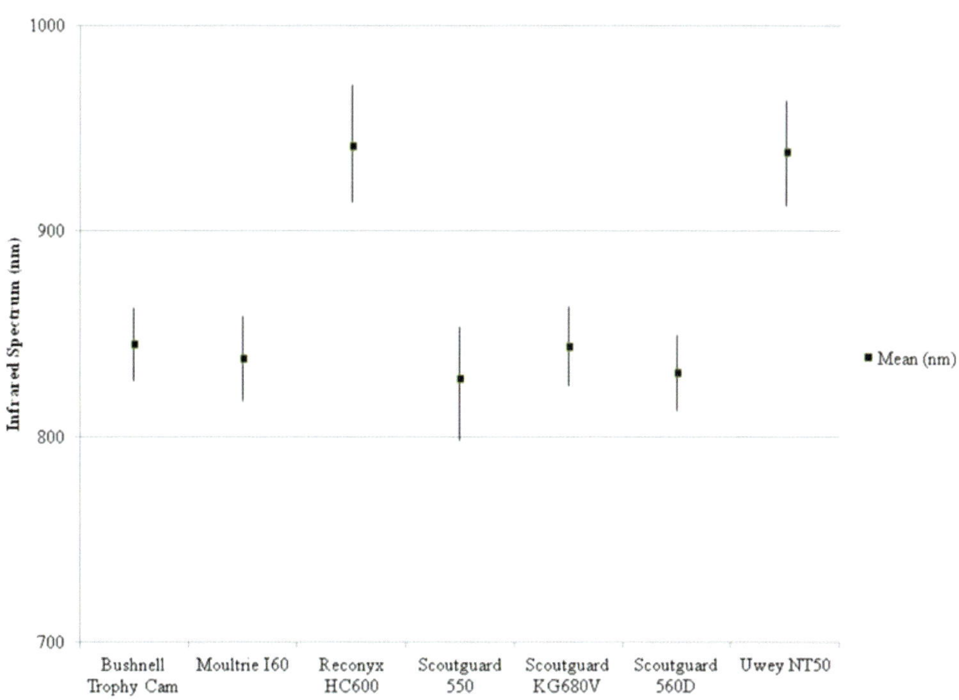

Figure 12. Mean infra-red wavelength illumination (nm) outputs for seven camera trap models showing the highest and lowest values.

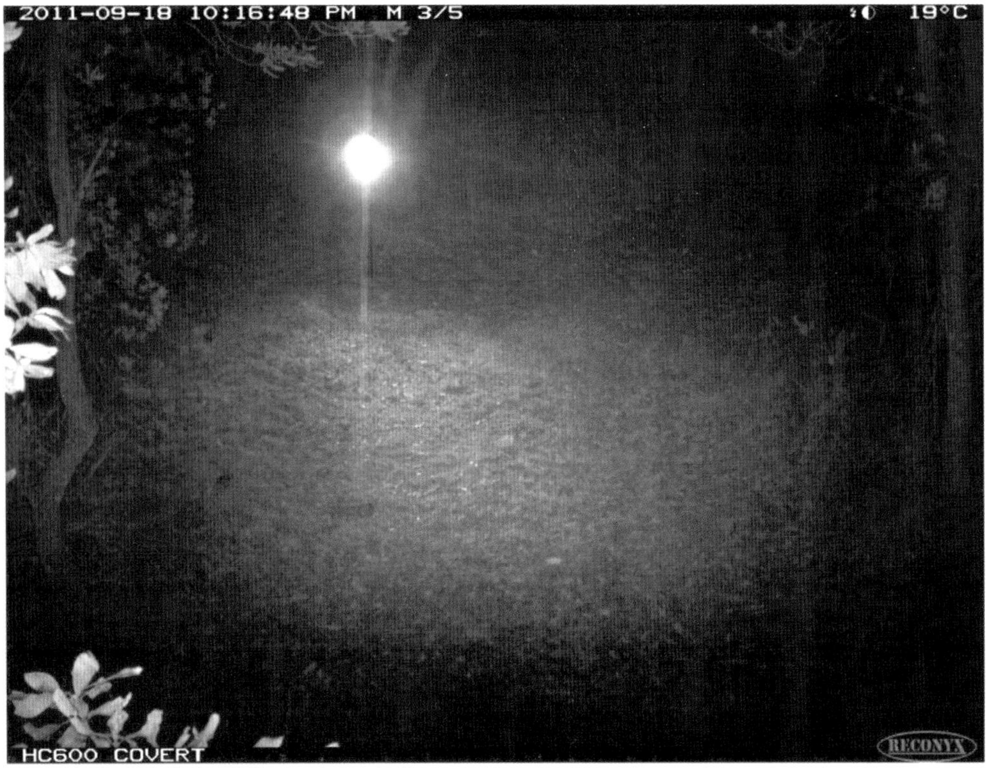

Figure 13. Infra red illumination of two opposing Reconyx HC600 camera traps simultaneously triggering.

frequency. The highest operational sound occurred at the lowest frequencies as well as the greatest variation and uncertainty between models.

A slight frequency dependent response was observed in the Moultrie MI65 (Fig. 7) around the mean, but the standard deviation estimate was highly frequency dependent with a pronounced peak occurring in the 0–3 kHz band and a general linear increase occurring from 4–20 kHz. The increasing width of the 95% confidence envelope as frequency increases reflects uncertainty with increasing frequency. This might be due to low sample sizes and our inability to establish whether or not the mean curve increases, remains stationary, or decreases at these frequencies. These data show that the sound level for the MI65 is higher than the MI40.

Estimates of the mean audio output and standard deviation were estimated as a function of frequency for four different camera models operating in video mode. All cameras appear to have frequency dependent operational characteristics and furthermore there appears to be differences in the mean sound levels between models. Importantly, the standard deviation curve estimates within a model appear greater or on similar magnitude to the mean differences between cameras. This could be due to the limited number of camera traps models, although this is unlikely because the analysis suggested wide variation in magnitude and form.

Comparisons between Video Modes and Background Sound

Our functional tests with multiple comparison corrections for background sound in video mode showed no significant difference (Table 4). There was however a difference in audio outputs between the MI40 and SG550 with a difference in the response around 1000 Hz but it was still within the range of the background sound (Fig. 8).

Except at very low frequencies and a slight ($t_{max}\approx 1$–1.5) variation around 1000 Hz, there were no significant differences in response across frequencies. The secondary peak at 1000 Hz is indicative of a difference in the functional mean estimates for these two cameras in video mode.

Comparisons between Still and Video Modes

There was no difference in still and video frequency response or between the four camera models (Scoutguard and Moultrie) (Table 5).

Ultrasonic recordings

Ultrasound frequencies tests on the five camera trap models confirm that camera traps do produce ultrasonic outputs each time a photo is taken (Table 6). Frequency ranges for Reconyx HC600 was 3–60 kHz with a median output of 52.5 kHz (SD = 13.4) directly in front of the device and 47.5 kHz (SD = 7.3) perpendicular to the device. Other models emitted outputs within a similar range. There was some variability within models due to the method of measuring the outputs; ANABAT detectors are designed to measure bat echolocation not low level ultrasonic sound.

Audio Outputs and Known Hearing Ranges of Animals

Our tests comparing Reconyx (HC600) camera trap outputs to the existing hearing ranges of 21 species (see http://psychology.utoledo.edu/showpage.asp?name=mammal_hearing, accessed 6 June 2014) found compelling evidence that camera trap sound outputs fall within the hearing range of most of the species (Fig. 9–11). In 9b, 9b and 9c we have presented data to show the relationship between the camera sound and the auditory threshold of the animal as a function of frequency. These data strongly suggest that dogs, cats and rats have the capacity to detect low frequency outputs (<20 kHz) from camera traps. Data presented in Figure 10 provide evidence that a further six mammals, including humans, have the capacity to detect camera traps in the lower frequency bandwidths. The hearing ranges in comparison to camera trap outputs for a further 12 mammals are provided in Figure S2.

Given the paucity of data on the known hearing range of red foxes we carried out a comparison on the minimal hearing range for this species based on their calling frequencies [25,45] (Fig. 11). This was based on the assumption that foxes must be able to hear the frequency of fox calls recorded at a minimum. From this analysis we derived an optimum hearing range for the red fox of around 8–12 kHz although this would be an under-estimation of their true range. Despite having to use call frequencies to model hearing range, the results show that red foxes can easily hear camera trap outputs.

The data presented provide robust evidence that mammals can detect the sound outputs of camera traps.

Infra-red Wavelength Outputs

The infra-red illumination ranges varied between models (Fig. 12) but there was no difference in wavelength outputs within models for the Reconyx HC600 (Mean = 940.5, SD = 1.8, 95% CI = 1.3), Scoutguard 550 (Mean = 828.3, SD = 4.7, 95% CI = 3.4) and Scoutguard 680 V (mean = 844.1, SD = 0.6, 95% CI = 0.5) camera traps.

Based on the data in Figure 12, camera traps that are advertised as "no glow" (HC600) or "black ops" (NT50) are clearly using infrared technology with wavelengths operating above 850 nm. These infrared LED's are emitting light that is nearly invisible to the human eye, but not some animals.

Discussion

In this study we tackled the first part of a two staged question; do camera traps have the capacity to project audio and optical stimuli to wildlife? Moreover, are these outputs different between and within models and recording modes (still or video)? We present these data on the audio and visual outputs of camera traps to highlight the importance of identifying the effects camera trapping may have on animal behaviour.

Animal Hearing

A wide range of comparisons were conducted to investigate the possibility of differences in operating audio outputs of different camera models in both still and video mode. In the vast majority of cases (except the Cuddeback) the operational sound was little different from the background sound in the sound laboratory. In some cases slight differences were found between models (e.g. MI40 and SG550 video) but were of such a low level that they were within the magnitude of the background sound. The noise created by two people being present in the anechoic chamber conducting the experiments probably produced sounds and affected the background sound envelope. If we were able to conduct the tests remotely there may have been a more significant difference between camera trap noise and background noise.

In comparing the auditory range of animals in contrast to our recorded outputs, we sourced sonagraph data for a range of species. There have not been any sonagraphs to determine the hearing ranges of foxes although it has been reported that red fox have an upper limit of 65 kHz [37]. While studies of 75 foxes [46] reported the frequency of a range of calls made by foxes to be less than 2 kHz, which is consistent with one other study [45] that reported calls all under 2.5 kHz. The foxes hearing capacity has been reported to have a reduced capacity between 5–11 kHz with a discernible reduction around 8.5 kHz, but reported that they hear sounds well at 10–14 kHz [25]. Given red fox calling frequencies, they would certainly hear some of the infra and ultra sounds emitted by camera traps. We report the first evidence that animals can detect the presence of camera traps due to the audio and optical outputs from these devices. This study determined that at certain frequencies, animal hearing (Table 2 and see http://www.lsu.edu/deafness/HearingRange.html, accessed 6 June 2014) can easily detect these sounds.

The results of our testing also provide conclusive evidence that camera traps do emit ultrasonic outputs, especially when battery levels are low. In a pilot trial we found that low powered batteries resulted in the ANABAT detecting an output but in subsequent tests with fully charged batteries, there was no audible signal suggesting that camera trap outputs vary with battery life. The use of a bat call monitoring device has been used previously to test LED lights being used in research on *Mustella* vision [17]. The authors were unable to detect any outputs by the lights, however in the case of camera traps there are a range of electrical and mechanical components apart from the LED circuitry that may be emitting sound.

Animal Vision

Information on the extent of infrared detection by other mammals is scant in the literature. There have been some investigations using behavioural methods that report some animals can see infrared light in the range 539–870 nm although the evidence is limited across the taxa. As such we were unable to conduct any comparative analysis of infrared flash light outputs with animal vision to test our hypotheses.

Research has established that Honey Possums (*Tarsipes rostrata*) are able to see light in the 557 nm range [18] while ferrets (*Mustela furo*) can see around 870 nm [17] and Tamar Wallaby (*Macropus eugenii*) peaked at 539 nm [20].

These data probably underestimate the extent of an animal's ability to detect infrared light since they are based on behavioural studies [38], not physiological analysis, because such technology is unavailable. As such, we are unable to state exactly what the limits of animal vision might be, and we believe that the range of infrared light presented in Figure 12 are likely seen by many species of animal. In support of this claim, one of the authors (PM) was able to see a faint red glow of a Reconyx HC600 in absolute darkness. Reports of humans detecting infrared (1064 nm) well above the illumination currently used in camera traps have been recorded [47,48]. This being the case, there is no doubt that nocturnal animals with vision sensitive to night light can see infrared illumination. The responses of animals to infrared flash are highly variable between species and individuals (Meek Unpub data; Ballard Unpub data). While we cannot measure exactly what animals see, they most likely see a similar image to the flash recorded by two camera traps triggered simultaneously, as shown in Figure 13.

Cats appear to detect the presence of camera traps more than other animals (Meek Unpub data; Ballard Unpub data), which is probably due to their retina sensitivity at 826 nm [49] and total vision field of view being 287° with binocular over lap of 130° [37]. This peripheral view combined with the very high sensitivity to infrared light at the higher end of the near infrared spectrum would make cats more than capable of easily detecting camera trap flashes; especially in models with light emissions below 800 nm (see Fig. 12).

The effects of white flash camera traps on animal behaviour have been recognised as an intrusive survey method because it has been shown to startle and cause animals to flee (7). Some authors have suggested that using infrared illumination may reduce this flight response [7,8,14], especially where infrared wavelengths exceed ~870 nm [17]. While there is little information on the detectable range of infrared wavelengths by most animals, one study did find that ferrets' (*Mustelo furo*) maximum observable range was about 870 nm [17]. Multiple images and corresponding footprint detecting plots from our research on feral cats, wild dogs and foxes in Australia over several years indicates that all three species can detect flash illumination from Reconyx HC600 camera traps (Meek Unpub data; Ballard Unpub data). In field trials where two HC600 were facing each other, we were able to accidentally trigger the cameras to simultaneously trigger showing visually what nocturnal animals may see when infra red illumination occurs (Fig. 13) [50].

Anecdotal reports of ship rats (*Rattus rattus*) and brush-tailed possums (*Trichosurus vulpecula*) from three unpublished studies describe avoidance of infrared illumination in these species (see [17]). Although there has not been any effect found on predator behaviour around ground-nesting bird nests from infrared camera traps used to detect visitation [51].

Despite wide spread belief that humans cannot see near infrared light, many authors have reported being able to detect infrared light during experiments and these descriptions have been described [17]. On the evidence presented in the literature and summarised here, we conclude that most nocturnal or arrhythmic (nocturnal with some diurnal activity) mammals can see the infrared illumination (flash) emitted by camera traps.

Conclusions

Hearing and vision work together to form what is referred to as auditory localisation acuity [22]; where an animal hears a sound and turns towards the sound using eye sight to focus in on the stimuli. This is probably the case in camera trapping, where a sound is heard by a passing animal and the device is further recognised by vision, thus enabling animals to detect the device.

With the constant sounds of the forest animals are unlikely to be hearing the camera traps constantly as the frequency and amplitude values are very similar. Furthermore, the audio outputs collected in the anechoic chamber were recorded at 50 cm, and it is reported that with every metre away from the camera a loss of 6 dB is expected [52]. Sound levels are affected by distance from the source, atmospheric attenuation, terrain, ground cover, wind and weather [53], forest density (a function of limb and trunk density) and foliage [54] and as such we acknowledge that this attenuation may reduce sounds from camera traps under field conditions. This is because unlike the pure sounds recorded by audiograms, complex sounds like those in a natural setting where multiple frequencies and background scatter exist are less likely to be detected by animals [55].

In some studies the target species' ability to detect a camera trap may not be important because the requirement is to detect presence only, so irrespective of whether the animal baulks and runs from a camera trap is of no importance. Where repeat visits to a site are imperative for analysis, i.e., mark recapture, photographic indexes, CPUE and activity indexes, the interference to behaviour and potential avoidance of the camera trap may introduce a bias on the probability of detection. An issue also raised by in one study [17] in regard to the potential for infrared light emitting surveillance devices or traps to cause avoidance by animals.

There is a convincing argument presented in this study to confirm that most mammals can hear the operational sounds generated by camera traps in both the infrasound and ultrasound ranges. Moreover, given the strong relationship between vision and hearing acuity [22], this study concludes that most mammals can see the infra-red illumination used in camera traps.

Supporting Information

Figure S1 The noise frequency outputs of twelve camera trap models and the background control.

Figure S2 The hearing range of an additional twelve animals in comparison to the noise outputs of a camera trap.

Table S1 The mean audio outputs of 12 camera trap models at different frequencies.

Acknowledgments

Thanks to the Schultz Foundation for their support and provision of some camera traps to use in our experiments. We greatly appreciate the technical assistance of Greg Stewart of the National Acoustic Laboratory and Keryn Lapidge of the Invasive Animals CRC. Thank you to Damien Byrne from Outdoor Cameras Australia and Nick Dexter of Jervis Bay National Park for lending us some camera traps. We appreciate the technical support and advice provided by Matt Dobson in recording the ultrasonic outputs. Thank you to Julian Partridge, Christa Neumeyer, Nathan Hart, Lyn Beazley, Catherine Arresse and Henry Heffner for their invaluable advice and opinions on animal hearing and vision.

Author Contributions

Conceived and designed the experiments: PM GB PF WW MS. Performed the experiments: PM GB PF WW MS. Analyzed the data: PM GF WW MS. Contributed reagents/materials/analysis tools: PM GB PF WW MS GF. Contributed to the writing of the manuscript: PM GB PF WW MS GF.

References

1. Caughley G (1977) Analysis of Vertebrate Populations. London: John Wiley & Son.
2. Swann DE, Hass CC, Dalton DC, Wolf SA (2004) Infrared-triggered cameras for detecting wildlife: an evaluation and review. Wildlife Society Bulletin 32: 357–365.
3. Cutler TL, Swann DE (1999) Using remote photography in wildlife ecology: a review. Wildlife Society Bulletin 27: 571–581.
4. Kucera TE, Barrett RH (2011) A History of Camera Trapping. In: O'Connell AF, Nichols JD, Karanth KU, editors. Camera Traps in Animal Ecology. New York: Springer. 9–26.
5. Long RA, MacKay P, Zielinski WJ, Ray JC (2008) Noninvasive Survey Methods for Carnivores. Washington DC, USA: Island Press.
6. Séquin ES, Jaeger MM, Brussard PF, Barrett RH (2003) Wariness of coyotes to camera traps relative to social status and territory boundaries. Canadian Journal of Zoology 81: 2015–2025.
7. Wegge P, Pokheral CP, Jnawali SR (2004) Effects of trapping effort and trap shyness on estimates of tiger abundance from camera trap studies. Animal Conservation 7: 251–256.
8. Schipper J (2007) Camera-trap avoidance by Kinkajous *Potos flavus*: rethinking the "non-invasive" paradigm. Small Carnivore Conservation, 36: 38–41.
9. Larrucea ES, Brussard PF, Jaeger MM, Barrett RH (2007) Cameras, Coyotes, and the Assumption of Equal Detectability. The Journal of Wildlife Management 71: 1682–1689.

10. Mahon PS, Bates PB, Dickman CR (1998) Population indices for wild carnivores: a critical study in sand-dune habitat, south-western Queensland. Wildlife Research 25: 217–217.
11. Caughley G, Sinclair ARE (1994) Wildlife Ecology and Management. Massachusetts: Blackwell Science.
12. Lehner PN, Krumm R, Cringan AT (1976) Tests for Olfactory Repellents for Coyotes and Dogs. 40: 145–150.
13. Windberg LA (1996) Coyote responses to visual and olfactory stimuli related to familiarity with an area. Canadian Journal of Zoology 74: 2248–2253.
14. Gibeau ML, McTavish C (2009) Not-So-Candid Cameras: how to prevent camera traps from skewing animal behaviour. The Wildlife Professional: 35–37.
15. Meek PD, Pittet A (2012) User-based design specifications for the ultimate camera trap for wildlife research. Wildlife Research 39: 649–660.
16. Neitz J, Geist T, Jacobs GH (1989) Color vision in the dog. Visual Neuroscience 3: 119–125.
17. Newbold HG, King CM (2009) Can a predator see 'invisible' light? Infrared vision in ferrets (*Mustela furo*). Wildlife Research 36: 309–318.
18. Sumner P, Arrese CA, Partridge JC (2005) The ecology of visual pigment tuning in an Australian marsupial: the honey possum *Tarsipes rostratus*. Journal of Experimental Biology 208: 1803–1815.
19. Arrese C, Archer M, Beazley LD (2002) Visual capabilities in a crepuscular marsupial, the honey possum (*Tarsipes rostratus*): a visual approach to ecology. Journal of Zoology 256: 151–158.
20. Hemmi JM, Maddess T, Mark RF (2000) Spectral sensitivity of photoreceptors in an Australian marsupial, the tammar wallaby (*Macropus eugenii*). Vision Research 40: 591–599.
21. Ebeling W, Natoli RC, Hemmi JM (2010) Diversity of Color Vision: Not All Australian Marsupials Are Trichromatic. PLoS ONE 5: e14231.
22. Heffner RS, Heffner HE (1992) Visual Factors in Sound Localization in Mammals. Journal of Comparative Neurology 317: 219–232.
23. Huang GT, Rosowski JJ, Ravicz ME, Peake WT (2002) Mammalian ear specializations in arid habitats: structural and functional evidence from sand cat (Felis margarita). Journal of Comparative Physiology a-Neuroethology Sensory Neural and Behavioral Physiology 188: 663–681.
24. Huang GT, Rosowski JJ, Peake WT (2000) Relating middle-ear acoustic performance to body size in the cat family: measurements and models. Journal of Comparative Physiology A 186: 447–465.
25. Isley TE, Gysel LW (1975) Sound-Source Localization by the Red Fox. Journal of Mammalogy 56: 397–404.
26. Webster DB, Webster M (1971) Adaptive value of hearing and vision in Kangaroo rat predator avoidance. Brain, Behavior and Evolution 4: 310–322.
27. Heffner RS, Heffner HE (1985) Hearing Range of the Domestic Cat. Hearing Research 19: 85–88.
28. Peterson EA, Heaton WC, Wruble SD (1969) Levels of Auditory Response in Fissiped Carnivores. Journal of Mammalogy 50: 566–578.
29. Heffner H, Masterton B (1980) Hearing in Glires: Domestic rabbit, cotton rat, feral house mouse, and kangaroo rat. Journal of Acoustic Society America 68: 1584–1599.
30. Heffner HE (1983) Hearing in large and small dogs: Absolute thresholds and size of the tympanic membrane. Behavioral Neuroscience 97: 310–318.
31. Aitkin LM, Nelson JE, Shepherd RK (1994) Hearing, Vocalization and the External Ear of a Marsupial, the Northern Quoll, *Dasyurus-Hallucatus*. Journal of Comparative Neurology 349: 377–388.
32. Heffner RS, Heffner HE (1983) Hearing in large mammals: Horses (*Equus caballus*) and cattle (*Bos taurus*). Behavioral Neuroscience 97: 299–309.
33. Heffner HE, Heffner RS (1985) Hearing in two cricetid rodents: Wood rat (*Neotoma floridana*) and grasshopper mouse (*Onychomys leucogaster*). Journal of Comparative Psychology 99: 275–288.
34. Jackson LL, Heffner HE, Heffner RS (1997) Audiogram of the fox squirrel (*Sciurus niger*). Journal of Comparative Psychology 111: 100–104.
35. Signal T, Foster TM, Temple W (2001) Determination of auditory thresholds in the brushtail possum (*Trichosurus vulpecula*). Physiology & Behavior 73: 195–200.
36. Heffner H, Ravizza RJ, Masterton B (1969) Hearing in primitive mammals, III: Tree shrew (*Tupaia glis*). Journal of Auditory Research 9: 12–18.
37. Ewer RF (1998) The Carnivores. New York, USA: Comstock Publishing Associates.
38. Jacobs GH (2010) The Verriest Lecture 2009: Recent progress in understanding mammalian color vision. Ophthalmic and Physiological Optics 30: 422–434.
39. Kelber A, Vorobyev M, Osorio D (2003) Animal colour vision – behavioural tests and physiological concepts. Biological Reviews 78: 81–118.
40. Sathyakumar S, Bashir T, Bhattacharya T, Poudyal K (2011) Assessing mammal distribution and abundance in intricate eastern Himalayan habitats of Khangchendzonga, Sikkim, India. Mammalia 75: 257–268.
41. Gunter r (1951) The absolute threshold for vision in the cat. Journal of Physiology 114: 8–15.
42. Cuevas A, Febrero M, Fraiman R (2006) On the use of the bootstrap for estimating functions with functional data. Computational Statistics & Data Analysis 51: 1063–1074.
43. Ramsay J, Hooker G, Graves S (2009) Functional Data Analysis with R and MATLAB.. New York.: Springer.
44. Benjamini Y, Hochberg Y (1995) Controlling the false discovery rate: a practical and powerful approach to multiple testing. Journal of the Royal Statistical Society Series B 57: 289–300.
45. Newton-Fisher N, Harris S, Green P, Jones G (1993) Structure and function of red fox *Vulpes vulpes* vocalisations. Bioacoustics 5: 1–31.
46. Gogoleva SS, Colodin JA, Volodinay V, Trutl N (2008) To bark or not to bark/ vocalisations by Red Foxes for tameness or aggressiveness towards humans. Bioacoustics 18: 99–132.
47. Griffin DR, Hubbard R, Wald G (1947) The Sensitivity of the Human Eye to Infra-Red Radiation. Journal of the Optical Society of America 37: 546–553.
48. Sliney DH, Wangemann RT, Franks JK, Wolbarsht ML (1976) Visual sensitivity of the eye to infrared laser radiation. Journal of the Optical Society of America 66: 339–341.
49. Gekeler F, Shinoda K, Blatsios G, Werner A, Zrenner E (2006) Scotopic threshold responses to infrared irradiation in cats. Vision Research 46: 357–364.
50. Meek PD, Ballard G-A, Fleming PJS (2012) A permanent security post for camera trapping. Australian Mammalogy 35: 123–127.
51. Sanders MD, Maloney RF (2002) Causes of mortality at nests of ground-nesting birds in the Upper Waitaki Basin, South Island, New Zealand: a 5-year video study. Biological Conservation 106: 225–236.
52. Bies DA, Hansen CH (1996) *Engineering Noise Control: Theory and Practice*, E & FN Spon, an imprint of Chapman & Hall, London
53. Pater L (2000) Defining Auditory Thresholds for Animal Species. In: Baker M, Belliveau G, editors. Terra Borealis; 2000; Labrador, Canada. Institute for Environmental Monitoring and Research. 22–25.
54. Price MA, Attenborough K, Heap NW (1988) Sound attenuation through trees: Measurements and models. The Journal of the Acoustical Society of America 84: 1836–1844.
55. Heffner HJ, Heffner HE (2010) The behavioural audiogram of whitetail deer (*Odocoileus virginianus*). The Journal of the Acoustical Society of America 127: EL111–EL114.

26

Self-Esteem in Hearing-Impaired Children: The Influence of Communication, Education, and Audiological Characteristics

Stephanie C. P. M. Theunissen[1]*, Carolien Rieffe[2,3], Anouk P. Netten[1], Jeroen J. Briaire[1], Wim Soede[1], Maartje Kouwenberg[2], Johan H. M. Frijns[1,4]

1 Department of Otorhinolaryngology and Head & Neck Surgery, Leiden University Medical Center, Leiden, The Netherlands, **2** Department of Developmental Psychology, Leiden University, Leiden, The Netherlands, **3** Dutch Foundation for the Deaf and Hard of Hearing Child, Amsterdam, The Netherlands, **4** Leiden Institute for Brain and Cognition, Leiden, The Netherlands

Abstract

Objective: Sufficient self-esteem is extremely important for psychosocial functioning. It is hypothesized that hearing-impaired (HI) children have lower levels of self-esteem, because, among other things, they frequently experience lower language and communication skills. Therefore, the aim of this study was to compare HI children's self-esteem across different domains with those of normal hearing (NH) children and to investigate the influence of communication, type of education, and audiological characteristics.

Methods: This large (N = 252) retrospective, multicenter study consisted of two age- and gender-matched groups: 123 HI children and 129 NH controls (mean age = 11.8 years). Self-reports were used to measure self-esteem across four domains: perceived social acceptance by peers, perceived parental attention, perceived physical appearance, and global self-esteem.

Results: HI children experienced lower levels of self-esteem regarding peers and parents than NH controls. Particularly HI children who attended special education for the deaf were at risk, even after correcting for their language development and intelligence. Yet, levels of global self-esteem and self-esteem involving physical appearance in HI children equalled those of NH controls. Furthermore, younger age at implantation and longer duration of having cochlear implants (CIs) were related to higher levels of self-esteem.

Conclusion: HI children experience lower levels of self-esteem in the social domains. Yet, due to the heterogeneity of the HI population, there is high variability in levels of self-esteem.

Discussion: Clinicians must always be aware of the risk and protective factors related to self-esteem in order to help individual patients reach their full potential.

Editor: Brett Thombs, McGill University, Canada

Funding: This research was supported by the Innovational Research Incentives Scheme (a VIDI grant) by The Netherlands Organisation for Scientific Research (NWO), no. 452-07-004 to Carolien Rieffe. The funders had no role in study design, data collection and analysis, decision to publish, or preparation of the manuscript.

Competing Interests: The authors have declared that no competing interests exist.

* E-mail: s.c.p.m.theunissen@lumc.nl

Introduction

Self-esteem refers to one's general evaluation or appraisal of the self, including feelings of self-worth [1]. Besides an evaluation of the self, self-esteem also denotes how one values oneself. This basic appreciation of the self has effects on multiple dimensions in our lives, such as our friendships, our successes, and our academic career. Moreover, individuals with higher levels of self-esteem are better able to cope with stressful life events [1], whereas lower levels of self-esteem are associated with more loneliness, peer rejection, aggression, delinquency, and psychopathology [2–6]. Hence, it is of the utmost importance to have a sufficient level of self-esteem.

One would assume that hearing-impaired (HI) individuals encounter more difficulties regarding their self-esteem because they often face multiple challenges, such as speech and language delays, communication problems, and less or no access to the sound-dominated world [7]. These problems could potentially harm HI children's level of self-esteem, resulting in for example less stable friendships and more bullying [8]. Well-developed language and communication skills have been linked to higher levels of self-esteem [9]. Nowadays, deaf children who can have no or minimal benefit from conventional hearing aids receive cochlear implants (CIs), which considerably change and often improved outcomes for them in the aforementioned domains [10,11]. Recently, CI recipients have been found to have levels of self-esteem that equal those of NH children [12,13], which emphasizes the importance of adequate language development for self-esteem.

Studies that looked at levels of self-esteem in a more heterogeneous group of HI children showed inconsistent results. When compared to normal hearing (NH) peers, some researchers reported lower self-esteem in children with mild to profound hearing losses [14–16], while others demonstrated that levels of self-esteem were similar to those of NH counterparts [12,13,17–19]. In the literature, no consensus has been reached for the effect of type of education on HI children's self-esteem: some researchers showed higher self-esteem in HI children attending mainstream education than the ones attending special education, whereas others found no difference [19–21]. Possibly, HI children evaluate their abilities differently in different school contexts. Whilst HI children attending special schools evaluate themselves within a compatible peer group, HI children in a mainstream setting will compare themselves with their hearing peers. [21]. Conversely, it could also be argued that HI children attending mainstream schools actually feel a higher self-worth, because they are able to fit in with hearing peers, which can be perceived as a major achievement.

Self-esteem is often conceptualized as being multidimensional, consisting of several specific domains that are related to various facets of life (e.g. perceived parental attention, social acceptance by peers and physical appearance), as well as a more general view of oneself, often called 'global self-esteem' [3,22]. Levels of self-esteem can vary considerably across these different domains, particularly during adolescence, as this is a transition phase marked by crucial emotional and behavioral changes [3,23]. Parents become less influential, while close friends' and classmates' judgments become increasingly important [24]. Attention to and perception of one's physical appearance also increase. A child may be at risk of low self-esteem in one specific domain but not in another [21]. Although it has been postulated that self-esteem interventions do not directly improve outcomes, being aware of these distinctions can support the caregiver when helping or counseling the child [2].

Besides the contrasting findings of past research regarding differences in HI and NH children's levels of global self-esteem, there is a paucity of data concerning the more specific domains of self-esteem in HI children compared to NH children. Only a few studies have reported on specific domains of self-esteem in HI children when compared to NH controls. These found that the HI children had more difficulties regarding peer acceptance and family relations although they felt equally confident about their physical appearance [15,19,25]. To the best of our knowledge, no other studies have been performed to date in which these specific domains were studied and compared in both HI and NH children.

Hence, our goal here was not only to investigate the level of global self-esteem in a large and diverse sample of HI and NH children and adolescents, but also to examine three more specific domains of self-esteem: perceived social acceptance by peers, perceived parental attention and perceived physical appearance. Secondly, we wanted to study whether language development and communication skills, type of education, and audiological characteristics would influence the level of self-esteem. Based on (the majority of) the existing literature, we expected that adequate communication skills would result in higher self-esteem [9,12,13] and that children attending special education would have lower self-esteem than children in mainstream education [19–21]. Concerning audiological factors, no recent studies were available on which to base our predictions. Therefore, we have performed several explorative analyses to see whether relations between these factors and the different domains of self-esteem exist.

Materials and Methods

Participants

A total of 252 children (Mean age = 11.8 years, *SD* = 1.7) participated in this study of which 123 were HI children and 129 were NH controls. All children had a nonverbal IQ of at least 80, and no other known learning problems. Children were not included if they experienced comorbidities such as visual impairment or Autism Spectrum Disorders. The HI children were included if they experienced a loss of at least 40 decibels in the best ear, which was detected prelingually (<3 years) or perilingually (3–5 years). Table 1 shows the characteristics of all included children. For the CI recipients specifically, the mean age at implantation was 3.8 years (*SD* = 2.7; range = 0.9–10.8 years). The mean duration of CI use was 8.3 years (*SD* = 2.6; range 0.8–13.0 years). Most CI users (*n* = 40; 76%) had one CI, and 13 (24%) children were bilaterally implanted.

Procedure

The NH controls were recruited from primary and secondary mainstream schools across the Netherlands to reach a geographically and socio-economically diverse sample. To collect a sample that represented the complete spectrum of HI children, we recruited from 14 (both primary and secondary) mainstream schools and special schools for the HI (schools that supported development of auditory and oral skills, with or without the use of signs), 2 hospitals, 5 Speech and Hearing centers or residential schools, and via newsletters in the Netherlands and the Dutch-speaking part of Belgium.

The questionnaire was administered on a laptop. Questions appeared one by one on the screen. Instructions for all tests were provided in the child's preferred mode of communication to ensure that the child understood. The HI children could choose between two versions of the questionnaire: the first version which comprised written items exclusively, and the second version in which each item was presented in written text and sign language simultaneously by means of a video clip in the upper right-hand corner of the screen. Translation from spoken language into sign language was performed by a qualified interpreter and back translation of all signed items showed good convergence with the original items.

Parents or caregivers were requested to complete a questionnaire assessing demographic variables such as net income and level of education. In the HI group, several audiological variables were derived from the child's medical and audiological notes after informed consent was given. SES was calculated as the mean of parental education, job, and net income. Unfortunately, due to privacy reasons, almost half of the parents did not fill out the question concerning net income, so these were not taken into account.

Ethics statement and privacy regulation

Approval for the study was obtained by the Medical Ethics Committee of the Leiden University Medical Center under number P10.137, and carried out in accordance with the standards set out by the Declaration of Helsinki. All parents or caregivers gave written consent for their child's participation prior to data collection. Next to parents and caregivers, all children aged 12 or older gave written consent as well. Before the assessment started, all children were assured that their responses would be processed anonymously.

Table 1. Characteristics of all participants.

	Total sample (N = 252)		HI sample (*n* = 123)	
	Controls	**HI**	**CI**	**Hearing aid**
Number of children – *n*	129	123	53	70
Age mean in years (*SD*)	11.6 (1.3)	12.0 (1.8)	11.9 (2.1)	12.0 (1.7)
Gender - *n* (%)				
Male	58 (45%)	60 (49%)	24 (45%)	36 (51%)
Female	71 (55%)	63 (51%)	29 (55%)	34 (49%)
Socioeconomic status mean (*SD*)[a]	12.1 (2.4)	11.5 (2.3)	11.7 (2.3)	11.3 (2.4)
Nonverbal IQ				
IQ norm score Picture arrangement (*SD*)	10.6 (3.4)	10.2 (3.5)	9.9 (3.5)	10.4 (3.5)
IQ norm score Block design (*SD*)	10.6 (3.0)	10.4 (3.1)	10.3 (2.8)	10.5 (3.4)
Spoken language skills[b]				
Sentence comprehension (*SD*)	7.1 (2.3)	6.6 (3.1)	6.6 (3.1)	6.7 (3.1)
Story comprehension (*SD*)	7.0 (2.5)	6.3 (2.8)	5.6 (3.0)	6.8 (2.6)
Sign language skills[c]				
Sentence comprehension (*SD*)	-	2.3 (0.9)	2.1 (1.0)	2.3 (1.0)
Story comprehension (*SD*)	-	2.6 (0.7)	2.8 (0.8)	2.5 (0.7)
Children's Communication Checklist[d]				
General Communication Composite (*SD*)	73.9 (18.2)	91.3 (18.2)[1]	91.9 (18.4)	90.8 (18.2)
Pragmatic Composite (*SD*)	36.2 (9.1)	46.6 (8.7)[1]	47.3 (9.1)	46.1 (8.5)
Audiological variables				
Degree of hearing loss - *n* (%)[e]				
Moderate (40–60 dB)	-	29 (24%)	0 (0%)	29 (41%)[1]
Severe (61–90 dB)	-	25 (20%)	1 (2%)	24 (34%)[1]
Profound (>90 dB)	-	61 (50%)	50 (94%)	11 (16%)[1]
Unknown	-	8 (6%)	2 (4%)	6 (9%)
Preferred mode of communication - *n* (%)				
Oral language only	-	88 (71%)	36 (68%)	52 (74%)
Sign-supported language	-	33 (27%)	17 (32%)	16 (23%)
Sign language only	-	2 (2%)	0 (0%)	2 (3%)
Type of education – *n* (%)				
Regular education	-	74 (60%)	32 (60%)	42 (60%)
Special education	-	49 (40%)	21 (40%)	28 (40%)
Mean age at onset in years (*SD*)	-	1.6 (1.3)	1.2 (0.9)	1.9 (1.5)[2]
Age at onset of hearing loss - *n* (%)				
Prelingual (<3 yrs)	-	104 (85%)	49 (93%)	55 (79%)[3]
Perilingual (3–5 yrs)	-	12 (10%)	2 (4%)	10 (14%)[3]
Unknown	-	7 (6%)	2 (4%)	5 (7%)
Mean age at 1st hearing aid in years (*SD*)	-	2.1 (1.4)	1.5 (0.9)	2.6 (1.5)[1]

[a]Socioeconomic status score was measured by parental education, job, and net income. (Unfortunately, due to privacy reasons, almost half of the parents did not fill out the question concerning the net income, so these were not taken into account.)
[b]Spoken language skills were derived from the Clinical Evaluation of Language Fundamentals; see Materials section for more information.
[c]Sign language skills were derived from the Assessment Instrument for Sign Language of the Netherlands; see Materials section for more information.
[d]Higher scores indicate more (social) language problems. More than 70% of the parents responded.
[e]Degree of hearing loss was calculated by averaging unaided hearing thresholds at 500, 1,000, and 2,000 Hertz.
[1]$p<.001$;
[2]$p<.01$;
[3]$p<.05$.

Self-esteem questionnaire

To assess self-esteem, the self-report *Children's Self-Confidence and Acceptance Scale* [26,27] was used, which had only been used in NH children previously. The scale showed a strong convergent validity with the CBSK, which is the well-established Dutch version of Harter's self-esteem scale (*The Self-Perception Profile for Children* [28,29]). Harter's scale was used because we wanted to address the different specific domains of self-esteem instead of the more general global self-esteem measured by the Rosenberg self-esteem scale [30]. The items of the questionnaire were formulated by a team of child psychologists, targeting key aspects of self-esteem. Sentences were formulated short and simple, so HI children with language comprehension problems would be able to understand these items and respond to them coherently. The reason for choosing a self-report instead of parent or teacher reports is that self-reports give the most accurate scores when measuring self-esteem [31,32].

The questionnaire represents three relevant domain-specific categories, and one overall category, that could be answered on a 3-point Likert scale:

1. The *perceived social acceptance by peers* ('peers', 5 items) domain examines the perception of the child of how well he or she is accepted by peers or feels popular (Example item: "Children ask to play with me").
2. The *perceived parental attention* ('parents', 7 items) domain assesses the self-perceived degree to which parents or caregivers are interested in and give support to the child's thoughts and needs ("My father or mother are happy with me").
3. The *perceived physical appearance* ('physical appearance', 5 items) domain reflects the child's idea of how good-looking or attractive he or she is ("Other children think my appearance is nice").
4. The *global self-esteem* ('global', 5 items) measures the child's perceptions of general statements concerning the self ("I am happy with myself"). These five items address comparable issues to those used in Rosenberg's self-esteem scale [30].

Children were asked to rate the items on a 3-point Likert-type scale (1 = *not true*, 2 = *sometimes true*, 3 = *often true*). The internal consistency was good for both the HI and the NH group (Table 2).

Language development and communication skills

Language development and communication skills were measured because of their known positive influence on self-esteem [9]. Two types of language development were assessed: *sentence comprehension* and *story comprehension*. HI children using spoken language and NH controls received two corresponding subtests of the Dutch version of the *Clinical Evaluation of Language Fundamentals - Fourth Edition* (CELF) [33,34]. HI children who use sign or sign-supported language received specific subtests of the *Assessment Instrument for Sign Language of the Netherlands* [35]. All original language scores were transformed to norm scores and these were corrected for chronological age. The sentence comprehension task was not administered to 10 HI and 16 controls and the story comprehension task was not administered to 5 HI and 16 NH controls.

The *Children's Communication Checklist version 2* was used to evaluate communication skills indicated by the parents or caregivers [36]. This questionnaire, consisting of 70 items, has been predominantly designed to assess social and pragmatic language of children aged 4 to 16, although it also assesses other qualitative aspects of language. The checklist contains eight scales: speech production, syntax, semantics, coherence, inappropriate initiation, stereotyped conversation, use of context, and non-verbal communication. Two composite scores are conventionally obtained from these scales: the general communication composite (GCC) and the pragmatic composite (PC). Each item can be scored from 0 (*never or less than once a week*) to 3 (*several times a day or always*). Higher scores indicate more (social) language problems. To the parents of the HI children using sign or sign-supported language, the speech production and syntax scales were not administered.

Intelligence

An index of the nonverbal intelligence was obtained with two tests from the *Wechsler Intelligence Scale for Children - Third Edition*: block design by copying geometric designs with cubes, and picture arrangement by sequencing pictures to make logical stories [37,38]. All raw scores were converted into age-equivalent norm scores based on Dutch standards (10 = average). A random sampling ($n = 23$) across HI children who were previously assessed with a complete intelligence test (either the Snijders-Oomen nonverbal intelligence test [39] or the WISC) showed a high correlation between the scores of our tests and the IQ score, $r = .79$, $p < .001$. The tasks were not administered to 8 HI and 17 NH children, due to time constraints.

Statistical analyses

First, in order to compare the levels of the specific domains of self-esteem between HI and NH children, Multivariate Analysis of Variance (MANOVA) and Multivariate Analysis of Covariance (MANCOVA) were used. In the MANCOVAs, several covariates were incorporated one by one, including intelligence, socio-economic status (SES) and language and communication skills. For the second and third research questions (i.e., influence of communication skills and type of education on the different domains of self-esteem, respectively) MANCOVAs were performed, and confounding variables were included one by one in case of group differences. Several continuous audiological factors (e.g., duration of CI use, age at implantation) and their association with the different domains of self-esteem were addressed by Pearson's correlations. Nominal variables (uni- or bilateral CI, pre-

Table 2. Psychometric properties of the four domains of self-esteem.

	Range	Number of items	Inter-item correlation	Cronbach's Alpha	
				HI	NH controls
Domains of self-esteem					
Perceived social acceptance by peers	1–3	5	.75	.74	.75
Perceived parental attention	1–3	7	.34	.76	.75
Perceived physical appearance	1–3	5	.46	.83	.78
Global self-esteem	1–3	5	.25	.66	.60

or perilingual onset of HI) were compared by means of MANOVAs. When a score or variable was not available, the participant was excluded from the analysis concerned. It was checked whether there were group differences on age, gender, SES, and type of hearing device between those who completed and those who did not complete all the questionnaires and this was not the case. The program *Statistical Packages for the Social Sciences* (version 20.0) was used.

Results

Self-esteem in HI versus NH children

Regarding global self-esteem, the scores of NH and HI children did not significantly differ ($\Delta = -.007$, $p = .881$). To compare the groups with respect to their specific domains of self-esteem, a MANOVA was carried out with group (NH or HI) as the between-subjects variable and the levels of self-esteem in each of the specific domains as the within-subjects variable. This analysis revealed a main effect for self-esteem $F_{HF}(1.62, 403.73) = 56.78$, $p < .001$ $\eta_p^2 = .19$, and for group $F(1, 250) = 11.77$, $p = .001$ $\eta_p^2 = .05$ which was qualified by a group x self-esteem interaction effect $F_{HF}(1.62, 403.73) = 6.16$, $p < .01$ $\eta_p^2 = .02$. Post-hoc t-tests showed that HI children had lower self-esteem than NH controls on two domains: the peers' domain ($\Delta = .20$, $p < .002$) and the parents' domain ($\Delta = .20$, $p < .001$) (Figure 1). For the physical appearance domain, no significant group difference was found. A MANCOVA was performed in which we controlled for several important variables (age, gender, intelligence, and SES). The above-described effects retained their significance, so these results were omitted from the results presented here.

When comparing children wearing HAs with those using CIs, the groups did not significantly differ on their level of global self-esteem ($\Delta = .086$, $p = .18$). A 2 (HA or CI) x 3 (domains of self-esteem) MANOVA also revealed no significant differences between the groups in the different domains of self-esteem $F(1, 121) = .014$, $p = .91$ $\eta_p^2 < .001$.

Language development, communication skills and self-esteem

As expected on the basis of past research, *t*-tests revealed that HI children had lower language and communication skills than NH children (story comprehension, $\Delta = .8$, $p < .038$, general communication composite, $\Delta = 17.4$, $p < .001$, and pragmatic composite, $\Delta = 10.4$, $p < .001$, respectively). Therefore, a 2 (group: HI or NH) x 3 (domains of self-esteem) MANCOVA corrected for language development and communication skills was carried out. Again a main effect for group was detected, which was qualified by a group x self-esteem interaction effect: *Wilks'* $\Lambda = .96$ $F(2, 165) = 3.80$ $p = .024$ $\eta_p^2 = .044$. Post-hoc MANCOVAs showed slightly different results than the MANOVAs: HI children still reported lower self-esteem with respect to the parents' domain $F(1, 216) = 4.89$ $p = .028$, whereas differences in the peers' domain were no longer statistically significant $F(1, 216) = .03$ $p = .86$.

Type of education and self-esteem

In order to properly examine levels of self-esteem between HI children in special education (for the HI or deaf) and in mainstream education, these two groups were compared on several factors: age, gender, intelligence, SES, and language and communication skills. HI children attending mainstream education had significantly better language skills ($\Delta = 3.17$, $p < .001$), higher intelligence scores ($\Delta = 2.22$, $p < .001$), and higher communication skills ($\Delta = -22.69$, $p < .001$) than children attending special education.

Regarding global self-esteem, the scores of HI children attending mainstream education did not significantly differ from those attending special education ($\Delta = .10$, $p = .14$). A 2 (type of school: special or mainstream) x 3 (domains of self-esteem) MANCOVA which corrected for language development, communication skills and intelligence revealed a significant difference in the parents' domain only, with children in mainstream education scoring higher then children attending special education: *Wilks'* $\Lambda = .82$ $F(3, 67) = 4.87$ $p = .004$ $\eta_p^2 = .18$.

Audiological factors

Finally, a series of Pearson's correlations were carried out to see which continuous audiological factors were associated with the specific domains of self-esteem (Table 3). For the peers' and physical appearance domains and for global self-esteem, no significant associations were detected. However, for the parents' domain, younger age at implantation, and consequent longer duration of having CIs, were related to higher self-esteem: $r(47) = -.359$ $p = .006$ and $r(47) = .376$ $p = .004$ respectively. These correlations remained significant when a correction for age and language development was performed, using partial correlation analyses: $r(41) = -.28$ $p = .035$ and $r(41) = .28$ $p = .034$ respectively. To analyze differences within the CI group between two nominal variables (i.e. uni- or bilateral implantation, and pre- or perilingual detection of hearing loss), a MANOVA was carried out for each variable. The independent variables were uni- or bilateral implantation and pre- or perilingual onset of hearing loss, and the dependent variables were the 3 specific domains of self-esteem. No differences between the groups were found: *Wilks'* $\Lambda = 1.0$ $F(3, 49) = .06$ $p = .98$ $\eta_p^2 = .004$ and *Wilks'* $\Lambda = .94$ $F(3, 112) = 2.37$ $p = .075$ $\eta_p^2 = .06$ respectively.

Discussion

Self-esteem is a principal prerequisite for healthy psychosocial development and enables children to adjust to stress or burdens [40]. HI children often face demanding situations, so it might be even more important for them to have sufficient levels of self-esteem. By tapping into self-esteem across a number of domains, a differentiated picture of self-esteem was obtained. First, we found that the levels of global self-esteem and perceived physical appearance of HI children did not significantly differ from those of NH controls, despite the former group wearing external amplification devices visible to those around them. This suggests that HI children do not feel more insecure about their looks than other teenagers around this age, which is a positive finding. However, HI children reported lower self-esteem in the domains of perceived social acceptance by peers and perceived parental attention when compared to NH peers. Adequate language development and communication skills can increase self-esteem in the peers' domain, but not in the parental domain.

The fact that HI children reported lower levels of self-esteem than NH children in the social domains indicates that HI children feel less liked and appreciated by parents and peers. This is in line with other studies with HI children [15,16,25]. The reasons for lower self-esteem involving parents could be subjective or objective. Children might perceive that their parents spend less time with them, while in fact parents might spend equal time with them as with their NH children. The quality of contact received by NH versus HI children could be different. Parents usually experience more stress and worries raising a HI than a NH child, because they have to adapt to a new situation which necessitates the investment of time, effort, and resources [41–44]. For example, an HI child requires frequent hospitals visits and involvement in

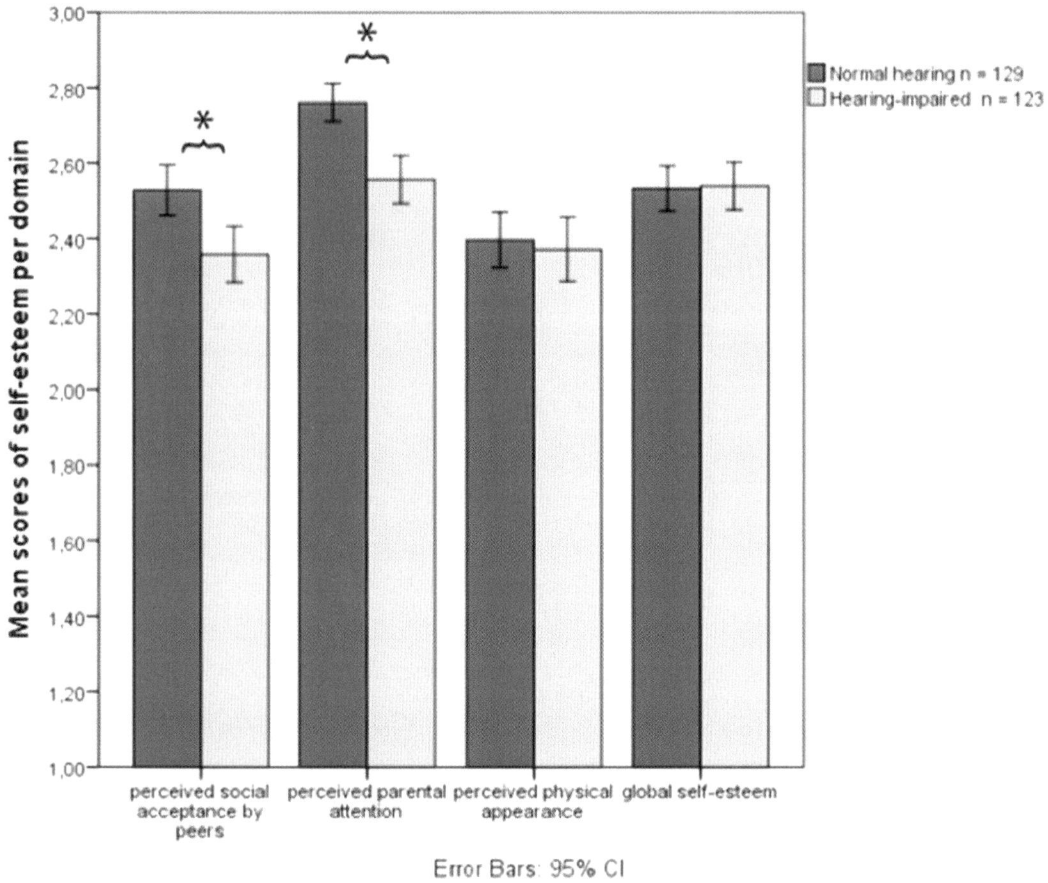

Figure 1. Mean scores of self-esteem per domain. $^{*}p<.05$.

intensive rehabilitation programs. Chronic parental stress can influence the child's functioning and development in a negative way (e.g., more behavioral problems and impaired psychological functioning) [8,45]. First of all, parents are a role model for their children. When parents have difficulties coping with stressful events, children will learn and apply these reactions as well. Secondly, more parental stress will also bring about a less positive atmosphere in the home, creating a less optimal environment for healthy development in children. Thirdly, parents might be focused on the impact of the hearing loss and medical site of this, overlooking the child's emotional need for support and guidance. Possibly, parents try hard to support their HI child by speaking slowly, helping with homework, or explaining difficult words [46]. Yet, HI children might interpret this extra attention as if they are failing or falling behind.

On the other hand, language development and communication skills influenced self-esteem in the peers' domain. This means that HI children's self-esteem regarding peers equals that of NH children when their language and communication skills are well-developed. Still, HI children are born into a sound-dominated world, where the focus lies on spoken language, resulting in less satisfactory communication. For example, making friends can be harder for HI children and they are also more neglected and less accepted by NH peers [16,47–50]. The communication barrier

Table 3. Pearson's correlations between the four domains of self-esteem and associated variables.

	Domains of self-esteem			
	Perceived social acceptance by peers	Perceived parental attention	Perceived physical appearance	Global self-esteem
Age of onset hearing loss	−.02	−.04	.06	−.04
Age at first hearing aid	−.02	.09	.04	−.10
Age at CI implantation	.16	−.36*	.20	−.08
Duration of CI use	−.21	.38**	−.07	−.07

$^{*}p<.05$;
$^{**}p<.01$ (two-tailed).

between HI and NH children can function as an obstacle for successful interpersonal relationships and may hamper these children in developing solid social networks [51,52]. This process may pave the way for social isolation and loneliness, with consequences for the child's self-esteem [53,54]. Hence, by improving language development and communication skills, the HI child might experience better contact with peers, which in turn would likely improve their self-esteem in this domain. In this respect, it has to be mentioned that language development and communication skills did not differ between hearing aided children and CI recipients in our sample. Though the literature often showed that CI recipients have better skills in this regard [10,55], most of the literature reports on early-implanted children, while our sample is mainly late-implanted. Therefore, we think that the next generation of CI recipients, with better language and communication will, in turn, have higher self-esteem.

Moreover, this research has revealed that children who attend special education for the HI or deaf have lower self-esteem concerning parents when compared to HI children attending mainstream education. Although we have to bear in mind that HI children with good language skills and/or higher intelligence are more easily referred to mainstream education [20,56–58], this study is the first to show that even after correcting for these variables, children in special education still have lower levels of self-esteem. It could be hypothesized that this stems from reasons related to discrimination or stigma. HI children often have to travel far to attend special education, which results in different environments: they have friends at school and different friends at home. Less contact with peers could hinder bonding and attachment, possibly resulting in lower self-esteem [59]. However, longitudinal studies are needed to reproduce these findings, because a cross-sectional study rules out drawing conclusions about causal relations. Additionally, such longitudinal studies must include larger samples in order to examine the influence of parental and friends' hearing statuses on the level of self-esteem.

A limitation of this study was missing data, especially concerning communication, intelligence and language development. It is possible that this missing data did not occur at random. For example, children who read slowly might not have had enough time to complete all the tests. Yet, comparison showed that the group for which information on these measures was missing did not differ from the group with no missing values on important other variables, including age, gender, SES, and the different domains for self-esteem. This seems to strengthen the basis for our conclusions, but future studies are needed to confirm these outcomes.

To conclude, self-esteem in HI children differs from NH children in the social domains only; the levels of perceived physical appearance and global self-esteem do not differ from those of NH children. Improving language development and communication skills could help to build up higher levels of self-esteem regarding peers. Unfortunately, irrespective of their language and communication skills, HI children in special education show lower levels of self-esteem in the parental domain. The aim of this research was to create more awareness concerning this vulnerable group of children, resulting in increased attention and monitoring by professionals, in order to promote good mental health in each HI child.

Acknowledgments

We gratefully acknowledge all children and their parents for participation in this study.

Author Contributions

Conceived and designed the experiments: ST, AN, CR, MK, WS, JB, JF. Performed the experiments: ST, MK. Analyzed the data: ST, AN, CR. Wrote the paper: ST, AN, CR, MK, WS, JB, JF.

References

1. Rosenberg M (1965) Society and the adolescent self-image. Princeton, NJ: Princeton University Press.
2. Baumeister RF, Campbell JD, Krueger JI, Vohs KD (2003) Does High Self-Esteem Cause Better Performance, Interpersonal Success, Happiness, or Healthier Lifestyles? Psychological science 4: 1–44.
3. Harter S (2006) Self-processes and developmental psychopathology. In: Cicchietti D, Cohen DJ, Developmental Psychopathology. Hoboken, NJ: Wiley & Sons. pp. 370–418.
4. Orth U, Robins RW, Roberts BW (2008) Low self-esteem prospectively predicts depression in adolescence and young adulthood. Journal of Personality and Social Psychology 95: 695–708.
5. Harper JF, Marshall E (1991) Adolescents' problems and their relationship to self-esteem. Adolescence 26: 799–807.
6. Donnellan MB, Trzesniewski KH, Robins RW, Moffitt TE, Caspi A (2005) Low self-esteem is related to aggression, antisocial behavior, and delinquency. Psychological Science 16: 328–335.
7. Polat F (2003) Factors Affecting Psychosocial Adjustment of Deaf Students. Journal of Deaf Studies and Deaf Education 8: 325–339.
8. Kouwenberg M, Rieffe C, Theunissen SCPM, de Rooij M (2012) Peer victimization experienced by Children and Adolescents who are Deaf or Hard of Hearing. PLoS ONE 7.
9. Hintermair M (2008) Self-esteem and satisfaction with life of deaf and hard-of-hearing people - a resource-oriented approach to identity work. Journal of Deaf Studies and Deaf Education 13: 278–300.
10. Tomblin JB, Spencer L, Flock S, Tyler R, Gantz B (1999) A comparison of language achievement in children with cochlear implants and children using hearing aids. J Speech Lang Hear Res 42: 497–509.
11. Theunissen SC, Rieffe C, Kouwenberg M, De Raeve LJ, Soede W, et al. (2013) Behavioral problems in school-aged hearing-impaired children: the influence of sociodemographic, linguistic, and medical factors. Eur Child Adolesc Psychiatry.
12. Percy-Smith L, Cay-Thomasen P, Gudman M, Jensen J, Thomsen J (2008) Self-esteem and social well-being of children with cochlear implant compared to normal-hearing children. International Journal of Pediatric Otorhinolaryngology 72: 1113–1120.
13. Sahli S, Belgin E (2006) Comparison of self-esteem level of adolescents with cochlear implant and normal hearing. International Journal of Pediatric Otorhinolaryngology 70: 1601–1608.
14. Bess FH, Dodd-Murphy J, Parker RA (1998) Children with minimal sensorineural hearing loss: prevalence, educational performance, and functional status. Ear and Hearing 19: 339–354.
15. Van Gent T, Goedhart AW, Knoors HET, Westenberg PM, Treffers PDA (2012) Self-concept and Ego Development in Deaf Adolescents: A Comparative Study. Journal of Deaf Studies and Deaf Education 17: 333–351.
16. Cappelli M, Daniels T, DurieuxSmith A, McGrath PJ, Neuss D (1995) Social development of children with hearing impairments who are integrated into general education classrooms. Volta Review 97: 197–208.
17. Cates JA (1991) Self-Concept in Hearing and Prelingual, Profoundly Deaf Students - a Comparison of Teachers Perceptions. American Annals of the Deaf 136: 354–359.
18. Eriks-Brophy A, Durieux-Smith A, Olds J, Fitzpatrick EM, Duquette C, et al. (2012) Communication, Academic, and Social Skills of Young Adults with Hearing Loss. Volta Review 112: 5–35.
19. Leigh IW, Maxwell-McCaw D, Bat-Chava Y, Christiansen JB (2009) Correlates of psychosocial adjustment in deaf adolescents with and without cochlear implants: a preliminary investigation. Journal of Deaf Studies and Deaf Education 14: 244–259.
20. Keilmann A, Limberger A, Mann W (2007) Psychological and physical well-being in hearing-impaired children. International Journal of Pediatric Otorhinolaryngology 71: 1747–1752.
21. Van Gurp S (2001) Self-concept of deaf secondary school students in different educational settings. Journal of Deaf Studies and Deaf Education 6: 54–69.
22. Blascovich J, Tomaka J (1991) Measures of self-esteem. In: Robinson JP, Shaver PR, Wrightsman LS, Measures of Personality and Social Psychological Attributes. San Diego, SA: Academic Press.
23. Cole DA, Maxwell SE, Martin JM, Peeke LG, Seroczynski AD, et al. (2001) The development of multiple domains of child and adolescent self-concept: A cohort sequential longitudinal design. Child Development 72: 1723–1746.
24. Coleman JS (1981) The adolescent society; Johnstone JWC, editor: Greenwood Press.

25. Loeb RC, Sarigiani P (1986) The impact of hearing impairment on self-perceptions of children. Volta Review 88: 89–100.
26. Rieffe C, Meerum Terwogt M, Bosch JD, Kneepkens CMF, Douwes AC, et al. (2007) Interaction between emotions and somatic complaints in children who did or did not seek medical care. Cognition and Emotion 21: 1630–1646.
27. Van Dijk P, Rieffe C (1999) Somatic complaints in children; a study on the influence of fear, self-esteem and concern on the reporting of physical complaints. Amsterdam: Vrije Universiteit. pp. 23.
28. Veerman JW, Straathof MAE, Treffers DA, Van den Bergh BRH, Brink LT (1997) Competentiebelevingsschaal voor Kinderen: Handleiding [Perceived competence scale for children: manual]. Lisse, The Netherlands: Swets & Zeitlinger.
29. Harter S (1985) Manual for the Self-perception Profile for Children. Denver, CO: University of Denver.
30. Rosenberg M (1979) Conceiving the self: Basic Books.
31. Robins RW, Hendin HM, Trzesniewski KH (2001) Measuring Global Self-Esteem: Construct Validation of a Single-Item Measure and the Rosenberg Self-Esteem Scale. Personality and Social Psychology Bulletin 27: 151–161.
32. Anmyr L, Larsson K, Olsson M, Freijd A (2012) Strengths and difficulties in children with cochlear implants - Comparing self-reports with reports from parents and teachers. International Journal of Pediatric Otorhinolaryngology 76: 1107–1112.
33. Kort W, Schittekatte M, Compaan E (2008) *CELF-4-NL: Clinical Evaluation of Language Fundamentals*: Pearson Assessment and Information B.V., Amsterdam.
34. Semel E, Wiig EH, Secord WA (1987) CELF: Clinical Evaluation of Language Fundamentals - revised; Corp TP, San Antonio, TX.
35. Hermans D, Knoors H, Verhoeven L (2010) Assessment of Sign Language Development: The Case of Deaf Children in the Netherlands. Journal of Deaf Studies and Deaf Education 15: 107–119.
36. Bishop DVM (1998) Development of the Children's Communication Checklist (CCC): A method for assessing qualitative aspects of communicative impairment in children. Journal of Child Psychology and Psychiatry and Allied Disciplines 39: 879–891.
37. Kort W, Schittekatte M, Compaan EL, Bosmans M, Bleichrodt N, et al. (2002) WISC-III NL. Handleiding. Nederlandse bewerking. London: The Psychological Corporation.
38. Wechsler D (1991) The Wechsler intelligence scale for children — third edition. San Antonio, TX: The Psychological Corporation.
39. Tellegen P, Laros J (1993) The Construction and Validation of a Nonverbal Test of Intelligence: the revision of the Snijders-Oomen tests. European Journal of Psychological Assessment 9: 147–157.
40. Dumont M, Provost MA (1999) Resilience in adolescents: Protective role of social support, coping strategies, self-esteem, and social activities on experience of stress and depression. Journal of Youth and Adolescence 28: 343–363.
41. Cohen MS (1999) Families coping with childhood chronic illness: A research review. Families, Systems, & Health 17: 149–164.
42. Quittner AL, Glueckauf RL, Jackson DN (1990) Chronic parenting stress: moderating versus mediating effects of social support. Journal of Personality and Social Psychology 59: 1266–1278.
43. Sach TH, Whynes DK (2005) Paediatric cochlear implantation: The views of parents. International Journal of Audiology 44: 400–407.
44. Quittner AL, Barker DH, Cruz I, Snell C, Grimley ME, et al. (2010) Parenting Stress Among Parents of Deaf and Hearing Children: Associations with Language Delays and Behavior Problems. Parenting: Science & Practice 10: 136–155.
45. Drotar D (1997) Relating parent and family functioning to the psychological adjustment of children with chronic health conditions: What have we learned? What do we need to know? Journal of Pediatric Psychology 22: 149–165.
46. Pinquart M (2013) Do the parent-child relationship and parenting behaviors differ between families with a child with and without chronic illness? A meta-analysis. J Pediatr Psychol 38: 708–721.
47. Nunes T, Pretzlik U, Olsson J (2001) Deaf children's social relationships in mainstream schools. Deafness & Education international 3: 123–136.
48. Wolters N, Knoors HE, Cillessen AH, Verhoeven L (2011) Predicting acceptance and popularity in early adolescence as a function of hearing status, gender, and educational setting. Research in Developmental Disabilities 32: 2553–2565.
49. Kluwin TN, Stinson MS, Colarossi GM (2002) Social processes and outcomes of in-school contact between deaf and hearing peers. Journal of Deaf Studies and Deaf Education 71: 1747–1752.
50. Davis JM, Elfenbein J, Schum R, Bentler RA (1986) Effects of Mild and Moderate Hearing Impairments on Language, Educational, and Psychosocial Behavior of Children. Journal of Speech and Hearing Disorders 51: 53–62.
51. Bat-Chava Y (1993) Antecedents of self-esteem in deaf people: A meta-analytic review. Rehabilitation Psychology 38: 221–234.
52. Calderon R, Greenberg MT (2003) Social and emotional development of deaf children: family, school and program effects. Marschark M, Spencer PE, editors. New York: Oxford University Press.
53. Rubin KH, Mills RSL (1988) The Many Faces of Social-Isolation in Childhood. Journal of Consulting and Clinical Psychology 56: 916–924.
54. Most T, Ingber S, Heled-Ariam E (2012) Social competence, sense of loneliness, and speech intelligibility of young children with hearing loss in individual inclusion and group inclusion. Journal of Deaf Studies and Deaf Education 17: 259–272.
55. Bond M, Mealing S, Anderson R, Elston J, Weiner G, et al. (2009) The effectiveness and cost-effectiveness of cochlear implants for severe to profound deafness in children and adults: a systematic review and economic model. Health Technology Assessment13: 1–+.
56. Van Eldik T (2005) Mental health problems of Dutch youth with hearing loss as shown on the Youth Self Report. American Annals of the Deaf 150: 11–16.
57. Stinson MS, Whitmire KA (2000) Adolescents who are deaf or hard of hearing: A communication perspective on educational placement. Topics in Language Disorders 20: 58–72.
58. Van Gent T, Goedhart A, Hindley P, Treffers PDA (2007) Prevalence and correlates of psychopathology in a sample of deaf adolescents. Journal of Child Psychology and Psychiatry and Allied Disciplines 48: 950–958.
59. Armsden GC, Greenberg MT (1987) The Inventory of Parent and Peer Attachment - Individual-Differences and Their Relationship to Psychological Well-Being in Adolescence. Journal of Youth and Adolescence 16: 427–454.

27

Phenotypic Characteristics of Hyperacusis in Tinnitus

Martin Schecklmann[1]*, Michael Landgrebe[2], Berthold Langguth[1], the TRI Database Study Group[¶]

1 Department of Psychiatry and Psychotherapy, University of Regensburg, Regensburg, Germany, 2 Department of Psychiatry and Psychotherapy, Social Foundation Bamberg, Bamberg, Germany

Abstract

Background: Many people with tinnitus also suffer from hyperacusis. Both clinical and basic scientific data indicate an overlap in pathophysiologic mechanisms. In order to further elucidate the interplay between tinnitus and hyperacusis we compared clinical and demographic characteristics of tinnitus patients with and without hyperacusis by analyzing a large sample from an international tinnitus patient database.

Materials: The default dataset import [November 1st, 2012] from the Tinnitus Research Initiative [TRI] Database was used for analyses. Hyperacusis was defined by the question "Do sounds cause you pain or physical discomfort?" of the Tinnitus Sample Case History Questionnaire. Patients who answered this question with "yes" were contrasted with "no"-responders with respect to 41 variables.

Results: 935 [55%] out of 1713 patients were characterized as hyperacusis patients. Hyperacusis in tinnitus was associated with younger age, higher tinnitus-related, mental and general distress; and higher rates of pain disorders and vertigo. In relation to objective audiological assessment patients with hyperacusis rated their subjective hearing function worse than those without hyperacusis. Similarly the tinnitus pitch was rated higher by hyperacusis patients in relation to the audiometrically determined tinnitus pitch. Among patients with tinnitus and hyperacusis the tinnitus was more frequently modulated by external noise and somatic maneuvers, i.e., exposure to environmental sounds and head and neck movements change the tinnitus percept.

Conclusions: Our findings suggest that the comorbidity of hyperacusis is a useful criterion for defining a sub-type of tinnitus which is characterized by greater need of treatment. The higher sensitivity to auditory, somatosensory and vestibular input confirms the notion of an overactivation of an unspecific hypervigilance network in tinnitus patients with hyperacusis.

Editor: Joel Snyder, UNLV, United States of America

Funding: The study was supported by the Tinnitus Research Initiative (TRI; www.tinnitusresearch.org). The funders had no role in study design, data collection and analysis, decision to publish, or preparation of the manuscript.

* E-mail: martin.schecklmann@medbo.de

¶ Membership of TRI Database Study Group is provided in the Acknowledgments

Introduction

Chronic tinnitus (ringing in the ears) is a widespread disorder affecting 5–15% of the population [1,2]. 10% of tinnitus patients are severely distressed and experience a distinct decline in their quality of life [1,2]. Concomitant symptoms are sleep disturbance, anxiety, depression, irritation, and concentration difficulties [3]. Furthermore, 40% of patients with tinnitus suffer from hyperacusis [4] while 86% of patients with hyperacusis have concomitant tinnitus [4]. Hyperacusis is described as hypersensitivity to sounds or the perception of ordinary sounds as louder as normal and with uncomfortable intensity [4–6].

The large overlap in prevalence between tinnitus and hyperacusis suggests that the two disorders share common pathophysiological mechanisms and risk factors. For tinnitus, hearing loss represents the main risk factor. It is assumed that the reduced peripheral auditory input causes alterations of the neural activity along the auditory pathway [7]. In addition, non-auditory areas of attention allocation, emotional processing and memory encoding are involved in the generation and maintenance of tinnitus [8,9]. The most efficient tinnitus therapies are tinnitus retraining and cognitive behavioural therapy by which quality of life can be significantly improved [10]. There is only very limited information available about hyperacusis. However, existing literature shows further similarities for both conditions in addition to the overlap in prevalence. Hyperacusis is also associated with hearing loss [11] and there is evidence for altered neural activity in auditory [12] and non-auditory cortical areas [13,14]. For both conditions, there is only a low correlation between audiometric measures and subjective ratings by visual analogue scales or questionnaires [15]. Due to these similarities, the same therapeutic approaches of tinnitus retraining and cognitive behavioural therapy have been suggested as treatment for hyperacusis [4,16].

Despite a clear overlap between tinnitus and hyperacusis, prevalence rates also indicate a population of patients who suffer from only one of the two conditions. A simplified definition of tinnitus is a "constant existent sound without external source" while hyperacusis is a "consistently exaggerated or inappropriate response to sounds that are neither threatening nor uncomfortably loud to a typical person" [17]. Thus, tinnitus might be related to increased spontaneous activity along the auditory pathway and hyperacusis to increased stimulus-related activity [12]. It is an open question if both hyperactive states are based on the same neurobiological condition [18,19], however there is clear clinical evidence that there is no complete overlap between tinnitus and hyperacusis. For example, hyperacusis, but not tinnitus, is a typical symptom of Williams syndrome, a hereditary disorder characterised by abnormal serotonergic metabolism [4]. There is also evidence that tinnitus and hyperacusis differ from each other in neural activity in the auditory pathway, specifically in the cingulate and orbitofrontal cortex [14,20].

Based on these observations one could postulate that the existence of comorbid hyperacusis defines a distinct subtype of chronic tinnitus. In this case one would expect that tinnitus patients with comorbid hyperacusis differ in their clinical and demographic characteristics from tinnitus patients without hyperacusis. Thus, the aim of the present study was the systematic evaluation of tinnitus patients with and without hyperacusis with respect to demographic, audiometric, and tinnitus characteristics, as well as tinnitus-related and general distress. High ecological validity was pursued by investigating a large sample from an international database [21].

Materials and Methods

The data presented in this study were derived from the Tinnitus Research Initiative (TRI) Database [22]. Data management was conducted according to the TRI Data Handling Plan (TRI-DHP V07, May 9th, 2011). Data analysis was performed according to the TRI Standard Operating Procedure (TRI-SA V01, May 9th, 2011), thereby following a study-specific Statistical Analysis Plan (SAP-009, Nov 22th 2012) that was written according to the TRI SAP template (TRI-SAP V01, May 9th, 2011). All documents can be accessed at http://database.tinnitusresearch.org/. Analysis details can be found at the end of the methods section.

The default dataset import (November 1st, 2012) from the TRI Database consisted of patients who were treated between 2005 and 2012 at tinnitus centres worldwide. Patients gave written informed consent to record their data in the database and for inclusion in analysis. The project was approved by the local ethics committee (Ethikkommission der Fakultät für Medizin der Universität Regensburg) at the location of the database, the University of Regensburg, Germany.

Hyperacusis was defined by the question "Do sounds cause you pain or physical discomfort?" of the Tinnitus Sample Case History Questionnaire (TSCHQ) [22]. Patients who did not answer this question (n = 620) or answered it with "I don't know" (n = 187) were excluded from analysis resulting in a sample of 1713 patients ("yes": n = 935; "no": n = 778). Thus, 55% of the patients were categorized as suffering from comorbid hyperacusis, which is a higher rate than indicated in the literature (40 (40%) [4]). Assessment was performed before the first consultation in the tinnitus clinics and included demographic and tinnitus-related questions (TSCHQ), questionnaires with respect to tinnitus, depression, and quality of life, and tinnitus-related numeric rating scales. An overview of all included variables can be seen in table 1. We also included audiology data (mean hearing level, minimal masking level, and tinnitus pitch), which were assessed at the first consultation in the different participating tinnitus centers. Mean hearing level was indicated by dB HL (hearing level) over all frequencies (0.125, 0.25, 0.5, 1, 2, 3, 4, 6, and 8kHz) in both ears; tinnitus loudness by minimal masking level (minimal volume of white noise to predominate the tinnitus percept); and the frequency of the tinnitus was assigned using pitch matching (for details see [23]). If no data were available from the screening visit (first consultation) we used data from the baseline visit of a clinical intervention. If both screening and baseline data were available we used the mean of the data at both time points.

For statistical analyses we contrasted tinnitus patients with and without hyperacusis using two-sided Student t-tests for continuous variables (e.g., age) and chi-square-tests for categorical variables (e.g., gender). In order to correct for the high number of dependent variables, significance threshold was set to a level of 0.001. We also reported the effect size Cohen's d [24]. Due to reasons of uniformity, chi-square Pearson r was transformed into Cohen's d by using the Statistical calculation spreadsheet "Converting effect sizes" at http://www.stat-help.com/based on a published converting formula [25]. Effect sizes are indicated as small with a range from 0.2 to 0.5, medium with values between 0.5 and 0.8, and high with values above 0.8. We relate the presentation of the results to significant effects ($p<0.001$) with at least small effect sizes since only these effects are considered as clinically meaningful.

Results

A detailed overview of the raw data and statistics is given in table 1. The result section is segmented according to the subgroups of variables as specified in table 1. There were significant differences between tinnitus patients with and without hyperacusis for age at tinnitus onset and age of treatment (small effect sizes). Patients with hyperacusis were younger (4 years on average). There was a significant effect for sex, but with a negligible effect size.

For many tinnitus-related characteristics we did not find significant group contrasts: tinnitus duration, laterality, character, day-to-day changes in loudness, intermittent/constant manifestation over time, or gradual/abrupt onset. However, patients with hyperacusis had a significantly higher probability to have pulsatile-like tinnitus, but with a negligible effect size. Spontaneous occurrence of tinnitus (without triggering events at tinnitus onset) was significantly less frequent in patients with hyperacusis (with small effect size).

For tinnitus-modulating factors, there were significant differences for all investigated variables except the ability to mask the tinnitus using music or sounds. The influence of sleep time and nap time was significant, but with negligible effect sizes. Hyperacusis patients could more frequently modulate their tinnitus with somatic maneuvers such as head movements, more frequently had a stress-sensitive tinnitus (all small effect sizes), and their tinnitus was more often influenced by noise (high effect size).

With respect to hearing function, hyperacusis patients had better hearing level in the pure tone audiometry (small effect size), but the patients' subjective assessment of hearing function was worse (significant, negligible effect size). A similar discrepancy between psychoacoustic measurements and subjective reports was observed for tinnitus pitch and loudness. Whereas minimal masking levels and tinnitus pitch match did not differ between groups, tinnitus patients with hyperacusis reported higher loudness ratings (significant, negligible effect size) and higher subjective pitch (significant, small effect size) of their tinnitus. Also in numeric rating scales, hyperacusis was related to higher tinnitus loudness, but also to reduced ability to ignore tinnitus and to increased discomfort, annoyance and unpleasantness (all with small effect sizes except for loudness which had negligible effect size).

Table 1. Descriptive values and statistics of group contrasts.

	tinnitus	tinnitus+hyperacusis	statistics
sample characteristics			
current age (years)	**54.3±12.9 (n=759)**	**50.7±13.2 (n=927)**	**T=5.640; df=1648; p<0.001; d=0.275**
age at tinnitus onset (years)	**45.3±13.9 (n=736)**	**41.6±13.7 (n=883)**	**T=5.352; df=1617; p<0.001; d=0.266**
gender (female/male)	245/533 (n=778); 32/68%	366/569 (n=935); 39/61%	χ^2=10.840; df=1; p<0.001; d=0.161
tinnitus characteristics			
duration (months)	98.6±108.3 (n=720)	100.6±106.2 (n=876)	T=−0.364; df=1594; p=0.716; d=0.018
tinnitus laterality (unilateral-right/ unilateral-left/elsewhere)	114/148/513 (n=775); 15/19/66%	96/161/675 (n=932); 10/17/72%	χ^2=9.824; df=2; p=0.007; d=0.152
pulsatile (no/yes)	650/118 (n=768); 85/15%	714/204 (n=918); 78/22%	χ^2=12.727; df=1; p<0.001; d=0.175
day-to-day changes of loudness (no/yes)	339/430 (n=769); 44/56%	354/570 (n=924); 38/62%	χ^2=5.782; df=1; p=0.016; d=0.116
manifestation over time (intermittent/constant)	121/650 (n=771); 16/84%	109/819 (n=928); 12/88%	χ^2=5.609; df=1; p=0.018; d=0.114
onset (gradual/abrupt)	381/373 (n=754); 50/49%	425/458 (n=883); 48/52%	χ^2=0.937; df=1; p=0.333; d=0.048
character (tone/noise/crickets/other)	415/153/132/68 (n=768); 54/20/17/9%	522/160/161/81 (n=924); 57/17/17/9%	χ^2=2.014; df=3; p=0.570; d=0.024
onset related event (none/one/multiple)	**149/515/113 (n=777); 19/66/15%**	**96/596/241 (n=933); 10/64/26%**	**χ^2=49.836; df=2; p<0.001; d=0.347**
modulating factors			
maskable by music or sound (no/yes)	173/489 (n=662); 26/74%	192/628 (n=820); 23/77%	χ^2=1.458; df=1; p=0.227; d=0.062
somatic modulation (no/yes)	**566/206 (n=772); 73/27%**	**562/355 (n=917); 61/38%**	**χ^2=27.341; df=1; p<0.001; d=0.256**
influence by noise (no/yes)	**388/257 (n=645); 60/40%**	**142/654 (n=796); 18/82%**	**χ^2=274.378; df=1; p<0.001; d=0.969**
influence by nap (worsens/reduces/no effect)	115/41/573 (n=729); 16/6/79%	144/99/622 (n=865); 17/11/72%	χ^2=17.811; df=2; p<0.001; d=0.100
influence by sleep (no/yes/don't know)	354/129/277 (n=760); 47/17/36%	324/220/357 (n=901); 36/24/40%	χ^2=23.349; df=2; p<0.001; d=0.155
influence by stress (worsens/reduces/no effect)	**423/11/316 (n=750); 56/2/42%**	**718/4/188 (n=910); 79/0/21%**	**χ^2=97.530; df=2; p<0.001; d=0.490**
hearing and tinnitus matching			
hearing level (dB HL mean of all frequencies)	**25.6±13.9 (n=596)**	**21.3±14.7 (n=698)**	**T=5.374; df=1292; p<0.001; d=0.299**
wearing of hearing aids (no/yes)	675/91 (n=766); 88/12%	788/130 (n=918); 86/14%	χ^2=1.906; df=1; p=0.167; d=0.068
subjective hearing problems (no/yes)	327/440 (n=767); 43/57%	308/613 (n=921); 33/67%	χ^2=15.067; df=1; p<0.001; d=0.189
minimal masking level (dB HL)	54.6±20.1 (n=429)	56.6±23.2 (n=505)	T=−1.394; df=932; p=0.164; d=0.091
tinnitus loudness	61.6±23.6 (n=745)	66.7±27.7 (n=894)	T=−3.959; df=1637; p<0.001; d=0.196
tinnitus pitch (Hz)	6329±3107 (n=436)	6669±3491 (n=514)	T=1.574; df=948; p=0.116; d=0.102
subjective tinnitus pitch (low, medium, high, very high)	**33/177/382/171 (n=763); 4/23/50/22%**	**15/155/478/272 (n=920); 2/17/52/30%**	**χ^2=27.545; df=3; p<0.001; d=0.250**
concomitant complaints and therapies			
suffering from headache (no/yes)	**526/242 (n=768); 68/31%**	**492/414 (n=906); 54/46%**	**χ^2=35.095; df=1; p<0.001; d=0.293**
suffering from temporomandibular joint complaints (no/yes)	**640/126 (n=766); 84/16%**	**672/236 (n=908); 74/26%**	**χ^2=22.321; df=1; p<0.001; d=0.232**
suffering from neck pain (no/yes)	**400/365 (n=765); 52/48%**	**351/565 (n=916); 38/62%**	**χ^2=32.909; df=1; p<0.001; d=0.283**
suffering from any other pain (no/yes)	**526/236 (n=762); 69/31%**	**486/421 (n=907); 54/46%**	**χ^2=41.389; df=1; p<0.001; d=0.318**
suffering from vertigo (no/yes)	**562/192 (n=754); 74/25%**	**534/368 (n=902); 59/41%**	**χ^2=43.147; df=1; p<0.001; d=0.326**

Table 1. Cont.

	tinnitus	tinnitus+hyperacusis	statistics
preceding tinnitus treatments (none/one/several)	**155/133/490 (n = 778); 20/17/63%**	**121/138/676 (n = 935); 13/15/72%**	**χ^2 = 19.728; df = 2; p<0.001; d = 0.215**
current psychiatric treatment (no/yes)	**696/80 (n = 776); 90/10%**	**738/186 (n = 924); 80/20%**	**χ^2 = 30.820; df = 1; p<0.001; d = 0.273**
questionnaires			
tinnitus questionnaire (0–84)	**35.8±17.1 (n = 544)**	**44.3±17.8 (n = 816)**	**T = −8.683; df = 1358; p<0.001; d = 0.471**
tinnitus handicap inventory (0–100)	**41.9±22.3 (n = 755)**	**53.6±23.0 (n = 918)**	**T = −10.466; df = 1671; p<0.001; d = 0.512**
Beck depression inventory (0–63)	**9.3±8.0 (n = 716)**	**12.8±9.4 (n = 867)**	**T = −7.922; df = 1581; p<0.001; d = 0.398**
quality of life: physical health (4–20)*	**15.0±3.0 (n = 572)**	**13.9±3.1 (n = 631)**	**T = 5.913; df = 1201; p<0.001; d = 0.341**
quality of life: psychological functions (4–20)*	**14.4±2.7 (n = 570)**	**13.5±2.9 (n = 634)**	**T = 5.648; df = 1202; p<0.001; d = 0.326**
quality of life: social relationships (4–20)*	14.7±3.0 (n = 568)	14.3±3.3 (n = 633)	T = 2.143; df = 1199; p = 0.032; d = 0.123
quality of life: environmental factors (4–20)*	15.8±2.6 (n = 572)	15.6±2.4 (n = 633)	T = 1.474; df = 1203; p = 0.141; d = 0.085
rating scales			
loudness (0–10)	6.1±2.3 (n = 752)	6.6±2.2 (n = 903)	T = −3.933; df = 1653; p<0.001; d = 0.193
discomfort (0–10)	**6.7±2.4 (n = 753)**	**7.3±2.2 (n = 906)**	**T = −5.110; df = 1657; p<0.001; d = 0.251**
annoyance (0–10)	**6.3±2.5 (n = 753)**	**6.9±2.4 (n = 908)**	**T = −5.285; df = 1659; p<0.001; d = 0.260**
ignorability (0–10)	**6.4±2.8 (n = 754)**	**7.0±2.6 (n = 907)**	**T = −4.770; df = 1659; p<0.001; d = 0.234**
unpleasantness (0–10)	**6.3±2.5 (n = 753)**	**6.9±2.4 (n = 99)**	**T = −5.058; df = 1660; p<0.001; d = 0.248**

Meaningful contrasts are defined by p<0.001 and d>0.2 and marked in bold font.
*High scores mean high functioning in quality of life in contrast to other questionnaires and rating scales.

With respect to comorbidities, hyperacusis was more frequently associated with headache, temporomandibular joint (TMJ) complaints, neck pain, general pain syndromes, and vertigo (all with small effect sizes). Hyperacusis was also related to an increased number of tinnitus treatment attempts and a current psychiatric treatment (both with small effect sizes).

Increased scores were found in the tinnitus questionnaire, the tinnitus handicap inventory, and the depression scale (small or medium effect sizes) for hyperacusis patients. In line, quality of life was significantly reduced for these patients with small effect sizes in the physical and psychological domain whereas there were no significant differences for quality of life in social relationships or environmental factors.

Discussion

We defined hyperacusis with the question ""Do sounds cause you pain or physical discomfort?". The main finding of our database analysis is, that tinnitus patients with and without hyperacusis differ in a large number of characteristics. In figure 1, all significant findings with at least small effect sizes are shown and grouped into different domains. The biggest effect size was found for the variable 'influence by noise' (brown box, figure 1), which means that patients with hyperacusis (82%) showed a higher probability that their tinnitus is influenced by external sounds and noise in contrast to patients without hyperacusis (40%). The finding that in people with both hyperacusis and tinnitus the sensitivity to sounds is directly related to the perception of tinnitus is an indication for an overlap in the pathophysiological mechanisms, as previously proposed [18,19,26,27]. Our finding also supports the notion of an abnormal increase of gain within the auditory system as a relevant mechanism for both tinnitus and hyperacusis [12,26]. The sensitivity to sound in some but not all tinnitus patients may represent a clinical criterion for pathophysiologically distinct subtypes of this disorder and may have important implications for the interpretation of imaging studies of tinnitus, which use auditory stimulation paradigms [20,28].

The next highest effect sizes were found for the questionnaires. Patients with comorbid hyperacusis showed increased scores in tinnitus and depression questionnaires and decreased scores in physical and psychological dimensions of quality of life. Along with this the numeric rating scales showed enhanced scores for tinnitus loudness, discomfort, annoyance and unpleasantness. The ability to ignore tinnitus was subjectively decreased in hyperacusis patients. These findings clearly confirm that comorbid hyperacusis increases the negative influence of tinnitus on quality of life [29,30]. Moreover the risk for comorbid depression is increased as demonstrated by both an increased amount of depressive symptoms and more frequent psychiatric treatment. Hyperacusis patients screened for mental conditions showed a high probability

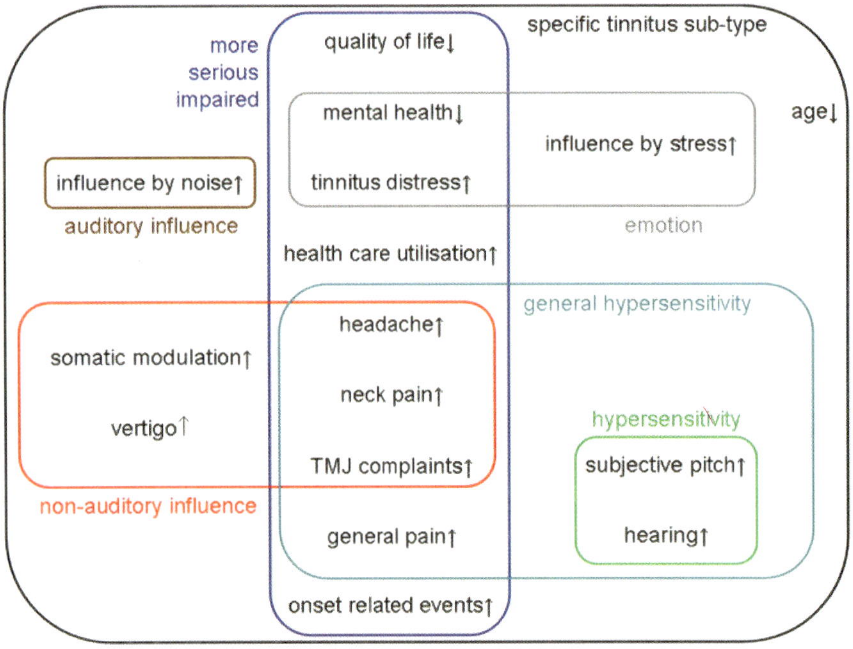

Figure 1. Illustrative overview of the Tinnitus Research Initiative Database analysis showing significant [p<0.001; d>0.2] effects for hyperacusis in tinnitus. Significant variables are subsumed for illustrative purposes in colored boxes.

for psychiatric comorbidity, especially anxiety disorders and neuroticism personality traits [31]. The higher overall number of tinnitus-related treatments, the higher number of reported events triggering tinnitus onset, and the high number of comorbid conditions can be summarized by the notion that tinnitus with hyperacusis is a more serious condition than tinnitus alone (blue box, figure 1).

Increased mental burden, increased tinnitus distress, reduced quality of life and increased modulation of tinnitus by stress in tinnitus patients with hyperacusis point to an increased role of brain circuits for emotional processing (grey box, figure 1) in patients with both hyperacusis and tinnitus. For tinnitus, there is clear evidence from neuroimaging studies of the involvement of emotion-related brain areas [8,9,32] in the pathology. For hyperacusis there are some suggestions of involvement of non-auditory areas. In a recent electroencephalography study, hyperacusis in tinnitus patients was related to increased activity in the auditory, anterior cingulate, and orbitofrontal cortex and increased connectivity between these areas [14]. The anterior cingulate and orbitofrontal cortex are brain areas which are related to vigilance and salience detection; pathalogically they are involved in anxiety disorders and may represent a "hypervigilance" or "hyperresponsive" network [14].

In addition to the increased relevance of emotional factors we also found evidence to suggest a more frequent involvement of somatosensoric aspects in tinnitus with comorbid hyperacusis (red box, figure 1). Increased prevalence of headache, neck pain, and TMJ complaints together with increased modulation of tinnitus by somatic manoeuvres all highlight the role of somatosensoric afferents. For TMJ disorder, there is clear evidence that TMJ complaints and tinnitus are inter-related. Severity of tinnitus is related to severity of TMJ pain [33]; tinnitus patients with subjectively or objectively assessed TMJ disorders can modulate their tinnitus with somatic manoeuvres [34,35] and the prevalence of tinnitus is increased in TMJ disorder [36]. This trigeminal influence might be mediated via the cochlear nucleus [37]. Both the hypersensitivity to somatic input and the increased prevalence of vertigo in tinnitus patients with hyperacusis could be the consequence of a generally increased sensitivity to sensory input, independent from the sensory modality (turquois box, figure 1). This would be in line with the notion of an overactivation of an unspecific hypervigilance network in people with hyperacusis [14].

Besides hypersensitivity to auditory, somatic and vestibular input, a divergence between subjective estimation and audiologic measures of tinnitus pitch, loudness and hearing level was found (green box, figure 1). Hyperacusis patients with tinnitus rate their hearing level as worse, their tinnitus as louder, and their tinnitus pitch as higher whereas the audiologic measurements do not show such a tendency for tinnitus patients with hyperacusis. These findings fit to the generalized hypervigilance hypothesis [38] which states that these patients have a "perceptual habit that involves subjective amplification of a variety of aversive sensations" [39]. This hypothesis was deduced from studies in fibromyalgia patients who showed increased perceived intensity and unpleasantness of cutaneous and auditory stimuli [39]. The notion of an unspecific hyperresponsive network is further supported by the investigation of people with subjective electromagnetic hypersensitivity, those who more frequently perceive tinnitus [40] and those who demonstrate an overactivation of the hyperresponsive network even in the absence of a real sensory stimulus [41].

It should be noted that tinnitus characteristics like duration, laterality, character, day-to-day changes in loudness, or intermittent/constant manifestation showed no relationship with hyperacusis. A possible hyperacusis subtype of tinnitus is not related to or a consequence of specific tinnitus characteristics. This makes it probable that hyperacusis is not a consequence but rather a predisposition for tinnitus. This notion is supported by animal studies, which have demonstrated behavioural changes suggestive of the development of hyperacusis, before the presence of tinnitus, after noise trauma [42]. Hypersensitivity might be relevant both for external sounds and for intermittent and chronic tinnitus percepts that cause difficulties in coping with the tinnitus.

A limitation of our study is the definition of hyperacusis. In the lack of internationally accepted diagnostic standards we defined hyperacusis by the answer to the question "Do sounds cause you pain and physical discomfort?". However, this question may focus particularly on one specific aspect of hyperacusis. Hyperacusis or decreased tolerance to sound might also exist without pain or physical discomfort. In addition, another aspect related to hyperacusis is the phenomenon of loudness recruitment which is the abnormally rapid increase in perceived loudness with increasing steps of presented sounds. Loudness recruitment is typically caused by sensorineural hearing loss and is restricted to frequencies of hearing loss [5,6]. It is suggested that hyperacusis and loudness recruitment represent different conditions which are not necessarily exclusive [4]. Another aspect is the missing precision of sounds. The question might be ambiguously interpreted and related not only to external sounds but also to the tinnitus. Based on these limitations we suggest that future studies should clearly describe the used definition of hyperacusis and should clearly consider related aspects of hyperacusis such as loudness recruitment. Furthermore it has to be mentioned that the conclusions of this analysis are limited to patients with hyperacusis and tinnitus. We are well aware that hyperacusis may also be present without tinnitus, but we cannot draw any conclusions about hyperacusis without tinnitus from our manuscript.

All these findings together with the fact that hyperacusis is related to an earlier onset and younger age at presentation at the clinic with an average of four years, affirm the assumption that hyperacusis constitutes a specific tinnitus subtype (black box, figure 1). This subtype is characterized by higher tinnitus related and general distress, decreased mental and somatic health, increased influence of sensory inputs and general hypersensitivity. However, we cannot exclude that the observed differences between tinnitus patients with and without hyperacusis all reflect increased severity in the hyperacusis group rather than a distinct mechanism of generating tinnitus. Increased severity might mediate the effects found for the other variables. Future studies should try to control for such spurious correlations. Independent of the interpretation, these findings highlight the importance of identifying comorbid hyperacusis both for clinical management and for neuroscientific tinnitus research.

Acknowledgments

We want to thank Susanne Staudinger, Sylvia Dorner-Mitschke, Sandra Pfluegl, Helene Niebling, and Jarmila Gerxhaliu-Holan for their help and effort in collecting and handling data. The TRI Database Study Group: Veronika Vielsmeier, Tobias Kleinjung, Astrid Lehner, Peter Kreuzer, Timm B. Poeppl, Ricardo Figueiredo, Andréia Azevedo, Ana Carolina Binetti, Ana Belén Elgoyhen, Marcelo Rates, Claudia Coelho, Sven Vanneste, Dirk de Ridder, Paul van de Heyning, Florian Zeman, Michael Koller.

Author Contributions

Conceived and designed the experiments: MS ML BL. Performed the experiments: ML BL. Analyzed the data: MS. Contributed reagents/materials/analysis tools: MS. Wrote the paper: MS ML BL. Contributed

References

1. Shargorodsky J, Curhan GC, Farwell WR (2010) Prevalence and characteristics of tinnitus among US adults. Am J Med 123[8]: 711–718.
2. Krog NH, Engdahl B, Tambs K (2010) The association between tinnitus and mental health in a general population sample: results from the HUNT Study. J Psychosom Res 69[3]: 289–298.
3. Langguth B (2011) A review of tinnitus symptoms beyond 'ringing in the ears': a call to action. Curr Med Res Opin 27[8]:1635–1643.
4. Baguley DM (2003) Hyperacusis. J R Soc Med 96[12]: 582–585.
5. Blasing L, Goebel G, Flotzinger U, Berthold A, Kroner-Herwig B (2010) Hypersensitivity to sound in tinnitus patients: an analysis of a construct based on questionnaire and audiological data. Int J Audiol 49[7]: 518–526.
6. Katzenell U, Segal S (2001) Hyperacusis: review and clinical guidelines. Otol Neurotol 22[3]: 321–326.
7. Eggermont JJ, Roberts LE (2004) The neuroscience of tinnitus. Trends Neurosci 27[11]: 676–682.
8. De Ridder D, Vanneste S, Weisz N, Londero A, Schlee W, et al. (in press) An integrative model of auditory phantom perception: Tinnitus as a unified percept of interacting separable subnetworks. Neurosci Biobehav Rev.
9. De Ridder D, Elgoyhen AB, Romo R, Langguth B (2011) Phantom percepts: tinnitus and pain as persisting aversive memory networks. Proc Natl Acad Sci U S A 108[20]: 8075–8080.
10. Cima RF, Maes IH, Joore MA, Scheyen DJ, El Refaie A, et al. (2012) Specialised treatment based on cognitive behaviour therapy versus usual care for tinnitus: a randomised controlled trial. Lancet 379[9830]: 1951–1959.
11. Nelson JJ, Chen K (2004) The relationship of tinnitus, hyperacusis, and hearing loss. Ear Nose Throat J 83[7]: 472–476.
12. Hebert S, Fournier P, Norena A (2013) The auditory sensitivity is increased in tinnitus ears. J Neurosci 33[6]: 2356–2364.
13. Hwang JH, Chou PH, Wu CW, Chen JH, Liu TC (2009) Brain activation in patients with idiopathic hyperacusis. Am J Otolaryngol 30[6]: 432–434.
14. Song JJ, De Ridder D, Weisz N, Schlee W, Van de Heyning P, et al. (in press) Hyperacusis-associated pathological resting-state brain oscillations in the tinnitus brain: a hyperresponsiveness network with paradoxically inactive auditory cortex. Brain Struct Funct.
15. Meeus OM, Spaepen M, Ridder DD, Heyning PH (2010) Correlation between hyperacusis measurements in daily ENT practice. Int J Audiol 49[1]: 7–13.
16. Jastreboff PJ, Jastreboff MM (2000) Tinnitus Retraining Therapy [TRT] as a method for treatment of tinnitus and hyperacusis patients. J Am Acad Audiol 11[3]: 162–177.
17. Klein AJ, Armstrong BL, Greer MK, Brown FR (1990) Hyperacusis and otitis media in individuals with Williams syndrome. J Speech Hear Disord 55[2]: 339–344.
18. Zeng FG (2013) An active loudness model suggesting tinnitus as increased central noise and hyperacusis as increased nonlinear gain. Hear Res 295: 172–179.
19. Norena AJ (2011) An integrative model of tinnitus based on a central gain controlling neural sensitivity. Neurosci Biobehav Rev 35[5]:1089–1109.
20. Gu JW, Halpin CF, Nam EC, Levine RA, Melcher JR (2010) Tinnitus, diminished sound-level tolerance, and elevated auditory activity in humans with clinically normal hearing sensitivity. J Neurophysiol 104[6]: 3361–3370.
21. Zeman F, Koller M, Schecklmann M, Langguth B, Landgrebe M (2012) Tinnitus assessment by means of standardized self-report questionnaires: psychometric properties of the Tinnitus Questionnaire (TQ), the Tinnitus Handicap Inventory (THI]), and their short versions in an international and multi-lingual sample. Health Qual Life Outcomes 10: 128.
22. Landgrebe M, Zeman F, Koller M, Eberl Y, Mohr M, et al. (2010) The Tinnitus Research Initiative (TRI) database: a new approach for delineation of tinnitus subtypes and generation of predictors for treatment outcome. BMC Med Inform Decis Mak 10: 42.
23. Schecklmann M, Vielsmeier V, Steffens T, Landgrebe M, Langguth B, et al. (2012) Relationship between Audiometric slope and tinnitus pitch in tinnitus patients: insights into the mechanisms of tinnitus generation. PLoS One 7[4]: e34878.
24. Cohen J (1988) Statistical Power Analysis for the Behavioral Sciences. 2. ed: Hillsdale: Lawrence Erlbaum Associates.
25. Rosenthal R (1994) Parametric measures of effect size. In: Cooper H, Hedges LV, editors. The Handbook of Research Synthesis: New York: Sage.
26. Jastreboff PJ, Hazell JW (1993) A neurophysiological approach to tinnitus: clinical implications. Br J Audiol 27[1]: 7–17.
27. Chen G, Lee C, Sandridge SA, Butler HM, Manzoor NF, et al. (2013) Behavioral evidence for possible simultaneous induction of hyperacusis and tinnitus following intense sound exposure. J Assoc Res Otolaryngol 14[3]:413–24.
28. Sereda M, Adjamian P, Edmondson-Jones M, Palmer AR, Hall DA (2013) Auditory evoked magnetic fields in individuals with tinnitus. Hear Res 302: 50–59.
29. Falkenberg ES, Wie OB (2012) Anxiety and depression in tinnitus patients: 5-year follow-up assessment after completion of habituation therapy. Int J Otolaryngol 2012: 375460.
30. Fioretti AB, Fusetti M, Eibenstein A (2013) Association between sleep disorders, hyperacusis and tinnitus: evaluation with tinnitus questionnaires. Noise Health 15[63]: 91–95.
31. Juris L, Andersson G, Larsen HC, Ekselius L (2013) Psychiatric comorbidity and personality traits in patients with hyperacusis. Int J Audiol 52[4]: 230–235.
32. Rauschecker JP, Leaver AM, Mühlau M (2010) Tuning out the noise: limbic-auditory interactions in tinnitus. Neuron 66[6]: 819–826.

33. Saldanha AD, Hilgenberg PB, Pinto LM, Conti PC (2012) Are temporomandibular disorders and tinnitus associated? Cranio 30[3]: 166–171.
34. Vielsmeier V, Strutz J, Kleinjung T, Schecklmann M, Kreuzer PM, et al. (2012) Temporomandibular joint disorder complaints in tinnitus: further hints for a putative tinnitus subtype. PLoS One 7[6]: e38887.
35. Vielsmeier V, Kleinjung T, Strutz J, Burgers R, Kreuzer PM, et al. (2011) Tinnitus with temporomandibular joint disorders: a specific entity of tinnitus patients? Otolaryngol Head Neck Surg. 2011 145[5]: 748–752.
36. Tuz HH, Onder EM, Kisnisci RS (2003) Prevalence of otologic complaints in patients with temporomandibular disorder. Am J Orthod Dentofacial Orthop 123[6]: 620–623.
37. Basura GJ, Koehler SD, Shore SE (2012) Multi-sensory integration in brainstem and auditory cortex. Brain Res 1485: 95–107.
38. McDermid AJ, Rollman GB, McCain GA (1996) Generalized hypervigilance in fibromyalgia: evidence of perceptual amplification. Pain 66[2–3]: 133–44.
39. Hollins M, Harper D, Gallagher S, Owings EW, Lim PF, et al. (2009) Perceived intensity and unpleasantness of cutaneous and auditory stimuli: an evaluation of the generalized hypervigilance hypothesis. Pain 141[3]: 215–221.
40. Landgrebe M, Frick U, Hauser S, Hajak G, Langguth B (2009) Association of tinnitus and electromagnetic hypersensitivity: hints for a shared pathophysiology? PLoS One 4[3]: e5026.
41. Landgrebe M, Barta W, Rosengarth K, Frick U, Hauser S, et al. (2008) Neuronal correlates of symptom formation in functional somatic syndromes: a fMRI study. Neuroimage 41[4]: 1336–1344.
42. Turner J, Larsen D, Hughes L, Moechars D, Shore S (2012) Time course of tinnitus development following noise exposure in mice. J Neurosci Res 90[7]: 1480–1488.

28

Optimal Dosage of Methylprednisolone for the Treatment of Sudden Hearing Loss in Geriatric Patients: A Propensity Score-Matched Analysis

Myoung Su Choi, Ho Yun Lee*, Chin Saeng Cho

Department of Otorhinolaryngology, Department of Otorhinolaryngology, Head & Neck Surgery, School of Medicine, Eulji University Medical Center, Eulji University, Daejeon, Korea

Abstract

We aimed to compare the treatment outcomes and the occurrence rates of adverse events associated with different steroid regimens in geriatric patients (aged 65 years or older) with unilateral idiopathic sudden sensorineural hearing loss (ISSNHL). After thorough medical chart reviews of 109 patients with ISSNHL between May 2006 and December 2013, we performed a propensity score-matched analysis using previously known prognostic factors, steroid regimens, and other cointerventions. Patients were divided based on their steroid regimens into group I (which initially received 48 mg of methylprednisolone daily with a subsequently tapered dose) and group II (which initially received 24 mg of methylprednisolone daily with a subsequently tapered dose). We compared final hearing and the occurrence of adverse events between the two groups. As a result, 20 pairs of propensity score-matched patients ($n = 40$) were enrolled. Group I patients showed better final hearing levels compared with group II patients (42.00 ± 22.35 dB and 57.38 ± 26.40 dB, respectively), although this difference was marginally significant ($p = 0.058$). Based on the comparative analysis of each of the frequencies in the final audiograms, lower hearing thresholds at 2 KHz were observed in group I ($p = 0.049$). There was no significant difference in the occurrence of adverse effects between the two groups ($p > 0.05$). In conclusion, conventional steroid regimens produced adverse event occurrence rates that were similar to those of low-dose treatment but may also have produced superior hearing recovery. The use of steroid dose reduction in geriatric patients with ISSNHL is not preferable to conventional steroid regimens.

Editor: Hanjun Liu, Sun Yat-sen University, China

Funding: This research was supported by EMBRI Grants 2013 EMBRI-DJ-0005 from Eulji University. The funders had no role in study design, data collection and analysis, decision to publish, and had a role in the preparation of the manuscript.

Competing Interests: The authors have declared that no competing interests exist.

* Email: hoyun1004@gmail.com

Introduction

According to recent guidelines, initial corticosteroid treatment can be administered to patients with idiopathic sudden sensorineural hearing loss (ISSNHL) [1]. Such treatment is commonly used on the basis of the hypothesis that it may affect the inner ear and induce suppression of the immune response, changes in microcirculation, and a decrease in endolymphatic pressure [2]. However, the effects of steroids on the treatment of sudden hearing loss remain unclear [3]. Although the adverse effects that occur after a 10- to 14-day course of steroids are usually acceptable and manageable [1], various symptoms may occur, including weight gain, gastritis, hypertension, hyperglycemia, cataracts, avascular necrosis of the hip, as well as changes in appetite, mood, sleep patterns, and even death [1,4,5].

A study of 18226 patients with diabetes revealed that patients with diabetes and chronic obstructive pulmonary disease who used high-dose corticosteroids were at a greater risk of diabetes-related hospitalization and suggested that the minimally effective corticosteroid dose should be used [6]. More than two-thirds of the geriatric population (aged 65 years or older) have hypertension and 22% to 33% have diabetes, which are associated with a high risk of major complications such as lower-extremity amputation, myocardial infarction, and visual impairment [7,8]. Therefore, the burden of complications associated with corticosteroid use may be larger in the elderly population than in younger patients.

Prednisone at a dose of 60 mg daily or methylprednisolone (MPD) at a dose of 48 mg for 7 to 14 days is frequently used as an initial medication in the treatment of ISSNHL, and the doses are subsequently tapered [1]. However, many clinicians use slightly different protocols in terms of the type of steroid, dosage, and duration in different clinical settings, and the number of comparative studies of different steroid protocols is limited [1,9].

Based on these findings, we assumed that, if treatment outcomes following low-dose steroid treatments were as effective as those following higher-dose steroid treatments, the low-dose treatments would be accompanied by a reduced risk of adverse effects and that the use of low-dose steroid treatments for ISSNHL in geriatric patients would be more rational.

In this study, we aimed to compare the treatment outcomes and the occurrence rates of adverse events according to different

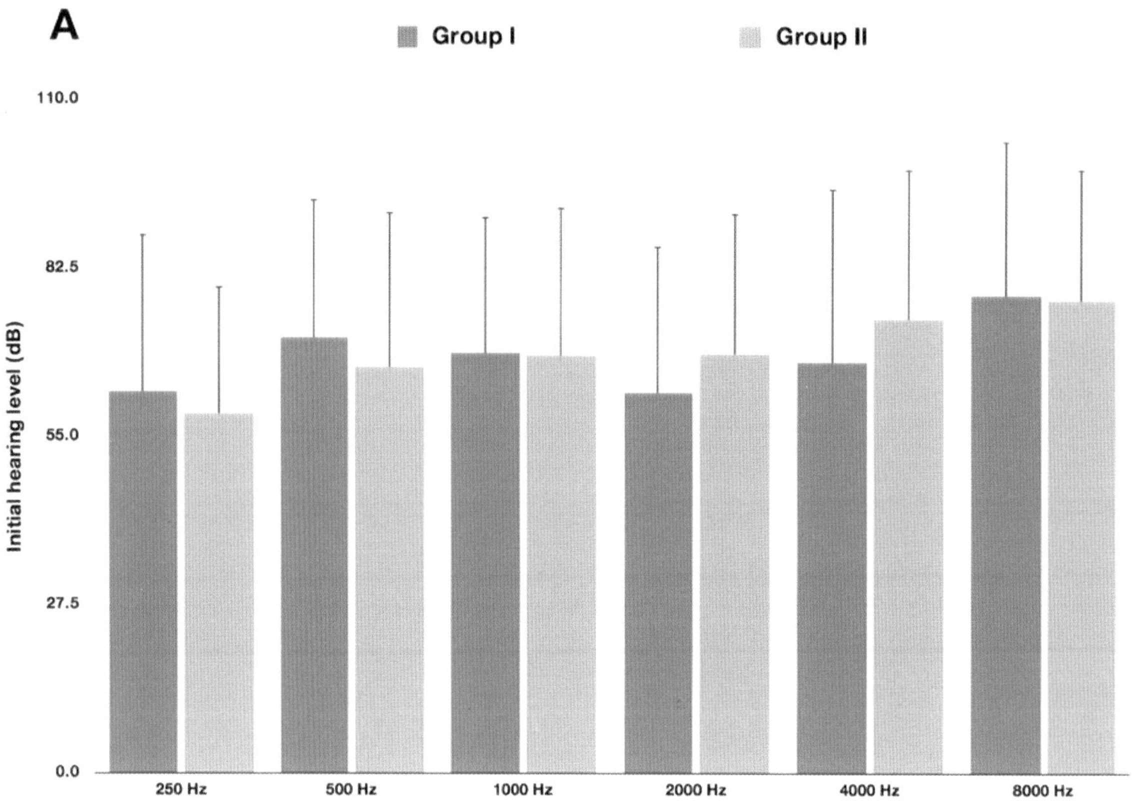
A
Group I
Group II
110.0
82.5
55.0
27.5
0.0
Initial hearing level (dB)
250 Hz
500 Hz
1000 Hz
2000 Hz
4000 Hz
8000 Hz

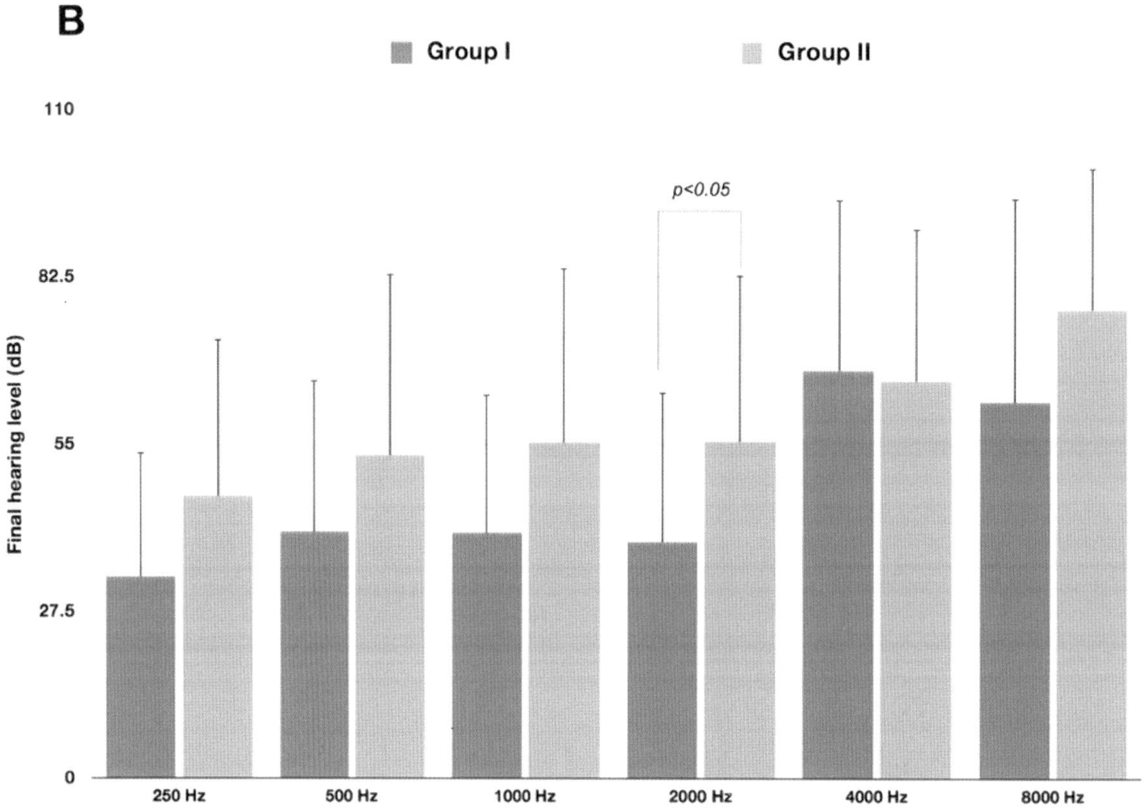
B
Group I
Group II
110
82.5
55
27.5
0
Final hearing level (dB)
p<0.05
250 Hz
500 Hz
1000 Hz
2000 Hz
4000 Hz
8000 Hz

Figure 1. Changes in hearing levels at each frequency before and after treatment in propensity-score matched population. (A) Comparison of the pretreatment hearing levels at each frequency. (B) Comparison of the posttreatment hearing levels at each frequency.

steroid regimens in ISSNHL patients aged 65 years or older by using a propensity score-matched (PSM) analysis.

Materials and Methods

Ethics Statement

This study was approved by the Institutional Review Board of the Eulji University (No. 2014-02-010). The Board granted a waiver of written informed consent for this retrospective study.

Patients

Based on retrospective medical chart reviews, we enrolled patients who were aged 65 years or older and had been diagnosed with ISSNHL and admitted to the university hospital between May 2006 and December 2013. The exclusion criteria were as follows: 1) concomitant meningitis, myelitis, vasculopathy, or neuropsychiatric disease; 2) a clinical observation period less than 3 months; 3) previous histories of sudden hearing loss and/or the possibility of Meniere's disease; and 4) uncontrolled hypertension or uncontrolled diabetes mellitus.

Age, sex, comorbid diabetes and hypertension, the presence of dizziness and/or tinnitus, the period of time from onset to treatment, the initial hearing levels of both ears, and the final hearing level of the affected side 3 months after the onset of treatment were documented.

Treatment Protocols

All patients were hospitalized for 1 week, and one of two types of treatment was provided using the time-variant differential approach: either oral MPD treatment or "low-dose" oral MPD treatment. Oral MPD treatment was administered between 2006 and 2008. Subsequently, oral "low-dose" MPD treatment became the mainstream treatment and was commonly used until 2010. From early 2011, an additional intratympanic dexamethasone injection (IT-DEX) administered as a salvage therapy following oral MPD treatment has been the main treatment for sudden deafness.

Patients who received the oral MPD treatment were treated with steroids for 10 days using the same recommended dosage protocol for MPD (48 mg/d for 4 days, followed by a taper of 8 mg every 2 days) [9]. The total cumulative dose of MPD was 432 mg (equivalent to 530 mg of prednisolone) over 14 days. These patients were classified as group I. Patients who received the oral "low-dose" MPD treatment were treated with a half-dose of oral MPD (24 mg/d for the first 4 days, followed by a taper by 8 mg every 2 days). The total cumulative dose of MPD was 144 mg (equivalent to 180 mg of prednisolone) over 8 days. These patients were classified as group II.

Moreover, for patients who required an additional cointervention, a continuous infusion of 10 μg/d of alprostadil over 7 days or daily intravenous infusions of 88 mg of zinc sulfate hydrate were provided.

Calculation of Hearing Levels and Estimation of Recoveries

Hearing levels were calculated using the arithmetic mean of the hearing levels at 500 Hz, 1 kHz, 2 kHz, and 4 kHz. Hearing improvement rates were calculated as the hearing gain divided by the initial hearing difference between the lesion side and the healthy side and then multiplied by 100 [10,11]. Complete recovery was defined by a final hearing level within 20 dB or equal to the hearing level of the unaffected ear [10,11]. Good recovery was defined as hearing gains greater than 30 dB [10,11]. Fair recovery was defined as hearing gains of 10 to 29 dB. Hearing

Table 1. Baseline clinical characteristics.

	Total population			Propensity-matched population		
	Group I (n = 66)	**Group II (n = 43)**	**p-value**	**Group I (n = 20)**	**Group II (n = 20)**	**p-value**
Age	72.52±5.00	70.49±5.24	0.045	71.45±5.56	71.10±5.15	0.816
Male	26 (59.1)	18 (58.1)	0.798	9 (45.0)	9 (45.0)	1.000
Body mass index (kg/m^2)	25.10±3.58	24.46±3.14	0.342	25.43±3.87	24.79±3.32	0.555
Diabetes mellitus	17 (25.8)	9 (20.9)	0.563	4 (20.0)	4 (20.0)	1.000
Hypertension	29 (43.9)	27 (62.8)	0.054	10 (50.0)	7 (35.0)	0.337
Days from onset to treatment	3.98±2.73	3.86±3.24	0.829	4.00±3.04	3.40±1.96	0.333
Right side	33 (50.0)	23 (53.5)	0.722	9 (45.0)	9 (45.0)	1.000
Dizziness	12 (18.2)	4 (9.3)	0.200	3 (15.0)	2 (10.0)	0.633
Tinnitus	43 (65.2)	33 (76.7)	0.198	16 (80.0)	15 (75.0)	0.705
Intratympanic injection	5 (7.6)	4 (9.3)	0.749	0 (0.0)	0 (0.0)	–
Alprostadil injection	48 (72.7)	30 (69.8)	0.738	15 (75.0)	18 (90.0)	0.212
Zinc injection	7 (10.6)	1 (2.3)	0.144	0 (0.0)	0 (0.0)	–
Initial hearing (dB)	65.70±23.34	73.92±22.51	0.071	67.38±22.16	69.38±22.25	0.800
Initial contralateral hearing (dB)	43.22±26.89	43.66±22.08	0.928	41.38±27.55	42.63±22.19	0.890
Final hearing (dB)	46.67±26.20	56.54±26.98	0.060	42.00±22.35	57.38±26.40	0.058

Data are presented as mean±standard deviation or number (percentage).

Table 2. Comparison of the posttreatment hearing levels at each frequency.

	250 Hz	500 Hz	1000 Hz	2000 Hz	4000 Hz	8000 Hz
Group I (dB)	33.25±20.28	40.75±24.83	40.50±22.65	39.00±24.53	67.25±28.03	62.00±33.50
Group II (dB)	46.50±25.76	53.25±29.84	55.25±28.72	55.50±27.38	65.50±24.92	77.25±23.25
p-value	0.096	0.142	0.065	0.049*	0.864	0.109

Data are presented as mean±standard deviation; *: $p<0.05$.

gains of less than 10 dB were defined as no change or deterioration [10,11].

Adverse Events

From the medical chart reviews, insomnia, abdominal discomfort, high blood pressure that occurred more than twice per day (systolic pressure, ≥150 mmHg, and/or diastolic pressure, ≥ 90 mmHg), and hyperglycemia for which insulin had been newly prescribed or increased were documented. Additionally, major complications such as myocardial infarction, gastrointestinal bleeding, and death were also documented.

Statistical Analyses

The details of the estimation of the propensity scores were as follows: (1) age, sex, accompanying hypertension and diabetes, presence of tinnitus or dizziness, initial hearing levels of the lesion and healthy sides, IT-DEX treatment, and other cointerventions (alprostadil or zinc injection) were selected as covariates based on the results of the previous studies [12–16]; (2) treatment assignment (group I or II) was used as the outcome variable; (3) logistic regression was performed, and propensity scores were calculated. The 1:1 nearest-neighbor method was used for matching. Next, a test of the balance of the covariates was performed, and the treatment effects were finally compared using paired t-tests and McNemar's tests. All statistical analyses were performed using the SPSS software (ver. 18.0, SPSS Inc., Chicago, IL, USA), and the level of statistical significance was set at a p-value of less than 0.05.

Results

A total of 109 patients were enrolled in this study, including 44 men (40.4%) and 65 women (59.6%), with a mean age of 71.72 years (range, 65–87 years) and mean ISSNHL duration (from the onset to treatment) of 3.94±2.93 days. Diabetes was reported in 26 patients (23.9%) and hypertension in 56 (51.4%). Of accompanying symptoms, 76 patients (69.7%) had tinnitus and 16 (14.7%) had dizziness. The mean initial hearing level was 68.95±23.26 dB and the initial contralateral hearing level was 43.39±25.00 dB. The baseline characteristics revealed marginally significant differences in age ($p=0.045$), accompanying hypertension ($p=0.054$), and initial hearing levels ($p=0.071$) between the steroid regimen groups.

After the PSM analysis, 20 pairs of patients were allocated either to group I or II (Table 1), and the balance test revealed that there were no significant differences in any of the covariates ($p>0.05$). The final hearing level in group I was 42.00±22.35 dB and that in group II was 57.38±26.40 dB ($p=0.058$, 95% confidence interval of the difference: −31.30 dB to 0.55 dB). Comparison of the individual frequencies in the PSM population revealed that the pretreatment audiograms were not different at any of the frequencies between the two groups (Figure 1A, $p>0.05$); however, the posttreatment audiograms showed marginally significant differences at 1000 Hz ($p=0.065$) and 2000 Hz ($p=0.049$) (Figure 1B, Table 2).

The hearing improvement rates did not differ between groups I and II (114.69±299.56% and 123.32±392.28%, respectively; $p=0.941$). Regarding hearing recovery, group I showed a tendency for better recovery compared with group II, but the difference was not significant (Table 3, $p>0.05$).

Table 3. Treatment outcomes according to different steroid regimens.

Total population (n = 109)	Total population			Propensity-matched population		
	Group I (n = 66)	Group II (n = 43)	p-value	Group I (n = 20)	Group II (n = 20)	p-value
Recovery, n (%)						
CR	7 (10.6)	1 (2.3)	0.144	2 (10.0)	1 (5.0)	0.370
CR+GR	25 (37.9)	11 (25.6)	0.182	8 (40.0)	3 (15.0)	0.109
CR+GR+FR	42 (63.6)	23 (53.5)	0.291	15 (75.0)	10 (50.0)	0.227
HIR	40.46±270.90	80.13±269.90	0.456	114.69±299.56	123.32±392.28	0.941
Adverse effects, n (%)						
Insomnia	5 (7.6)	1(2.3)	0.400	2 (10.0)	1(5.0)	1.000
Abdominal discomfort	14 (21.2)	12 (27.9)	0.493	3(15.0)	6(15.0)	0.375
High BP	17 (25.8)	15 (34.9)	0.309	7 (35.0)	6 (30.0)	1.000
Hyperglycemia	17 (25.8)	6 (14.0)	0.140	7 (35.0)	4 (20.0)	0.453

CR: complete recovery; GR: good recovery; FR: fair recovery; HIR: hearing improvement rate; BP: blood pressure.

Regarding severe adverse events during treatment, one patient in group II experienced pulmonary edema and upper gastrointestinal bleeding. However, other major complications, such as myocardial infarction and death, did not occur in any of the groups.

Regarding minor adverse events, the PSM analysis revealed that patients in group I complained of insomnia (10% of the patients), abdominal discomfort (15%), high blood pressure (35%), and hyperglycemia (35%). However, the occurrence rates of these adverse events were not significantly different between the two groups (Table 3).

Discussion

Our study showed that patients receiving conventional steroid treatment had slightly better hearing recovery than patients who received reduced steroid doses, although the difference was marginally significant. Similar trends were found when the final audiograms at all frequencies were compared, with the exception of the 4 kHz frequency. No significant differences in the occurrence rates of adverse effects were found between the two groups.

These findings may suggest that steroid dose reduction is not preferable to the conventional steroid regimen in geriatric patients with ISSNHL.

In contrast, a prospective randomized trial reported that therapeutic outcomes did not differ between 7-day prednisolone and 300 mg dexamethasone pulse therapies [17]. The colleagues of those authors also reported newly developed myocardial infarctions in patients following the pulse therapy and urged clinicians to consider the severe risks of steroid treatment [18]. These findings suggest that the potential benefits of high-dose pulse therapy may not exceed the risks of severe complications. In addition, the duration of steroid use as well as the dosage may be important variables, both of which determine the cumulative steroid dose that may affect the hearing outcome or occurrence of adverse events. The relatively short-term duration of treatment in group II (8 days) compared with that in group I (14 days) might have affected the treatment outcome in our study. A recent survey conducted in the United States reported that 32.2% of the physicians preferred a 14-day steroid treatment, 33.2%, 10-day treatment, and 16.1%, 7-day treatment [19]. This may be attributed to the fact that the optimal dosage and duration of steroid treatment, particularly in elderly population with comorbidities, have not been determined.

With aging, liver function, which is primarily responsible for the metabolism of steroids, is mostly maintained, but phase I metabolism catalyzed by cytochrome P450 tends to decrease, and an increase in interindividual variability is distinctive [20]. Moreover, the affinities of the receptor protein for dexamethasone and corticosterone tend to decrease [21]. Therefore, the use of higher steroid doses might be more rational than lower-dose steroid treatment; however, excessively high-dose steroid treatments have failed to show additional benefits [17]. Based on these findings, we suggest that further studies comparing a greater range of steroid regimens for the treatment of ISSNHL should be performed to identify the optimal dose because we still do not have many options other than steroid treatment [9].

Apart from systemic steroid treatment, intratympanic steroid injection is currently recommended after the failure of the initial treatment [1]. Other possible treatment options include hyperbaric oxygen therapy, and a significant improvement in hearing was reported in the acute stage of ISSNHL following this therapy [22]. The mechanism of action in this therapy is now thought to be the control of cochlear ischemia by increasing oxygen partial pressure. However, in most hospitals, this therapy is not available because it requires a specific sealed chamber. Moreover, it is an expensive and time-consuming treatment method. Other possible options include medications such as antiviral agents [23], vasodilators (such as carbogen, alprostadil, naftidrofuryl, and low-molecular-weight dextran) [24], high-dose vitamins [25,26], and zinc supplementation [27]. However, the effects of these agents have not been sufficiently studied and there is no evidence to support their use.

To reduce the confounding effects between diverse treatment options and the observed baseline characteristics, we performed the PSM analysis [28,29]. Selection bias was decreased as far as possible by controlling for the diverse prognostic factors and cointerventions that may have influenced the treatment outcomes. As a result, we were able to compare the intervention effects of the examined steroid regimens by the PSM analysis in order to overcome the limitations of the retrospective, observational study design [29].

Our study has several limitations. It seems unnatural to include covariates such as IT-DEX, alprostadil, and zinc, which may act as confounding factors to the outcome, in the PSM analysis. However, the exclusion of all patients who were treated with cointerventions could result in insignificant conclusions owing to a small sample size. Therefore, we controlled cointerventions as covariates to be able to evaluate the sole effect of steroid dose by minimizing the between-group difference.

In conclusion, conventional steroid regimens produced the occurrence rates of adverse events that were similar to those of low-dose treatment but may also have produced better recoveries. The use of steroid dose reduction in geriatric patients with ISSNHL is not preferable to conventional steroid regimen.

Author Contributions

Conceived and designed the experiments: HYL CSC. Performed the experiments: MSC HYL. Analyzed the data: MSC HYL. Contributed reagents/materials/analysis tools: MSC HYL. Wrote the paper: MSC HYL.

References

1. Stachler RJ, Chandrasekhar SS, Archer SM, Rosenfeld RM, Schwartz SR, et al. (2012) Clinical practice guideline: sudden hearing loss. Otolaryngol Head Neck Surg 146(3 Suppl): S1-35.
2. Schreiber BE, Agrup C, Haskard DO, Luxon LM (2010) Sudden sensorineural hearing loss. Lancet 375: 1203–1211.
3. Wei BP, Stathopoulos D, O'Leary S (2013) Steroids for idiopathic sudden sensorineural hearing loss. Cochrane Database Syst Rev 7: CD003998.
4. Rauch SD, Halpin CF, Antonelli PJ, Babu S, Carey JP, et al. (2011) Oral vs intratympanic corticosteroid therapy for idiopathic sudden sensorineural hearing loss: a randomized trial. JAMA 305: 2071–2079.
5. Ogino-Nishimura E, Nakagawa T, Tateya I, Hiraumi H, Ito J (2013) Systemic steroid application caused sudden death of a patient with sudden deafness. Case Rep Otolaryngol 3: 734131–7341312. doi:10.1155/2013/734131
6. Caughey GE, Preiss AK, Vitry AI, Gilbert AL, Roughead EE (2013) Comorbid diabetes and COPD: impact of corticosteroid use on diabetes complications. Diabetes Care 36: 3009–3014. doi:10.2337/dc12-2197
7. Lionakis N, Mendrinos D, Sanidas E, Favatas G, Georgopoulou M (2012) Hypertension in the elderly. World J Cardiol 4: 135–147.
8. Kirkman MS, Briscoe VJ, Clark N, Florez H, Haas LB, et al. (2012) Diabetes in older adults. Diabetes Care 35: 2650–2664.
9. Rauch SD (2008) Clinical practice. Idiopathic sudden sensorineural hearing loss. N Engl J Med 359: 833–840.
10. Kanzaki J, Taiji H, Ogawa K (1988) Evaluation of hearing recovery and efficacy of steroid treatment in sudden deafness. Acta Otolaryngol Suppl 456: 31–36.
11. Suzuki H, Hashida K, Nguyen KH, Hohchi N, Katoh A, et al. (2012) Efficacy of intratympanic steroid administration on idiopathic sudden sensorineural hearing

loss in comparison with hyperbaric oxygen therapy. Laryngoscope 122: 1154–1157.
12. Xenellis J, Karapatsas I, Papadimitriou N, Nikolopoulos T, Maragoudakis P, et al. (2006) Idiopathic sudden sensorineural hearing loss: prognostic factors. J Laryngol Otol 120: 718–724.
13. Cvorović L, Deric D, Probst R, Hegemann S (2008) Prognostic model for predicting hearing recovery in idiopathic sudden sensorineural hearing loss. Otol Neurotol 29: 464–469.
14. Hikita-Watanabe N, Kitahara T, Horii A, Kawashima T, Doi K, et al. (2010) Tinnitus as a prognostic factor of sudden deafness. Acta Otolaryngol 130: 79–83.
15. Yang CH, Ko MT, Peng JP, Hwang CF (2011) Zinc in the treatment of idiopathic sudden sensorineural hearing loss. Laryngoscope 121: 617–621. doi:10.1002/lary.21291 Epub 2010 Oct 6.
16. Kim MG, Jung YG, Eun YG (2011) Effect of steroid, carbogen inhalation, and lipoprostaglandin E1 combination therapy for sudden sensorineural hearing loss. Am J Otolaryngol 32: 91–95. doi:10.1016/j.amjoto.2009
17. Westerlaken BO, de Kleine E, van der Laan B, Albers F (2007) The treatment of idiopathic sudden sensorineural hearing loss using pulse therapy: a prospective, randomized, double-blind clinical trial. Laryngoscope 117: 684–690.
18. Free RH, Smale ND, de Kleine E, van der Laan BF (2009) Side effects of oral dexamethasone pulse therapy for idiopathic sudden sensorineural hearing loss. Otol Neurotol 30: 691.
19. Coelho DH, Thacker LR, Hsu DW (2011) Variability in the management of idiopathic sudden sensorineural hearing loss. Otolaryngol Head Neck Surg 145: 813–817.
20. Schmucker DL (2001) Liver function and phase I drug metabolism in the elderly: a paradox. Drugs Aging 18: 837–851.
21. Bolla R (1980) Age-dependent changes in rat liver steroid hormone receptor proteins. Mech Ageing Dev 12: 249–259.
22. Bennett MH, Kertesz T, Perleth M, Yeung P, Lehm JP (2012) Hyperbaric oxygen for idiopathic sudden sensorineural hearing loss and tinnitus. Cochrane Database Syst Rev 17: CD004739.
23. Awad Z, Huins C, Pothier DD (2012) Antivirals for idiopathic sudden sensorineural hearing loss. Cochrane Database Syst Rev 15: CD006987.
24. Agarwal L, Pothier DD (2009) Vasodilators and vasoactive substances for idiopathic sudden sensorineural hearing loss. Cochrane Database Syst Rev 7: CD003422.
25. Kaya H, Koç AK, Sayın I, Güneş S, Altıntaş A, et al. (2014) Vitamins A, C, and E and selenium in the treatment of idiopathic sudden sensorineural hearing loss. Eur Arch Otorhinolaryngol. doi:10.1007/s00405-014-2922-9 Epub ahead of print.
26. Kang HS, Park JJ, Ahn SK, Hur DG, Kim HY (2013) Effect of high dose intravenous vitamin C on idiopathic sudden sensorineural hearing loss: a prospective single-blind randomized controlled trial. Eur Arch Otorhinolaryngol 270: 2631–2636.
27. Yang CH, Ko MT, Peng JP, Hwang CF (2011) Zinc in the treatment of idiopathic sudden sensorineural hearing loss. Laryngoscope 121: 617–621.
28. Stuart EA (2010) Matching methods for causal inference: A review and a look forward. Stat Sci 25: 1–21.
29. Austin PC, Laupacis A (2011) A tutorial on methods to estimating clinically and policy-meaningful measures of treatment effects in prospective observational studies: a review. Int J Biostat 7: 6. doi:10.2202/1557-4679.1285

Whole-Exome Sequencing Identifies a Novel Genotype-Phenotype Correlation in the Entactin Domain of the Known Deafness Gene *TECTA*

Byung Yoon Choi[1]¶, Jiwoong Kim[2]¶, Juyong Chung[3], Ah Reum Kim[4], Sue Jean Mun[4], Seong Il Kang[4], Sang-Heon Lee[2,5], Namshin Kim[2,5]*, Seung-Ha Oh[4]*

1 Department of Otorhinolaryngology, Seoul National University Bundang Hospital, Seongnam, South Korea, **2** Korean Bioinformation center, Korea Research Institute of Bioscience and Biotechnology (KRIBB), Daejeon, South Korea, **3** Department of Otolaryngology, Ajou University School of Medicine, Suwon, South Korea, **4** Department of Otorhinolaryngology, Seoul national University College of Medicine, Seoul, South Korea, **5** Department of Bioinformatics, University of Science and Technology, Daejeon, South Korea

Abstract

Postlingual progressive hearing loss, affecting primarily the high frequencies, is the clinical finding in most cases of autosomal dominant nonsyndromic hearing loss (ADNSHL). The molecular genetic etiology of ADNSHL is extremely heterogeneous. We applied whole-exome sequencing to reveal the genetic etiology of high-frequency hearing loss in a mid-sized Korean family without any prior linkage data. Whole-exome sequencing of four family members (two affected and two unaffected), together with our filtering strategy based on comprehensive bioinformatics analyses, identified 21 potential pathogenic candidates. Sanger validation of an additional five family members excluded 20 variants, leaving only one novel variant, *TECTA* c.710C>T (p.T237I), as the strongest candidate. This variant resides in the entactin (ENT) domain and co-segregated perfectly with non-progressive high-frequency hearing loss in the family. It was absent among 700 ethnically matched control chromosomes, and the T237 residue is conserved among species, which supports its pathogenicity. Interestingly, this finding contrasted with a previously proposed genotype-phenotype correlation in which variants of the ENT domain of *TECTA* were associated with mid-frequency hearing loss. Based upon what we observed, we propose a novel "genotype to phenotype" correlation in the ENT domain of *TECTA*. Our results shed light on another important application of whole-exome sequencing: the establishment of a novel genotype-phenotype in the molecular genetic diagnosis of autosomal dominant hearing loss.

Editor: Mathias Toft, Oslo University Hospital, Norway

Funding: This study was supported by the Korea Healthcare Technology R&D Project, Ministry for Health, Welfare and Family Affairs, Republic of Korea (Nos. A080588 and A111377), and the National Research Foundation of Korea grant funded by the Korean government (Ministry of Education, Science, and Technology; No. 20120009215). The funding bodies had no role in study design, data collection and analysis, decision to publish, or preparation of the manuscript.

Competing Interests: The authors have declared that no competing interests exist.

* E-mail: n@rna.kr (NSK); shaoh@snu.ac.kr (SHO)

¶ These authors contributed equally to this work.

Introduction

Postlingual progressive hearing loss, primarily affecting higher frequencies, is the clinical finding in most cases of autosomal dominant nonsyndromic hearing loss (ADNSHL) [1]. ADNSHL is extremely heterogeneous. To date, 64 loci and 27 autosomal genes have been identified (http://hereditaryhearingloss.org). Mutation screening is rarely offered to patients, owing to the extreme clinical and genetic heterogeneity of ADNSHL. Regarding this heterogeneity, *TECTA* has been identified as the causative gene for DFNA8/12 [2,3] as well as DFNB21 [4]. Alpha-tectorin, a major non-collagenous component of the tectorial membrane, is encoded by the *TECTA* gene located on human chromosome 11q22-24 [3,5,6]. Alpha-tectorin has several functional domains: the entactin (ENT)-like domain, the large zonadhesin region containing four von Willebrand factor–like type D domains, and the zona pellucida domain [5,7,8]. Autosomal dominant missense mutations in *TECTA* give rise to various hearing loss phenotypes, depending on the protein domains in which the mutations reside, in contrast with autosomal recessive mutations that show similar phenotypes [3,9-20].

TECTA is a highly polymorphic gene [10], and functional analyses of the variants of *TECTA* are not achieved easily, except in limited cases [21,22]. Therefore, confirming that the detected variant of *TECTA* truly accounts for hearing loss and excluding other genes that may be responsible for the phenotype are extremely difficult without proper linkage data. However, many families are too small for linkage studies to be undertaken. To overcome this limitation, researchers have proposed audioprofiling as a method of categorizing phenotypic data to make genotypic correlations [18]. Recent advances in DNA enrichment, followed by next-generation sequencing technologies, have allowed the rapid and cost-effective sequencing of all the exons in the genome, to identify the causative alleles responsible for Mendelian disorders [23,24]. This technique is expected to be useful for identifying the molecular genetic etiology of deafness, because most genetic hearing loss is caused by monogenic lesions [25]. Indeed, numerous new causative genes for hearing loss have recently been identified successfully using next-generation sequencing [26-33].

We applied whole-exome sequencing to reveal the molecular genetic etiology of high-frequency hearing loss segregating in one mid-sized Korean family, SNUBH18 (Seoul National University Bundang Hospital 18). In this study, whole-exome sequencing and further sequence analyses clearly identified a genetic defect underlying the hearing loss within the ENT domain of *TECTA*, defying a conventional genotype-phenotype correlation and establishing a diverse correlation in the ENT domain of the gene.

Methods

Human subjects

All procedures in this study were approved by the institutional review boards at Seoul National University Hospital (IRBY-H-0905-041-281) and Seoul National University Bundang Hospital (SNUBH: IRB-B-1007-105-402). Written informed consent was obtained from all individuals or guardians. The pedigree comprised 16 individuals, nine of whom were willing to join the study. Nine members (SB18 I-1, II-1, 2, 3, 4, 5, III-1, 2 and 3) from the SNUBH18 family were identified and evaluated at the Seoul National University Hospital and SNUBH for this study (see Fig. 1). Phenotype evaluations included medical and developmental history interviews, physical examinations, and pure-tone audiometry.

Audiometric evaluation

Pure-tone audiometry with air and bone conduction at frequencies ranging from 250–8000 Hz was carried out on the recruited subjects, according to standard protocols. The hearing loss range was described as follows, depending on the pure-tone audiometry results: low frequency, 250–500 Hz; mid frequency, 1–2 kHz; and high frequency, 4–8 kHz [34]. First-visit pure-tone audiograms for eight individuals and the auditory steady state response (ASSR) results for a 9-month-old child (SB18 III-3) are shown in Fig. 1. We calculated the mean level of hearing loss over all frequencies and at each frequency based upon the pure tone audiograms. We also calculated the mean hearing level of low frequencies, mid frequencies, and high frequencies. Temporal bone computed tomography was obtained from subjects II-4 and III-1 to identify any inner ear anomalies related to hearing loss in this family.

Whole-exome sequencing

DNA from four of the nine recruited subjects (two affected and two unaffected) were selected for a commercial whole-exome sequencing service (Otogenetics, Norcross, GA, USA; Fig. 1). In total, 32–69 million short reads (90-bp paired-end reads) were obtained via whole-exome sequencing. More than 85% of the target exon regions were covered by at least five sequence reads. Alignment of the exome sequences was performed using the Burrows Wheeler Aligner (http://bio-bwa.sourceforge.net/). Picard software (http://picard.sourceforge.net/) was used to remove duplicates, and mate information was corrected using the FixMateInformation and MarkDuplicates modules. Regions around short indels were realigned using IndelRealigner, and base quality scores were recalibrated using the CountCovariates and TableRecalibration modules of the Genome Analysis Toolkit [35].

SNPs and short indels were identified and filtered using the UnifiedGenotyper and VariantFiltration modules, and annotated using the VariantAnnotator module of the Genome Analysis Toolkit. Finally, all variants were compared and tagged using the Single Nucleotide Polymorphism database (dbSNP build 138) and an in-house database, an independent cohort comprising 54 normal Korean individuals. Multigenome conservation scores (phyloP) across 46 vertebrate species from the University of California, Santa Cruz genome browser (http://genome.ucsc.edu) were also used to find variants of the conserved chromosome region. The detected novel variants have been submitted to the publicly available Leiden Open Variation Database repository (https://grenada.lumc.nl/LOVD2/Usher_montpellier/variants.php?select_db = TECTA&action = view&view = 0003658). We utilized another cohort comprising 280 normal Korean control subjects to exclude rare *TECTA* variants.

Results

Auditory phenotype

Pure-tone audiograms of four affected individuals showed bilateral, moderate, symmetrical, and stable sensorineural hearing loss, most significantly that involving high frequencies (Fig. 1). The mean ± standard deviation (SD) levels of hearing impairment at 250, 500, 1000, 2000, 4000, and 8000 Hz from three older subjects were described (Table 1). The mean threshold level of 4 kHz was the lowest among the six frequencies, followed by that of 8 kHz, most significantly involving high frequencies. This indicated that the hearing impairment was most severe at high frequencies, followed by mid frequencies and then low frequencies. Insufficient follow-up time precluded serial audiograms in the affected subjects to detect any progression of hearing loss. Therefore, we compared the audiograms among the three affected SB18 subjects with their ages being roughly three decades apart. Progression of hearing loss did not seem to be significant, because the average aggravation rate (0.64 dB/yr) did not exceed 1 dB/yr for 1 kHz, which showed the most prominent aggravation among those at other frequencies in the affected subjects. The aggravation rates for 0.5 kHz, 2 kHz, and 4 kHz were 0.28, 0.24, and 0.20 dB/yr, respectively. Subjects II-4 and I-1 recollected that they noticed mild hearing loss and abnormal pronunciation during their early teens. They denied experiencing rapid progression of hearing loss. Subject III-1 (F/8yr) did not complain of hearing loss, however her pronunciation was mildly abnormal. All subjects denied any exposure to risk factors such as drugs or loud noise. No syndromic features were detected in the physical examination. Subject II-4 was reluctant to wear a hearing aid; however, subject III-2 (F/6yr) had begun wearing a hearing aid.

Exome sequencing data analysis

Ninety percent of the reads were mapped onto a human reference genome, achieving 20.7–45.4× coverage (44% on target reads; Table S1). Each individual contained 259–431 novel single-nucleotide polymorphisms (SNPs) and 3–28 novel short indels, which were used to detect novel pathogenic mutations in this family. Of these variants, approximately 65% of the novel SNPs were predicted, using SIFT software, to be deleterious mutations [36]. In total, 70 SNPs and three indels were selected as primary candidate alleles inherited by the affected daughter (III-1) from the affected mother (II-4), and which did not exist in individuals II-1 and II-5. Next, we prioritized 21 candidates (20 SNPs and one insertion) determined as deleterious using the following criteria: a phyloP score of at least 1.5 and a prediction of "damaging" by the SIFT software. Additional software analyses (Polyphen-2 [37], MutationTaster [38], and MutationAssessor [39]) gave similar overall predictions based on their own parameters. Finally, Sanger

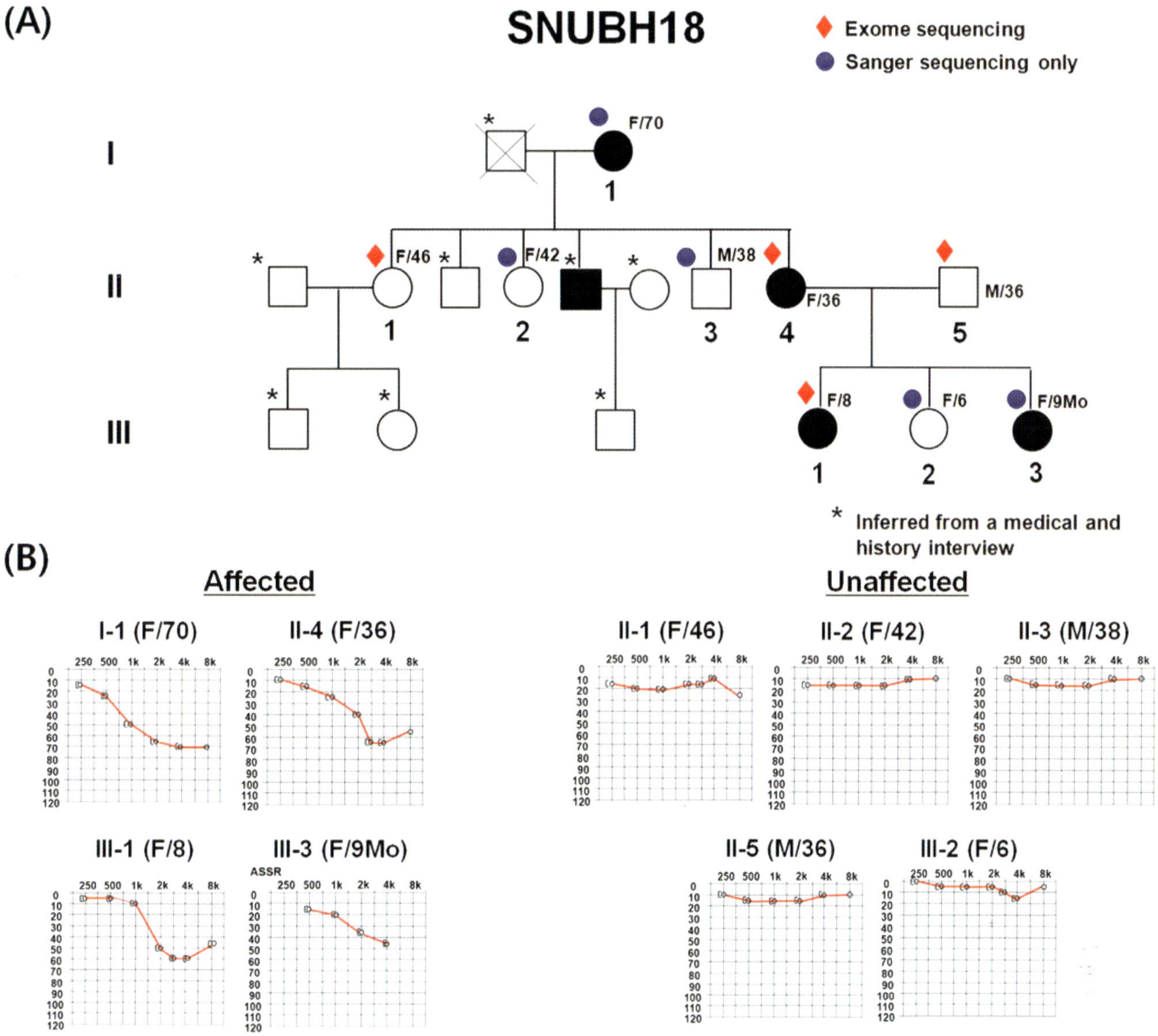

Figure 1. Pedigree and pure tone audiograms of the family SNUBH18. (A) Whole exome sequencing was performed for two affected (III-1 and II-4) and two unaffected individuals (II-5 and II-1) (red diamond). An additional five individuals (two affected and three unaffected) (blue) were recruited for Sanger validation and further filtering. (B) Individuals I-1, II-4, III-1, and III-3 showed typical high frequency hearing loss, while the others showed a normal hearing threshold over all frequencies.

validation of an additional five individuals (I-1, II-2, II-3, III-2, and III-3; Fig. 1) and a control study from two independent cohorts were adequate for identifying one causative SNP, *TECTA* c.710 C>T (p.T237I) (Table 1). This *TECTA* variant was absent in a control population of 280 Koreans (560 chromosomes). The *TECTA* gene in this family harbors four intronic SNPs (rs681311, rs504626, rs2186747, and rs543577), as well as three missense SNPs (rs612969, rs520805, and rs526433) and three silent SNPs (rs536069, rs586473, and rs2155369; Table S2). These 10 SNPs, which apparently do not affect hearing loss, were also present in our in-house database. The sequence variant c.710 C>T resides in the nidogen (NIDO)-like domain, formerly known as the ENT domain (Table S3) (Fig. 2B). This variant (p.T237I) on the ENT domain co-segregated with high-frequency hearing loss in this study, as shown in Fig. 2A.

Protein structure homology modeling and conservation

The protein structure of *TECTA* is not yet known, but we performed homology modeling using the *E. coli* chain A, L-fucose isomerase (1FUI_A). However, insufficient information was available due to the large differences between the human and *E.coli* protein sequences. A contact-map inferred from the DISTIL utility (http://distill.ucd.ie) predicted that the mutant residue would be exposed to the surface when the residue was converted from threonine to isoleucine. In contrast, the wild type threonine residue was embedded in the structure, suggesting a significant effect of p.T237I on protein structure (Fig. S1). Amino acid conservation within the NIDO domain indicated that the p.T237 residue was well-conserved among vertebrate species, with threonine (TECTA and SNED1 proteins) and serine (NID1 and NID2 proteins) polar, uncharged side chains (Fig. 2).

Table 1. The mean ± standard deviation (SD) level of hearing impairment at 250, 500, 1000, 2000, 4000, and 8000 Hz from three older subjects.

Frequency (Hz)	Hearing threshold (dB)(mean + standard deviation) Right	Left
Low frequency		
250Hz	10.0 ± 5.0	11.7 ± 5.7
500Hz	15.0 ± 10.0	18.3 ± 11.5
	12.5 ± 7.5	*15.0 ± 8.9*
Mid frequency		
1000Hz	28.3 ± 20.2	31.7 ± 20.2
2000Hz	51.6 ± 12.6	53.3 ± 10.4
	40 ± 19.7	*42.5 ± 18.6*
High frequency		
4000Hz	65.0 ± 5.0	65.0 ± 8.7
8000Hz	56.7 ± 12.6	55.0 ± 15.0
	60.8 ± 9.7	*60 ± 12.2*
Total (all frequencies)	**37 ± 23.9**	**39.2 ± 23.1**

Discussion

The majority of missense mutations that cause hearing loss related to *TECTA* reside in the zona pellucida and zonadhesin domains of the gene [16]. Previous studies have discovered only four probable pathogenic mutations within the ENT domain (Fig. 2). Two truncation mutations, c.266delT (p.L89Rfs*34) and c.649insC (p.N218Qfs*31), have been found in autosomal recessive nonsyndromic hearing loss. These two frameshift recessive mutations are associated with mid-frequency and all-frequency sensorineural hearing loss, respectively [17,40]. The autosomal dominant missense mutations c.632T>C (p.F211S) and c.589G>A (p.D197N) in the NIDO domain have been clearly associated with mid-frequency sensorineural hearing loss [16], suggesting a genotype-phenotype correlation between mutations in the NIDO domain of *TECTA* and mid-frequency sensorineural hearing loss.

However, this study revealed that carriers of the variant c.710 C>T (p.T237I) in the NIDO domain showed definitive high-frequency hearing loss, arguing against the previously proposed genotype-phenotype correlation. It would not have been possible to ascertain this without whole-exome sequencing. Whole-exome sequencing and further validation excluded other genes as possible causes of hearing loss in the family SNUBH18, thereby leaving p.T237I of *TECTA* as the only candidate. Of course, it is possible that genes that fell within the low- or no-coverage region on whole-exome sequencing might harbor a causative variant. Regardless, the variant c.710 C>T (p.T237I) was considered pathogenic and causative of the phenotype of SNUBH18 for the following reasons. First, SIFT and Polyphen prediction software consistently suggested that this variant was "damaging" (Table 2). Second, this variant was undetected in 334 (54+280) ethnically matched Korean control subjects and in 1,000 genomes. Third, p.T237 is well-conserved among species. Last, the same variant (c.710 C>T [p.T237I]) was detected in another Korean family, segregating with similar high-frequency hearing loss in an autosomal dominant fashion (personal communication with Dr. Hong-Joon Park).

Hildebrand et al. (2001) observed that homozygous mutant mice with a targeted deletion of the ENT domain of the alpha-tectorin gene display severe elevation of the mid-frequency hearing threshold (5–20 kHz) [41], which supported their genotype-phenotype correlation. However, the mouse model likely reflects a null status of alpha-tectorin, not the effect of an autosomal dominant mutation, because heterozygous knockout mutant mice showed no phenotype [41]. A diverse genotype-phenotype correlation for the mutations may be located in the NIDO domain of *TECTA*, depending on the exact location in the domain. The NIDO domain of alpha-tectorin has been predicted to facilitate the assembly and modeling of the extracellular matrix of the tectorial membrane, interacting with laminin and type IV collagen [42-44]. Generation of a knock-in mouse model of the p.T237I mutation and evaluation of the mechanotransduction of mid and high frequencies may reveal the reason for this phenotypic difference between the previously reported mutations and the mutation discovered in this study in the same domain. Our result clearly shows that a diverse genotype-phenotype correlation can exist, even within the same domain of the protein, proposing a possible "variant to phenotype correlation" beyond "gene to phenotype" or "domain to phenotype" correlations. Verification of the various effects of the mutations on either the structure or the function of alpha-tectorin, as suggested by the different phenotypes, will further the understanding of the role of the tectorial membrane.

The tectorial membrane is formed during development, and tectorin is not usually replaced, based on the expression profile of tectorin in the developing cochlea [7,8,45]. This feature is compatible with the stable nature of most of the DFNA8/12 cases, except those in which a cysteine residue is mutated [12,13,16]. The progressive nature of hearing loss due to *TECTA* mutations appears to be correlated with a progressive loss of outer hair cells, as suggested by transient-evoked otoacoustic emission data from subjects carrying p.Cys1837Gly [16]. In contrast, this pathology has not been reported in mutant mice carrying a p.Tyr1870Cys mutation responsible for non-progressive stable hearing loss [41,46]. It would have been very interesting to examine the distortion product-evoked otoacoustic or transient-

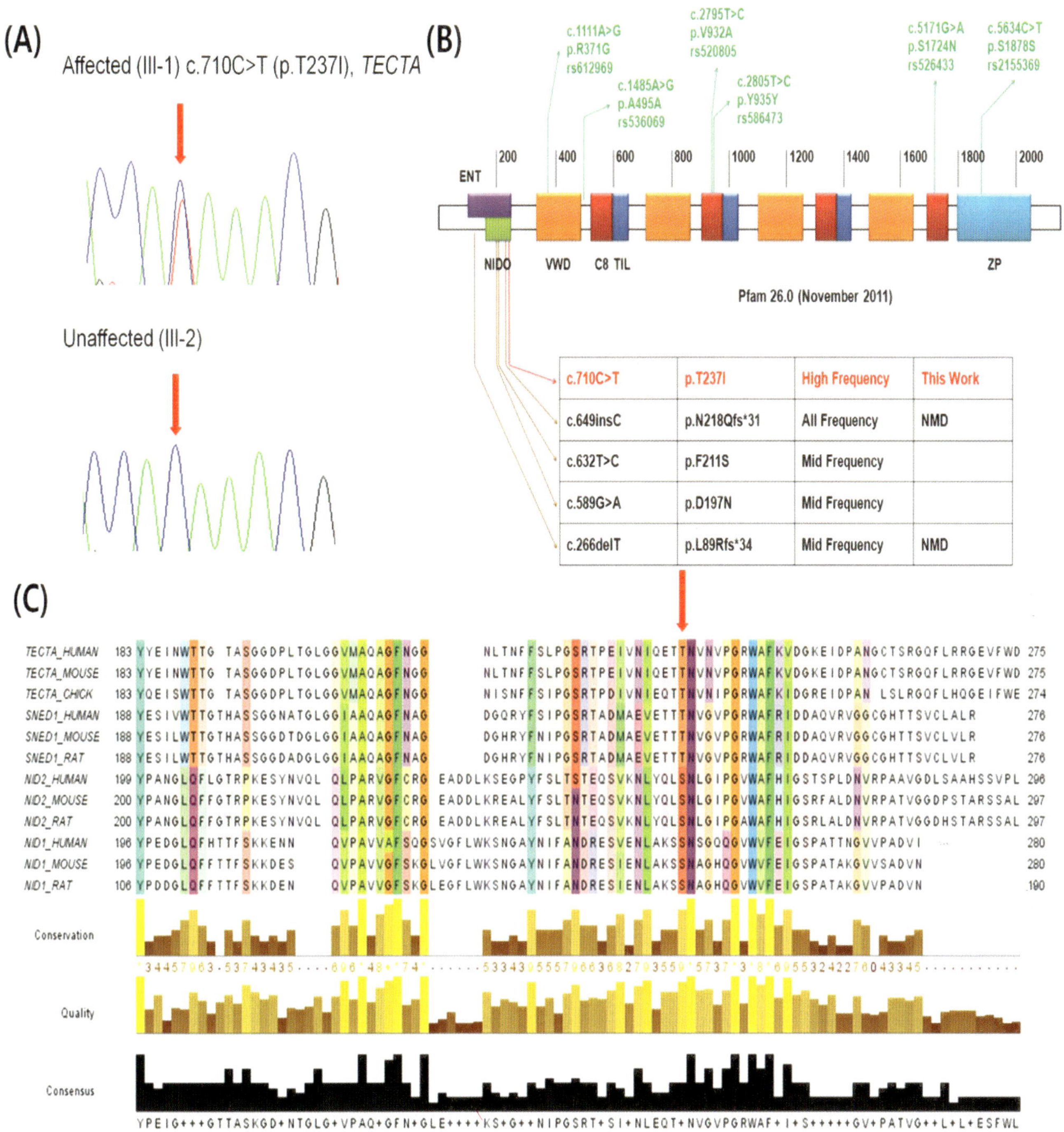

Figure 2. p.T237I variant of *TECTA* in SNUBH18. (A) Sanger sequencing traces of the p.T237I heterozygote and the wildtype. (B) Sequence variants related to hearing loss in the ENT domain of the *TECTA* gene. *TECTA* has five protein domains (NIDO, VWD, C8, TIL and ZP). To date, two missense and two frameshift indel variants related to mid- and all-frequency hearing loss have been discovered in the ENT domain. In contrast, p.T237I in the ENT domain is associated with high-frequency hearing loss. (C) Protein conservation of NIDO proteins among vertebrate species. p.T237 is well-conserved with threonine in Tecta and serine in NIDO proteins.

evoked otoacoustic emission results from subjects II-4 and III-1, who carry p.T237I of the *TECTA* gene. However, these subjects refused the test, leaving the status of their outer hair cells unknown.

Although next-generation per-base sequencing costs have become relatively low, the cost of sequencing the entire human genomes remains high. Whole-genome sequencing is unnecessary for many diagnostic and research applications, because the protein-coding regions of genes (exons) constitute an estimated 1% of the genome but harbor 85% of the mutations, which have large effects on disease [23]. After evaluating whole-exome sequencing from four family members and performing subsequent Sanger sequencing validation in an additional five family members, we are almost confident that this *TECTA* variant is

Table 2. Whole filtering process to identify a causative variant of deafness from SNUBH18.

Gene Symbol	Variant Type	Exome Sequencing				Sanger Sequencing					Control Group		Functional impact prediction of nonsynonymous SNPs				
		III-1†	**II-4**†	II-5	II-1	**I-1**†	**III-3**†	II-2	II-3	III-2	Cohort #1 (70)	Cohort #2 (210)	PhyloP score	SIFT	Polyphen-2	Mutation Taster	Mutation Assessor
ARHGAP31	c.4211C>G	Het	Het	.	.	O		O	X				2.200	Y	Y	Y	Low
	p.T1404R missense													0.00			0.895
FAM214A	c.1064C>G	Het	Het	.	.	O			O				4.194	N/A	N/A	Y	N/A
	p.S355X nonsense																
GPRC5B	c.805G>A	Het	Het	.	.	O		X	O				4.071	Y	Y	Y	Medium
	p.D269N missense													0.01			2.685
ITCH	c.17C>T	Het	Het	.	.	X		X	X				1.938	Y	N	Y	Low
	p.S6L missense													0.01			1.590
MICAL3	c.74G>T	Het	Het	.	.	O	X	X	X	O	N.D.‡	N.D. ‡	4.393	Y	Y	N	Low
	p.C25F missense													0.03			1.720
PCDP1	c.1751T>C	Het	Het	.	.	O	X	X	X	O	N.D.‡	N.D.‡	2.403	Y	Y	Y	Low
	p.I584T missense													0.01			1.445
TECTA	c.710C>T	Het	Het	.	.	O	O	X	X	X	N.D.‡	N.D.‡	4.045	Y	Y	N	Medium
	p.T237I													0.01			2.955
	missense																
TPRG1	c.721G>A	Het	Het	.	.	X			X				4.269	Y	Y	Y	Medium
	p.V241M missense													0.00			2.275
WDR12	c.959A>G	Het	Het	.	.	O		O	X				5.143	Y	Y	Y	Neutral
	p.H320R missense													0.00			0.675

†III-1, II-4, I-1 and III-3 in bold: Affected, ‡N.D.: not detected.

the causative variant. A mutation in a neighboring gene that fell within the no- or low-coverage region on the whole-exome sequence might account for the high-frequency hearing loss in this family, and p.T237I in *TECTA* may have coincidentally been in linkage disequilibrium with the true causative gene. However, a significant effect of p.T237I upon protein structure as predicted by homology modeling makes the hypothesis least likely.

We may find additional rare variants through further exome sequencing endeavors, but we are certain that the whole-exome sequencing covered at least 85% (depth $\geq$ 5) of the target enrichment region. Moreover, most rare nonpathogenic variants in exome sequences reside outside of coding sequences owing to the efficiency of microarray cross-hybridization. Furthermore, most disease-causing mutations are located in highly conserved regions, which exome sequencing is expected to cover.

Conclusion

We identified a novel variant of *TECTA* and a phenotype that disputes a previously proposed genotype-phenotype correlation in the ENT domain of this gene. Because we acquired a thorough roadmap from whole-exome sequencing of five family members and undertook a subsequent segregation study using Sanger sequencing from an additional four members, we propose a novel genotype-phenotype correlation.

Supporting Information

Figure S1 The protein structure of the chain A, L-fucose isomerase (1FUI_A 499–568) fragment (A) p.T559 of 1FUI_A is equivalent to p.T237. Yellow circle denotes p.T559. (B) View of the predicted protein structure from various angles when threonine is converted into isoleucine: yellow arrows denote the isoleucine residue, and a contact-map using the DISTIL utility (http://distill.ucd.ie/) indicates that the mutant residue is likely to be exposed to the surface, while the wildtype threonine residue (white arrow) is embedded in the structure (C).

Table S1 Statistics of whole exome sequencing data for four individuals from SNUBH18.

Table S2 Mutation profile of *TECTA* gene (located on chr11).

Table S3 Pfam domain and Amino Acid Position.

Author Contributions

Conceived and designed the experiments: BYC NK SO. Performed the experiments: BYC JK JC ARK SJM SHL NK. Analyzed the data: BYC JK JC SJM SIK. Contributed reagents/materials/analysis tools: BYC JK JC ARK SJM SHL NK. Wrote the paper: BYC JK. Recruited patients and analyzed the clinical test results: SJM ARK JC. Performed the bioinformatics analyses: JK SL NK. Substantial input on the the manuscript: SJM JC SIK ARK JK SHL SHO. Supervised the study: NK. All authors contributed to and approved the final manuscript for publication: BYC JK JC ARK SJM SIK SHL NK SHO.

References

1. Huygen PL, Pauw RJ, Cremers CW (2007) Audiometric profiles associated with genetic non-syndromal hearing impairment: a review and phenotype analysis. In: I. A M., editor editors. Genes, Hearing and Deafness. London: Informa Healthcare. pp. 185–204.
2. Govaerts PJ, De Ceulaer G, Daemers K, Verhoeven K, Van Camp G, et al. (1998) A new autosomal-dominant locus (DFNA12) is responsible for a nonsyndromic, midfrequency, prelingual and nonprogressive sensorineural hearing loss. Am J Otol 19: 718–723.
3. Verhoeven K, Van Laer L, Kirschhofer K, Legan PK, Hughes DC, et al. (1998) Mutations in the human alpha-tectorin gene cause autosomal dominant non-syndromic hearing impairment. Nat Genet 19: 60–62.
4. Mustapha M, Weil D, Chardenoux S, Elias S, El-Zir E, et al. (1999) An alpha-tectorin gene defect causes a newly identified autosomal recessive form of sensorineural pre-lingual non-syndromic deafness, DFNB21. Hum Mol Genet 8: 409–412.
5. Legan PK, Rau A, Keen JN, Richardson GP (1997) The mouse tectorins. Modular matrix proteins of the inner ear homologous to components of the sperm-egg adhesion system. J Biol Chem 272: 8791–8801.
6. Verhoeven K, Van Camp G, Govaerts PJ, Balemans W, Schatteman I, et al. (1997) A gene for autosomal dominant nonsyndromic hearing loss (DFNA12) maps to chromosome 11q22-24. Am J Hum Genet 60: 1168–1173.
7. Maeda Y, Fukushima K, Kasai N, Maeta M, Nishizaki K (2001) Quantification of TECTA and DFNA5 expression in the developing mouse cochlea. Neuroreport 12: 3223–3226.
8. Rau A, Legan PK, Richardson GP (1999) Tectorin mRNA expression is spatially and temporally restricted during mouse inner ear development. J Comp Neurol 405: 271–280.
9. Alloisio N, Morle L, Bozon M, Godet J, Verhoeven K, et al. (1999) Mutation in the zonadhesin-like domain of alpha-tectorin associated with autosomal dominant non-syndromic hearing loss. Eur J Hum Genet 7: 255–258.
10. Balciuniene J, Dahl N, Jalonen P, Verhoeven K, Van Camp G, et al. (1999) Alpha-tectorin involvement in hearing disabilities: one gene-two phenotypes. Hum Genet 105: 211–216.
11. Iwasaki S, Harada D, Usami S, Nagura M, Takeshita T, et al. (2002) Association of clinical features with mutation of TECTA in a family with autosomal dominant hearing loss. Arch Otolaryngol Head Neck Surg 128: 913–917.
12. Moreno-Pelayo MA, del Castillo I, Villamar M, Romero L, Hernandez-Calvin FJ, et al. (2001) A cysteine substitution in the zona pellucida domain of alpha-tectorin results in autosomal dominant, postlingual, progressive, mid frequency hearing loss in a Spanish family. J Med Genet 38: E13.
13. Pfister M, Thiele H, Van Camp G, Fransen E, Apaydin F, et al. (2004) A genotype-phenotype correlation with gender-effect for hearing impairment caused by TECTA mutations. Cell Physiol Biochem 14: 369–376.
14. Plantinga RF, de Brouwer AP, Huygen PL, Kunst HP, Kremer H, et al. (2006) A novel TECTA mutation in a Dutch DFNA8/12 family confirms genotype-phenotype correlation. J Assoc Res Otolaryngol 7: 173–181.
15. Alasti F, Sanati MH, Behrouzifard AH, Sadeghi A, de Brouwer AP, et al. (2008) A novel TECTA mutation confirms the recognizable phenotype among autosomal recessive hearing impairment families. Int J Pediatr Otorhinolaryngol 72: 249–255.
16. Hildebrand MS, Morin M, Meyer NC, Mayo F, Modamio-Hoybjor S, et al. (2011) DFNA8/12 caused by TECTA mutations is the most identified subtype of nonsyndromic autosomal dominant hearing loss. Hum Mutat 32: 825–834.
17. Meyer NC, Alasti F, Nishimura CJ, Imanirad P, Kahrizi K, et al. (2007) Identification of three novel TECTA mutations in Iranian families with autosomal recessive nonsyndromic hearing impairment at the DFNB21 locus. Am J Med Genet A 143A: 1623–1629.
18. Meyer NC, Nishimura CJ, McMordie S, Smith RJ (2007) Audioprofiling identifies TECTA and GJB2-related deafness segregating in a single extended pedigree. Clin Genet 72: 130–137.
19. Sagong B, Park HJ, Lee KY, Kim UK (2012) Identification and functional characterization of novel compound heterozygotic mutations in the TECTA gene. Gene 492: 239–243.
20. Sagong B, Park R, Kim YH, Lee KY, Baek JI, et al. (2010) Two novel missense mutations in the TECTA gene in Korean families with autosomal dominant nonsyndromic hearing loss. Ann Clin Lab Sci 40: 380–385.
21. Collin RW, de Heer AM, Oostrik J, Pauw RJ, Plantinga RF, et al. (2008) Mid-frequency DFNA8/12 hearing loss caused by a synonymous TECTA mutation that affects an exonic splice enhancer. Eur J Hum Genet 16: 1430–1436.
22. Lezirovitz K, Batissoco AC, Lima FT, Auricchio MT, Nonose RW, et al. (2012) Aberrant transcript produced by a splice donor site deletion in the TECTA gene is associated with autosomal dominant deafness in a Brazilian family. Gene 511: 280–284.
23. Choi M, Scholl UI, Ji W, Liu T, Tikhonova IR, et al. (2009) Genetic diagnosis by whole exome capture and massively parallel DNA sequencing. Proc Natl Acad Sci U S A 106: 19096–19101.
24. Ng SB, Buckingham KJ, Lee C, Bigham AW, Tabor HK, et al. (2010) Exome sequencing identifies the cause of a mendelian disorder. Nat Genet 42: 30–35.
25. Hilgert N, Smith RJ, Van Camp G (2009) Forty-six genes causing nonsyndromic hearing impairment: which ones should be analyzed in DNA diagnostics? Mutat Res 681: 189–196.

26. Schraders M, Haas SA, Weegerink NJ, Oostrik J, Hu H, et al. (2011) Next-generation sequencing identifies mutations of SMPX, which encodes the small muscle protein, X-linked, as a cause of progressive hearing impairment. Am J Hum Genet 88: 628–634.
27. Walsh T, Shahin H, Elkan-Miller T, Lee MK, Thornton AM, et al. (2010) Whole exome sequencing and homozygosity mapping identify mutation in the cell polarity protein GPSM2 as the cause of nonsyndromic hearing loss DFNB82. Am J Hum Genet 87: 90–94.
28. Rehman AU, Santos-Cortez RL, Morell RJ, Drummond MC, Ito T, et al. (2014) Mutations in TBC1D24, a gene associated with epilepsy, also cause nonsyndromic deafness DFNB86. Am J Hum Genet 94: 144–152.
29. Yariz KO, Duman D, Seco CZ, Dallman J, Huang M, et al. (2012) Mutations in OTOGL, encoding the inner ear protein otogelin-like, cause moderate sensorineural hearing loss. Am J Hum Genet 91: 872–882.
30. Schraders M, Ruiz-Palmero L, Kalay E, Oostrik J, del Castillo FJ, et al. (2012) Mutations of the gene encoding otogelin are a cause of autosomal-recessive nonsyndromic moderate hearing impairment. Am J Hum Genet 91: 883–889.
31. Delmaghani S, Aghaie A, Michalski N, Bonnet C, Weil D, et al. (2012) Defect in the gene encoding the EAR/EPTP domain-containing protein TSPEAR causes DFNB98 profound deafness. Hum Mol Genet 21: 3835–3844.
32. Tekin M, Chioza BA, Matsumoto Y, Diaz-Horta O, Cross HE, et al. (2013) SLITRK6 mutations cause myopia and deafness in humans and mice. J Clin Invest 123: 2094–2102.
33. Santos-Cortez RL, Lee K, Azeem Z, Antonellis PJ, Pollock LM, et al. (2013) Mutations in KARS, encoding lysyl-tRNA synthetase, cause autosomal-recessive nonsyndromic hearing impairment DFNB89. Am J Hum Genet 93: 132–140.
34. King KA, Choi BY, Zalewski C, Madeo AC, Manichaikul A, et al. (2010) SLC26A4 genotype, but not cochlear radiologic structure, is correlated with hearing loss in ears with an enlarged vestibular aqueduct. Laryngoscope 120: 384–389.
35. McKenna A, Hanna M, Banks E, Sivachenko A, Cibulskis K, et al. (2010) The Genome Analysis Toolkit: a MapReduce framework for analyzing next-generation DNA sequencing data. Genome Res 20: 1297–1303.
36. Sim NL, Kumar P, Hu J, Henikoff S, Schneider G, et al. (2012) SIFT web server: predicting effects of amino acid substitutions on proteins. Nucleic Acids Res 40: W452–457.
37. Adzhubei IA, Schmidt S, Peshkin L, Ramensky VE, Gerasimova A, et al. (2010) A method and server for predicting damaging missense mutations. Nat Methods 7: 248–249.
38. Schwarz JM, Rodelsperger C, Schuelke M, Seelow D (2010) MutationTaster evaluates disease-causing potential of sequence alterations. Nat Methods 7: 575–576.
39. Reva B, Antipin Y, Sander C (2011) Predicting the functional impact of protein mutations: application to cancer genomics. Nucleic Acids Res 39: e118.
40. Naz S, Alasti F, Mowjoodi A, Riazuddin S, Sanati MH, et al. (2003) Distinctive audiometric profile associated with DFNB21 alleles of TECTA. J Med Genet 40: 360–363.
41. Legan PK, Lukashkina VA, Goodyear RJ, Kossi M, Russell IJ, et al. (2000) A targeted deletion in alpha-tectorin reveals that the tectorial membrane is required for the gain and timing of cochlear feedback. Neuron 28: 273–285.
42. Chung AE, Dong LJ, Wu C, Durkin ME (1993) Biological functions of entactin. Kidney Int 43: 13–19.
43. Durkin ME, Chakravarti S, Bartos BB, Liu SH, Friedman RL, et al. (1988) Amino acid sequence and domain structure of entactin. Homology with epidermal growth factor precursor and low density lipoprotein receptor. J Cell Biol 107: 2749–2756.
44. Dziadek M, Paulsson M, Timpl R (1985) Identification and interaction repertoire of large forms of the basement membrane protein nidogen. EMBO J 4: 2513–2518.
45. Knipper M, Richardson G, Mack A, Muller M, Goodyear R, et al. (2001) Thyroid hormone-deficient period prior to the onset of hearing is associated with reduced levels of beta-tectorin protein in the tectorial membrane: implication for hearing loss. J Biol Chem 276: 39046–39052.
46. Legan PK, Lukashkina VA, Goodyear RJ, Lukashkin AN, Verhoeven K, et al. (2005) A deafness mutation isolates a second role for the tectorial membrane in hearing. Nat Neurosci 8: 1035–1042.

A Novel Mutation in the *TECTA* Gene in a Chinese Family with Autosomal Dominant Nonsyndromic Hearing Loss

Yu Su[1,2], Wen-Xue Tang[3], Xue Gao[1,4], Fei Yu[1], Zhi-Yao Dai[5], Jian-Dong Zhao[1], Yu Lu[1], Fei Ji[1], Sha-Sha Huang[1], Yong-Yi Yuan[1], Ming-Yu Han[1,2], Yue-Shuai Song[1,2], Yu-Hua Zhu[1], Dong-Yang Kang[1], Dong-Yi HAN[1*], Pu Dai[1,2*]

1 Department of Otorhinolaryngology, Head and Neck Surgery, PLA General Hospital, Beijing, P. R. China, **2** Department of Otorhinolaryngology, Hainan Branch of PLA General Hospital, Sanya, P. R. China, **3** Department of Otolaryngology, Emory University School of Medicine, Atlanta, Georgia, **4** Department of Otorhinolaryngology, the Second Artillery General Hospital, Beijing, P. R. China, **5** Department of Otorhinolaryngology, the First Affiliated Hospital of PLA General Hospital, Beijing, P. R. China

Abstract

TECTA-related deafness can be inherited as autosomal-dominant nonsyndromic deafness (designated DFNA) or as the autosomal-recessive version. The α-tectorin protein, which is encoded by the *TECTA* gene, is one of the major components of the tectorial membrane in the inner ear. Using targeted DNA capture and massively parallel sequencing (MPS), we screened 42 genes known to be responsible for human deafness in a Chinese family (Family 3187) in which common deafness mutations had been ruled out as the cause, and identified a novel mutation, c.257–262CCTTTC>GCT (p. Ser86Cys; p. Pro88del) in exon 3 of the *TECTA* gene in the proband and his extended family. All affected individuals in this family had moderate down-sloping hearing loss across all frequencies. To our knowledge, this is the second *TECTA* mutation identified in Chinese population. This study demonstrates that targeted genomic capture, MPS, and barcode technology might broaden the availability of genetic testing for individuals with undiagnosed DFNA.

Editor: Berta Alsina, Universitat Pompeu Fabra, Spain

Funding: This work was supported by Chinese National Nature Science Foundation Research Grant (81070792), the National Basic Research Program of China (973 Program) (#2013CB945402) to HD. The Project of the National Natural Science Foundation of China (Grant No. 81230020), a grant from State 863 High Technology R&D Key Project of China (2011AA02A112), a grant from Natural Science Foundation of Beijing (Grant No 7122172), a grant from Minister of Science and Technology of China (2012BAI09B02) and a grant from Minister of Health of China (201202005) to PD, China postdoctoral granted financial support and speccial financial grant (No. 20120481482 & 201104779) to YS. The funders had no role in study design, data collection and analysis, decision to publish, or preparation of the manuscript.

Competing Interests: The authors have declared that no competing interests exist.

* E-mail: hdy301@263.net (DYH); daipu301@vip.sina.com (PD)

These authors contributed equally to this work.

Introduction

Hearing loss is one of the most common sensory disorders in humans. Genetic factors account for more than 50% of the cases with congenital or prelingual hearing loss, with autosomal-recessive (77%), autosomal-dominant (22%), and X-linked (1%) inheritance [1]. Single-gene defects are responsible for over half of these cases and most are thought to affect the cochlea [2]. A common clinical scenario is the identification of a child with partial hearing loss who then slowly progresses to deafness over a period of years. Identification of the responsible mutation in families with autosomal-dominant nonsyndromic hearing loss (ADNSHL) is difficult because mutations in 27 different genes have been identified as causing this common form of deafness (Hereditary Hearing Loss Homepage). Although certain gene mutations affect inner ear-specific proteins and can be linked to progressive hair cell degeneration, the mechanisms behind most common causes of progressive hearing loss in childhood are unknown [3].

Mutations in the *TECTA* gene at the DFNA8/12 (OMIM 601543) and DFNB21 (OMIM 603629) loci result in ADNSHL and the autosomal-recessive version, respectively [4–17] (Table1, 2). The *TECTA* gene encodes alpha (α)-tectorin, a major extracellular protein in the tectorial membrane (TM), a ribbon-like strip of extracellular matrix that lies over the stereocilia of the hair cells and is critical for the mechanical transmission and amplification of sound [18]. α-Tectorin is a large modular glycoprotein that contains several protein-protein interaction domains: the entactin domain (ENT), the large zonadhesin region (ZA) containing three full and two partial von Willebrand factor (vWF) type D repeats, an N-terminal entactin G1-like domain, a C-terminal zona pellucida (ZP) domain, and three trypsin inhibitor-like cysteine-rich domains [19–21].

Mutations in *TECTA* (*DFNA8/12*) can cause either stable or progressive hearing loss, depending on the affected protein domain [22]. Mutations in the ZP domain are commonly associated with stable hearing loss, whereas mutations within the vWF domains tend to manifest as progressive hearing loss [15]. *TECTA* null mice are deaf because the TM is detached completely from the organ of Corti; consequently, vibrations of the basilar membrane associated with the traveling wave do not lead to the deflection of outer hair cell (OHC) or inner hair cell (IHC) stereocilia [23]. Mice carrying a mutation in the ZP domain have congenital hearing loss because they have a misshapen TM that stimulates OHCs normally, but under-stimulates IHCs [24].

Table 1. *TECTA* mutations described in DFNA8/12 families, including those identified in this study.

Exon	Mutation	Protein change	Domain	Time of onset	Progression	Frequencies	Ethnic origin	Reference
3	c.257–262CCTTTC>GCT	p. Ser 86Cys p. Pro88del	ENT	Postlingual	Stable	High	Chinese	This study
4	c.589G>A	p.Asp197Asn	ENT	Postlingual	Stable	Mid	American	[7]
5	c.632T>C	p.Phe211Ser	ENT	Postlingual	Stable	Mid	Spanish	[7]
6	c.950T>A	p.Val317Glu	ZA (none)	Postlingual	Unknown	High	Korean	[17]
6	c.1084A>T	p.Ser362Cys	ZA (VWFD1)	Postlingual	Unknown	Mid	American	[7]
6	c.1124delT	p.Val375Alafs*4	ZA (VWFD1)	Postlingual	Unknown	Mid	Spanish	[7]
7	c.1395T>G	p.Asn465Lys	ZA (VWFD1)	Postlingual	Progressive	Mid	Belgian	[7]
7	c.1685C>T	p.Thr562Met	ZA (none)	Postlingual	Unknown	Mid	American	[7]
9	c.2444C>T	p.Thr815Met	ZA (VWFD2)	Prelingual	Unknown	Mid	American	[7]
9	c.2657A>G	p.Asn886Ser	ZA (VWFD2)	Prelingual	Progressive	High	UK	[7]
10	c.3107G>A	p.Cys1036Tyr	ZA (TIL2)	Postlingual	Stable	Mid	Spanish	[7]
10	c.3169T>A	p.Cys1057Ser	ZA (none)	Postlingual	Progressive	High	Swedish	[31]
10	c.3293C>T	p.Ala1098Val	ZA (none)	Postlingual	Unknown	High	Spanish	[7]
10	c.3406G>C	p.Asp1136His	ZA (VWFD3)	Postlingual	Unknown	High	Spanish	[7]
11	c.3743C>T	p.Pro1248Leu	ZA (VWFD3)	Prelingual	Unknown	High	Spanish	[7]
13	c.4525T>G	p.Cys1509Gly	ZA (VWFD4)	Unknown	Progressive	High	Turkish	[22]
13	c.4549T>C	p.Cys1517Arg	ZA (VWFD4)	Postlingual	Progressive	High	Spanish	[7]
14	c.4856G>C	p.Cys1619Ser	ZA (VWFD4)	Postlingual	Progressive	High	French	[32]
16	c.5331G>A	p.Leu1777Leu	ZA (none)	Prelingual	Stable	Mid	Dutch	[5]
16	c.5372C>G	p.Pro1791Arg	ZA (none)	Prelingual	Unknown	Mid	American	[7]
	c.5383+2T>G		ZA (none)	Prelingual	Stable	Mid	Spanish	[7]
	c.5383+5del GTGA		ZA (none)	Prelingual	Progressive	High	UK	[7]
17	c.5458C>T	p.Leu1820Phe	ZP	Postlingual	Stable	Mid	Belgian	[18]
17	c.5471G>A	p.Gly1824Asp	ZP	Postlingual	Stable	Mid	Belgian	[18]
17	c.5509T>G	p.Cys1837Gly	ZP	Postlingual	Progressive	Mid	Spanish	[33]
17	c.5509T>G	p.Cys1837Gly	ZP	Postlingual	Progressive	Mid	Spanish	[7]
17	c.5509T>C	p.Cys1837Arg	ZP	Postlingual	Progressive	Mid	American	[34]
18	c.5597C>T	p.Thr1866Met	ZP	Postlingual	Stable	Mid	Korean	[17]
18	c.5597C>T	p.Thr1866Met	ZP	Postlingual	Progressive, Unknown	Mid	Spanish, American	[7]
18	c.5600A>G	p.His1867Arg	ZP	Postlingual	Progressive	Mid	Spanish	[7]
18	c.5609A>G	p.Tyrl870Cys	ZP	Prelingual	Stable	Mid	Austrian	[18]
18	c.5668C>T	p.Arg1890Cys	ZP	Prelingual	Stable	Mid	Dutch	[15]
18	c.5668C>T	p.Arg1890Cys	ZP	Prelingual	Stable	Mid	Spanish American	[7]
18	c.5692T>C	p.Cys1898Arg	ZP	Postlingual	Unknown	Mid	American	[7]
19	c.5839C>T	p.Arg1947Cys	ZP	Postlingual	Unknown	Mid	American	[7]
19	c.5945C>A	p.Ala1982Asp	ZP	Prelingual	Progressive	Mid	Chinese	[35]
20	c.6026T>C	p.Ile2009Thr	ZP	Postlingual	Stable	High	Spanish	[7]
20	c.6062G>A	p.Arg2021His	ZP	Prelingual	Stable	Mid	Japanese	[9]

Massively parallel sequencing (MPS), also known as next-generation sequencing (NGS), produces large amounts of genomic sequence information in an incomparably more rapid and less expensive manner than before [25]. Given its large capacity to survey the entire genome without bias, NGS is suited for discovering the causative mutations of hereditary hearing loss with genetic heterogeneity. Novel genes for non-syndromic [26,27] and syndromic [28] hearing loss were identified recently using a targeted NGS approach. In this study, we first identified ADNSHL in Chinese Family 3187 caused by the c.257–262CCTTTC>GCT (p. Ser86Cys; p. Pro88del) mutation of *TECTA* using targeted capture of 42 deafness genes and MPS. To exclude the possibility that the mutation is a polymorphism in the Chinese population, we sequenced the mutation directly (c.257–262CCTTTC>GCT (p. Ser86Cys; p. Pro88del)) in 100 ethnicity-matched, unrelated controls. The c.257–262CCTTTC>GCT (p. Ser86Cys; p. Pro88del) variant co-segregated with the phenotype and was absent in the 100 ethnicity-matched controls.

Table 2. DFNB21 *TECTA* mutations and the associated phenotypes.

Exon	Mutation	Protein change	Domain	Time of onset	Progression	Frequencies	Ethnic origin	Reference
3	c.266delT	p.Leu89Argfs*34	ENT	Prelingual	Stable	Mid	Iranian	[11]
5	c.651dupC	p.Asn218Glnfs*31	ENT	Prelingual	Stable	All freq	Iranian	[14]
	c.2941+1G>A		ZA	Prelingual	ND	All freq		[36]
	9.6 Kb	del	ZA	Prelingual	Stable	Mid	Iranian	[11]
15	c.5211C>A	p.Tyr1737*	ZA	Prelingual	Stable	Mid	Iranian	[11]
20	c.6037delG	p.Glu2013Argfs*6	ZP	Prelingual	Stable	Mid	Pakistani	[14]
21	c.6203–6218del	p.Lys2068Argfs*38	ZP	Prelingual	Stable	All freq	Iranian	[4]

This is the first report of *TECTA* c.257–262CCTTTC>GCT (p. Ser86Cys; p. Pro88del) as a gene causing ADNSHL in Chinese families with hereditary deafness.

Materials and Methods

Subjects and Ethics Statement

We enrolled six cases of ADNSHL from Family 3187, a large ethnic Han Chinese family, through the Otolaryngology Department of the General Hospital of People's Liberation Army,

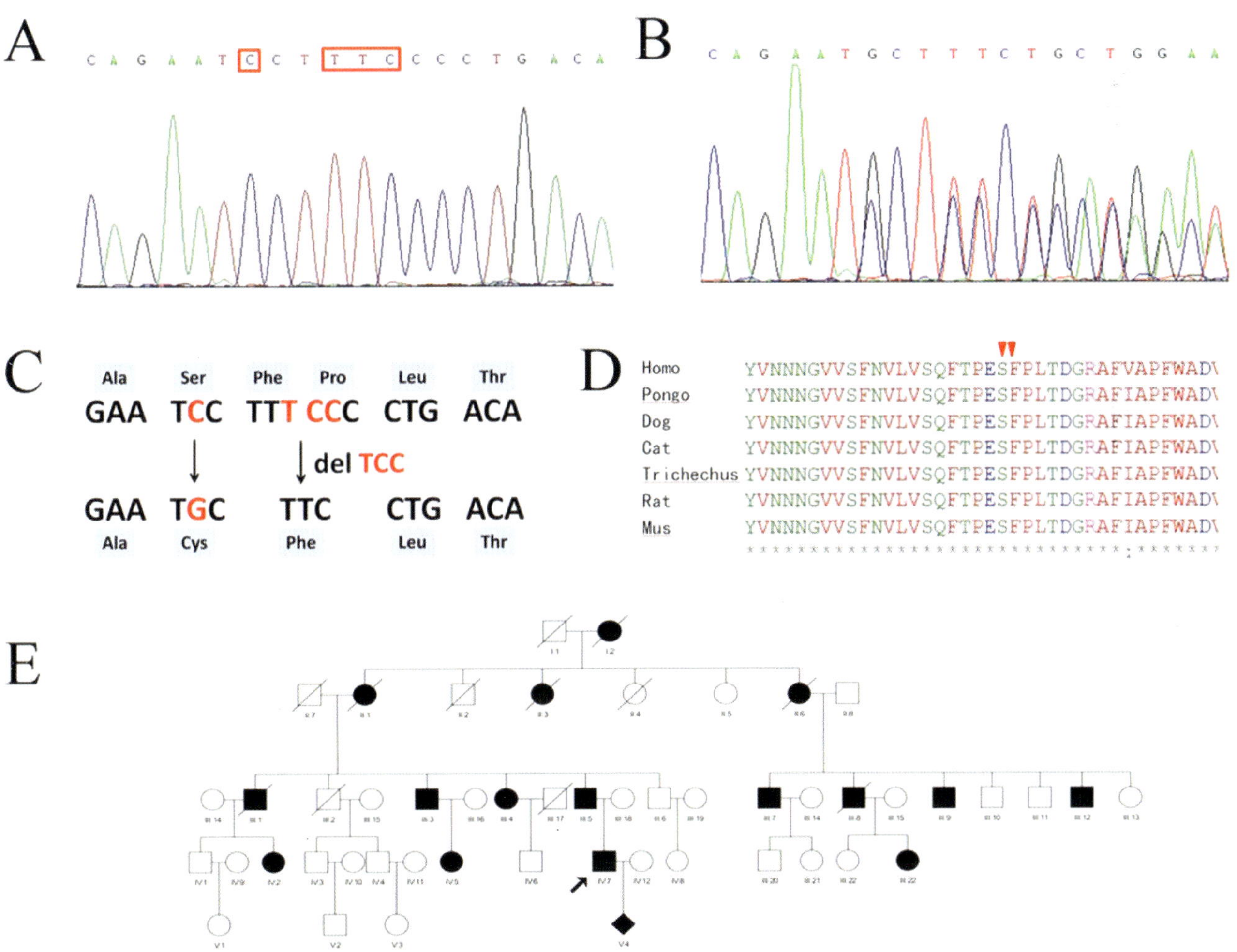

Figure 1. The c.257–262CCTTTC>GCT mutation detected in Family 3187. (**A**) Partial DNA sequences of the *TECTA* gene in a normal family member and (**B**) the c.257–262CCTTTC>GCT mutation (in family members IV:2, IV:7, III:4, III:5, III:3, IV:5). (**C**) The amino acid changes caused by the changes in the DNA sequence. (**D**) Alignment of the α-tectorin and homologous sequences in the N-terminal ENT-like interdomain. The arrow marks the position of the c.257–262CCTTTC>GCT mutation (p. Ser86Cys; p. Pro88del). The ENT-like domain is highly conserved in different species. (**E**) The pedigree of Family 3187 for the c.257–262CCTTTC>GCT mutation. The solid symbols indicate affected individuals.

Beijing, China clinical evaluations, temporal bone imaging results, audiograms, and other relevant clinical information were collected for each member. The proband had no obvious syndromic symptoms, and *GJB2* mutations, *SLC26A4* hotspot mutations, and mtDNA1494 and 1555 mutations were excluded.

Pure-tone audiometry was performed in a sound-controlled room at frequencies ranging from 250 to 8000 Hz, according to standard protocols. Audiograms were available for 6 of the 10 affected members (IV:2, IV:7, III:4, III:5, III:3, IV:5) and 6 unaffected individuals (III:6, III:18, IV:1, IV:3, IV:4, IV:6) (Fig. 1c). The audiology results were characterized in terms of hearing level and audiogram shape.

The study was approved by the Chinese PLA General Hospital Research Ethics Committee. After obtaining written informed consent, blood samples were obtained from 12 family members. Consent was attained from each subject or their guardians.

Target Enrichment, Capture Libraries, MPS

The quality of the genomic DNA (gDNA) was examined by checking the optical density ratio (260/280 ratio) and performing gel electrophoresis. High-molecular-weight gDNA (~5 μg) was fragmented ultrasonically with a Covaris E210 DNA shearing instrument (Covaris, Woburn, MA) to an average size of 200 base pairs (bp). The Covaris protocol was set as follows: 3 min total duration, duty cycle 10%, intensity 5, and 200 cycles per burst.

The exons and flanking 50 bp of 42 known human deafness genes were selected for capture and NGS sequencing with an Illumina Genome Analyzer IIX (Solexa). Hybridization probes (0.5~1.6 kilobase pairs) for these genes were generated from either cDNA clones of the genes or by polymerase chain reaction (PCR) amplification of targeted gDNA regions. To ensure reliable capture of shorter exons, we specifically generated longer hybridization probes from gDNA for those exons that were shorter than 50 bp by including about 100 bp gDNA flanking the exons on both sides. All PCR products (10 ng of each) were cleaned using the QIAquick PCR Purification Kit (QIAGEN, Valencia, CA) before use. More details of capture probe validation and preparation can be found in a previous report [29].

Fragmented gDNA libraries for Illumina GAII sequencing were prepared with the NEBNext™ DNA Sample Prep Master Mix set (E6040, New England Biolabs, Ipswich, MA). End repair of DNA fragments, the addition of a 3′ adenine (A), adaptor ligation, and reaction clean-up were carried out following the manufacturer's protocol. The libraries were cleaned and size-selected using the AMPure DNA Purification kit (Beckman Agencourt, Danvers, MA). The ligated product (20 ng) was amplified for 14 PCR cycles with Illumina PCR primers InPE1.0, InPE2.0, and indexing primers, following the manufacturer's instructions.

For targeted enrichment of deafness genes, the Illumina library DNA was purified with a QIAquick MinElute column and eluted into 50 μL hybridization buffer (HB, Roche NimbleGen, Madison, WI). The barcoded Illumina gDNA libraries (5 μg) were incubated in 16 μL HB on the surface of hybridization glass slides on a hybridization station (BioMicro Systems, Salt Lake City, UT) at 42°C for 72 h. Nonspecific DNA fragments were removed after six washing steps in washing buffer (Roche NimbleGen, Madison, WI). The DNA bound to the probes was eluted by incubating it with NaOH (425 mL, 125 mM) for 10 min. The eluted solution was transferred to a 1.5 mL Eppendorf tube containing 500 μL neutralization buffer (QIAGEN PBI buffer). The neutralized DNA was desalted and concentrated on a QIAquick MinElute column and eluted into 30 μL EB buffer. To increase the yield, we amplified 5 μL eluted solution with 12 PCR cycles using Illumina PCR primers InpE1.0 and InpE2.0. The enrichment of targeted deafness genes was examined by quantitative PCR (qPCR), comparing the growth curves of captured and non-captured samples [30]. Twelve barcoded libraries of captured samples were pooled and paired-end Illumina sequencing was performed with the Illumina HiSeq system (Illumina, San Diego, CA). Details of the bioinformatic analysis methods were previously published [29]. Sequence read data of the patient in this article has been deposited into Sequence Read Archive (http://www.ncbi.nlm.nih.gov/sra webcite; accession number SRR1106702).

Sanger Sequencing

After filtering against multiple databases, Sanger sequencing was used to determine if any of the potential novel mutations in known genes causing ADNSHL co-segregated with the disease phenotype in this family. Sequencing was performed using the ABI 3130 Avant capillary electrophoresis system.

Prenatal Diagnosis

After confirming the genetic defect in Family 3187, we performed prenatal diagnosis for the proband's wife in the 11th week of pregnancy. After obtaining informed consent from the proband and his wife, we performed transabdominal chorion villus sampling under ultrasound guidance. The DNA from the chorion was extracted using a chorion DNA extraction kit (TianGen, Beijing, China). PCR amplification and sequencing of TECTA from the chorion was performed under the same conditions as those used for the blood samples.

Results

Mutation Analysis of the TECTA Gene

We identified a novel mutation (c.257–262CCTTTC>GCT [p. Ser86Cys; p. Pro88del]) in exon 3 (Fig. 1A) of the *TECTA* gene in Family 3187, and confirmed the two mutations at the same allele. The mutation in the coding region of *TECTA* results in two amino acid substitutions: serine to cysteine at position 86 and a deletion of phenylalanine at position 87. The affected members in this family (Fig. 1C) were heterozygous for this mutation, while the mutation was not observed in family members with normal hearing or in 100 unrelated subjects. This mutation was located in the N-terminal region, upstream from the ENT-like domain (Fig. 2), which is highly conserved across species (Fig. 1B). The inheritance pattern of hearing loss in this family is autosomal dominant. This evidence supports the inference that c.257–262CCTTTC>GCT is a pathogenic mutation rather than a rare polymorphism.

The prenatal diagnosis results revealed that the fetus (P0818374) carried the mutation *TECTA* (c.257–262CCTTTC>GCT [p. Ser86Cys; p. Pro88del]) and was predicted to inherit his father's hearing (3187–1).

Audiological Features

In Family 3187, the affected members developed progressive down-sloping bilateral hearing loss beginning in their teens. All six subjects had bilaterally symmetrical hearing loss with average thresholds of 0.5, 1, 2, and 4 kHz (4FA) of 61~70 dB hearing loss in both ears, demonstrating severe hearing impairment according to the WHO 1997 criteria (Table 3). None of the affected subjects had a history or evidence of any other cause of hearing loss (Fig. 3).

Discussion

According to the second nationwide survey of the disabled Chinese population performed in 2006, there were 27.80 million

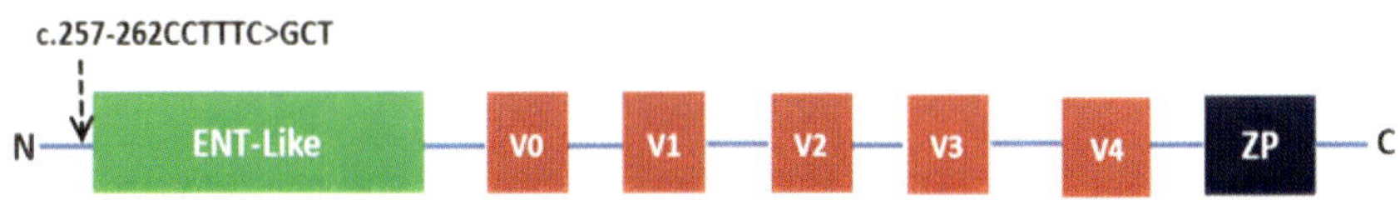

Figure 2. Domain structure of *TECTA*. The mutation lies within the N-terminal region, upstream from the ENT-like domain.

people with hearing and speech disabilities in China; of these, 20.04 million have simple hearing disabilities, with genetic factors accounting for about 50% of the Chinese deaf population of Han ethnicity [37]. Of these cases, almost 80% show autosomal-recessive inheritance. In China, routine clinical diagnostic tests for deafness have consisted of the GJB2 [38,39], SLC26A4 [40], and mitochondrial 12S rRNA genes [41,42]. So far, there is no clinical genetic diagnosis for ADNSHL in China.

ADNSHL is a common and often progressive sensory deficit. There are currently 64 mapped loci for this condition, but only 25 causative genes have been identified. In general, the ADNSHL phenotypes are postlingual hearing loss mostly affecting the high frequencies, although some hereditary hearing loss involves mainly low or intermediate frequencies. The latter is seen in cases with mutations at the DFNA8/12, DFNA13, DFNA21, DFNA31, DFNA44, and DFNA49 loci. In the majority of these traits, some progression is observed. DFNA8/12 hearing loss is caused by mutations in the *TECTA* gene, which encodes the TM protein α-tectorin. Depending on the exons carrying the mutation and thus the protein domains affected, *TECTA* mutations cause either mid- or high-frequency hearing loss. Michael et al. (2011) completed unbiased screening for *TECTA* mutations in a Spanish cohort of 372 probands from ADNSHL families and identified 20 novel mutations in 23 *TECTA* mutations, more than doubling the number of reported *TECTA* ADNSHL mutations from 13 to 33. They postulated that DFNA8/12 hearing loss is one of the most common forms of ADNSHL in the Spanish population and suggested that its global prevalence is about 4% of all ADNSHL [7].

We discovered a novel mutation in exon 3 of the *TECTA* gene in Family 3187: c.257–262CCTTTC>GCT (p. Ser86Cys; p. Pro88del). This was implicated as a pathogenic mutation causing hearing loss. In families with *TECTA* ADNSHL, all reported changes are missense mutations that cause a dominant-negative effect. The mutation c.257C>G located within exon 3 in the N-terminal region of *TECTA*, upstream from the ENT-like domain, resulted in a single amino acid substitution: serine to cysteine. The mutation c.260delTTC results in the deletion of phenylalanine at position 87. Two mutations in this domain have been reported: c.266delT and c.248C>T (p.T83M). Meyer et al. [11] identified three novel homozygous *TECTA* gene mutations in Iranian families, including one frameshift mutation (266delT) in exon 3 that creates a stop codon at position 122 of the protein (122X). Plantinga et al. [43] detected two changes (p.R1890C and p.T83M) in α-tectorin in a family with autosomal-dominant middle-frequency hearing impairment. The mutation c.248C>T (p.T83M) was not in a specific domain and seemed to be a relatively mild amino acid substitution according to the Dayhoff table. However, because this change was not present in controls, it might have affected the phenotype of these patients or even acted synergistically with the p.R1890C mutation [15].

Mutations of the ENT-like domain may cause sensorineural hearing loss. Exon 3 has 287 nucleotides and encodes 96 amino acids (66–162). Together with type IV collagen, laminin, and heparin sulfate proteoglycans, entactin is a major component of basement membranes where it facilitates cell adhesion by binding to calcium ions [44]. Entactin is predicted to interact with laminin and type IV collagen by acting as a bridge and inducing their deposition in the extracellular matrix [45,46]. Therefore, it is possible that the entactin domain of *TECTA* facilitates the assembly and modeling of the extracellular matrix of the TM and that the identified mutations could drastically affect its role during the mechanotransduction of sound.

The *TECTA* gene encodes α-tectorin, which plays an important role in the structure and function of the TM. In mice, targeted deletion of the *TECTA* gene results in complete detachment of the TM from the organ of Corti [23]. In humans, nearly all recessive DFNB21 mutations in *TECTA* result in premature stop codons that may result in either truncated α-tectorin protein products or nonsense-mediated degradation of the *TECTA* mRNA, and are considered loss-of-function mutations [11,14,36]. The DFNA8/12 mutations in *TECTA*, which cause dominant hearing loss, all substitute highly conserved amino acids. The various missense mutations in *TECTA* that cause DFNA8/12 can be subdivided into classes with a clear genotype/phenotype correlation.

The phenotype associated with dominant *TECTA* mutations usually depends on the affected α-tectorin domain. Structural variation in the ZP and ZA domains is common, and most of it likely causes functional problems in α-tectorin. Mutations that affect the vWFD2-D3 inter-repeat connector or vWFD4 repeat from the ZA domain are associated with progressive hearing loss at high frequencies [7]. Conversely, mutations in regions other than the ZA, entactin, or ZP domains, with few exceptions, are associated with mid-frequency hearing loss and result in a flat-to-shallow U-shaped audiometric profile [7,15]. This type of correlation does not exist in familial ADNSHL.

All of our affected subjects had audiogram configurations showing mild ski-slope loss, with greater hearing loss at high frequencies than at low frequencies. The average hearing thresholds at low frequencies of 0.25to 1 kHz were in the range of 40–60 dB hearing loss, whereas those at frequencies higher than 2 kHz were in the range of 60–80 dB hearing loss. The tympanograms were type A, indicating normal function of the middle ear and Eustachian tube. Recruitment was revealed in the subjects by the lower dynamic range between hearing and stapedial acoustic reflex thresholds, which indicated that the

Table 3. Grades of hearing impairment (WHO1997).

Grade of impairment	Corresponding audiometric ISO value
0– None	25 dB or better
1– Slight	26–40 dB
2– Moderate	41–60 dB
3– Severe	61–80 dB
4– Profound, including deafness	81 dB or greater

Grades 2 to 4 are classified as disabling hearing impairment. The audiometric ISO values are averages of values at 500, 1000, 2000, 4000 Hz.

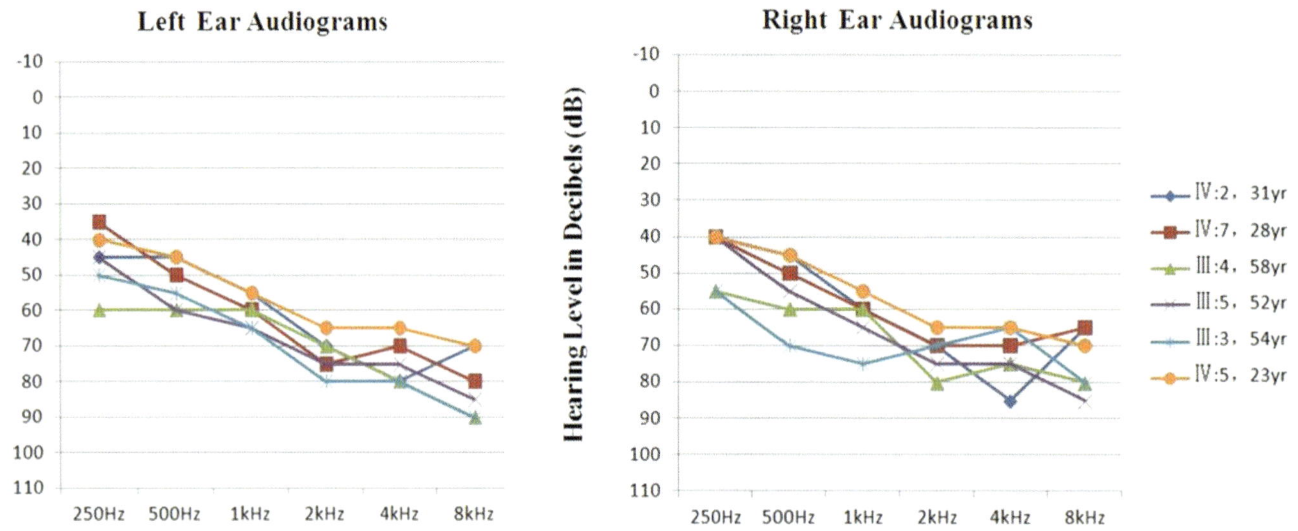

Figure 3. Pure-tone audiograms for the left and right ears of six affected individuals (IV:2, IV:7, III:4, III:5, III:3, IV:5). The numbers to the right are the individuals' ages.

lesions were in cochlea. The patients had absent distortion-product otoacoustic emissions at all frequencies, while auditory brainstem responses were present with normal inter-peak latencies. These results demonstrate that the nonlinear compression function of the cochlea was impaired and suggest that the lesion was near the outer hair cells. The *TECTA* gene encodes the α-tectorin protein in the striated sheet matrix, whereas the TM is an acellular gelatinous structure that contacts the hair cells in the organ of Corti; therefore, mutation of the *TECTA* gene leads to hearing loss.

Worldwide, of the 33 reported DFNA8/12 mutations, only 4 (p.Cys1036Tyr, p.Cys1837Gly, p.Thr1866Met, and p.Arg1890Cys) have been observed in multiple unrelated families. It is difficult to research ADNSHL in depth because of the cost and time involved. In the past few years, NGS technologies have made great strides in both basic and clinical research, providing deeper insights into the complex genomic landscapes of many diseases. Due to the high genetic heterogeneity of hearing loss, targeted DNA capture and MPS appear to be ideal tools for investigating this disease.

The English in this document has been checked by at least two professional editors, both native speakers of English. For a certificate, please see:

http://www.textcheck.com/certificate/sTwy8P.

Author Contributions

Conceived and designed the experiments: PD DYH YS. Performed the experiments: YS WXT XG FY ZYD JDZ YL. Analyzed the data: YS WXT FJ SSH YYY MYH. Contributed reagents/materials/analysis tools: YHZ DYK YSS. Wrote the paper: YS PD.

References

1. Friedman TB, Griffith AJ (2003) Human nonsyndromic sensorineural deafness. Annu Rev Genomics Hum Genet 4: 341–402.
2. Steel KP, Brown SD (1996) Genetics of deafness. Curr Opin Neurobiol 6: 520–525.
3. Cristobal R, Oghalai JS (2008) Hearing loss in children with very low birth weight: current review of epidemiology and pathophysiology. Arch Dis Child Fetal Neonatal Ed 93: F462–468.
4. Alasti F, Sanati MH, Behrouzifard AH, Sadeghi A, de Brouwer AP, et al. (2008) A novel TECTA mutation confirms the recognizable phenotype among autosomal recessive hearing impairment families. Int J Pediatr Otorhinolaryngol 72: 249–255.
5. Collin RW, de Heer AM, Oostrik J, Pauw RJ, Plantinga RF, et al. (2008) Mid-frequency DFNA8/12 hearing loss caused by a synonymous TECTA mutation that affects an exonic splice enhancer. Eur J Hum Genet 16: 1430–1436.
6. de Heer AR, Pauw RJ, Huygen PL, Collin RW, Kremer H, et al. (2009) Flat threshold and mid-frequency hearing impairment in a Dutch DFNA8/12 family with a novel mutation in TECTA. Some evidence for protection of the inner ear. Audiol Neurootol 14: 153–162.
7. Hildebrand MS, Morin M, Meyer NC, Mayo F, Modamio-Hoybjor S, et al. (2011) DFNA8/12 caused by TECTA mutations is the most identified subtype of nonsyndromic autosomal dominant hearing loss. Hum Mutat 32: 825–834.
8. Hughes DC, Legan PK, Steel KP, Richardson GP (1998) Mapping of the alpha-tectorin gene (TECTA) to mouse chromosome 9 and human chromosome 11: a candidate for human autosomal dominant nonsyndromic deafness. Genomics 48: 46–51.
9. Iwasaki S, Harada D, Usami S, Nagura M, Takeshita T, et al. (2002) Association of clinical features with mutation of TECTA in a family with autosomal dominant hearing loss. Arch Otolaryngol Head Neck Surg 128: 913–917.
10. Lezirovitz K, Batissoco AC, Lima FT, Auricchio MT, Nonose RW, et al. (2012) Aberrant transcript produced by a splice donor site deletion in the TECTA gene is associated with autosomal dominant deafness in a Brazilian family. Gene 511: 280–284.
11. Meyer NC, Alasti F, Nishimura CJ, Imanirad P, Kahrizi K, et al. (2007) Identification of three novel TECTA mutations in Iranian families with autosomal recessive nonsyndromic hearing impairment at the DFNB21 locus. Am J Med Genet A 143A: 1623–1629.
12. Moreno-Pelayo MA, Goodyear RJ, Mencia A, Modamio-Hoybjor S, Legan PK, et al. (2008) Characterization of a spontaneous, recessive, missense mutation arising in the Tecta gene. J Assoc Res Otolaryngol 9: 202–214.
13. Moteki H, Nishio SY, Hashimoto S, Takumi Y, Iwasaki S, et al. (2012) TECTA mutations in Japanese with mid-frequency hearing loss affected by zona pellucida domain protein secretion. J Hum Genet 57: 587–592.
14. Naz S, Alasti F, Mowjoodi A, Riazuddin S, Sanati MH, et al. (2003) Distinctive audiometric profile associated with DFNB21 alleles of TECTA. J Med Genet 40: 360–363.
15. Plantinga RF, de Brouwer AP, Huygen PL, Kunst HP, Kremer H, et al. (2006) A novel TECTA mutation in a Dutch DFNA8/12 family confirms genotype-phenotype correlation. J Assoc Res Otolaryngol 7: 173–181.
16. Sagong B, Park HJ, Lee KY, Kim UK (2012) Identification and functional characterization of novel compound heterozygotic mutations in the TECTA gene. Gene 492: 239–243.
17. Sagong B, Park R, Kim YH, Lee KY, Baek JI, et al. (2010) Two novel missense mutations in the TECTA gene in Korean families with autosomal dominant nonsyndromic hearing loss. Ann Clin Lab Sci 40: 380–385.

18. Verhoeven K, Van Laer L, Kirschhofer K, Legan PK, Hughes DC, et al. (1998) Mutations in the human alpha-tectorin gene cause autosomal dominant non-syndromic hearing impairment. Nat Genet 19: 60–62.
19. Legan PK, Rau A, Keen JN, Richardson GP (1997) The mouse tectorins. Modular matrix proteins of the inner ear homologous to components of the sperm-egg adhesion system. J Biol Chem 272: 8791–8801.
20. Maeda Y, Fukushima K, Kasai N, Maeta M, Nishizaki K (2001) Quantification of TECTA and DFNA5 expression in the developing mouse cochlea. Neuroreport 12: 3223–3226.
21. Rau A, Legan PK, Richardson GP (1999) Tectorin mRNA expression is spatially and temporally restricted during mouse inner ear development. J Comp Neurol 405: 271–280.
22. Pfister M, Thiele H, Van Camp G, Fransen E, Apaydin F, et al. (2004) A genotype-phenotype correlation with gender-effect for hearing impairment caused by TECTA mutations. Cell Physiol Biochem 14: 369–376.
23. Legan PK, Lukashkina VA, Goodyear RJ, Kossi M, Russell IJ, et al. (2000) A targeted deletion in alpha-tectorin reveals that the tectorial membrane is required for the gain and timing of cochlear feedback. Neuron 28: 273–285.
24. Legan PK, Lukashkina VA, Goodyear RJ, Lukashkin AN, Verhoeven K, et al. (2005) A deafness mutation isolates a second role for the tectorial membrane in hearing. Nat Neurosci 8: 1035–1042.
25. Metzker ML (2010) Sequencing technologies - the next generation. Nat Rev Genet 11: 31–46.
26. Rehman AU, Morell RJ, Belyantseva IA, Khan SY, Boger ET, et al. (2010) Targeted capture and next-generation sequencing identifies C9orf75, encoding taperin, as the mutated gene in nonsyndromic deafness DFNB79. Am J Hum Genet 86: 378–388.
27. Walsh T, Shahin H, Elkan-Miller T, Lee MK, Thornton AM, et al. (2010) Whole exome sequencing and homozygosity mapping identify mutation in the cell polarity protein GPSM2 as the cause of nonsyndromic hearing loss DFNB82. Am J Hum Genet 87: 90–94.
28. Pierce SB, Walsh T, Chisholm KM, Lee MK, Thornton AM, et al. (2010) Mutations in the DBP-deficiency protein HSD17B4 cause ovarian dysgenesis, hearing loss, and ataxia of Perrault Syndrome. Am J Hum Genet 87: 282–288.
29. Tang W, Qian D, Ahmad S, Mattox D, Todd NW, et al. (2012) A low-cost exon capture method suitable for large-scale screening of genetic deafness by the massively-parallel sequencing approach. Genet Test Mol Biomarkers 16: 536–542.
30. de Lau W, Barker N, Low TY, Koo BK, Li VS, et al. (2011) Lgr5 homologues associate with Wnt receptors and mediate R-spondin signalling. Nature 476: 293–297.
31. Balciuniene J, Dahl N, Jalonen P, Verhoeven K, Van Camp G, et al. (1999) Alpha-tectorin involvement in hearing disabilities: one gene–two phenotypes. Hum Genet 105: 211–216.
32. Alloisio N, Morle L, Bozon M, Godet J, Verhoeven K, et al. (1999) Mutation in the zonadhesin-like domain of alpha-tectorin associated with autosomal dominant non-syndromic hearing loss. Eur J Hum Genet 7: 255–258.
33. Moreno-Pelayo MA, del Castillo I, Villamar M, Romero L, Hernandez-Calvin FJ, et al. (2001) A cysteine substitution in the zona pellucida domain of alpha-tectorin results in autosomal dominant, postlingual, progressive, mid frequency hearing loss in a Spanish family. J Med Genet 38: E13.
34. Meyer NC, Nishimura CJ, McMordie S, Smith RJ (2007) Audioprofiling identifies TECTA and GJB2-related deafness segregating in a single extended pedigree. Clin Genet 72: 130–137.
35. Li Z, Guo Y, Lu Y, Li J, Jin Z, et al. (2013) Identification of a Novel TECTA mutation in a Chinese DFNA8/12 family with prelingual progressive sensorineural hearing impairment. PLoS One 8: e70134.
36. Mustapha M, Weil D, Chardenoux S, Elias S, El-Zir E, et al. (1999) An alpha-tectorin gene defect causes a newly identified autosomal recessive form of sensorineural pre-lingual non-syndromic deafness, DFNB21. Hum Mol Genet 8: 409–412.
37. Han DY (2010) [Strengthen the research on prevention and treatment of sensorineural hearing loss in China]. Zhonghua Er Bi Yan Hou Tou Jing Wai Ke Za Zhi 45: 265–268.
38. Estivill X, Fortina P, Surrey S, Rabionet R, Melchionda S, et al. (1998) Connexin-26 mutations in sporadic and inherited sensorineural deafness. Lancet 351: 394–398.
39. Dai P, Yu F, Han B, Liu X, Wang G, et al. (2009) GJB2 mutation spectrum in 2,063 Chinese patients with nonsyndromic hearing impairment. J Transl Med 7: 26.
40. Smith RJ, Robin NH (2002) Genetic testing for deafness–GJB2 and SLC26A4 as causes of deafness. J Commun Disord 35: 367–377.
41. Zhu Y, Li Q, Chen Z, Kun Y, Liu L, et al. (2009) Mitochondrial haplotype and phenotype of 13 Chinese families may suggest multi-original evolution of mitochondrial C1494T mutation. Mitochondrion 9: 418–428.
42. Kupka S, Bodden-Kamps B, Baur M, Zenner HP, Pfister M (2004) [Mitochondrial A1555G mutation. Molecular genetic diagnosis in sporadic cases of non-syndromic hearing impairment]. HNO 52: 968–972.
43. National Biomedical Research Foundation., Dayhoff MO (1978) Protein segment dictionary 78 : from the Atlas of protein sequence and structure, volume 5, and supplements 1, 2, and 3. Silver Spring, Md.Washington, D.C.: National Biomedical Research Foundation; Georgetown University Medical Center. vii, 470 p.
44. Chung AE (1993) Embryonal carcinoma and the basement membrane glycoproteins laminin and entactin. Int J Dev Biol 37: 141–150.
45. Dziadek M, Paulsson M, Timpl R (1985) Identification and interaction repertoire of large forms of the basement membrane protein nidogen. EMBO J 4: 2513–2518.
46. Dziadek M, Timpl R (1985) Expression of nidogen and laminin in basement membranes during mouse embryogenesis and in teratocarcinoma cells. Dev Biol 111: 372–382.

31

Relation between Speech-in-Noise Threshold, Hearing Loss and Cognition from 40–69 Years of Age

David R. Moore[1,2,3]*, Mark Edmondson-Jones[1,4], Piers Dawes[5], Heather Fortnum[1,4], Abby McCormack[1,2,4], Robert H. Pierzycki[1,4], Kevin J. Munro[5,6]

1 NIHR Nottingham Hearing Biomedical Research Unit, Nottingham, United Kingdom, **2** MRC Institute of Hearing Research, University Park, Nottingham, United Kingdom, **3** Cincinnati Children's Hospital Medical Center and Department of Otolaryngology, University of Cincinnati College of Medicine, Cincinnati, Ohio, United States of America, **4** Otology and Hearing Group, Division of Clinical Neuroscience, School of Medicine, University of Nottingham, Nottingham, United Kingdom, **5** School of Psychological Sciences, University of Manchester, Manchester, United Kingdom, **6** Central Manchester University Hospitals NHS Foundation Trust, Manchester Academic Health Science Centre, Manchester, United Kingdom

Abstract

Background: Healthy hearing depends on sensitive ears and adequate brain processing. Essential aspects of both hearing and cognition decline with advancing age, but it is largely unknown how one influences the other. The current standard measure of hearing, the pure-tone audiogram is not very cognitively demanding and does not predict well the most important yet challenging use of hearing, listening to speech in noisy environments. We analysed data from UK Biobank that asked 40–69 year olds about their hearing, and assessed their ability on tests of speech-in-noise hearing and cognition.

Methods and Findings: About half a million volunteers were recruited through NHS registers. Respondents completed 'whole-body' testing in purpose-designed, community-based test centres across the UK. Objective hearing (spoken digit recognition in noise) and cognitive (reasoning, memory, processing speed) data were analysed using logistic and multiple regression methods. Speech hearing in noise declined exponentially with age for both sexes from about 50 years, differing from previous audiogram data that showed a more linear decline from <40 years for men, and consistently less hearing loss for women. The decline in speech-in-noise hearing was especially dramatic among those with lower cognitive scores. Decreasing cognitive ability and increasing age were both independently associated with decreasing ability to hear speech-in-noise (0.70 and 0.89 dB, respectively) among the population studied. Men subjectively reported up to 60% higher rates of difficulty hearing than women. Workplace noise history associated with difficulty in both subjective hearing and objective speech hearing in noise. Leisure noise history was associated with subjective, but not with objective difficulty hearing.

Conclusions: Older people have declining cognitive processing ability associated with reduced ability to hear speech in noise, measured by recognition of recorded spoken digits. Subjective reports of hearing difficulty generally show a higher prevalence than objective measures, suggesting that current objective methods could be extended further.

Editor: Joel Snyder, UNLV, United States of America

Funding: DRM was supported by the Intramural Programme of the Medical Research Council [Grant U135097130] and by Cincinnati Children's Hospital. The Nottingham Hearing Biomedical Research Unit is funded by the National Institute for Health Research. This paper presents independent research funded in part by the National Institute for Health Research (NIHR). The views expressed are those of the authors and not necessarily those of the NHS, the NIHR or the Department of Health. This research was facilitated by the NIHR Manchester Biomedical Research Centre. The funders had no role in study design, data collection and analysis, decision to publish, or preparation of the manuscript.

Competing Interests: The authors have declared that no competing interests exist.

* Email: david.moore2@cchmc.org

Introduction

The detection of quiet tones of varying frequency, has for >70 years been the gold standard test of hearing [1]. However, the most frequent complaint expressed by people about their hearing is inability to follow speech in noisy environments [2]. Pure-tone audiograms, measures of tone detection threshold across frequency [2], and speech perception measured in the quiet [3], do not predict well the handicap produced by hearing loss. These principles were first recognized long ago [4–7], as was the finding that speech-in-noise (SiN) hearing ability decreases with age [3], even while the audiogram may remain relatively stable [4]. SiN measures that use familiar speech correlate with the average level of hearing based on the pure-tone audiogram (the 'pure tone average', PTA [8–10]) and may offer an alternative gold standard more relevant to everyday hearing. Despite much research, SiN hearing has until recently received little attention in large population studies and limited clinical application. However, the development of the Digit Triplets Test (DTT [11]), a measure of SiN hearing that can be administered without specialist supervision and in any quiet room (go to actiononhearingloss.org.uk for a demonstration and test), enabled inclusion in UK Biobank [12,13]. UK Biobank is an internationally accessible data resource based on a very large-scale, ongoing, longitudinal study across England, Scotland and Wales of many aspects of health, starting in middle age (40–69 year olds; www.ukbiobank.ac.uk).

We report here on the baseline UK Biobank DTT data, compared in the same participants with other UK Biobank data on cognitive ability and self-reported hearing, and with other large, audiogram-based studies [14–18]. Paraphrasing Neisser [19], cognition is the transformation of sensory information into meaning. It may refer to a broad range of constructs relevant to hearing including attention, memory, intelligence, learning, processing speed and language. Language skills were not tested directly in UK Biobank, but they undoubtedly contributed to some extent to the self-report questions on hearing, the DTT, and all the cognitive tests, especially some items in the test of Fluid Intelligence (Fig. S3 in Results S1).

We first asked whether the increase in tone threshold with age, previously measured by the audiogram and by sentences in noise [20], is paralleled by an increase in DTT speech reception threshold (DTT SRT). Given the presumed greater cognitive demand of DTT, involving speech recognition and working memory, we predicted that an increase in DTT SRT with age would be greater than the relative increase in PTA because of a combination of reduced audibility and reduced cognition [21]. This prediction bears on a fundamental clinical issue, how best to measure and treat hearing impairment. This is a timely issue because of the increase of hearing-related problems in an aging population [21] and the large proportion of middle age people with significant and treatable hearing loss who currently remain untreated [22].

Sensitivity to high frequency tones begins to decline in most people by 30–40 years old [16,18] then spreads to lower frequencies from 40 years onwards (Fig. 1B, C). Overall, 21% of UK 40–69 year olds had clinical hearing loss (PTA>20 dB hearing level, HL, 0.5–4.0 kHz in better ear) in the mid-1980s [14], the last time it was measured in a large UK population. The version of the DTT used in UK Biobank, like the original telephone test, has a high frequency limit of 4.0 kHz, so is a suitable test for comparison with those historical data. Cognitive function is most commonly measured using IQ, processing speed and working memory tests [23]. In UK Biobank, cognition is assessed using visually delivered measures of fluid intelligence, processing speed, executive function, number storage (digit span), and visuospatial working memory (shape pairs matching). It is not currently known which aspects of cognition are most closely related to hearing but the broad cognitive categories tested in UK Biobank have all been implicated [24,25]. We report here the relationships between those categories and DTT SRT in middle age.

SiN hearing varies significantly in difficulty, and everyday relevance, with the nature of both the speech (typically syllables, words or sentences) and the noise (e.g. 'white', speech-shaped, modulated, or real, competing speakers). The DTT choice of single digit words promotes easy understanding and the opportunity to 'fill-in' missed acoustic information, while steady-state, speech-shaped noise enables masking across the speech range, but does not allow the 'glimpsing' that can reduce masking in more complex noise. Overall, DTT performance correlates more closely with PTA than do some other SiN tests [10]. The DTT is reproducible, easy to standardize, available in several languages, does not require a sound booth, and may be delivered through the internet. However, it has been suggested [9,10] that it may not be as sensitive to cognitive function as some other SiN tests.

Self-report of hearing difficulties, using questionnaire instruments or often only one or two questions, has commonly been used to assess the prevalence of hearing loss in large epidemiological studies [14,26]. Some studies [14,27] have reported the relationship of self-report with audiometric measures but only rarely have self-report data been validated against standard audiometric measures [28–30]. Self-report assessed by a single question ('Do you feel you have a hearing loss?') has been reported to demonstrate high sensitivity and specificity. A multi-question hearing handicap inventory had lower sensitivity but higher specificity and a positive predictive value. Both question and inventory were recommended for assessing burden but could not measure hearing loss [28].

In this study we investigated the relation between DTT SRT and cognitive ability as a function of age, sex, socioeconomic status, and noise exposure. The results were compared with self-report of hearing difficulties and findings from other studies, including some previously unpublished data from the NIH Toolbox [18,23], of age-related changes in tone sensitivity and cognitive performance. It was predicted that DTT SRT would decline with age more rapidly than tone sensitivity and that the decline in DTT SRT would be more closely associated with increased self-reported hearing difficulty.

Methods

Complete details of all UK Biobank procedures are available at www.ukbiobank.ac.uk.

Ethics statement

This research was covered by the UK Biobank ethics agreement. Within England, UK Biobank has approval from the North West Multi-centre Research Ethics Committee (MREC). All participants provided written informed consent.

Population and setting

Participants (n = 502,642; Table 1) volunteered between March 2007 and July 2010 following invitation letters to 9.2 million eligible UK residents [12]. Data were gathered at 22 assessment centres in England, Scotland and Wales. Participants attended a two-hour appointment during which they answered, via a touch-screen, questions about their life history, lifestyle and health, including their hearing. They also completed a hearing test and several tests of cognitive ability. Participants were free to opt out of the study at any time, either during the assessment or subsequently. Further details of UK Biobank recruitment, the DTT, and prevalence of hearing loss are presented elsewhere [31].

Hearing tests

All participants (Table 1) were asked "Do you have any difficulty with your hearing?" and "Do you find it difficult to follow a conversation if there is background noise (such as TV, radio, children playing)?" Possible answers were 'Yes'; 'No'; 'Do not know'; 'Prefer not to answer'. About one third of the participants were also asked "Have you ever worked in a noisy place where you had to shout to be heard?" and "Have you ever listened to music for more than 3 hours per week at a volume which you would need to shout to be heard or, if wearing headphones, someone else would need to shout for you to hear them?" Possible answers for these noise and music exposure questions were 'Yes, for more than 5 years'; 'Yes, for around 1–5 years'; 'Yes, for less than a year'; 'No'; 'Do not know'; 'Prefer not to answer'.

Guided by a video demonstration (see http://biobank.ctsu.ox.ac.uk/crystal/videos/hearing.swf), about one third of the participants (Table 1) completed a truncated DTT with fifteen (monosyllabic single digit) triplets (e.g. 5-0-8) presented separately to each ear via circumaural headphones (Sennheiser D25 [31]. A noise, shaped spectrally to the complete set of 9 digits, was played

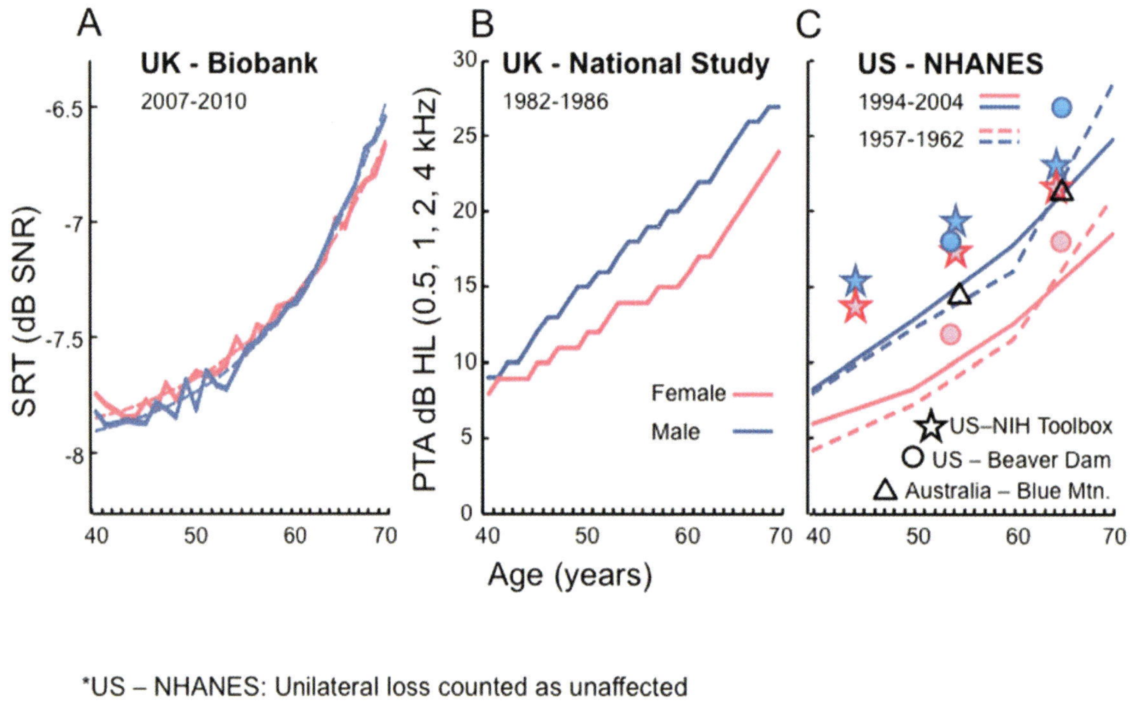

Figure 1. Hearing declines from 40–69 years of age. (A) UK Biobank: Mean DTT speech reception threshold (SRT; better ear) data, corrected for differences in socio-economic between samples. Exponential functions with an additive constant are fitted to the data. (B) National Study of Hearing (UK [14]): Mean pure tone average (PTA) thresholds (0.5, 1, 2, 4 kHz; better ear). (C) National Health and Nutrition Examination Survey (NHANES, US [16]): Mean PTA thresholds (0.5–4 kHz). Other data points from NIH Toolbox (US, 2011 [18]), Beaver Dam Epidemiology of Hearing Loss Study (US, 1993 [15]), Blue Mountains Hearing Study (Australia, 1997–2000 [17]).

Table 1. Characteristics of UK Biobank participants.

Demographics	Female		Male		All	
	N (%)	mean±sd % +ve	N (%)	mean±sd % +ve	N (%)	mean±sd % +ve
Gender	273,448 (54%)	-	229,194 (46%)	-	502,642 (100%)	-
Age	273,448 (100%)	56.3±8.0 yrs	229,194 (100%)	56.7±8.2 yrs	502,642 (100%)	56.5±8.1 yrs
Auditory tests/questions						
SRT (better ear; dB)	87,650 (32%)	−7.4±1.6 dB	73,305 (32%)	−7.4±1.8 dB	160,955 (32%)	−7.4±1.7 dB
Hearing difficulty	258,576 (95%)	21%	219,120 (96%)	31%	477,696 (95%)	26%
Hearing in noise	266,966 (98%)	33%	224,032 (98%)	43%	490,998 (98%)	38%
Noisy workplace exposure	92,881 (34%)	11%	77,501 (34%)	37%	170,382 (34%)	23%
Loud music exposure	92,424 (34%)	9%	77,109 (34%)	17%	169,533 (34%)	12%
Cognitive tests						
Fluid Intelligence	90,202 (33%)	5.9±2.1 correct	75,306 (33%)	6.1±2.2 correct	165,508 (33%)	6.0±2.2 correct
Prospective Memory	93,382 (34%)	76%	78,219 (34%)	77%	171,601 (34%)	76%
Visual Memory	270,996 (99%)	4.7±3.7 pairs	227,054 (99%)	4.7±3.9 pairs	498,050 (99%)	4.7±3.8 pairs
Reaction Time	270,470 (99%)	567±117 ms	226,412 (99%)	551±116 ms	496,882 (99%)	560±117 ms
Digit Span	28,179 (10%)	6.4±1.8 digits	23,637 (10%)	6.6±1.9 digits	51,816 (10%)	6.5±1.8 digits

Number and performance of participants completing each auditory and cognitive measure. Percentages for each N other than gender are corrected for missing data. Mean ± sd: descriptive statistics for age, SRT, cognitive tests. % +ve: percent positive responses to each question. Cognitive test performance shows number of questions correctly answered (FI), % correct responses (PM), and number of incorrectly chosen pairs (VM).

simultaneously. Both noise and (suprathreshold) speech levels were initially adjusted together to a comfortable level. The speech level was then fixed and noise level was varied adaptively after each triplet, dependent on the listener's correct touchscreen response to all three digits, to obtain criterion performance of 50% correct. The measure of hearing, the DTT SRT, was the mean signal-to-noise ratio from the last eight triplets. Testing of each ear took ~4 minutes.

Participants were asked about several other aspects of hearing, including their use of hearing aids or cochlear implants. If they used hearing aids they were asked to remove them prior to completing the DTT. If they used cochlear implants they were asked not to attempt the test. Further studies using the UK Biobank resource and dealing in detail with associations and predictions between hearing and hearing aids [32], tinnitus [33], visual impairment and dual sensory problems [34], cigarette smoking and alcohol consumption [35], have or will be published elsewhere.

Cognitive tests

Variable numbers of participants completed each test (Table 1), primarily due to the introduction of different tests at different stages during the UK Biobank project. The Fluid Intelligence test comprised thirteen questions designed to test logic and reasoning ability (e.g. If Truda's mother's brother is Tim's sister's father, what relation is Truda to Tim?; Fig. S3 in Results S1). The Prospective (long-term) Memory test presented the following instruction early in the cognitive test battery: "At the end of the games we will show you four coloured shapes and ask you to touch the Blue Square. However, to test your memory, we want you to actually touch the Orange Circle instead." In two rounds, the Visual (short-term) Memory ('Pairs matching') test presented a matrix (1st round: 2×3; 2nd round: 3×4) of cards showing 3 and 6 pairs of shapes, respectively. The shapes were concealed and the participant was required to recall locations of matching shape pairs. Correct responses were confirmed. The Reaction Time test of processing speed sequentially presented twelve pairs of shapes. The participant pressed a button as quickly as possible if a pair of shapes matched. Finally, in the Digit Span ('Numeric memory') test of verbal working memory participants were initially presented on the screen with two digits and were required to key in the digits in reverse order. After each correct response the digit sequence was increased by one. The task ended after two incorrect responses. Raw score was the maximum number of correctly recalled and ordered digits. Performance on the Prospective Memory, Reaction Time and Digit Span tests additionally depended on executive function and all tests depended on alerting and orienting attention.

Analysis and reporting

Analysis of self-report measures used binary logistic regression. Standardised scores, which each maximised the variability within the sampled population, were derived for each cognitive test using principal components analysis. A composite score was defined as a simple sum of the five standardised scores. Both individual and composite cognitive scores were standardised to have zero mean and unit standard deviation, such that higher values corresponded to higher ability. Scores were grouped into deciles for analysis. Regression modelling techniques accounting for sex, socio-economic deprivation (Townsend score, a proxy measure of socioeconomic status [31]), noise exposure (work and music), and interaction of socio-economic deprivation and noise with sex, were used to dissociate decline in hearing from decline in cognition with increasing age. Age at which full-time education was completed was not accounted for in these models but varied little between women (mean = 16.68, s.d. = 2.17) and men (mean = 16.76 years; s.d. = 2.52). Modelling that included cognitive scores was restricted to the 40,655 participants who completed all auditory and cognitive tests and questions. Data were assumed to be missing completely at random, as the primary reason for absent responses was the phased introduction of test components.

Results

Hearing

Age-related decline of hearing differs between test measures (Fig. 1). DTT SRT, averaged across participants, declined exponentially with age, starting from a low (sensitive) level in the 40 s (Fig. 1A). Both the absolute level and the rate of age-related decline of DTT SRT in men and women advanced in close parallel as individuals in the population became older, although SRT was slightly better in younger men than in younger women, and slightly better in older women than in older men. Tone sensitivity (indexed by the PTA, [9]) has also been shown in several studies across a 50 year time span to decline with age (Figs. 1B,C). However, in contrast to DTT SRT, tone sensitivity has previously been shown to decline rapidly through the 40 s, at least among men. Men had markedly poorer sensitivity than women at all ages >40, but women's sensitivity started to deteriorate in parallel with that of men when they reached their 60 s. A reduction in the rate of declining tone sensitivity with advancing age has been noted in some more recent studies (Fig. 1C [16,18,36]), but high frequency sensitivity remains much more susceptible to aging and clearly poorer in men (Fig. S1 in Results S1).

In UK Biobank, more men reported having problems with their hearing than did women (Fig. 2). Reported problems for both sexes grew linearly with age. By 69 y.o., men were reporting hearing difficulties, and difficulties in noise, at 40–60% higher prevalence than women. This increasing difference between men and women with age was not paralleled by objective measures of either speech or tone hearing (Fig. 1), nor by direct comparison between the prevalence of reported difficulty and DTT hearing (Fig. S2 in Results S1). Responses to questions about workplace noise (Table 2) showed the same relationship for women and men between increasing duration of noise exposure and the objective measure of decreased DTT SRT. Note, however, that the maximum effect size (mean 0.19 dB loss of SRT for >5 years exposure) was relatively small compared with age-related hearing loss (Fig. 1A; Table 3). No difference was found between the sexes for the effect of workplace noise on DTT SRT, and no significant effect of music exposure on DTT SRT was found. In contrast, both workplace noise and music exposure were significantly related to subjective reports of 'difficulty hearing' (Table 2) and 'hearing in noise' (Table S1 in Results S1). But while a far higher proportion of men than women reported exposure both to a noisy workplace and to loud music (Table 1), there was not a consistent dose-response difference between the sexes (Table 2). Men who experienced shorter noisy workplace exposure were less likely than women to report difficulty with their hearing, whereas men who experienced longer exposure were more likely than women to report difficulty. For music, there was no significant difference between the sexes.

Cognition

Cognitive performance, like hearing, decreased with advancing age on all tests (Fig. 3, Table 3). For four tests, the pattern of decline was relatively simple and monotonic. However, Fluid Intelligence did not begin to decline until 60 y.o., then declined

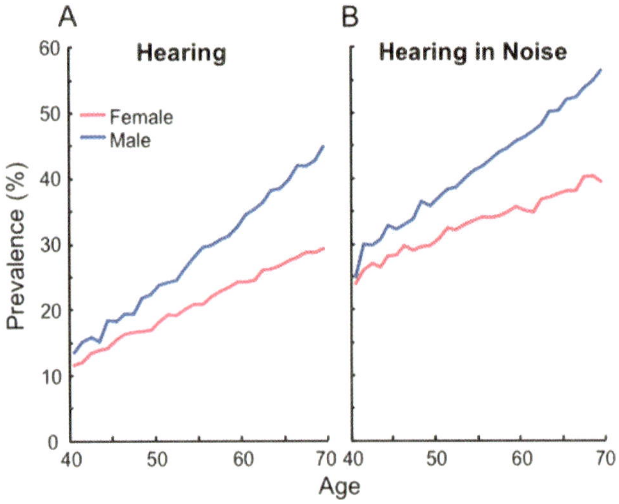

Figure 2. Men report greater difficulty hearing than women. Prevalence of self-report of (A) hearing difficulty and (B) difficulty hearing speech-in-noise in women and men from 40–70 y.o., corrected for socio-economic.

linearly for ages >60. Responses to individual Fluid Intelligence questions suggested this was due to a decline in both verbal and non-verbal performance from about this age (Fig. S3 in Results S1). Men performed better than women on all tests except prospective memory. The mean gap between the sexes increased with age on Reaction Time and Digit Span. Correlation between scores on individual tests varied from r = 0.19–0.38 (Table S2 in Results S1).

Relation between hearing and cognition

Better DTT SRT was associated with better cognitive ability. Fig. 4 shows cognitive ability on each test, plotted as deciles from 1 (lowest) to 10 (highest), as a function of DTT SRT. DTT SRT decreased by about 0.7 dB across the range of ability (i.e. from decile 1 to 10) on each cognitive test. This was similar in size to the increase in average DTT SRT across the 40–69 year age range (women: 0.75 dB, men: 1.05 dB; Table 3). DTT SRT differences were greatest at the lower end of cognitive ability. These results suggested that the ability to compensate for impaired DTT SRT depended strongly on cognitive performance, especially at the lower end of the spectrum. However, DTT SRT declined with age across the cognitive spectrum (Fig. S5 in Results S1).

Discussion

Hearing in quiet and in noise

We found that, on average, DTT SRT declines substantially during late middle age, confirming earlier studies [11,20]. However, we also found little decline in DTT SRT until the 50 s, whereas declining PTA, based on the same frequency range used in the DTT, begins in the 30 s [14,16,18]. These differences may be due to the high 'redundancy' of the DTT speech signal relative to a single tone. Digits are a closed set of overlearned words. A listener can access many auditory tone channels, only some of which need be fully functional, to gain cues to digit identity. For example, many English digits can be distinguished using only vowels. Small changes in sensitivity to higher frequency tones in the 30 s and 40 s can therefore over-estimate real-life difficulty with speech, even when there is little or no contextual information, as in the DTT. At later ages, deficits in DTT SRT escalate rapidly and, by the early 60 s, are advancing relatively more rapidly than loss of tone sensitivity, presumably due to both more widespread loss of tone sensitivity and reduced auditory processing in the brain. Historically, tone sensitivity studies have also reported that men's hearing begins to deteriorate before that of women, particularly at high sound frequencies, and that the difference is maintained into old age. Some recent evidence [18] suggests that disparity may be declining, at least in the main speech range of hearing. Nevertheless, the UK Biobank data are notable in showing a close similarity between the DTT hearing of men and women across most of the age range studied, but with men showing a slightly greater decline in the late 60 s.

The different patterns of age-related hearing loss revealed by the two measures is evidence that DTT SRT utilizes different or additional mechanisms to those revealed by audiometry. One candidate mechanism may be an age-related loss of inner hair cell afferent synapses, as recently reported in mice [37]. In that example of supra-threshold hearing loss, mid-frequency pure tone thresholds measured by wave I of the auditory brainstem response were still normal in older (64–80 week old) mice when supra-threshold response amplitude was reduced relative to younger (4–16 week old) mice. The results suggest a loss of the number and synchrony of functional cochlear nerve fibres. In a human parallel of these findings, cochlear nerve neuron (spiral ganglion) cell bodies appear to be lost continually from a young age (<20 years [38]) when, again, auditory thresholds and otoacoustic emissions are normal, signifying intact hair cells. However, no differences in this process were seen between the sexes or across the length of the cochlea. Because aging men typically have poorer high frequency, but may not have poorer low frequency hearing than women (Fig. 1B; Fig. S1 in Results S1 [39]), we also suggest that the high redundancy of the speech signals enables men to identify the digits used in the current study based on the lower frequency cues (e.g. vowels) they can hear.

Subjective reports of hearing difficulty were predictable from DTT SRT, but did not match the pattern of decline in DTT SRT (or PTA [14–18]) with increasing age. A surprisingly high proportion of 40–50 y.o. people with normal DTT SRT indicated that they had difficulty hearing. That proportion rose with age and reduced DTT SRT, as expected, but the proportion of men reporting difficulty was markedly higher than that of women at nearly all ages. Two explanations for these phenomena are that the tests did not capture the handicap experienced, or that people misperceived their hearing to be worse than it really was. We think both these factors contributed to the results. Challenges to making realistic measures of speech hearing include the variety of situations encountered in everyday life and the variety of speech hearing to which individual brains are 'tuned'. For example, we do most of our listening in reverberant rooms having a wide range of acoustic characteristics known to affect speech intelligibility [40]. Accents can be remarkably variable both between older, established communities and within modern, multi-ethnic urban centres, making calibration difficult, both for the audiologist and for the listener. The band-limited (<4 kHz) UK Biobank DTT probably captures some, but not all hearing loss that affects suprathreshold listening. Newly-developed, internet-deliverable SiN hearing tests that have shown greater sensitivity to high frequency hearing loss than the UK Biobank DTT [41,42], may help further in meeting these challenges, and other SiN tests may capture additional relevant properties of the acoustic environment. For example, a modified version of the widely used QuickSIN [43] sentence-in-noise test incorporates separately measurable audiovi-

Table 2. Noisy workplace and music exposure: objective and subjective effects on hearing.

Objective (SRT)	Female (dB)	p	Male (dB)	p	All (dB)	p	Factor (p)	Sex (p)
Noisy workplace	-	-	-	-	-	-	<0.001	0.572
<1year	-	-	-	-	0.05	0.10		
1–5 years	-	-	-	-	0.08	0.01		
>5 years	-	-	-	-	0.19	<0.001		
Music exposure	-	-	-	-	-	-	0.24	0.79
Subjective ('Difficulty')	Female (OR)	p	Male (OR)	p	All (OR)	p	Factor (p)	Sex (p)
Noisy workplace	-	-	-	-	-	-	<0.001	<0.001
<1year	1.72	<0.001	1.33	<0.001	-	-		
1–5 years	1.76	<0.001	1.84	<0.001	-	-		
>5 years	2.19	<0.001	2.89	<0.001	-	-		
Music exposure	-	-	-	-	-	-	<0.001	0.11
<1year	-	-	-	-	1.50	<0.001		
1–5 years	-	-	-	-	1.87	<0.001		
>5 years	-	-	-	-	1.98	<0.001		

Objective (SRT): General linear modelling of better ear speech reception threshold (dB) based on number of years workplace noise exposure relative to no exposure. Factor: Main effect for noise/music exposure. Sex: Interaction with gender. The model also includes terms for age, sex and cognition (Table 3).

Subjective ('Difficulty hearing'): Logistic modelling of question association yielding odds ratios (OR) between no exposure and number of years indicated. Other details as for objective test. Similar results were obtained for 'Difficulty hearing in noise' (Table S1 in Results S1).

Table 3. Modelling speech-in-noise.

	Female		Male		All		Factor	Sex
	dB	**p**	**dB**	**p**	**dB**	**p**	**p**	**p**
Gender (Female)								
Male	-	-	-	-	−0.16	<0.001		
Age (40–44)	0	-	-	-	-	-	<0.001	<0.001
45–49	0.03	0.48	0.02	0.60	-	-		
50–54	0.12	0.001	0.16	<0.001	-	-		
55–59	0.31	<0.001	0.39	<0.001	-	-		
60–64	0.52	<0.001	0.66	<0.001	-	-		
65–69	0.75	<0.001	1.05	<0.001	-	-		
Deprivation	-	-	-	-	-	-	0.37	0.47
Cognition (1 = poor)	-	-	-	-	0	-	<0.001	0.39
2	-	-	-	-	−0.31	<0.001		
3	-	-	-	-	−0.43	<0.001		
4	-	-	-	-	−0.45	<0.001		
5	-	-	-	-	−0.51	<0.001		
6	-	-	-	-	−0.59	<0.001		
7	-	-	-	-	−0.59	<0.001		
8	-	-	-	-	−0.63	<0.001		
9	-	-	-	-	−0.63	<0.001		
10 = good	-	-	-	-	−0.70	<0.001		

General linear modelling of better ear speech reception threshold (dB) based on gender, age, socio-economic, and cognition. Gender, Age and Cognition reference levels were females, the youngest quintile, and the poorest performers, respectively. Factor: Main effect for Age/Deprivation/Cognition. Sex: Interaction with gender.

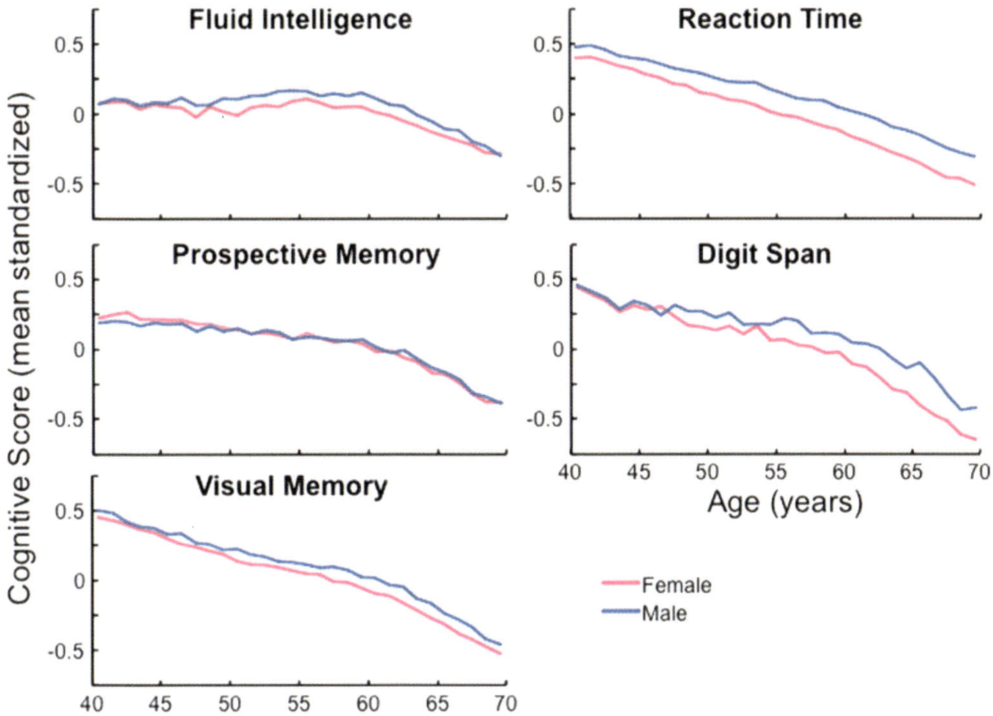

Figure 3. Cognitive performance declines with age. Cognitive performance of men and women in the UK Biobank study expressed as a mean standardized (z) score for ease of comparison between different tests.

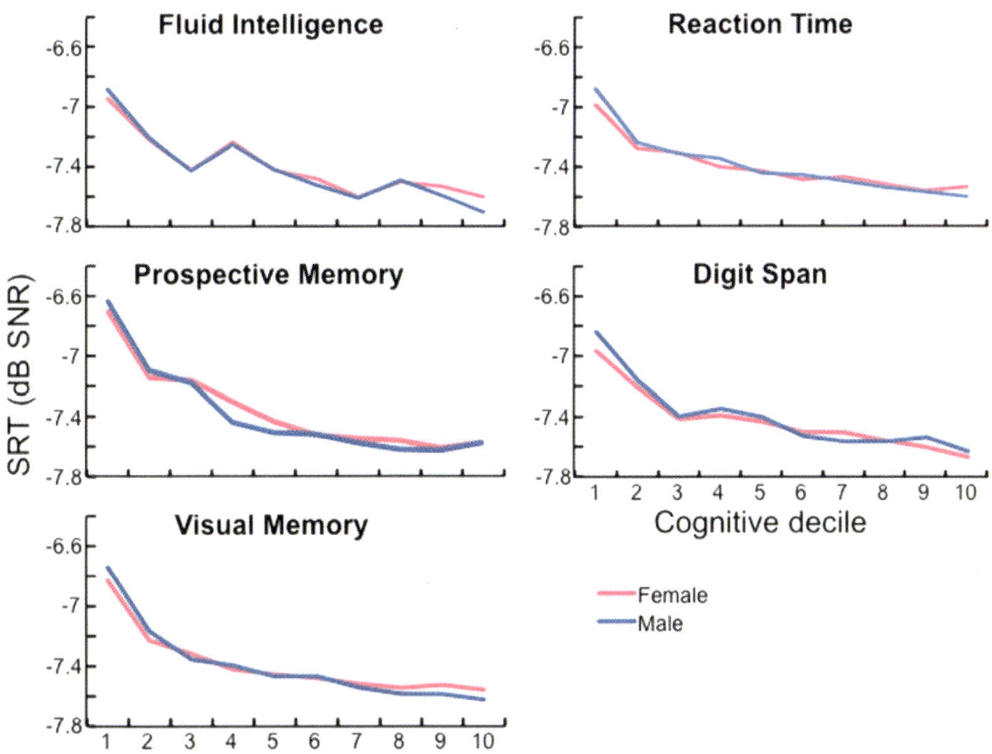

Figure 4. Better cognition is associated with better hearing. Relation between mean SRT and mean performance on each cognitive test (by decile of standardized score from 1 = low to 10 = high), all ages (40–69 y.o.) combined.

sual, reverberation, and spatial cues, and a speeded speech condition [44] (see [45] for a review of SiN tests). Nevertheless, self-report remains an important 'reality check' on the usefulness of any measure of hearing.

This raises the second possibility, that people misperceive their degree of handicap. Everyone has difficulty hearing in some circumstances, and those circumstances are typically in a busy, noisy, reverberant room, such as a bar [40]. The UK Biobank data suggest this 'baseline' rate for perceived difficulty hearing in noise is around 25% for women and 35% for men (Fig. S2 in Results S1). There are many possible reasons why men may both have high estimates of their degree of handicap and have poorer tone sensitivity. One is that they may operate in noisier environments than women. In fact, more men than women reported spending time in noisy environments, both at work and at leisure, and men having longer exposure to noise also reported more difficulty hearing. Nevertheless, the DTT SRT of men did not differ significantly from exposure-matched women who made fewer reports of hearing difficulties, possibly because the men had an increased prevalence of auditory pathology that was not captured by the DTT SRT. Self-reported difficulty in relation to music exposure, which was significant, had quite high odds ratios, and did not differ between the sexes, was similarly not matched by any significant change in DTT SRT.

Cognition and hearing

DTT SRT was found to decline with decreasing cognitive ability, consistent with previous reports using other SiN tests [46,47]. If some aspect(s) of cognition (e.g. long-term memory [48]) was more important than others for speech-in-noise hearing and listening, that aspect should associate more strongly than others with DTT SRT. However, the decline was seen on each cognitive test used, to about the same extent, suggesting that some general cognitive factor may have been responsible. It has been suggested that reduced tone sensitivity is the 'primary predictor' of speech intelligibility with advancing age [49] and that age-related changes in cognitive function are mediated by age-related changes in 'global sensory processing' (hearing, vision, touch composite [47]). The current data suggest a much more prominent role for cognition in hearing, at least for the DTT. Other data from the NIH Toolbox, reported here for the first time, even suggest that poor cognitive function plays a role, albeit a relatively minor one, in reduced PTA (Fig. S4 in Results S1; [18]).

A critical question is whether decreasing tone sensitivity, decreasing cognitive function, both, or another factor (e.g. 'common cause' [50]) is primarily responsible for age-related decline of DTT SRT. Our analysis showed that, across the ages examined, better cognitive function was associated independently with a 0.7 dB reduction in DDT SRT. The effect of increasing age was additive to that effect, leading to a 0.7 (female) to 1.0 dB (male) increase in DDT SRT. In auditory terms, the decline in DTT SRT with age could be due to both peripheral and central factors. Peripheral hearing loss certainly contributes, since we know that tone sensitivity declines with age, even in the most cognitively able [50]. But declining central function may also contribute. For example, there is recent evidence that age-related decline in the maximum speed of auditory temporal processing includes a specifically central mechanism [51]. It is currently unknown whether this is operative within the central auditory system, which includes extensive sub-cortical networks, or within higher level processing areas that include those with multimodal cognitive functions. In either case, such a mechanism could have a marked effect on speech perception, since reduced temporal fine structure can reduce consonant discrimination [52]. Because of the high reliance of auditory processing on precise timing, auditory processing may prove a sensitive model for testing the 'Processing speed theory' of cognitive decline [53], according to which declining processing speed is the common cause of cognitive decline.

Clinical significance

It is clear that cognitive factors play a major role in speech perception. Although even tone sensitivity is influenced by cognition (e.g. motivation, learning [54]), that influence is not strong, so there is an argument for the addition of tests of speech perception to routine audiometric assessment. Among the older population, differences in the cognitive abilities of the most and least able become more extreme [55] and reports of difficulties hearing speech in noisy environments become more common, as shown here and elsewhere [2]. SiN assessment may help identify those individuals who are likely to benefit from different interventions. Among middle-aged people, who do not typically seek assistance for their hearing loss [22], poorer SiN ability could be a first warning of a need for intervention. Unlike the audiogram, the DTT and some other SiN hearing tests can be delivered remotely for unsupervised, user-based testing via the internet, and are already being used for widespread hearing screening (e.g. visit actiononhearingloss.org.uk). A DTT (the Dutch Digits-in-Noise, DIN, test) has recently been suggested as a clinical diagnostic test [9]. Despite the close association with cognition demonstrated here, DTTs that use steady noise masking have been suggested to be less cognitively demanding than other SiN tests (e.g. using speech maskers [7]). However, this view has been questioned by DTT data [9] showing an extremely high correlation ($r = 0.96$, following level correction) with performance on Plomp and Mimpen [20] sentences. In contrast to other SiN tests, DTTs are also readily transferrable across cultural and even language groups (www.HearCom.eu [42], [10]). Together, these findings suggest the possibility of a DTT as an international standard for SiN testing.

Supporting Information

Results S1 This file contains Table S1, Table S2, and Figure S1–Figure S5. Table S1, Noisy workplace and music exposure: Relation to 'Hearing in noise' question. Table S2, Pairwise Pearson correlation coefficients between cognitive test measures. Figure S1. Average (PTA) tone detection thresholds declined from 18–85 years (NIH Toolbox data [13]). Figure S2, Reported difficulty hearing increased with declining DTT hearing. Figure S3, Fluid intelligence varied with question, age and gender. Figure S4, PTA did not vary substantially with cognitive ability. Figure S5, Hearing declined with both cognitive ability and age.

Acknowledgments

Disclaimer: This paper presents independent research funded in part by the National Institute for Health Research (NIHR). The views expressed are those of the authors and not necessarily those of the NHS, the NIHR or the Department of Health.

This research has been conducted using the UK Biobank resource. Funding to support the present research was provided by the National Institute of Health Research, the Medical Research Council, the University of Manchester, the Central Manchester University Hospitals NHS Foundation Trust, and Cincinnati Children's Hospital. Additional data were obtained from the NIH Toolbox standardization project [18]. We thank the participants of the UK Biobank resource and NIH Toolbox project for donating their time.

Author Contributions

Conceived and designed the experiments: DRM. Analyzed the data: DRM MEJ PD KJM. Contributed reagents/materials/analysis tools: DRM MEJ PD. Wrote the paper: DRM MEJ PD HF AMC RHP KJM. Liaised with UK Biobank: DRM MEJ PD HF AMC RHP KJM.

References

1. Johnson EW (1970) Tuning forks to audiometers and back again. Laryngoscope 80: 49–68.
2. Vermiglio AJ, Soli SD, Freed DJ, Fisher LM (2012) The relationship between high-frequency pure-tone hearing loss, hearing in noise test (HINT) thresholds, and the articulation index. J Am Acad Audiol 23: 779–788.
3. Plomp R (1986) A signal-to-noise ratio model for the speech-reception threshold of the hearing impaired. J Speech Hear Res 29: 146–154.
4. Bergman M (1971) Hearing and aging. Implications of recent research findings. Audiology 10: 164–171.
5. CHBBC (1988) Speech understanding and aging. Working Group on Speech Understanding and Aging. Committee on Hearing, Bioacoustics, and Biomechanics, Commission on Behavioral and Social Sciences and Education, National Research Council. J Acoust Soc Am 83: 859–895.
6. Gordon-Salant S, Frisina RD, Fay RR, Popper AN, editor (2009) The Aging Auditory System. New Yor: Springer.
7. Humes LE, Kidd GR, Lentz JJ (2013) Auditory and cognitive factors underlying individual differences in aided speech-understanding among older adults. Front Syst Neurosci 7: 55.
8. Smits C, Kapteyn TS, Houtgast T (2004) Development and validation of an automatic speech-in-noise screening test by telephone. Int J Audiol 43: 15–28.
9. Smits C, Theo Goverts S, Festen JM (2013) The digits-in-noise test: assessing auditory speech recognition abilities in noise. J Acoust Soc Am 133: 1693–1706.
10. Jansen S, Luts H, Dejonckere P, van Wieringen A, Wouters J (2013) Efficient Hearing Screening in Noise-Exposed Listeners Using the Digit Triplet Test. Ear Hear 34: 773–778.
11. Smits C, Houtgast T (2005) Results from the Dutch speech-in-noise screening test by telephone. Ear Hear 26: 89–95.
12. Allen N, Sudlow C, Downey P, Peakman T (2012) UK Biobank: Current status and what it means for epidemiology. Health Policy and Technology 1: 123–126.
13. Collins R (2012) What makes UK Biobank special? Lancet 379: 1173–1174.
14. Davis A (1995) Hearing in Adults: Whurr Publishers limited. 1011 p.
15. Cruickshanks KJ, Wiley TL, Tweed TS, Klein BE, Klein R, et al. (1998) Prevalence of hearing loss in older adults in Beaver Dam, Wisconsin. The Epidemiology of Hearing Loss Study. Am J Epidemiol 148: 879–886.
16. Hoffman HJ, Dobie RA, Ko CW, Themann CL, Murphy WJ (2010) Americans hear as well or better today compared with 40 years ago: hearing threshold levels in the unscreened adult population of the United States, 1959–1962 and 1999–2004. Ear Hear 31: 725–734.
17. Chia EM, Wang JJ, Rochtchina E, Cumming RR, Newall P, et al. (2007) Hearing impairment and health-related quality of life: the Blue Mountains Hearing Study. Ear Hear 28: 187–195.
18. Gershon R, Beaumont J (2012) NIH Toolbox norming study data set: Sensation [data file] Version 1.0. Chicago, IL: Northwestern University and National Institutes of Health.
19. Neisser U (1967) Cognitive Psychology. New York: Appleton-Century-Crofts.
20. Plomp R, Mimpen AM (1979) Speech-reception threshold for sentences as a function of age and noise level. J Acoust Soc Am 66: 1333–1342.
21. Moore DR, Fullgrabe C (2012) Cognitive contributions to hearing in older people. J Hear Sci 2: 58–60.
22. Davis A, Smith P, Ferguson M, Stephens D, Gianopoulos I (2007) Acceptability, benefit and costs of early screening for hearing disability: a study of potential screening tests and models. Health Technol Assess 11: 1–294.
23. Weintraub S, Dikmen SS, Heaton RK, Tulsky DS, Zelazo PD, et al. (2013) Cognition assessment using the NIH Toolbox. Neurology 80: S54–64.
24. Moore DR, Ferguson MA, Edmondson-Jones AM, Ratib S, Riley A (2010) Nature of auditory processing disorder in children. Pediatrics 126: e382–390.
25. Sorqvist P, Stenfelt S, Ronnberg J (2012) Working memory capacity and visual-verbal cognitive load modulate auditory-sensory gating in the brainstem: toward a unified view of attention. J Cogn Neurosci 24: 2147–2154.
26. Rosenhall U, Pedersen K, Moller MB (1987) Self-assessment of hearing problems in an elderly population. A longitudinal study. Scand Audiol 16: 211–217.
27. Wilson DH, Walsh PG, Sanchez L, Davis AC, Taylor AW, et al. (1999) The epidemiology of hearing impairment in an Australian adult population. Int J Epidemiol 28: 247–252.
28. Sindhusake D, Mitchell P, Smith W, Golding M, Newall P, et al. (2001) Validation of self-reported hearing loss. The Blue Mountains Hearing Study. Int J Epidemiol 30: 1371–1378.
29. Clark K, Sowers M, Wallace RB, Anderson C (1991) The accuracy of self-reported hearing loss in women aged 60–85 years. Am J Epidemiol 134: 704–708.
30. Nondahl DM, Cruickshanks KJ, Wiley TL, Tweed TS, Klein R, et al. (1998) Accuracy of self-reported hearing loss. Audiology 37: 295–301.
31. Dawes P, Fortnum H, Moore DR, Emsley R, Norman P, et al. (2014) Hearing in middle age: a population snapshot of 40- to 69-year olds in the United Kingdom. Ear Hear 35: e44–51.
32. Dawes P, Emsley R, Cruickshanks KJ, Moore DR, Fortnum H, et al. (In revision) Hearing loss and cognitive decline: the role of hearing aids, social isolation and depression.
33. McCormack A, Edmondson-Jones M, Fortnum H, Dawes P, Middleton H, et al. (2014) The prevalence of tinnitus and the relationship with neuroticism in a middle-aged UK population. J Psychosom Res 76: 56–60.
34. Dawes P, Dickinson C, Emsley R, Bishop P, Cruickshanks K, et al. (2014) Vision impairment and dual sensory problems in middle age. Ophthalmic Physiol Opt 34: 479–488.
35. Dawes P, Cruickshanks K, Moore DR, Edmondson-Jones M, McCormack A, et al. (2014) Cigarette smoking, passive smoking, alcohol consumption and hearing loss. J Assoc Res Otolaryngol 15: 663–674.
36. Zhan W, Cruickshanks KJ, Klein BE, Klein R, Huang GH, et al. (2010) Generational differences in the prevalence of hearing impairment in older adults. Am J Epidemiol 171: 260–266.
37. Sergeyenko Y, Lall K, Liberman MC, Kujawa SG (2013) Age-related cochlear synaptopathy: an early-onset contributor to auditory functional decline. J Neurosci 33: 13686–13694.
38. Makary CA, Shin J, Kujawa SG, Liberman MC, Merchant SN (2011) Age-related primary cochlear neuronal degeneration in human temporal bones. J Assoc Res Otolaryngol 12: 711–717.
39. Dubno JR, Eckert MA, Lee FS, Matthews LJ, Schmiedt RA (2013) Classifying human audiometric phenotypes of age-related hearing loss from animal models. J Assoc Res Otolaryngol 14: 687–701.
40. Bronkhorst AW (2000) The cocktail party phenomenon: A review of research on speech intelligibility in multiple-talker conditions. Acta Acustica united with Acustica 86: 117–128.
41. Leensen MC, de Laat JA, Snik AF, Dreschler WA (2011) Speech-in-noise screening tests by internet, part 2: improving test sensitivity for noise-induced hearing loss. Int J Audiol 50: 835–848.
42. Vlaming MSMG, MacKinnon RC, Jansen M, Moore DR (2014) Automated screening for high-frequency hearing loss. Ear Hear 35 epub ahead of print.
43. Killion MC, Niquette PA, Gudmundsen GI, Revit LJ, Banerjee S (2004) Development of a quick speech-in-noise test for measuring signal-to-noise ratio loss in normal-hearing and hearing-impaired listeners. J Acoust Soc Am 116: 2395–2405.
44. Brungart DS, Sheffield BM, Kubli LR (2014) Development of a test battery for evaluating speech perception in complex listening environments. J Acoust Soc Am in the press.
45. Houtgast T, Festen JM (2008) On the auditory and cognitive functions that may explain an individual's elevation of the speech reception threshold in noise. Int J Audiol 47: 287–295.
46. Pichora-Fuller MK, Schneider BA, Daneman M (1995) How young and old adults listen to and remember speech in noise. J Acoust Soc Am 97: 593–608.
47. Humes LE, Busey TA, Craig J, Kewley-Port D (2013) Are age-related changes in cognitive function driven by age-related changes in sensory processing? Atten Percept Psychophys 75: 508–524.
48. Ronnberg J, Lunner T, Zekveld A, Sorqvist P, Danielsson H, et al. (2013) The Ease of Language Understanding (ELU) model: theoretical, empirical, and clinical advances. Front Syst Neurosci 7: 31.
49. Akeroyd MA (2008) Are individual differences in speech reception related to individual differences in cognitive ability? A survey of twenty experimental studies with normal and hearing-impaired adults. Int J Audiol 47 Suppl 2: S53–71.
50. Baltes PB, Lindenberger U (1997) Emergence of a powerful connection between sensory and cognitive functions across the adult life span: a new window to the study of cognitive aging? Psychol Aging 12: 12–21.
51. Dobreva MS, O'Neill WE, Paige GD (2011) Influence of aging on human sound localization. J Neurophysiol 105: 2471–2486.
52. Rosen S (1992) Temporal information in speech: acoustic, auditory and linguistic aspects. Philos Trans R Soc Lond B Biol Sci 336: 367–373.
53. Salthouse TA (1996) The processing-speed theory of adult age differences in cognition. Psychol Rev 103: 403–428.
54. Zwislocki J, Maire F, Feldman AS, Rubin H (1958) On the effect of practice and motivation on the threshold of audibility. Journal of the Acoustical Society of America 30: 254–262.
55. Rabbitt P (1993) Does it all go together when it goes? The Nineteenth Bartlett Memorial Lecture. Q J Exp Psychol A 46: 385–434.

32

Cross-Modal Re-Organization in Adults with Early Stage Hearing Loss

Julia Campbell[1], Anu Sharma[1,2]*

1 University of Colorado at Boulder, Department of Speech, Language and Hearing Sciences, Boulder, Colorado, United States of America, 2 University of Colorado at Boulder, Institute of Cognitive Science, Boulder, Colorado, United States of America

Abstract

Cortical cross-modal re-organization, or recruitment of auditory cortical areas for visual processing, has been well-documented in deafness. However, the degree of sensory deprivation necessary to induce such cortical plasticity remains unclear. We recorded visual evoked potentials (VEP) using high-density electroencephalography in nine persons with adult-onset mild-moderate hearing loss and eight normal hearing control subjects. Behavioral auditory performance was quantified using a clinical measure of speech perception-in-noise. Relative to normal hearing controls, adults with hearing loss showed significantly larger P1, N1, and P2 VEP amplitudes, decreased N1 latency, and a novel positive component (P2′) following the P2 VEP. Current source density reconstruction of VEPs revealed a shift toward ventral stream processing including activation of auditory temporal cortex in hearing-impaired adults. The hearing loss group showed worse than normal speech perception performance in noise, which was strongly correlated with a decrease in the N1 VEP latency. Overall, our findings provide the first evidence that visual cross-modal re-organization not only begins in the early stages of hearing impairment, but may also be an important factor in determining behavioral outcomes for listeners with hearing loss, a finding which demands further investigation.

Editor: Giuseppe Biagini, University of Modena and Reggio Emilia, Italy

Funding: This work was supported by the National Institutes of Health (RO106257 to A.S., F31DC011970 to J.C.). The funders had no role in study design, data collection and analysis, decision to publish, or preparation of the manuscript.

Competing Interests: The authors have declared that no competing interests exist.

* E-mail: anu.sharma@colorado.edu

Introduction

A basic tenet of neuroplasticity is that central pathways will re-organize following long-term sensory deprivation. There is ample evidence from animal and human studies of cross-modal re-organization of the cortex that occurs in both blindness [1,2,3,4,5,6,7], and congenital deafness [8,9,10,11,12,13,14,15,16,17,18,19,20,21,22,23]. For example, congenitally deaf white cats show enhanced motion processing and localization in the visual periphery, and recruit higher-order auditory cortex for improved performance in these tasks [19,24]. Similarly, congenitally and post-lingually deaf humans (with and without cochlear implants) demonstrate activation of auditory cortical areas during processing of visual motion and complex visual pattern changes, which is not seen for normal hearing control subjects [15,17,25,26,27]. Although cross-modal recruitment serves to enhance behavioral performance for the recruiting modality [19,28], it has been linked to a decrease in performance of the recruited modality. In deaf adults fitted with cochlear implants, cross-modal recruitment (measured by event-related potentials) has been correlated with decreased performance on speech perception tasks [25,26,29]. All of the studies mentioned above have been conducted on individuals in the most advanced stage of hearing loss (i.e., profound deafness). However, most post-lingual deafened adults show a gradual decline in hearing, which typically progresses through the mild, moderate, severe and profound stages of hearing loss [30,31]. Thus, the degree of sensory deprivation necessary to induce cross-modal cortical plasticity remains unclear. Given the potential impact on clinical outcomes, it would be useful to determine whether cross-modal cortical changes begin during early stages of hearing decline or whether these changes are limited to the near-total sensory deprivation that accompanies deafness. In this study, we examined visual evoked potentials (VEP) using high-density electroencephalography and auditory behavioral outcome using a clinical test of speech perception in noise in persons with adult-onset mild-moderate hearing loss and normal hearing control subjects.

Materials and Methods

Participants and Ethics Statement

Seventeen adults between the ages of 37 to 68 years participated in this study. The study was approved by the University of Colorado at Boulder Institutional Review Board, and all participants provided written consent. Subjects were recruited via advertisements in the community, and hearing was tested for all subjects using standard clinical audiometric procedures prior to speech-in-noise and EEG measurements. Eight of the subjects (mean age and standard deviation: 50.5+/−6.2 years; range: 37.4–57 years) revealed clinically normal hearing thresholds (i.e., below 25 dB Hearing Level) for frequencies ranging from 250 Hz to 8000 Hz. Nine of the subjects demonstrated hearing loss (mean age and standard deviation: 56.9+/−8.9 years; range: 38.4–68.2 years). On average, this group showed normal hearing from 250 Hz through 1000 Hz and a mild-to-moderate sensorineural hearing loss bilaterally from 2000 Hz to 8000 Hz. Average audiograms for the two groups are shown in Figure 1. None of the participants with hearing loss were receiving clinical intervention at the time of enrollment. However, many participants suspected a possible hearing loss prior to diagnosis. Subjects who were diagnosed with hearing loss through the study received counseling from a state-licensed clinical audiologist (first author) and referrals to audiology clinics for possible consideration of amplification. EEG testing sessions took place on separate days for those diagnosed with hearing loss unless otherwise requested. The participants in the normal hearing (NH) group and hearing loss (HL) group showed no difference in age between groups ($t(15) = -1.69$, $p > 0.05$). All participants reported no issues with visual acuity and no neurological impairment.

Auditory Behavioral Testing: Test of Speech Perception-in-noise

Speech perception in background noise was measured using the QuickSIN™ test [32], a clinical assessment of auditory acuity in background noise. Participants faced a speaker at 0° azimuth and were instructed to repeat two recorded sentence lists (six sentences each) presented at 65 dB Hearing Level (HL). Background noise was varied to determine the signal-to-noise ratio (SNR) required by the participant to accurately repeat 50% of the sentences. The SNR values began at 25 dB and decreased in 5 dB increments to 0 dB. The SNR score from the two lists was computed and averaged for each participant. Overall, the lower the SNR score, the better the performance on the test.

EEG Procedures

Visual stimuli. Participants were shown a high contrast sinusoidal concentric grating that morphs into a radially modulated grating or circle-star pattern [25,33,34] on a 26-inch flat-screen LCD television at a viewing distance of approximately 42 inches. The circle and star figures were presented 150 times. The star figure was presented on the screen for 600 ms, then immediately followed by the circle figure, also lasting for 600 ms. This presentation method provided the percept of apparent motion and shape change to the viewer. A total of 300 stimulus presentations (sweeps) were presented, for a testing time of three minutes. The VEP was time-locked to the onset of each individual star and circle presentation. Participants were instructed to direct their gaze to the center of the star/circle at a black dot and to not shift gaze during the three minutes.

EEG Recording and Analyses

Participants were fitted with a 128-channel EEG electrode recording net (Electrical Geodesic, Inc.) and seated in a comfortable reclining chair in an electro-magnetically shielded sound booth. All stimuli were presented via E-Prime® 2.0, stimulus software compatible with Net Station 4 (Electrical Geodesic, Inc). The sampling rate for the EEG recordings was 1 kHz, with a band-pass filter set at 0.1–200 Hz.

Data were band-pass filtered offline at 1–30 Hz and segmented according to the EEG activity surrounding the stimulus presentation (epochs), with 100 ms pre-stimulus and 495 ms post-stimulus time. EEG recordings were corrected to the pre-stimulus baseline, and eye-blink artifact recorded at designated eye channels was removed if greater than $+/-100$ μV, unless adjusted for individual subjects. Bad channels were removed from the recording and replaced with interpolated data from the remaining channels via a spline interpolation algorithm. Remaining data were averaged and re-referenced using common average reference. Individual waveform averages were averaged together for each of the two groups (i.e., the normal hearing and hearing loss group) to compute a grand-averaged waveform. Amplitudes and latencies for individual participants were recorded for all three obligatory visual evoked potential (VEP) peaks (i.e., P1, N1 and P2). The P1 peak component was observed as the first positive-going peak occurring approximately within a latency window of 90 to 130 ms, the N1 component was observed as the second peak or first negative-going peak occurring approximately between 135 ms to 200 ms, and the P2 component was observed as the third peak or second positive-going peak occurring approximately within 200

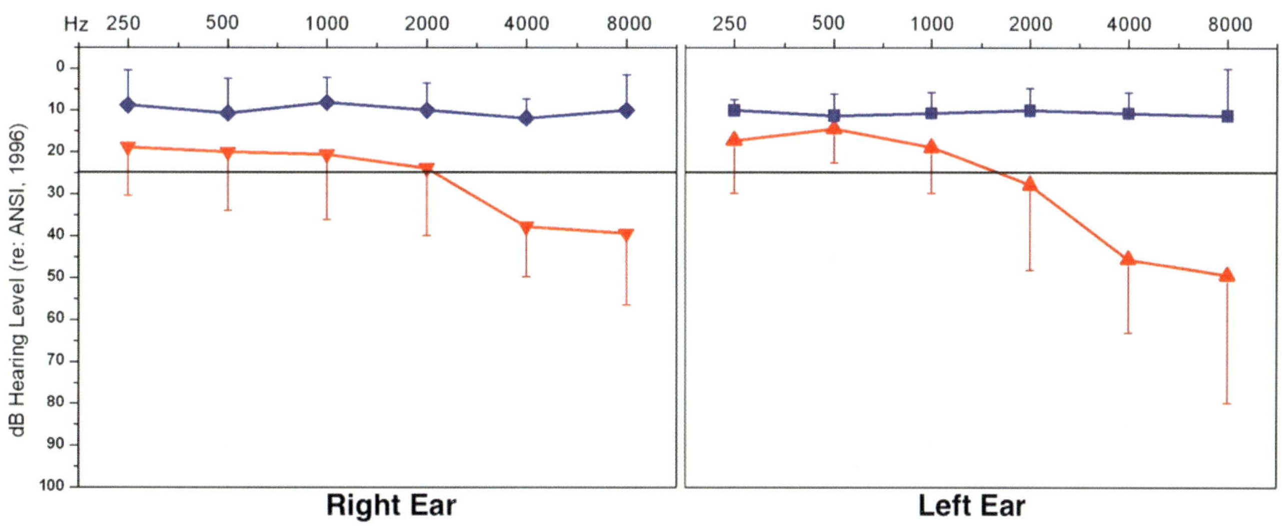

Figure 1. Mean audiometric subject thresholds. Auditory thresholds are shown for right and left ears for the standard audiometric frequencies from 250 Hz to 8000 Hz. Thresholds for the normal hearing (NH) group are depicted in blue; the hearing loss (HL) group in red. The positive-going blue bars illustrate the standard deviation for the average threshold at the designated frequency for the NH group, and negative-going red bars illustrate the standard deviation for the HL group. The solid black line illustrates the criterion for normal hearing, at 25 dB HL.

to 300 ms. If a peak component occurred outside of the described latency ranges, it was still marked and included according to the order of appearance (e.g., the first large positive component at 80 ms was marked as P1). P1 amplitudes were defined as the onset to peak value, N1 amplitudes as the peak of the N1 component to peak of the P2 component, and P2 amplitudes as peak of the P2 component to offset value. Latencies were chosen at the highest amplitude of the peak.

First we created a two-dimensional voltage map using Net Station 4 (Electrical Geodesic, Inc), which allowed us to examine regions of interest (ROI) around the occipital midline [25,29], focusing on the greatest group differences for visual stimuli. Using planned comparisons with the Bonferroni correction, electrodes within the ROI were then chosen for statistical analysis according to the largest mean group differences for the amplitude and latency of each VEP component.

Source Localization Analysis (Current Density Reconstructions)

EEG data for individual participants were exported from Net Station and imported into EEGLAB [35] using MatLab® (The MathWorks®, Inc., 2010). The data were corrected to the baseline of a pre-stimulus interval of 100 ms and sweeps greater than +/− 100 μV were rejected as artifacts. The sampling rate was down-sampled to 250 Hz to reduce processing, altering the post-stimulus time to 492 ms. The first step in creating source models was to prune the concatenated EEG sweeps or trials for each subject through independent component analysis (ICA) [36,37]. This statistical procedure allows for observation of the spatially fixed and temporally independent components that underlie the evoked potential [38], and is useful in precise source modeling in EEG, including for deeper generators [37,39,40,41]. EEGLAB was chosen specifically for preliminary source localization analysis in order to utilize the ICA algorithm that provides for optimal cortical source localization, and to perform ICA on concatenated EEG sweeps [36,37,42]. Once the independent components that accounted for greatest percent variance in the evoked potential were identified in the designated timeframe for a peak component of interest (e.g., P1, N1, P2), the remaining independent components were regarded as artifact/noise and discarded. The pruned potential waveforms for each subject were then grand averaged for each group (NH and HL) and exported into CURRY® Scan 7 Neuroimaging Suite (Compumedics Neuroscan™) for source modeling. In CURRY®, an additional ICA was run on the VEP mean global field power (MGFP) (incorporating all 128 channel EEG data), with only components showing a signal-to-noise ratio (SNR) of 2.0 or greater accepted. The third VEP component in the HL group (P2') was pruned and averaged as an individual component as it was present in a subset of this group.

Peak components for the VEP MGFP waveforms were selected separately for current density reconstruction (CDR) via sLORETA, with no a-priori restrictions placed on the model. The selected head model was standardized using the boundary element method (BEM) [43]. sLORETA, or standardized low-resolution brain electromagnetic tomography, is a specific statistical method that estimates CDR [44,45]. The CDR is represented by a graded color scale image placed on an average MRI of 100 people. Sagittal MRI slices were selected to illustrate the greatest differences in cortical activation between the groups. Montreal Neurological Institute (MNI) co-ordinates (in millimeters) illustrate the three dimensional physical locations of each slice.

Results

Visual Evoked Potentials

Waveforms for the two groups across the whole head (128 channels) are shown in Figure 2. Three obligatory cortical VEP components elicited in response to the visual stimulus were analyzed: the P1 (occurring at approximately 100 ms), the N1 (occurring at approximately 150 ms), and the P2 (occurring at approximately 230 ms). We compared amplitude and latencies for these components between NH and HL groups at electrodes in the occipital ROI. A one-way ANOVA was computed to compare group differences. Post-hoc planned comparison of means using the Bonferroni correction was completed to describe significant differences between electrodes (see Figure 2).

P1 amplitude was larger for the HL group ($F(1, 285) = 6.265$, $\rho < 0.05$). N1 amplitude was larger for the HL group ($F(1, 285) = 9.865$, $\rho < 0.01$). N1 latency was decreased for the HL group ($F(1, 285) = 7.684$, $\rho < 0.01$). Finally, P2 amplitudes were increased for the HL group ($F(1, 285) = 8.983$, $\rho < 0.01$). Overall, this trend of decreased latencies and increased amplitudes for obligatory VEP components for HL listeners is consistent with previous results, which showed evidence of cross-modal recruitment in deaf subjects [13,25,26,46].

An unexpected finding was the visual identification of a positive component following the P2 (occurring between approximately 295 and 395 ms) in the HL group (see Figure 2C). We labeled this component P2'. While a possible component similar to this is observed by Doucet and colleagues [25], it was not analyzed or discussed in that study. Figure 2 shows the evoked potential waveforms for both groups at the described electrodes, with mean bar graphs illustrating significant differences.

Cortical Source Localization

Cortical source localization, or current density reconstruction (CDR), was performed in order to visualize anatomical regions of possible cross-modal re-organization in the HL group. The sLORETA algorithm provided by CURRY® Scan 7 Neuroimaging Suite was applied to the three VEP peak components (Figure 3). The activations were superimposed on an average MRI (sagittal slice view) and the MNI co-ordinates are shown beneath each slice. The scale of the F distribution, indicating the strength of the activations, is also shown.

As expected, for the NH group, the visual stimuli elicited all three VEP components and activated visual processing regions, including multiple cerebellar areas, which have been shown to respond to visual motion [47,48] (Figure 3). Higher-order visual cortical regions such as Brodmann areas 18 and 19, and the fusiform region, were also activated. These findings are consistent with previous studies, which used stimuli generally similar to ours in NH subjects [34,47,48,49]. The P1 component showed similar cortical and cerebellar activation for both groups. However, for the N1 and P2 components, the HL group showed greater activation along the ventral visual stream in temporal areas, which are traditionally associated with auditory processing (including superior temporal gyrus (STG), medial temporal gyrus (MTG), and inferior temporal gyrus (ITG)). This result is consistent with previous reports of cross-modal activation of temporal areas in deaf\ subjects [15,17,27]. Figure 3 shows the current density reconstructions for the NH and HL groups. A table is provided in Figure 3 describing activated regions corresponding to each of the peak components. Interestingly, the P2' component (seen only in the HL group) showed activation of both cerebellar/occipital regions as well as temporal areas. This response pattern suggests

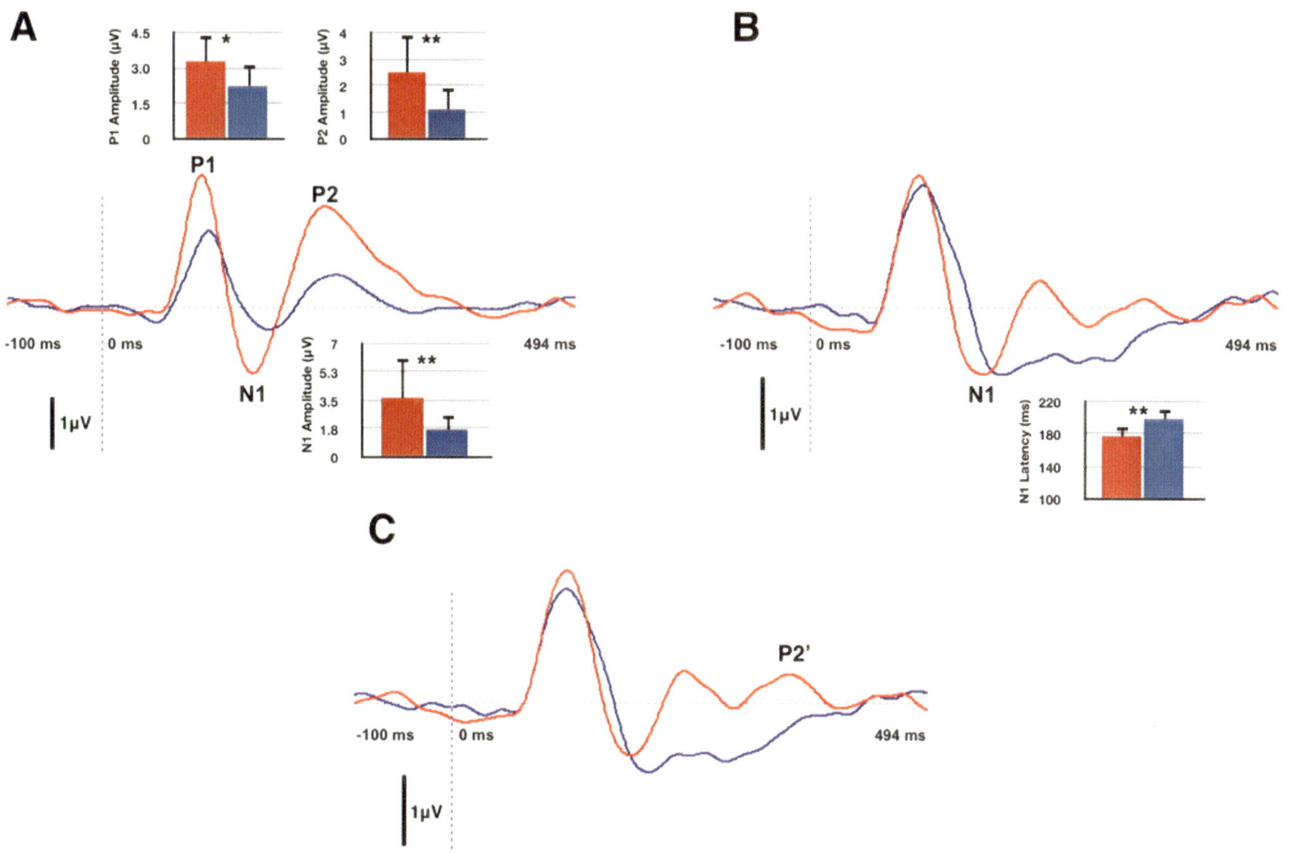

Figure 2. Occipital Region of Interest (ROI) cortical visual evoked potentials (VEPs). A. Peak components P1, N1, and P2 amplitudes are significantly larger for the adult Hearing Loss (HL) group (red) in comparison to the adult Normal Hearing group (blue). Mean group differences are illustrated in corresponding mean bar graphs for each component. One asterisk indicates significance at $p < 0.05$; two asterisks indicate significance at $p < 0.01$. B. The N1 component latency is significantly decreased in the HL group as compared to the NH group, also illustrated in the mean bar graph. C. A third positive peak component, denoted as P2', has been found in a subset of the HL group.

that an additional processing step may take place within the ventral visual stream in listeners with hearing loss.

Behavioral Performance

Speech perception-in-noise acuity was measured for both groups using the QuickSIN^{TM} clinical test [32]. The results of the QuickSIN^{TM} are reported as a signal-to-noise ratio (SNR) threshold; therefore a lower score reflects better performance. Mean scores for the NH and HL groups are shown in Figure 4A. A Mann-Whitney U Test revealed a significant difference between the two groups ($U = 10.5$, $Z = -2.46$, $p < 0.05$). This difference in auditory performance in background noise between normal hearing listeners and listeners with mild-to-moderate hearing loss is consistent with Killion et al. [32] and Wilson et al. [50].

The N1 VEP component has been suggested as a marker of cross-modal re-organization in deafness [13,26,46,51]. Therefore, we correlated the latency of the N1 with QuickSIN^{TM} scores for the subjects. Due to hearing loss consisting of a gradual increase in auditory threshold from 0 dB HL, we included the N1 latency values and QuickSIN scores of all 17 participants in the correlation analysis. Mean QuickSIN^{TM} scores and N1 VEP latencies were tested for normal distribution, and a Spearman's rank-order correlation was computed due to the non-normal distribution of the data. As seen in Figure 4B, a negative correlation was observed between N1 latency and QuickSIN scores ($r = -0.701$, $\rho = 0.001$). That is, a shorter N1 latency was associated with higher scores (i.e., worse performance) on the QuickSIN^{TM} test. Overall, our results reflecting differences in speech-in-noise perception between the NH and HL groups as a function of visual evoked potentials are consistent with previous studies in deaf subjects showing cross-modal re-organization in subjects with poor speech perception [25,26]. N1 latency changes also showed a significant negative correlation with the pure tone threshold averages (PTA) at 500, 1000, and 2000 Hz, which is a clinically relevant indicator of audiometric function (right ear, $r = -0.446$, $\rho < 0.05$; left ear, $r = -0.540$, $\rho < 0.05$). That is, as the degree of hearing loss increased, there was a corresponding decrease in N1 latency.

Discussion

We sought to examine whether cross-modal recruitment is evident in early stages of hearing decline or whether cross-modal plasticity is limited to the near-total sensory deprivation that accompanies profound deafness. We recorded high-density EEG in response to a visual stimulus in adults with normal hearing in the low frequencies and a mild-to-moderate hearing loss in the high frequencies. A group of age-matched normal hearing adults served as the control group. All participants were administered the QuickSIN, a test of speech-in-noise perception which is used to document clinical outcomes in patients with hearing loss.

A

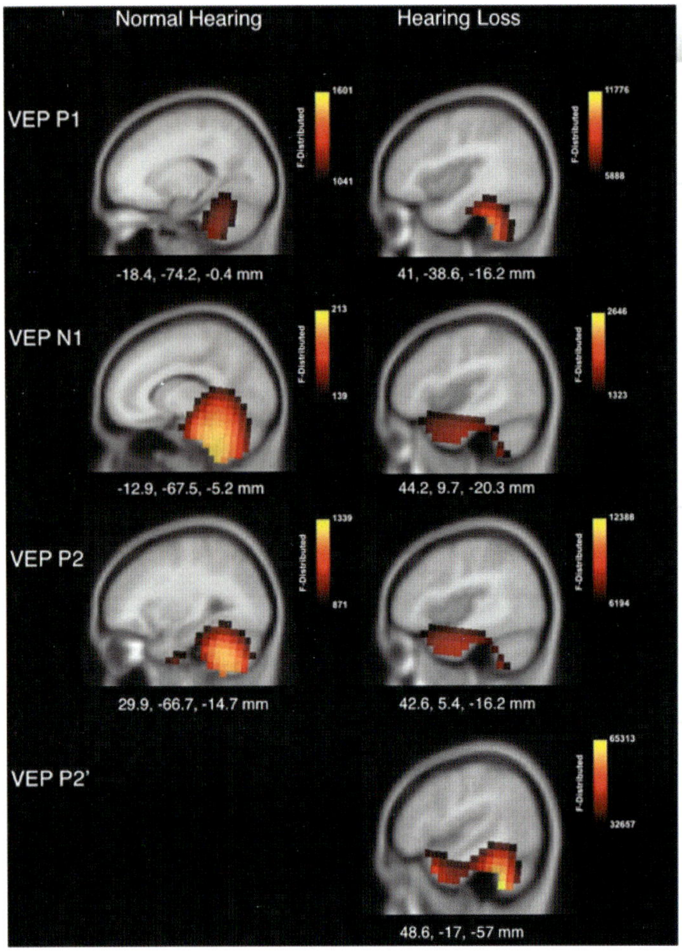

B

	Normal Hearing	Hearing Loss
VEP P1	Cerebellum, Brodmann Area 19	Cerebellum, Brodmann Areas 20, 36, Fusiform gyrus
VEP N1	Cerebellum, Brodmann Areas 18, 19, 30, Lingual Gyrus	Inferior Temporal Gyrus, Brodmann Area 20, Fusiform Gyrus, Medial Temporal Gyrus, Brodmann Area 21, Superior Temporal Gyrus, Brodmann Area 38, Cerebellum, Inferior Frontal Gyrus, Brodmann Area 47
VEP P2	Cerebellum, Brodmann Areas 36, 35, Fusiform Gyrus, Brodmann Areas 19, 20, 37, 38, Superior Temporal Gyrus	Inferior Temporal Gyrus, Brodmann Area 21, Medial Temporal Gyrus, Fusiform Gyrus, Brodmann Area 20, Superior Temporal Gyrus, Brodmann Area 38, Cerebellum, Inferior Frontal Gyrus, Brodmann Areas 36, 47
VEP P2'		Cerebellum, Brodmann Area 36, Superior Temporal Gyrus, Brodmann Area 38, Fusiform Gyrus, Brodmann Area 20, Medial Temporal Gyrus, Brodmann Areas 21, 37, Inferior Temporal Gyrus, Inferior Frontal Gyrus, Brodmann Area 47

Figure 3. Current source density reconstructions for the NH and HL groups. A. The cortical activation at the P1, N1 and P2 VEP peak components using sagittal magnetic resonance imaging (MRI) slices. The scale of the F Distribution is shown in a scale the upper right corner ranging from red to yellow (where yellow reflects the greater strength of activation). The Montreal Neurological Institute (MNI) coordinates are listed beneath each MRI slice. B. The table describing the activated cortical regions for the VEP components for the NH and HL groups, listed in approximate order of highest level of activation.

Relative to normal hearing controls, adults with mild-to-moderate hearing loss showed: (i) increased amplitude of the P1, N1 and P2 VEP components, (ii) presence of an additional positive VEP component (P2') occurring after the P2, (iii) decreased latency of the N1 VEP, (iv) cortical re-organization as evidenced by increased activation of auditory temporal areas elicited by visual stimulation, (iv) poorer speech perception scores in noise, (v) a significant negative correlation between the degree of hearing loss and N1 VEP latency, and (vi) a strong negative correlation between speech-in-noise perception and N1 VEP latency. Overall, this pattern of results in our listeners with mild hearing loss is consistent with previous findings in deaf subjects suggesting visual cross-modal recruitment in deafness [13,25,26,51].

Consistent with our findings, significantly increased amplitudes of N1 and P2 VEPs with hearing loss are well-documented in deafness [13,46,51]. More recently, changes in visual shift of form and motion have been shown to elicit larger N1 and P2 responses correlated with poor speech perception in deaf, cochlear-implanted adults, respectively [25,26]. Interestingly, smaller than normal amplitude of the visual P1 component has recently been reported in cochlear-implanted adults [29]. However, Sandmann and colleagues used a stimulus consisting of four separate checkerboard reversal patterns at varying luminance ratios, which is a more complex pattern of stimulation relative to the one used in this study. The checkerboard pattern is therefore more likely to tap into a different stage of visual processing than is evident in this study [29]. Typically, decreased latencies and increased amplitudes of evoked potential components are considered to be reflective of faster processing [52,53] suggesting that HL subjects recruit additional cortical areas to subserve processing speed and/or efficiency. To this end, we identified the P2' VEP component (following the P2) only in the HL group, possibly indicating a new or additional generator facilitating visual processing in the HL group.

Current source density reconstructions (CDR) were compared between NH and HL listeners. As expected, for the visual stimulus, NH listeners showed cerebellar/occipital activation for the P1, N1 and P2 VEP components (Figure 3). Responsive regions included Brodmann areas 18 and 19, which comprise higher-order visual cortex. Visual stimuli comparable in both shape and appearance of motion to the one used in the present study have been shown to

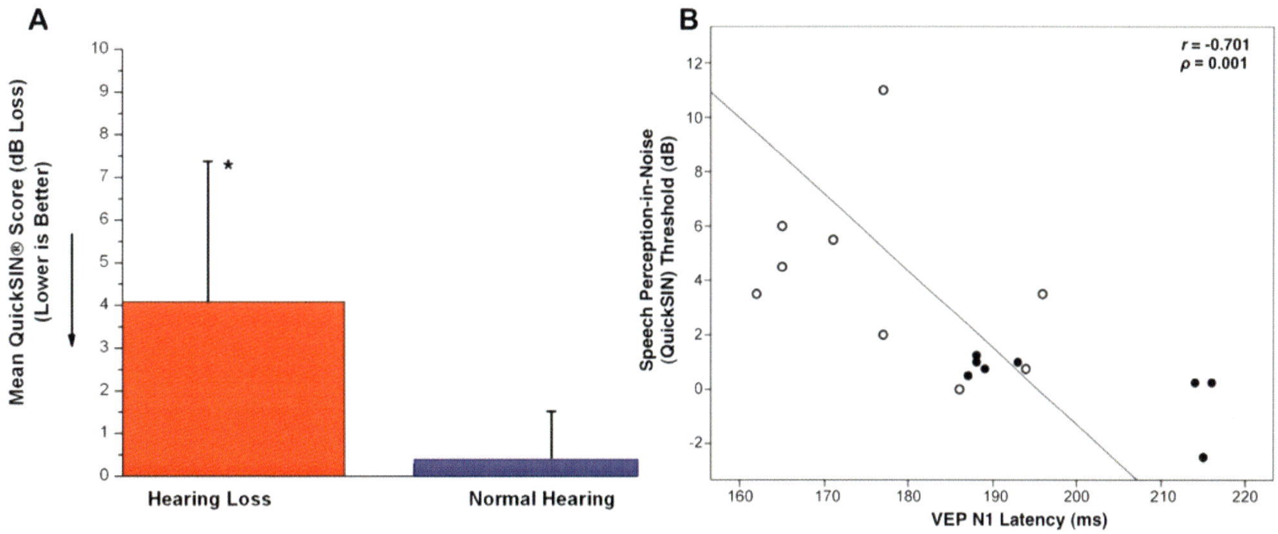

Figure 4. Mean scores on the QuickSIN test for the NH and HL groups, (A). Error bars are shown as vertical black lines. The asterisk reflects significant differences at $\rho < 0.05$. B. QuickSIN scores are shown on the vertical axis and N1 VEP component latencies on the horizontal axis. Values are shown as closed circles for the NH group and open circles for the HL group. The Spearman's rho value (-0.7) and significance at $\rho = 0.001$ are indicated on the upper right hand corner.

activate similar cortical regions in VEP and fMRI imaging studies [34,47,54].

The HL group showed occipital/cerebellar activation comparable to the NH group, as was evident in the CDR for the P1 response. However, higher-order processing as reflected by the CDR for the N1 and P2 components showed clear evidence of cortical re-organization. Cortical activation for these components showed an emphasis in ventral stream processing within temporal cortex, including temporal gyri (ITG, MTG and STG), which are typically associated with auditory cortical processing [55,56]. The P2' component, identified in only the HL group, showed underlying activation of both cerebellar/occipital areas and temporal areas, suggestive of a possible new generator in temporal cortex subserving visual processing.

In a recent study, Campbell and Sharma [57] examined cortical responses to auditory stimulation in adults with mild-moderate hearing loss. The authors reported a change in cortical resource allocation, including decreased temporal activation in STG and increased frontal activation in response to passive auditory stimulation in mild-moderate hearing loss. Taken together with the present results, this suggests that a decreased temporal activation to sound in mild-moderate hearing loss may be coincidental with the increased visual activation of temporal areas in this study.

Overall, the CDR findings are strongly suggestive of cortical re-organization facilitating cross-modal recruitment for visual processing in adults with mild-moderate hearing loss. The shift of activation to temporal cortex represents activation of the ventral visual stream, which is typically responsive to visual object form or shape changes, and is located within temporal cortex in proximity to auditory areas. The ventral stream has been implicated in the processing of facial and mouth movements [58,59]. Thus, our results may be suggestive of compensatory plasticity as HL listeners begin to rely on facial information as a strategy to compensate for their hearing impairment [60,61,62,63,64]. Because the ventral stream is largely responsible for processing object and face information, a heavier processing load may be imposed on this stream when listeners with hearing loss begin to pay more attention to lip and facial cues. Indeed, visual attention is a modulatory influence for compensatory plasticity, and congruent visual input has shown to enhance auditory speech perception performance in cochlear-implanted adults [18,65]. A recent study by Strelnikov and colleagues suggests that increased intra-modal compensatory activity in occipital cortex predicts better outcomes for post-lingually deaf adults after cochlear implantation, presumably due to the synergy of the visual system in deciphering auditory information and ultimately increasing the ability for auditory discrimination when sound is re-introduced via implantation [65]. However, similar to the present study, increased cross-modal re-organization in superior temporal sulcus (STS) appears to predict poor outcomes for both pre- and post-lingually deaf implant users [65,66,67].

Hearing loss is most consistently associated with poor outcomes in recognizing speech in background noise, a skill essential for everyday listening [30,68,69,70]. Consistent with previous research in hearing-impaired listeners, our results show that listeners with even mild-to-moderate hearing loss demonstrate a significant deficit when listening to speech in background noise [71,72]. A strong negative correlation was observed between speech perception-in-noise performance on the QuickSIN test and N1 VEP latency. That is, a shorter N1 latency was associated with higher scores (i.e., worse performance) on the QuickSIN™ test. While hearing loss is a well-known contributor to decreased speech in noise performance [73,74], our results suggest that cross-modal plasticity may also be an important factor that should be considered in the decreased auditory performance in background noise of listeners with hearing loss. If we assume that cross-modal plasticity implies a greater reliance on lip-reading, then it might possibly serve as a facilitatory compensation in noisy situations where congruent visual input enhances auditory processing [65]. A decrease in N1 latency was also correlated with higher audiometric thresholds, suggesting a possible increase in cross-modal recruitment as hearing loss gets worse. Future studies should systematically describe the extent of cross-modal recruitment as a function of hearing loss ranging from mild to profound, as well as investigate the possible contribution of cross-modal plasticity on speech perception performance.

Overall, the VEP and behavioral results that we describe are strongly indicative of visual cross-modal re-organization in adults with mild-moderate hearing loss. This is a new finding as previous reports of cross-modal plasticity have been confined to adults with deafness, which was congenital or pre-lingual, and/or in cochlear-implanted adults [13,25,27,51,65,75,76]. The mechanisms of cross-modal plasticity in both deafness and moderate hearing loss have been explored in animal studies. Recent studies suggest that only those cortical areas involved in the sharing of multi-modal information are recruited, and still maintain the functional specificity of the original sensory modality [19,24]. That is, higher-order, multi-modal areas are more susceptible to recruitment when a shared modality is no longer receiving appropriate input. Furthermore, this cross-modal plasticity has been found to take place as a result of moderate hearing loss, and not just profound sensory deprivation [77]. In humans, both audition and vision share object recognition functions in the ventral stream [78,79], and are thus primed for compensatory plasticity in hearing loss. When the listening environment becomes challenging, as in background noise, greater attention to visual objects in the form of processing of faces and lips, may facilitate auditory object recognition. Along these same lines, activation of the ventral stream in adults who have experienced late-onset blindness has been correlated with poor performance in an auditory spatial task [80]. Similarly, resting state studies of pre-lingually deaf cochlear implanted children and post-lingually deaf cochlear implanted children and adults showed ventral activation in patients who had poor speech perception outcomes [66,67]. Thus, it appears that compensatory activation, in either modality, of the cortical auditory-visual ventral stream may be associated with poorer auditory performance.

Summary and Conclusion

Our study provides new evidence of cross-modal cortical re-organization in adult-onset mild-moderate hearing loss. Increased amplitudes of P1, N1 and P2 VEP components, decreased N1 latency, a novel P2' component and current source density reconstructions reflecting a ventral shift in activation were observed for adults with mild to moderate hearing loss relative to normal hearing controls. Furthermore, we observed a strong negative correlation between cross-modal re-organization (as reflected by decreased N1 latency) and speech perception in noise. Future studies are needed to outline the detailed trajectory of cross-modal changes as hearing declines from a mild hearing loss to deafness. Prospective longitudinal studies will provide important information concerning the timeline of cross-modal re-organization according to severity of hearing loss, including a quantification of the degree or severity of re-organization. In addition, such studies may indicate the effect of clinical interventions, such as amplification or cochlear implantation, in reversing cross-modal re-organization.

Acknowledgments

We would like to acknowledge Teresa Mitchell, Ph.D, for her comments on a draft of the manuscript.

Author Contributions

Conceived and designed the experiments: JC AS. Performed the experiments: JC. Analyzed the data: JC AS. Contributed reagents/materials/analysis tools: JC AS. Wrote the paper: JC AS.

References

1. Kujala T, Alho K, Naatanen R (2000) Cross-modal reorganization of human cortical functions. Trends Neurosci 23(3): 115–20.
2. Roder B, Stock O, Bien S, Neville H, Rosler F (2002) Speech processing activates visual cortex in congenitally blind humans. Eur J Neurosci 16(5): 930–6.
3. Voss P, Gougoux FDR, Lassonde M, Zatorre RJ, Lepore F (2006) A positron emission tomography study during auditory localization by late-onset blind individuals. NeuroReport 17(4): 383–8.
4. Collignon O, Lassonde M, Lepore F, Bastien D, Veraart C (2007) Functional cerebral reorganization for auditory spatial processing and auditory substitution of vision in early blind subjects. Cereb Cortex 17(2): 457–65.
5. Collignon O, Vandewalle G, Voss P, Albouy G, Charbonneau G, et al. (2011) Functional specialization for auditory–spatial processing in the occipital cortex of congenitally blind humans. Proc Natl Acad Sci U S A 108(11): 4435–4440.
6. Watkins KE, Shakespeare TJ, O'Donoghue MC, Alexander I, Ragge N, et al. (2013) Early auditory processing in area V5/MT+ of the congenitally blind brain. J Neurosci 13; 33(46): 18242–18246.
7. Kupers R, Ptito M (2013). Compensatory plasticity and cross-modal reorganization following early visual deprivation. Neurosci Biobehav Rev S01497634(13)00191–197.
8. Sharma A, Dorman MF, Kral A (2005) The influence of a sensitive period on central auditory development in children with unilateral and bilateral cochlear implants. Hear Res 203(1–2): 134–143.
9. Sharma A, Gilley PM, Dorman MF, Baldwin R (2007) Deprivation-induced cortical reorganization in children with cochlear implants. Int J Audiol 46(9): 494–499.
10. Sharma A, Nash AA, Dorman M (2009) Cortical development, plasticity and re-organization in children with cochlear implants. J Commun Disord 42(4): 272–279.
11. Sharma A, Dorman M (2011) Central auditory system development and plasticity after cochlear implantation. In F-G Zeng et al. (Eds.), *Auditory Prostheses: New Horizons* (233–255). Springer Handbook of Auditory Research 39. New York: Springer.
12. Sharma A, Mitchell T (2013) The impact of deafness on the human central auditory and visual systems. In A Kral et al. (Eds.), *Deafness* (189–215). Springer Handbook of Auditory Research 47. New York: Springer.
13. Neville HJ, Lawson D (1987) Attention to central and peripheral visual space in a movement detection task: an event-related potential and behavioral study. II. Congenitally deaf adults. Brain Res 405(2): 268–83.
14. Bavelier D, Tomann A, Hutton C, Mitchell T, Corina D, et al. (2000) Visual attention to the periphery is enhanced in congenitally deaf individuals. J Neurosci 20(17): RC93.
15. Finney EM, Fine I, Dobkins KR (2001) Visual stimuli activate auditory cortex in the deaf. Nat Neurosci 4(12): 1171–3.
16. Neville HJ, Bavelier D (2001) Effects of auditory and visual deprivation on human brain development. Clin Neurosci Res 1(4): 248–57.
17. Finney EM, Clementz BA, Hickok G, Dobkins KR (2003) Visual stimuli activate auditory cortex in deaf subjects: evidence from MEG. NeuroReport 14(11): 1425–7.
18. Bavelier D, Hirshorn EA (2010) I see where you're hearing: how cross-modal plasticity may exploit homologous brain structures. Nat Neurosci 13(11): 1309–11.
19. Lomber SG, Meredith MA, Kral A (2010) Cross-modal plasticity in specific auditory cortices underlies visual compensations in the deaf. Nat Neurosci 13(11): 1421–7.
20. Kral A, Sharma A (2012) Developmental neuroplasticity after cochlear implantation. Trends Neurosci 35(2): 111–22.
21. Meredith MA, Allman BL (2012) Early hearing-impairment results in cross-modal reorganization of ferret core auditory cortex. Neural Plast 2012: 601591.
22. Gilley PM, Sharma A, Dorman MF (2008) Cortical reorganization in children with cochlear implants. Brain Res 1239: 56–65.
23. Kral A (2013) Auditory critical periods: a review from system's perspective. Neuroscience 5; 247: 117–133.
24. Meredith MA, Kryklywy J, McMillan AJ, Malhotra S, Lum-Tai R, et al. (2011) Crossmodal reorganization in the early deaf switches sensory, but not behavioral roles of auditory cortex. Proc Natl Acad Sci U S A 108(21): 8856–61.
25. Doucet ME, Bergeron F, Lassonde M, Ferron P, Lepore F (2006) Cross-modal reorganization and speech perception in cochlear implant users. Brain 129(Pt 12): 3376–83.
26. Buckley KA, Tobey EA (2011) Cross-modal plasticity and speech perception in pre- and postlingually deaf cochlear implant users. Ear Hear (1): 2–15.
27. Vachon P, Voss P, Lassonde M, Leroux J-M, Mensour B, et al. (2013) Reorganization of the auditory, visual and multimodal areas in early deaf individuals. Neuroscience 15; 245: 50–60.
28. Bosworth RG, Dobkins KR (2002) The effects of spatial attention on motion processing in deaf signers, hearing signers, and hearing nonsigners. Brain Cogn 49(1): 152–69.

29. Sandmann P, Dillier N, Eichele T, Meyer M, Kegel A, et al. (2012) Visual activation of auditory cortex reflects maladaptive plasticity in cochlear implant users. Brain 135(2): 555–68.
30. Lazard DS, Vincent C, Venail F, Van de Heyning P, Truy E, et al. (2012) Pre-, per- and postoperative factors affecting performance of postlinguistically deaf adults using cochlear implants: a new conceptual model over time. PLoS ONE 7(11): e48739.
31. Lazard DS, Innes-Brown H, Barone P (2014) Adaptation of the communicative brain to post-lingual deafness. Evidence from functional imaging. Hear Res 307: 136–143.
32. Killion MC, Niquette PA, Gudmundsen GI, Revit LJ, Banerjee S (2004) Development of a quick speech-in-noise test for measuring signal-to-noise ratio loss in normal-hearing and hearing-impaired listeners. J Acoust Soc Am 116(4 Pt 1): 2395–405.
33. Doucet ME, Gosselin F, Lassonde M, Guillemot JP, Lepore F (2005) Development of visual evoked potentials to radially modulated concentric patterns. NeuroReport 16(16): 1753–6.
34. Bertrand J-A, Lassonde M, Robert M, Nguyen DK, Bertone A, et al. (2012) An intracranial event-related potential study on transformational apparent motion. Does its neural processing differ from real motion? Exp Brain Res 216(1): 145–53.
35. Delorme A, Makeig S (2004) EEGLAB: an open source toolbox for analysis of single-trial EEG dynamics including independent component analysis. J Neurosci Methods 134(1): 9–21.
36. Debener S, Ullsperger M, Siegel M, Engel AK (2006) Single-trial EEG fMRI reveals the dynamics of cognitive function. Trends Cogn. Sci 10(12): 558–63.
37. Debener S, Hine J, Bleeck S, Eyles J (2008) Source localization of auditory evoked potentials after cochlear implantation. Psychophysiology 45(1): 20–4.
38. Makeig S, Jung TP, Bell AJ (1997) Blind separation of auditory event-related brain responses into independent components Proc Natl Acad Sci U S A 94(20): 10979–10984.
39. Makeig S, Delorme A, Westerfield M, Jung TP, Townsend J, et al. (2004) Electroencephalographic brain dynamics following manually responded visual targets. PLoS Biol 2(6): e176.
40. Hine J, Debener S (2007) Late auditory evoked potentials asymmetry revisited. Clin Neurophysiol 118(6): 1274–85.
41. Joos K, Vanneste S, De Ridder D (2012) Disentangling depression and distress networks in the tinnitus brain. PLoS ONE 7(7): e40544.
42. Delorme A, Palmer J, Onton J, Oostenveld R, Makeig S (2012) Independent EEG sources are dipolar. PLoS ONE 7(2): e30135.
43. Fuchs M, Kastner J, Wagner M, Hawes S, Ebersole JS (2002) A standardized boundary element method volume conductor model. Clin Neurophysiol 113(5): 702–12.
44. Pascual-Marqui RD (2002) Standardized low-resolution brain electromagnetic tomography (sLORETA): technical details. Methods Find Exp Clin Pharmacol 24(Suppl. D): 5–12.
45. Grech R, Cassar T, Muscat J (2008) Review on solving the inverse problem in EEG source analysis. JNER 5: 25.
46. Armstrong BA, Neville HJ, Hillyard SA, Mitchell TV (2002) Auditory deprivation affects processing of motion, but not color. Brain Res Cogn Brain Res 14(3): 422–34.
47. Dupont P, Sary G, Peuskens H, Orban GA (2003) Cerebral regions processing first- and higher order motion in an opposed-direction discrimination task. Eur J Neurosci 17(7): 1509–17.
48. Kellermann T, Regenbogen C, De Vos M, Mößnang C, Finkelmeyer A, et al. (2012) Effective connectivity of the human cerebellum during visual attention. J Neurosci 32(33): 11453–60.
49. Wilkinson F, James TW, Wilson HR, Gati JS, Menon RS, et al. (2000) An fMRIstudy of the selective activation of human extrastriate form vision areas by radial and concentric gratings. Curr Biol 10(22): 1455–8.
50. Wilson RH, McArdle RA, Smith SL (2007) An Evaluation of the BKB-SIN, HINT, QuickSIN, and WIN Materials on Listeners With Normal Hearing and Listeners With Hearing Loss. J Speech Lang Hear Res 50(4): 844–56.
51. Neville HJ, Schmidt A, Kutas M (1983) Altered visual-evoked potentials in congenitally deaf adults. Brain Res 266(1): 127–32.
52. Tong Y, Melara RD, Rao A (2009) P2 enhancement from auditory discrimination training is associated with improved reaction times. Brain Res 1297: 80–8.
53. George EM, Coch D (2011) Music training and working memory: an ERP study. Neuropsychologia 49(5): 1083–1094.
54. Allison T, Puce A, Spencer DD, McCarthy G (1999) Electrophysiological studies of human face perception. I: Potentials generated in occipitotemporal cortex by face and non-face stimuli. Cereb Cortex 9(5): 415–30.
55. Andics A, McQueen JM, Petersson KM, Gál V, Rudas G, et al. (2010) Neural mechanisms for voice recognition. NeuroImage 52(4): 1528–40.
56. Pasley BN, David SV, Mesgarani N, Flinker A (2012) Reconstructing speech from human auditory cortex. PLoS biology 10(1): e1001251.
57. Campbell J, Sharma A (2013) Compensatory changes in cortical resource allocation in adults with hearing loss. Front Syst Neurosci 7: 71.
58. Puce A, Allison T, McCarthy G (1999) Electrophysiological studies of human face perception. III: Effects of top-down processing on face-specific potentials. Cereb Cortex 9(5): 445–458.
59. Nasr S, Tootell RBH (2012) Role of fusiform and anterior temporal cortical areas in facial recognition. NeuroImage 63(3): 1743–53.
60. McCullough S, Emmorey K, Sereno M (2005) Neural organization for recognition of grammatical and emotional facial expressions in deaf ASL signers and hearing nonsigners. Brain Res Cogn Brain Res 22(2): 193–203.
61. Sadato N, Okada T, Honda M, Matsuki K, Yoshida M, et al. (2005) Cross modal integration and plastic changes revealed by lip movement, random-dot motion and sign languages in the hearing and deaf. Cereb Cortex 15(8): 1113–22.
62. Woodhouse L, Hickson L (2009) Review of visual speech perception by hearing and hearing-impaired people: clinical implications. Int J Lang Commun Disord 44(3): 253–70.
63. Letourneau SM, Mitchell TV (2011) Gaze patterns during identity and emotion judgments in hearing adults and deaf users of American Sign Language. Perception 40: 563–575.
64. Rouger J, Lagleyre S, Démonet J-F, Fraysse B, Deguine O, et al. (2012) Evolution of crossmodal reorganization of the voice area in cochlear-implanted deaf patients. Hum Brain Mapp 33(8): 1929–40.
65. Strelnikov K, Rouger J, Demonet JF, Lagleyre S, Fraysse B, et al. (2013) Visual activity predicts auditory recovery from deafness after adult cochlear implantation. Brain 136(12): 3682–3695.
66. Giraud AL, Lee HJ (2007) Predicting cochlear implant outcome from brain organisation in the deaf. Restor Neurol Neurosci 25(3–4): 381–90.
67. Lee HJ, Giraud AL, Kang E, Oh SH, Kang H, et al. (2007) Cortical activity at rest predicts cochlear implantation outcome. Cereb Cortex 17(4): 909–17.
68. Souza PE, Boike KT, Witherell K, Tremblay K (2007) Prediction of Speech Recognition from Audibility in Older Listeners with Hearing Loss: Effects of Age, Amplification, and Background Noise. J AM Acad Audiol 18: 54–65.
69. Anderson S, Kraus N (2010) Sensory-Cognitive Interaction in the Neural Encoding of Speech in Noise: A Review. J AM Acad Audiol 21(9): 575–85.
70. Gifford RH, Revit LJ (2010) Speech perception for adult cochlear implant recipients in a realistic background noise: effectiveness of preprocessing strategies and external options for improving speech recognition in noise. J AM Acad Audiol 21(7): 441-51-quiz487-8.
71. Dubno JR (1984) Effects of age and mild hearing loss on speech recognition in noise. J Acoust Soc Am 76(1): 87–96.
72. Vermiglio AJ, Soli SD, Freed DJ, Fisher LM (2012) The relationship between high frequency pure-tone hearing loss, hearing in noise test (HINT) thresholds, and the articulation index. J AM Acad Audiol 23(10): 779–88.
73. Hornsby BW, Johnson EE, Picou E (2011) Effects of degree and configuration of hearing loss on the contribution of high- and low-frequency speech information to bilateral speech understanding. Ear Hear 32(5): 543–55.
74. Moore BC (1996) Perceptual consequences of cochlear hearing loss and their implications for the design of hearing aids. Ear Hear 17(2): 133–61.
75. Lazard DS, Lee HJ, Gaebler M, Kell CA, Truy E, et al. (2010) Phonological processing in post-lingual deafness and cochlear implant outcome. NeuroImage 49(4): 3443–51.
76. Lazard DS, Lee HJ, Truy E, Giraud AL (2013) Bilateral reorganization of posterior temporal cortices in post-lingual deafness and its relation to cochlear implant outcome. Hum Brain Mapp 34(5): 1208–1219.
77. Meredith MA, Keniston LP, Allman BL (2012) Multisensory dysfunction accompanies crossmodal plasticity following adult hearing impairment. Neuroscience 214: 136–48.
78. Rauschecker JP (2012) Ventral and dorsal streams in the evolution of speech and language. Front Evol Neurosci 4: 7.
79. Schirmer A, Fox PM, Grandjean D (2012) On the spatial organization of sound processing in the human temporal lobe: a meta-analysis. NeuroImage 63(1): 137–47.
80. Voss P, Gougoux F, Zatorre RJ, Lassonde M, Lepore F (2008) Differential occipital responses in early- and late-blind individuals during a sound-source discrimination task. NeuroImage 40: 746–758.

Permissions

All chapters in this book were first published in PLOS ONE, by The Public Library of Science; hereby published with permission under the Creative Commons Attribution License or equivalent. Every chapter published in this book has been scrutinized by our experts. Their significance has been extensively debated. The topics covered herein carry significant findings which will fuel the growth of the discipline. They may even be implemented as practical applications or may be referred to as a beginning point for another development.

The contributors of this book come from diverse backgrounds, making this book a truly international effort. This book will bring forth new frontiers with its revolutionizing research information and detailed analysis of the nascent developments around the world.

We would like to thank all the contributing authors for lending their expertise to make the book truly unique. They have played a crucial role in the development of this book. Without their invaluable contributions this book wouldn't have been possible. They have made vital efforts to compile up to date information on the varied aspects of this subject to make this book a valuable addition to the collection of many professionals and students.

This book was conceptualized with the vision of imparting up-to-date information and advanced data in this field. To ensure the same, a matchless editorial board was set up. Every individual on the board went through rigorous rounds of assessment to prove their worth. After which they invested a large part of their time researching and compiling the most relevant data for our readers.

The editorial board has been involved in producing this book since its inception. They have spent rigorous hours researching and exploring the diverse topics which have resulted in the successful publishing of this book. They have passed on their knowledge of decades through this book. To expedite this challenging task, the publisher supported the team at every step. A small team of assistant editors was also appointed to further simplify the editing procedure and attain best results for the readers.

Apart from the editorial board, the designing team has also invested a significant amount of their time in understanding the subject and creating the most relevant covers. They scrutinized every image to scout for the most suitable representation of the subject and create an appropriate cover for the book.

The publishing team has been an ardent support to the editorial, designing and production team. Their endless efforts to recruit the best for this project, has resulted in the accomplishment of this book. They are a veteran in the field of academics and their pool of knowledge is as vast as their experience in printing. Their expertise and guidance has proved useful at every step. Their uncompromising quality standards have made this book an exceptional effort. Their encouragement from time to time has been an inspiration for everyone.

The publisher and the editorial board hope that this book will prove to be a valuable piece of knowledge for researchers, students, practitioners and scholars across the globe.

List of Contributors

Yoon-Hyeong Choi
Department of Preventive Medicine, Gachon University Graduate School of Medicine, Incheon, Korea

KyooSang Kim
Occupational Safety and Health Research Institute, Korea Occupational Safety and Health Agency, Incheon, Korea

James R. Engle
Evelyn F. McKnight Brain Institute and ARL Division of Neural Systems, Memory and Aging, University of Arizona, Tucson, Arizona, United States of America
Center for Neuroscience, University of California Davis, Davis, California, United States of America

Steve Tinling
Department of Otolaryngology, University of California Davis, Davis, California, United States of America

Gregg H. Recanzone
Center for Neuroscience, University of California Davis, Davis, California, United States of America
Department of Neurobiology, Physiology and Behavior, University of California Davis, Davis, California, United States of America

Berthold Langguth, Michael Landgrebe and Martin Schecklmann
Department of Psychiatry and Psychotherapy, University of Regensburg, Regensburg, Germany
Interdisciplinary Tinnitus Clinic, University of Regensburg, Regensburg, Germany

Veronika Vielsmeier
Interdisciplinary Tinnitus Clinic, University of Regensburg, Regensburg, Germany
Department of Otorhinolaryngology, University of Regensburg, Regensburg, Germany

Thomas Steffens
Department of Otorhinolaryngology, University of Regensburg, Regensburg, Germany

Tobias Kleinjung
Interdisciplinary Tinnitus Clinic, University of Regensburg, Regensburg, Germany
Department of Otorhinolaryngology, University of Regensburg, Regensburg, Germany
Department of Otorhinolaryngology, University of Zurich, Zurich, Switzerland

Katarzyna Iwanicka-Pronicka, Agnieszka Pollak, Urszula Lechowicz, Mariusz Furmanek, Maciej Rzeski, Lech Korniszewski and Henryk Skarżyński
Institute of Physiology and Pathology of Hearing, Warsaw, Poland
World Hearing Center, Kajetany, Poland

Rafał Płoski
Department of Medical Genetics, Medical University of Warsaw, Poland

Agata Skórka
Department of Paediatrics, Medical University of Warsaw, Poland

Magdalena Pajdowska
Department of Biochemistry and Experimental Medicine, The Children's Memorial Health Institute, Warsaw, Poland

Ashok R. Asthagiri, Keaton Morgan and Russell R. Lonser
Surgical Neurology Branch, National Institute of Neurological Disorders and Stroke, National Institutes of Health, Bethesda, Maryland, United States of America

Raul A. Vasquez
Surgical Neurology Branch, National Institute of Neurological Disorders and Stroke, National Institutes of Health, Bethesda, Maryland, United States of America
Department of Neurological Surgery, University of Florida, Gainesville, Gainesville, Florida, United States of America

John A. Butman
Radiology and Imaging Sciences, The Clinical Center at the National Institutes of Health, National Institutes of Health, Bethesda, Maryland, United States of America

Tianxia Wu
Clinical Neurosciences Program, National Institute of Neurological Disorders and Stroke, National Institutes of Health, Bethesda, Maryland, United States of America

Carmen C. Brewer, Kelly King and Chris Zalewski
Audiology Unit, Otolaryngology Branch, National Institute on Deafness and Other Communication Disorders, National Institutes of Health, Bethesda, Maryland, United States of America

H. Jeffrey Kim
Office of the Clinical Director, National Institute on Deafness and Other Communication Disorders, National Institutes of Health, Bethesda, Maryland, United States of America

Vera G. Pshennikova and Natalya A. Solovyeva
Department of Molecular Genetics, Yakut Scientific Centre of Complex Medical Problems, Siberian Branch of the Russian Academy of Medical Sciences, Yakutsk, Russian Federation

Nikolay A. Barashkov, Fedor M. Teryutin and Sardana A. Fedorova
Department of Molecular Genetics, Yakut Scientific Centre of Complex Medical Problems, Siberian Branch of the Russian Academy of Medical Sciences, Yakutsk, Russian Federation
Laboratory of Molecular Biology, Institute of Natural Sciences, M.K. Ammosov North-Eastern Federal University, Yakutsk, Russian Federation

Aisen V. Solovyev
Laboratory of Molecular Biology, Institute of Natural Sciences, M.K. Ammosov North-Eastern Federal University, Yakutsk, Russian Federation

Leonid A. Klarov and Nikolay V. Luginov
Department of Radiology, Republican Hospital #2-Center of Emergency Medicine, Ministry of Public Health of the Sakha Republic, Yakutsk, Russian Federation

Andrei A. Kozhevnikov
Republican Centre of Professional Pathology, Republican Hospital #2- Center of Emergency Medicine, Ministry of Public Health of the Sakha Republic, Yakutsk, Russian Federation

Lena M. Vasilyeva and Elvira E. Fedotova
Audiology-Logopaedic Center, Republican Hospital #1- National Medical Centre, Ministry of Public Health of the Sakha Republic, Yakutsk, Russian Federation

Maria V. Pak
Department of Pediatric, Medical Institute, M.K. Ammosov North-Eastern Federal University, Yakutsk, Russian Federation

Sargylana N. Lekhanova
Department of Normal and Abnormal Anatomy, Operative Surgery with Topographic Anatomy and Forensic Medicine, Medical Institute, M.K. Ammosov North-Eastern Federal University, Yakutsk, Russian Federation

Elena V. Zakharova
Institute of Foreign Philology and Regional Studies, M.K. Ammosov North-Eastern Federal University, Yakutsk, Russian Federation

Kyunney E. Savvinova and Nyurgun N. Gotovtsev
Laboratory of Molecular Biology, Institute of Natural Sciences, M.K. Ammosov North-Eastern Federal University, Yakutsk, Russian Federation
Institute of Natural Sciences, M.K. Ammosov North-Eastern Federal University, Yakutsk, Russian Federation

Adyum M. Rafailo
Institute of Natural Sciences, M.K. Ammosov North-Eastern Federal University, Yakutsk, Russian Federation

Anatoliy N. Alexeev
Institute of Humanitarian Research and Indigenous Peoples of the North, Siberian Branch of the Russian Academy of Sciences, Yakutsk, Russian Federation

Olga L. Posukh
Institute of Cytology and Genetics, Siberian Branch of the Russian Academy of Sciences, Novosibirsk, Russian Federation
Novosibirsk State University, Novosibirsk, Russian Federation

Lilya U. Dzhemileva
Department of Genomics, Institute of Biochemistry and Genetics, Ufa Scientific Centre, Russian Academy of Sciences, Ufa, Russian Federation

Elza K. Khusnutdinova
Department of Genomics, Institute of Biochemistry and Genetics, Ufa Scientific Centre, Russian Academy of Sciences, Ufa, Russian Federation
Department of Genetics and Fundamental Medicine, Bashkir State University, Ufa, Russian Federation

Ying-Chang Lu and Chuan-Jen Hsu
Department of Otolaryngology, National Taiwan University Hospital, Taipei, Taiwan

Chen-Chi Wu
Department of Otolaryngology, National Taiwan University Hospital, Taipei, Taiwan
Department of Medical Genetics, National Taiwan University Hospital, Taipei, Taiwan

Yin-Hung Lin
Department of Otolaryngology, National Taiwan University Hospital, Taipei, Taiwan

Graduate Institute of Molecular Medicine, National Taiwan University College of Medicine, Taipei, Taiwan

Pei-Jer Chen
Graduate Institute of Clinical Medicine, National Taiwan University College of Medicine, Taipei, Taiwan
Department of Internal Medicine, National Taiwan University Hospital, Taipei, Taiwan

Wei-Shiung Yang
Department of Medical Genetics, National Taiwan University Hospital, Taipei, Taiwan
Graduate Institute of Clinical Medicine, National Taiwan University College of Medicine, Taipei, Taiwan
Department of Internal Medicine, National Taiwan University Hospital, Taipei, Taiwan
Research Center for Developmental Biology and Regenerative Medicine, National Taiwan University, Taipei, Taiwan

Pei-Lung Chen
Department of Medical Genetics, National Taiwan University Hospital, Taipei, Taiwan
Department of Internal Medicine, National Taiwan University Hospital, Taipei, Taiwan
Research Center for Developmental Biology and Regenerative Medicine, National Taiwan University, Taipei, Taiwan
Graduate Institute of Medical Genomics and Proteomics, National Taiwan University College of Medicine, Taipei, Taiwan

Peter M. Kreuzer, Martin Schecklmann, Susanne Staudinger and Berthold Langguth
Department of Psychiatry and Psychotherapy, University of Regensburg, Regensburg, Germany

Michael Landgrebe
Department of Psychiatry and Psychotherapy, University of Regensburg, Regensburg, Germany
Department of Psychiatry, Psychosomatic Medicine and Psychotherapy, Sozialstiftung Bamberg, Bamberg, Germany

Wendy Hutchison
Murdoch Childrens Research Institute, Royal Children's Hospital, Melbourne, Australia

Hans-Henrik M. Dahl
Murdoch Childrens Research Institute, Royal Children's Hospital, Melbourne, Australia
Department of Pediatrics, University of Melbourne, Melbourne, Australia

Sanna Hou, Mark Seeto, Jessica Sjahalam-King and Teresa Y.C. Ching
National Acoustic Laboratories, Sydney, Australia
HEARing Cooperative Research Centre, Melbourne, Australia

Lisa E. Wolber, Claire J. Steves, Tim D. Spector and Frances M. K. Williams
Department of Twin Research and Genetic Epidemiology, King's College London, London, United Kingdom

Dorothea Wendt, Thomas Brand and Birger Kollmeier
Medizinische Physik and Cluster of Excellence Hearing4all, Universita¨t Oldenburg, Oldenburg, Germany

So Young Kim, Kyu-Hee Han and Ahreum Kim
Department of Otorhinolaryngology-Head and Neck Surgery, Seoul National University Hospital, Seoul National University College of Medicine, Seoul, Korea

Gibeom Park
Department of Biomedical Sciences, Seoul National University College of Medicine, Seoul, Korea

Byung Yoon Choi and Ja-Won Koo
Department of Otorhinolaryngology-Head and Neck Surgery, Seoul National University Bundang Hospital, Seoul National University College of Medicine, Seongnam, Korea
Sensory Organ Research Institute, Seoul National University Medical Research Center, Seoul, Korea

Sun O. Chang and Seung Ha Oh
Department of Otorhinolaryngology-Head and Neck Surgery, Seoul National University Hospital, Seoul National University College of Medicine, Seoul, Korea
Sensory Organ Research Institute, Seoul National University Medical Research Center, Seoul, Korea

Woong-Yang Park
Department of Molecular Cell Biology, Sungkyunkwan University School of Medicine, Suwon, Korea
Translational Genomics Laboratory, Samsung Genome Institute, Samsung Medical Center, Seoul, Korea

Jae Woong Bae, Dong-Bin Kim, Seung-Hyun Bae and Un-Kyung Kim
Department of Biology, College of Natural Sciences, Kyungpook National University, Daegu, South Korea

Jae Young Choi
Department of Otorhinolaryngology, Yonsei University College of Medicine, Seoul, South Korea

Hong-Joon Park
Soree Ear Clinic, Seoul, South Korea

Jong Dae Lee
Department of Otorhinolaryngology-Head and Neck Surgery, Soonchunhyang University College of Medicine, Bucheon, South Korea

Dong Gu Hur
Department of Otorhinolaryngology-Head and Neck Surgery, Gyeongsang National University Hospital, Jinju, South Korea

Kyu Yup Lee, Da Jung Jung and Sang Heun Lee
Department of Otolaryngology, College of Medicine, Kyungpook National University, Daegu, South Korea

Marianna Cavinato, Jessica Rigon, Chiara Volpato and Francesco Piccione
San Camillo Foundation, Institute of Care and Research, Venice, Italy

Carlo Semenza
San Camillo Foundation, Institute of Care and Research, Venice, Italy
Department of Neuroscience, University of Padova, Padova, Italy

Samer Khateb, Lina Zelinger, Saul Merin, Eyal Banin and Dror Sharon
Department of Ophthalmology, Hadassah - Hebrew University Medical Center, Jerusalem, Israel

Tamar Ben-Yosef
Genetics Department, Rappaport Faculty of Medicine, Technion – Israel Institute of Technology, Haifa, Israel

Ornit Crystal-Shalit
Department of Ophthalmology, Meir Medical Center, Kfar-Saba, Israel

Menachem Gross
Department of Otolaryngology - Head and Neck Surgery, Hadassah - Hebrew University Medical Center, Jerusalem, Israel

Elvira Perez and Barrie A. Edmonds
National Biomedical Research Unit in Hearing, National Institute for Health Research (NIHR), Nottingham, United Kingdom
School of Clinical Sciences, University ofNottingham, Nottingham, United Kingdom

Martin Schecklmann, Elmar Frank, Rainer Rupprecht, Philipp G. S, Peter Eichhammer Berthold and Langguth
Department of Psychiatry and Psychotherapy, University Regensburg, Regensburg, Germany

Michael Landgrebe and Göran Hajak
Department of Psychiatry, Psychosomatic Medicine and Psychotherapy Social Foundation Bamberg, Bamberg, Germany

Tobias Kleinjung
Department of Otorhinolaryngology, University of Zurich, Zurich, Switzerland

Isabelle Pia Maiditsch and Friedrich Ladich
Department of Behavioural Biology, University of Vienna, Vienna, Austria

Jennifer R. Prentice, Christopher S. Blackwell and J. Mark Wilkinson
Department of Human Metabolism, University of Sheffield, Sheffield, South Yorkshire, United Kingdom,

Naz Raoof
Department of Ophthalmology, Sheffield Teaching Hospitals NHS Foundation Trust, Sheffield, South Yorkshire, United Kingdom,

Paul Bacon and Jaydip Ray
Department of Otolaryngology, Sheffield Teaching Hospitals NHS Foundation Trust, Sheffield, South Yorkshire, United Kingdom

Simon J. Hickman
Department of Neurology, Sheffield Teaching Hospitals NHS Foundation Trust, Sheffield, South Yorkshire, United Kingdom

Dayong Wang, Liang Zong, Feifan Zhao, Wei Shi, Lan Lan, Hongyang Wang, Qian Li, Bing Han and Qiuju Wang
Chinese PLA Institute of Otolaryngology, Chinese PLA General Hospital, Beijing, China

Yali Zhao
Chinese PLA Institute of Otolaryngology, Chinese PLA General Hospital, Beijing, China
Beijing Institute of Otorhinolaryngology, Beijing Tongren Hospital, Capital Medical University, Beijing, China

Liping Guan, Peng Zhang, Jian Wang and Jun Wang
BGI-Shenzhen, Shenzhen, China

Xin Jin
BGI-Shenzhen, Shenzhen, China
School of Bioscience and Biotechnology, South China University of Technology, Guangzhou, China

Ling Yang
BGI-Tianjin, Tianjin, China

Qiuju Wang, Hongyang Wang, Yali Zhao, Yun Gao, Qiong Liu, Dayong Wang, Qian Li, Lan Lan, Na Li, Jing Guan, Zifang Yin, Bing Han, Feifan Zhao, Liang Zong, Wenping Xiong and Lan Yu
Institute of Otolaryngology, Chinese PLA General Hospital, Medical School of Chinese PLA, Beijing, China

Yuting Yi, Lijie Song, Xin Yi and Ling Yang
BGI-Tianjin, Tianjin, China

Christine Petit
Unité de Génétique et Physiologie de l'Audition, Institut Pasteur, Paris, France
UMRS 1120, Institut National de la Santéet de la Recherche Médicale (INSERM), Paris, France
Université Pierreet Marie Curie (Paris VI), Paris, France
Collège de France, Paris, France

Fan-Gang Zeng, Qing Tang and Thomas Lu
Center for Hearing Research, Departments of Anatomy and Neurobiology, Biomedical Engineering, Cognitive Sciences, and Otolaryngology - Head and Neck Surgery, University of California Irvine, Irvine, California, United States of America

Rainer Huber
Centre of Competence HörTech gGmbH, Oldenburg, Germany
Cluster of Excellence Hearing4All, Oldenburg and Hannover, Germany

Vijay Parsa and Susan Scollie
National Centre for Audiology, Western University, London, Canada
Ann-Cathrine Lindblad, Åke Olofsson and Björn Hagerman
Department of Clinical Science, Intervention and Technology, Division of Ear, Nose and Throat Diseases, Unit of Technical and Experimental Audiology, Karolinska Institutet, Stockholm, Sweden

Ulf Rosenhall
Department of Clinical Science, Intervention and Technology, Division of Ear, Nose and Throat Diseases, Karolinska Institutet; and Department of Audiology and Neurotology, Karolinska University Hospital, Stockholm, Sweden

Paul D. Meek and Guy-Anthony Ballard
Invasive Animals CRC, Coffs Harbour, New South Wales, Australia
Vertebrate Pest Research Unit, NSW Department Primary Industries, Armidale, New South Wales, Australia
School of Environmental and Rural Sciences, University of New England, Armidale, New South Wales, Australia

Peter J. S. Fleming
Invasive Animals CRC, Coffs Harbour, New South Wales, Australia
School of Environmental and Rural Sciences, University of New England, Armidale, New South Wales, Australia
Vertebrate Pest Research Unit, NSW Department Primary Industries, Orange, New South Wales, Australia

Greg Falzon
Invasive Animals CRC, Coffs Harbour, New South Wales, Australia
School of Science and Technology, University of New England, Armidale, New South Wales, Australia

Michael Schaefer
School of Environmental and Rural Sciences, University of New England, Armidale, New South Wales, Australia
Marine and Atmospheric Research, CSIRO, Canberra, Australian Capital Territory, Australia

Warwick Williams
National Acoustic Laboratory, Sydney, New South Wales, Australia

Stephanie C. P. M. Theunissen, Jeroen J. Briaire, Wim Soede and Anouk P. Netten
Department of Otorhinolaryngology and Head & Neck Surgery, Leiden University Medical Center, Leiden, The Netherlands

Johan H. M. Frijns
Department of Otorhinolaryngology and Head & Neck Surgery, Leiden University Medical Center, Leiden, The Netherlands
Leiden Institute for Brain and Cognition, Leiden, The Netherlands

Maartje Kouwenberg
Department of Developmental Psychology, Leiden University, Leiden, The Netherlands

Carolien Rieffe
Department of Developmental Psychology, Leiden University, Leiden, The Netherlands
Dutch Foundation for the Deaf and Hard of Hearing Child, Amsterdam, The Netherlands

Martin Schecklmann and Berthold Langguth
Department of Psychiatry and Psychotherapy, University of Regensburg, Regensburg, Germany

Michael Landgrebe
Department of Psychiatry and Psychotherapy, Social Foundation Bamberg, Bamberg, Germany

Myoung Su Choi, Ho Yun Lee and Chin Saeng Cho
Department of Otorhinolaryngology, Department of Otorhinolaryngology, Head & Neck Surgery, School of Medicine, Eulji University Medical Center, Eulji University, Daejeon, Korea

Byung Yoon Choi
Department of Otorhinolaryngology, Seoul National University Bundang Hospital, Seongnam, South Korea

Jiwoong Kim
Korean Bioinformation center, Korea Research Institute of Bioscience and Biotechnology (KRIBB), Daejeon, South Korea

Sang-Heon Lee and Namshin Kim
Korean Bioinformation center, Korea Research Institute of Bioscience and Biotechnology (KRIBB), Daejeon, South Korea
Department of Bioinformatics, University of Science and Technology, Daejeon, South Korea

Juyong Chung
Department of Otolaryngology, Ajou University School of Medicine, Suwon, South Korea

Seung-Ha Oh, Ah Reum Kim, Sue Jean Mun and Seong Il Kang
Department of Otorhinolaryngology, Seoul national University College of Medicine, Seoul, South Korea

Fei Yu, Jian-Dong Zhao, Yu Lu, Fei Ji, Sha-Sha Huang, Yong-Yi Yuan, Yu-Hua Zhu, Dong-Yang Kang and Dong-Yi HAN
Department of Otorhinolaryngology, Head and Neck Surgery, PLA General Hospital, Beijing, P. R. China

Ming-Yu Han, Yue-Shuai Song, Pu Dai and Yu Su
Department of Otorhinolaryngology, Head and Neck Surgery, PLA General Hospital, Beijing, P. R. China
Department of Otorhinolaryngology, Hainan Branch of PLA General Hospital, Sanya, P. R. China

Xue Gao
Department of Otorhinolaryngology, Head and Neck Surgery, PLA General Hospital, Beijing, P. R. China
Department of Otorhinolaryngology, the Second Artillery General Hospital, Beijing, P. R. China

Wen-Xue Tang
Department of Otolaryngology, Emory University School of Medicine, Atlanta, Georgia

Zhi-Yao Dai
Department of Otorhinolaryngology, the First Affiliated Hospital of PLA General Hospital, Beijing, P. R. China

David R. Moore
NIHR Nottingham Hearing Biomedical Research Unit, Nottingham, United Kingdom
MRC Institute of Hearing Research, University Park, Nottingham, United Kingdom
Cincinnati Children's Hospital Medical Center and Department of Otolaryngology, University of Cincinnati College of Medicine, Cincinnati, Ohio, United States of America

Abby McCormack
NIHR Nottingham Hearing Biomedical Research Unit, Nottingham, United Kingdom
MRC Institute of Hearing Research, University Park, Nottingham, United Kingdom
Otology and Hearing Group, Division of Clinical Neuroscience, School of Medicine, University of Nottingham, Nottingham, United Kingdom

Mark Edmondson-Jones, Heather Fortnum and Robert H. Pierzycki
NIHR Nottingham Hearing Biomedical Research Unit, Nottingham, United Kingdom
Otology and Hearing Group, Division of Clinical Neuroscience, School of Medicine, University of Nottingham, Nottingham, United Kingdom

Piers Dawes
School of Psychological Sciences, University of Manchester, Manchester, United Kingdom

Kevin J. Munro
School of Psychological Sciences, University of Manchester, Manchester, United Kingdom
Central Manchester University Hospitals NHS Foundation Trust, Manchester Academic Health Science Centre, Manchester, United Kingdom

Julia Campbell
University of Colorado at Boulder, Department of Speech, Language and Hearing Sciences, Boulder, Colorado, United States of America

Anu Sharma
University of Colorado at Boulder, Department of Speech, Language and Hearing Sciences, Boulder, Colorado, United States of America
University of Colorado at Boulder, Institute of Cognitive Science, Boulder, Colorado, United States of America

Index